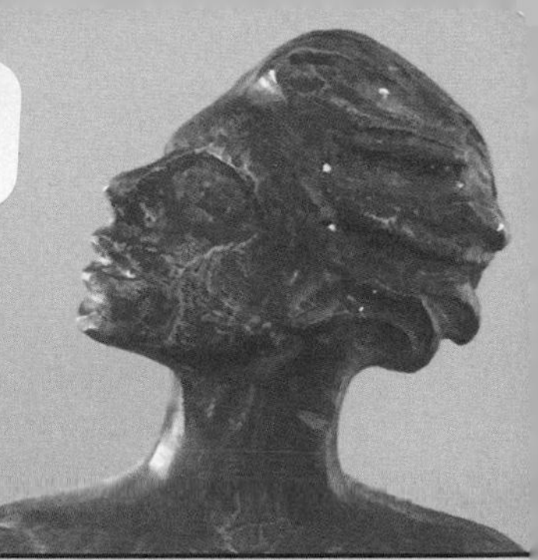

FIFTH EDITION

Kielhofner's

Model of Human Occupation:

THEORY AND APPLICATION

Renée R. Taylor, PhD
Director, UIC Model of Human Occupation Clearinghouse
Professor of Occupational Therapy
Vice Provost for Faculty Affairs
The University of Illinois at Chicago
Chicago, Illinois

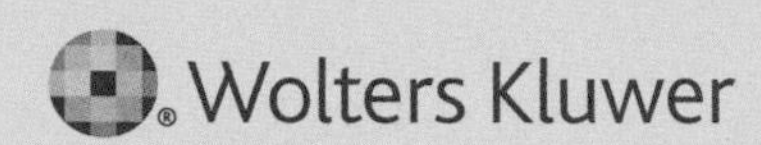

Philadelphia • Baltimore • New York • London
Buenos Aires • Hong Kong • Sydney • Tokyo

Acquisitions Editor: Michael Nobel
Product Development Editor: Linda G. Francis
Marketing Manager: Shauna Kelley
Production Editor: Kim Cox
Design Coordinator: Holly McLaughlin
Artist: Christine Mercer-Vernon
Compositor: S4Carlisle Publishing Services

Fifth Edition

9 8 7 6 5 4 3 2 1

Printed in China

Library of Congress Cataloging-in-Publication Data

Names: Taylor, Ren?ee R., 1970– editor. | Preceded by (work): Kielhofner, Gary, 1949– Model of human occupation
Title: Kielhofner's model of human occupation: theory and application / [edited by] Rene Taylor.
Other titles: Model of human occupation
Description: Fifth edition. | Philadelphia: Wolters Kluwer Health, [2017] | Preceded by Model of human occupation: theory and application / Gary Kielhofner. 4th ed. 2008. | Includes bibliographical references and index.
Identifiers: LCCN 2016051255 | ISBN 9781451190342
Subjects: | MESH: Occupational Therapy | Models, Psychological
Classification: LCC RM735 | NLM WB 555 | DDC 615.8/515—dc23 LC record available at https://lccn.loc.gov/2016051255

LWW.com

RRS1701

This edition is dedicated to the memory of Professor Gary Kielhofner, whose work defined and revolutionized the art, practice, and science of occupational therapy as we know it today.

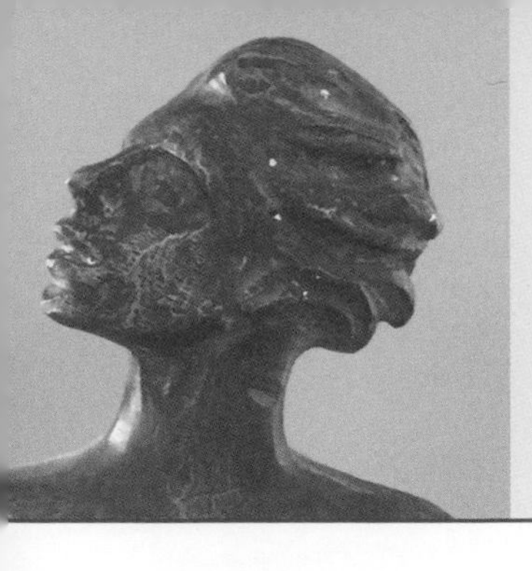

Contributors

Judith Abelenda, MSc/OT, Certificate in Advanced Practice, Autism
Occupational Therapist
Uutchi Desarrollo Infantil
Vitoria-Gasteiz, Spain

Patricia Bowyer, EdD, MS, OTR, FAOTA
Associate Professor and Associate Director
School of Occupational Therapy—Houston
College of Health Sciences
Texas Women's University
Texas Medical Center
Houston, Texas

Susan M. Cahill, OTR/L, PhD
Associate Professor and Associate Director of the Doctorate of Health Sciences Program
Occupational Therapy Program
College of Health Sciences
Midwestern University
Downers Grove, Illinois

John Cooper, BSc/OT
Occupational Therapist
2gether National Health Service Foundation Trust
Gloucester, England

Nichola Duffy, BSc/OT
Senior Occupational Therapist
Cumbria Partnership
National Health Services Foundation Trust
Voreda, Portland Place, Penrith
Cumbria, England

Elin Ekbladh, MSc/OT, PhD
Senior Lecturer
Department of Social and Welfare Studies
Section of Occupational Therapy
Linkoping University
Linkoping, Sweden

Anette Erikson, OT, PhD
Associate
Division of Occupational Therapy
Department of Neurobiology, Care Sciences and Society
Karolinska Institutet
Stockholm, Sweden

Mandana Fallaphour, OT (reg), PhD
Lecturer
Division of Occupational Therapy
Department of Neurobiology, Care Sciences and Society
Karolinska Institutet
Stockholm, Sweden

Chia-Wei Fan, MSc/OT, PhD
Departmental Affiliate
Department of Occupational Therapy
College of Applied Health Sciences
University of Illinois at Chicago
Chicago, Illinois

Gail Fisher, MPA, OTR/L, FAOTA
Clinical Associate Professor
Department of Occupational Therapy
University of Illinois at Chicago
Chicago, Illinois

Kirsty Forsyth, BSc/OT, MSc/OT, PhD
Professor
Department of Occupational Therapy and Arts Therapies
School of Health Sciences
Queen Margaret University
Edinburgh, Scotland

Sylwia Gorska, BSc/OT
Research Practitioner
Department of Occupational Therapy and Arts Therapies
School of Health Sciences
Queen Margaret University
Edinburgh, Scotland

Lena Haglund, PhD, MScOT, OT (Reg)
Associate Professor
Department of Social and Welfare Studies
Linköping University
Linköping, Sweden

Michele Harrison, BSc/OT
Lead Research Practitioner
Department of Occupational Therapy and Arts Therapies
School of Health Sciences
Queen Margaret University
Edinburgh, Scotland

Helena Hemmingsson, MSc/OT, PhD
Professor and Section Head
Department of Social and Welfare Studies
Section of Occupational Therapy
Linkoping University
Linkoping, Sweden

Carmen-Gloria de las Heras de Pablo, MS, OTR
Independent MOHO Consultant
Santiago de Chile
Región Metropolitana, Chile

Roberta P. Holzmueller, PhD
Associate Professor of Psychology in Psychiatry
Department of Psychiatry
University of Illinois at Chicago
Chicago, Illinois

Riitta Keponen, MSc, OTR
Lecturer
Metropolia University of Applied Health Sciences
Department of Occupational Therapy
Helsinki, Finland

Jessica Kramer, PhD, OTR/L
Department of Occupational Therapy
College of Health and Rehabilitation Sciences
Boston University
Boston, Massachusetts

Patricia Lavedure, BCP, OTR/L, OTD
Assistant Professor, Director of Fieldwork
Department of Occupational Therapy
Virginia Commonwealth University
Richmond, Virginia

Sun Wook Lee, PhD, OTR/L
Assistant Professor
Department of Occupational Therapy
Daegu University
Republic of Korea

Donald Maciver, BSc/OT, PhD
Reader
Department of Occupational Therapy and Arts Therapies
School of Health Sciences
Queen Margaret University
Edinburgh, Scotland

Alice Moody, BSc (Hons)/OT
Occupational Therapist
Mental Health Services for Older People
Gloucestershire Partnership Trust
Cheltenham, England

Jane Melton, PhD, MSc, DipCOT, FCOT
Director of Engagement and Integration
2gether NHS Foundation Trust
Gloucestershire, England, United Kingdom

Kelly Munger, PhD
Department of Occupational Therapy
College of Applied Health Sciences
University of Illinois at Chicago
Chicago, Illinois

Lauro Munoz, MOT, OTR, C/NDT
Rehabilitation Regulatory Supervisor
Department of Occupational Therapy
MD Anderson Cancer Center
Houston, Texas

Hiromi Nakamura-Thomas, OT, PhD
Department of Occupational Therapy
Saitama Prefectural University
Japan

Louise Nygard, OT (reg), PhD
Professor of Occupational Medicine
Division of Occupational Therapy
Department of Neurobiology, Care Sciences and Society
Karolinska Institutet
Stockholm, Sweden

Jane C. O'Brien, PhD, OTR/L, FAOTA
Professor
Department of Occupational Therapy
University of New England
Portland, Maine

Ay-Woan Pan, MSc/OT, OTR (USA), OTC (Taiwan), PhD
Associate Professor
School of Occupational Therapy
College of Medicine
National Taiwan University
Taipei, Taiwan

Sue Parkinson, BSc/OT
Occupational Therapist
Derbysire, England

Genevieve Pépin, BSc/OT, MSc/OT, PhD
Faculty of Health—Occupational Therapy
Deakin University
Geelong, Victoria, Australia

Susan Prior, BSc/OT, PhD
Senior Lecturer
Department of Occupational Therapy and Arts Therapies
School of Health Sciences
Queen Margaret University
Edinburgh, Scotland

Laura Quick, BSc/OT, PgDIP
Clinical Specialist, Occupational Therapist
Gloucestershire Partnership
National Health Services Foundation Trust
Charlton Lane Centre
Gloucestershire, England

Christine Raber, PhD, OTR/L
Master of Occupational Therapy Program
Department of Rehabilitation and Sports Professions
Shawnee State University
Portsmouth, Ohio

Jan Sandqvist, BSc/OT, Reg. OT, PhD
Senior Lecturer
Department of Social and Welfare Studies
Linköping University
Linköping, Sweden

Patricia J. Scott, PhD, MPH, OT, FAOTA
Associate Professor
Department of Occupational Therapy
Indiana University
Indianapolis, Indiana

Rebecca Shute, BSc/OT
Head of Profession for Occupational Therapy
2gether National Health Service Foundation Trust
Gloucester, England

Meghan Suman, MSc
Occupational Therapist in Practice
Naperville, Illinois

Renée R. Taylor, PhD
Director, UIC Model of Human Occupation Clearinghouse
Professor of Occupational Therapy
Vice Provost for Faculty Affairs
The University of Illinois at Chicago
Chicago, Illinois

Kerstin Tham, BSc/OT, Reg. OT, PhD
Professor, Department of Neurobiology, Care Sciences and Society
Karolinska Institutet
Stockholm, Sweden

Marjon ten Velden, OT (reg), PhD
Docent in Ergotherapy
Centre for Applied Research on Education
Amsterdam University of Applied Sciences
Amsterdam, Holland

Takashi Yamada, PhD, OTR
Professor, Department of Occupational Therapy
Faculty of Health Science
Professor and Director
Graduate School of Rehabilitation
Mejiro University
Tokyo, Japan

Preface and Editorial Introduction to the Fifth Edition

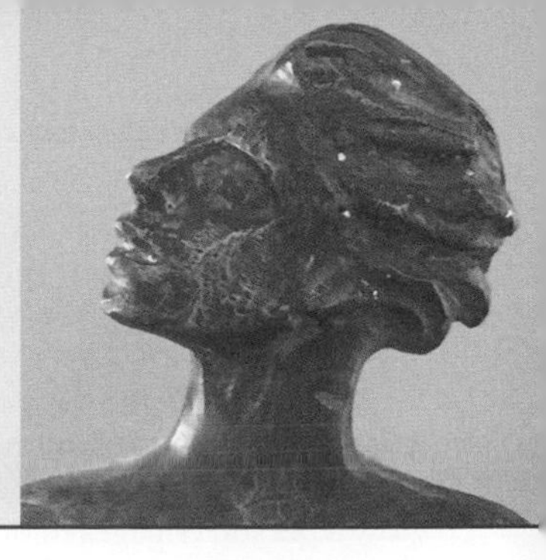

As a widely used conceptual practice model that has been subjected to nearly four decades of scientific inquiry, *Kielhofner's Model of Human Occupation* echoes the voices of occupational therapy clients, educators, practitioners, and scientists from across the globe. Contributors to this fifth edition are largely educators, applied researchers, practitioners, and clients with a wide range of knowledge and practical familiarity with the Model of Human Occupation (MOHO). They range from those who have been following the work since its emergence, to those who are relatively new to the model, and many somewhere in between.

We all rely upon our private motivations for learning and using the model to guide our teaching, practice, and research. Some of us recognize its power from having applied its concepts and measures to address an obstacle within our personal lives. Most have learned the benefits of its use by witnessing a marked improvement in clients. The researchers among us value the vast and consistently strong evidence base that demonstrates the relevance and effectiveness of this model in today's practice settings.

As students and practitioners of MOHO, we develop personalized understandings and practical interpretations of the model that allow us to shape our craft from a more liberated ideological foundation. For me, MOHO is a model that inspires personal epiphany and psychic freedom from the boundaries of institutionalized meanings, mores, and rituals that currently envelop the inevitably pathologizing health care settings and practices that I find myself and many students and colleagues practicing within today.

The Four Elements of MOHO

People new to the model will inevitably ask, ***what is MOHO?***

MOHO is about volition. As a client-centered, occupation-focused model, MOHO emphasizes the understanding of what motivates a client to action. MOHO is about accessing that place within ourselves in which our own interest and curiosity in another person comes alive. MOHO is about being real. It is about humility. As therapists, this allows us to develop a keen awareness of another person's interests, sense of abilities, and values. This is referred to as empathic understanding. This understanding allows us to learn how a client views their ability to contribute and enact meaning in the world. Quite simply, MOHO is about knowing the other.

MOHO is about habituation. It is about how a therapist utilizes this knowledge to understand the existing capacities and new potentials for a client to form a habit pattern that supports their interests, self-perception, and values toward an occupation. It is about understanding the social relevance of these habits and how they are organized across time and space to form roles. It is about understanding the relative importance of these roles to the individual at any given time point.

MOHO is about performance capacity. MOHO carries a deep respect for a person's lived and subjective experience of the body in interaction with its environment. Performance is conceived uniquely as a simultaneous experience of the body and of the mind. Performance capacity is viewed as objectively observable, measurable, and quantifiable but, most importantly, as lived, or subjectively experienced, by the client. Approaching a client's body with a respect for this sense of subjectivity offers a novel, client-centered conceptualization in which endless possibilities for occupational performance and participation exist, particularly within facilitative physical and social environments.

MOHO is about the environment. MOHO relies upon numerous physical, social, and occupational variables within the client's immediate, local, and global contexts as powerful influences on occupational engagement, performance, and participation. Equally, MOHO views clients that are enduring even the most severe difficulties as having a capacity to also influence these variables within these respective contexts. Environmental variables include, but are not limited to, the actions of meaning that are widely recognized within a given context, the person or persons with which one interacts, and the physical spaces, objects, and occupations that are available for engagement. Other aspects that influence a client include the cultural context, political conditions, and economic conditions. Aspects of the environment create both demands (which offer opportunities for action and behavior) and constraints (that limit or restrict action and behavior).

What is MOHO? Quite simply, MOHO encompasses these four elements (volition, habituation, performance capacity, and environment) and explains how a person engages in occupation as a result of the dynamic and reciprocal interaction between them.

Over a lifetime, we develop skills that enable us to perform tasks and activities and participate in occupational roles. Successful and consistent experiences with participation over time allow us to develop an occupational identity, which corresponds with our feelings of occupational competence regarding certain roles and activities.

When the circumstance of an impairment interrupts this dynamic, a client must be reengaged via an intensive intervention focusing on one or more of the four elements of MOHO (volition, habituation, performance capacity, and the environment), and ideally upon all four. This reengagement will offer revised opportunities for occupational participation and performance, feeding one's original sense of identity and competence, and thus defining the hallmark process of occupational adaptation.

MOHO-Oriented Practice

The perennial question that might follow is, ***What does it mean to practice from a MOHO-based orientation?***

Put otherwise, what does it mean to be a "MOHO therapist?" Being a MOHO therapist acknowledges a tendency for a therapist to constantly strive to understand a client from these multiple perspectives. It means locating each of these aspects of the person and the relevant aspects of the client's environment as they interact in synchronous and nonsynchronous ways. MOHO also connotes an earnest curiosity to learn about a client by listening to her life story and by hearing her perception of her own experience of participation within her unique personal constraints and environmental conditions. In some cases, this involves dissecting the events that form a client's plot and arriving at a central metaphor that defines her life experience.

A MOHO therapist is a deeply feeling, sensate, and organized thinker who not only reasons with precise attention to the model's moving parts but also intuits and feels her way through the therapy relationship, always prioritizing a client's sense of autonomy, dignity, desires, values, and capacity. A MOHO therapist can adapt to the changing dynamics of this process within the context of learning and knowing the client's experience of her own changed circumstances. A MOHO therapist can change an object, like a shirt button, into something of meaning, like a spaceship, so that a child is motivated to manipulate it into closure. A MOHO therapist can change a common activity like putting on a shirt into a habituated one that facilitates engagement with the social environment in a psychologically important activity, with the ultimate outcome being meeting a new friend.

A MOHO therapist can notice a client's most subtle change in gaze in response to a particular sound, person, or object of interest and tailor a significant greeting that acknowledges a client's fledgling demonstration of volition. Being a MOHO therapist means seeking to understand and contemplate a person's lived experience of disability. When you meet a MOHO therapist, you will see a spontaneity of thought, a candor, a true interest in others, and an artist. You will meet a person who will strive to understand you and your experience, in the context of your world. The MOHO therapist provides clients with opportunities to explore their environments while supporting them in testing out their own approaches to doing things. The therapist knows how to let go of the client in the precise moments when this letting go is needed most.

ORGANIZATION OF THIS BOOK

This book is organized into four sections, relying on case examples and case composites from actual practice situations throughout. The first section articulates each component of MOHO and provides an overarching viewpoint of MOHO as a conceptual practice model. The second section covers the application of MOHO in practice, including therapeutic reasoning, MOHO-based assessments, and planning and documenting therapy. The third section illustrates this application in focal client populations, emphasizing the use of MOHO with children and older adults. The fourth section provides resources for the use of MOHO in practice and research.

FEATURES

This book includes the following features to enhance learning.

- Learning Outcomes at the beginning of each chapter list the concepts readers should expect to understand by the end of the chapter.
- Case Examples illustrate application of the essential aspects of MOHO to practice.
- MOHO Problem-Solver Cases illustrate the power of MOHO in addressing an existing clinical dilemma or problematic case context.
- Quiz Questions and Homework Assignments allow for the assessment of learning, retention, and application of MOHO concepts and practices.

About Gary Kielhofner

The primary founder and developer of the Model of Human Occupation was Dr. Gary Kielhofner (b. 1949–d. 2010), an occupational therapist and scholar whose work lives on to sustain a high global impact on the practice, teaching, and research of occupational therapy.

Though it is the most evidence-based, occupation-focused, and client-centered OT conceptual practice model in the world, Kielhofner's model was born directly out of practice and lives deeply within practice, throughout the world, today. Originally developed from Kielhofner's work with U.S. military veterans with spinal cord injuries resulting from combat during the Vietnam War, MOHO continues to exist today as a quintessential foundation for the field of occupational therapy.

The fifth edition of this book is dedicated to Professor Gary Kielhofner. This edition was edited with an intention to preserve as much of Dr. Kielhofner's original voice and contributions in its pages as possible, while updating the concepts and their uses in today's practice environment. Without his contributions, many of which took shape within the context of MOHO, occupational therapy would be a very different field of practice today.

As editor, I am personally grateful to you, the reader, for your interest in this model and for your willingness to explore opportunities to use, disseminate, and advance the model. I hope that the contents of this edition will stimulate and inspire you to continue to transform your practice and/or research in creative and unprecedented ways, with the ultimate objective being improvement in the lived experiences of your clients.

Renée R. Taylor, PhD
Director, UIC Model of Human Occupation Clearinghouse
Professor of Occupational Therapy
Vice Provost for Faculty Affairs
The University of Illinois at Chicago
Chicago, Illinois

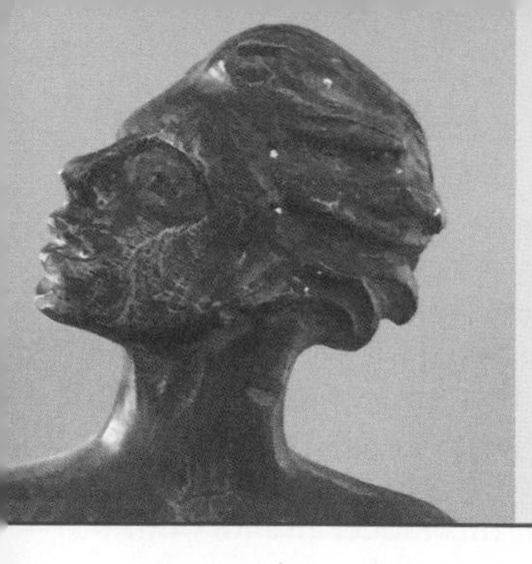

Table of Contents

PART I

EXPLAINING HUMAN OCCUPATION

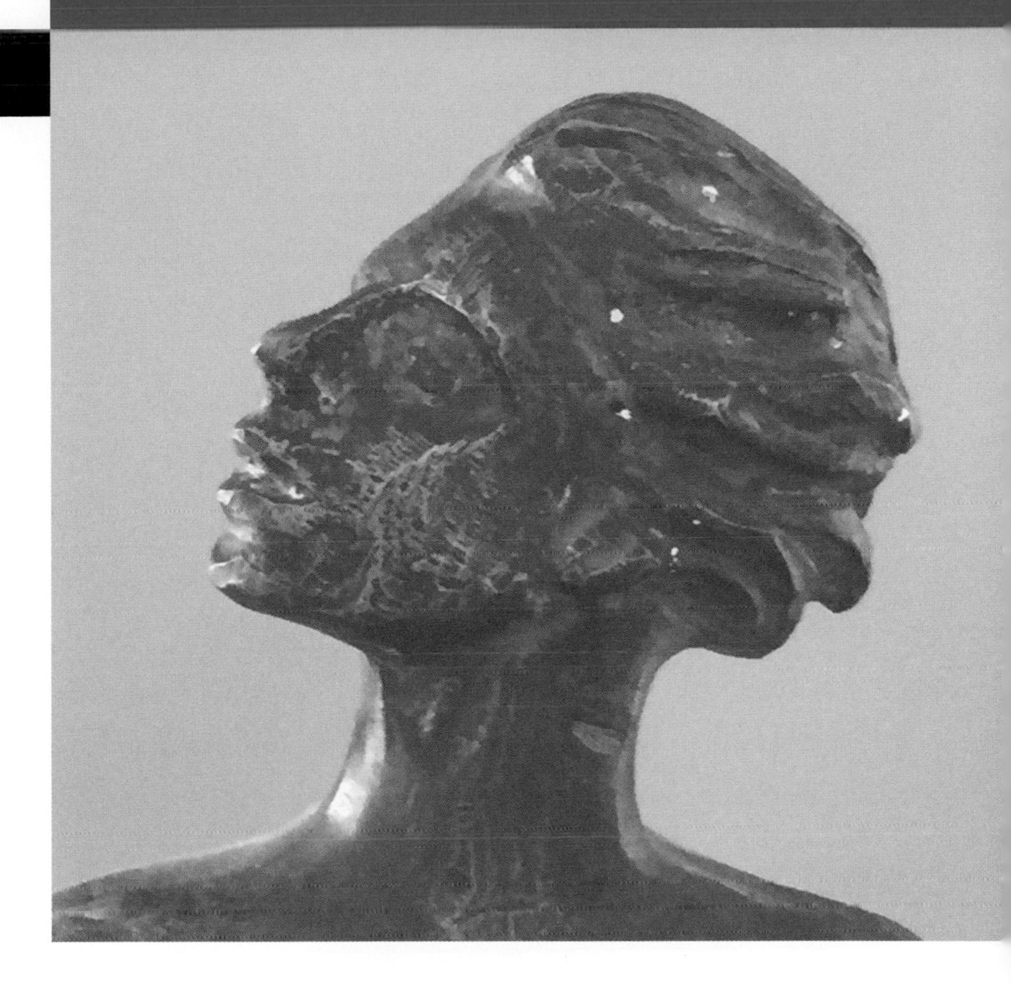

Introduction to the Model of Human Occupation

Renée R. Taylor and Gary Kielhofner (posthumous)

CHAPTER 1

EXPECTED LEARNING OUTCOMES

Upon completion of this chapter, readers will be able to:

1. List and define each of the four components of the model of human occupation (MOHO).
2. Provide an example of the MOHO from your everyday life and/or from your practice.
3. Define the seven elements of the MOHO that characterize its vision for advancing occupational therapy practice.
4. Describe the extent of use of the MOHO in occupational therapy practice.
5. Understand Kielhofner's vision for the MOHO in occupational therapy.

MOHO Problem-Solver: Alicia

A modest beechwood piano sits vacant within a gazebo in the middle of a town square. An innocent and lively redheaded child runs up to the piano and plays a few stiff and awkward-sounding notes. They seem to reflect a song from the popular musical *Frozen*. The girl's playing catches the ear of Alicia, an ungroomed woman in her late 60s standing isolated and idle by a streetlight as she waits for the van from her community living center to return her home from a shopping trip. Once a concert pianist and music teacher, Alicia had not touched a piano in over 10 years. A moderate traumatic brain injury, followed by a mild stroke, had permanently affected her executive functioning and her stability of mood. When she was first injured 10 years ago, an occupational therapist tried to reacquaint her with the piano through simulation exercises on a personal computer. However, the therapist's efforts had failed at the time because Alicia was simply not motivated to engage in the exercises, finding them to be too artificial.

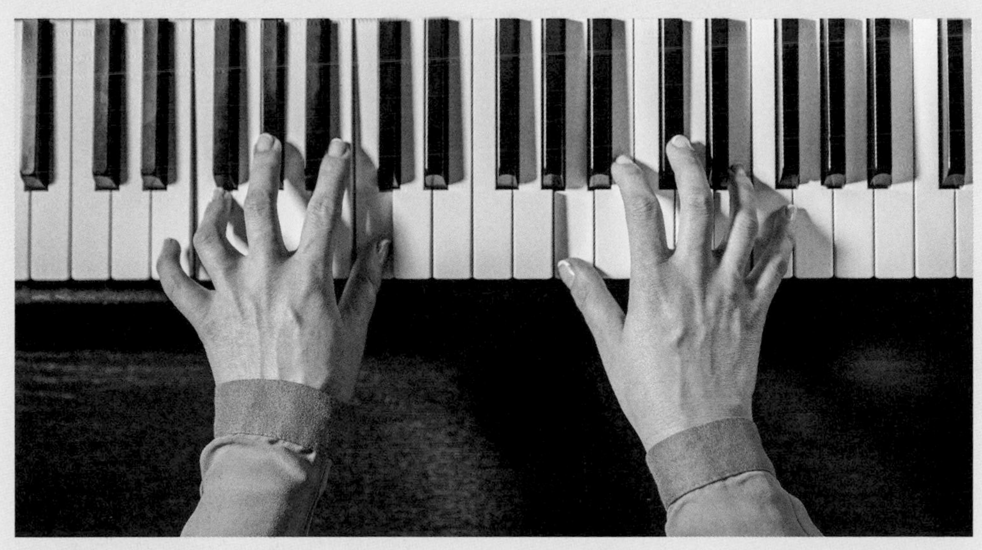

Alicia playing the piano

On returning to the group home from her shopping trip, Alicia spontaneously feels compelled to sit at the piano in the basement. She begins to play a few notes from *Frozen* by ear. The occupational therapist at the facility notices her playing and recognizes the piece. The next day, the sheet music for the entire soundtrack of *Frozen* arrives in Alicia's mailbox—a gift from the therapist. The therapist then makes sure to listen for the times that she hears Alicia playing. As Alicia practices, it is obvious that her mind becomes completely and unitarily organized and focused in a way that is not observed during other activities of daily living. Soon, Alicia's housemates begin to show up at her practice sessions. Knowing they will be there, she begins to practice more readily and habitually. Alicia senses that a new level of respect is developing from her peers, and she has even been named "the musician" by a newer tenant at the home.

Two and a half months later, Alicia shows up in the town square, sits down at the piano, and brilliantly plays the entire soundtrack to *Frozen* by memory. A crowd soon gathers, stunned and in praise of the woman's gift of music. Alicia is gradually becoming reacquainted with her occupational identity as a musician.

This scenario depicts an example of Kielhofner's **model of human occupation** (MOHO; Kielhofner, 2008). Specifically, it highlights the compelling role of the social and physical environment (i.e., the red-headed child playing a piece from *Frozen* on a piano in a public space) in influencing a client's motivation to reawaken an internalized role and perform a cherished activity of interest and value.

MOHO explains how people are motivated to perform occupations (**volition**) and repeat their performance over time (**habituation**). As occupations are repeated, the individual's subjective perception of his or her own capacity changes, as does the therapist's objective evaluation of it (**performance capacity**). This entire process unfolds within a social and physical context (**environment**) that facilitates the occupational engagement.

Quite simply, MOHO encompasses these four elements (volition, habituation, performance capacity, and environment) and explains how a person engages in occupation as a result of the dynamic and reciprocal interaction between them. MOHO explains how a disabled individual becomes motivated to engage in an occupation, how habits and roles are formed to support the occupation, and how an individual's self-perception of his or her own ability develops and articulates with objective assessments thereof, such as the therapist's opinion. These elements interact synergistically with each other and within an environmental context that, ideally, includes physical and social facilitators (Fig. 1-1).

The primary founder and developer of the MOHO was Dr. Gary Kielhofner (1949–2010), an occupational therapist and scholar whose work lives on to sustain

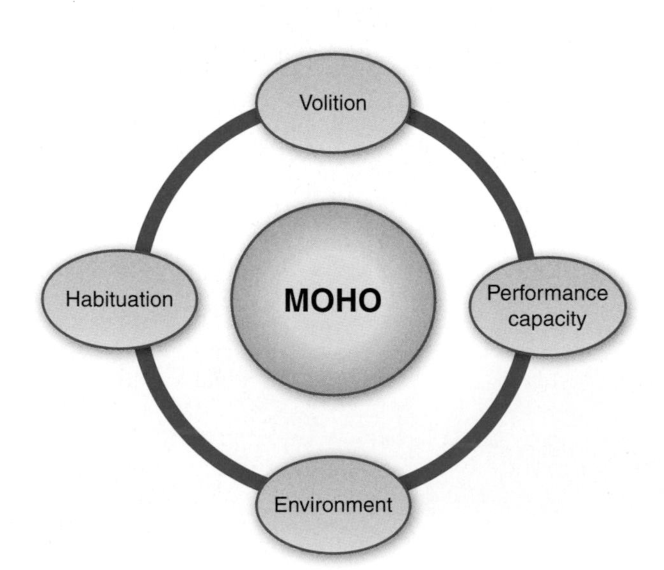

FIGURE 1-1 The Four Elements of the Model of Human Occupation.

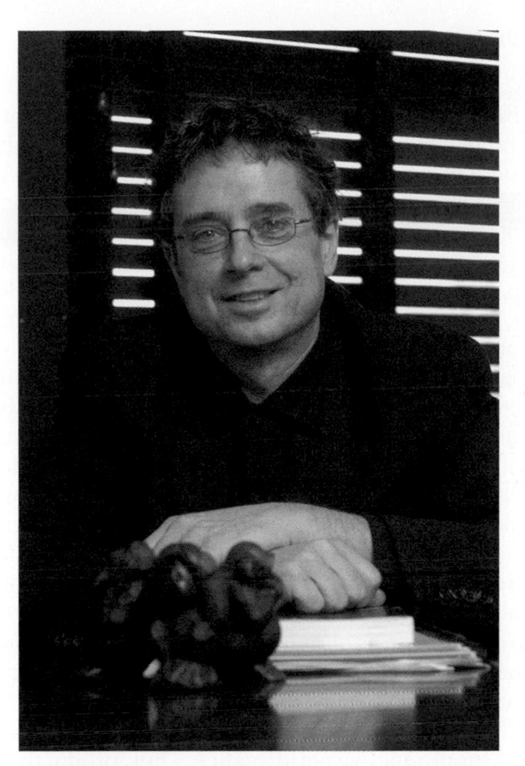

Dr. Gary Kielhofner

a high global impact on the practice, teaching, and research of occupational therapy. Born directly from its founder's work with US military veterans with spinal cord injuries resulting from combat during the Vietnam War, the MOHO continues to exist today as a quintessential foundation for the field of occupational therapy.

MOHO is an evidence-based conceptual practice model that explains how people adapt to severe disability and rediscover satisfying and meaningful ways to live their lives. The model's first concepts were developed and published in a series of four articles by three practitioners (Kielhofner, 1980a, 1980b; Kielhofner & Burke, 1980; Kielhofner, Burke, & Heard, 1980). Dr. Gary Kielhofner extended, refined, and researched these concepts over a four-decade period, ultimately making the model a relevant, straightforward, and contemporary guide for occupational therapy practitioners and educators.

Since that time, countless practitioners and researchers from around the world have enriched and expanded the application of MOHO concepts in practice, and continue to do so today. These individuals have contributed to a broad evidence base that exceeds a large and growing body of peer-reviewed research articles covering a wide range of treatment areas. Using a case-based approach, this book provides an overview of the model's theory and updated information about current, evidence-based assessment and treatment approaches using the model.

A number of research studies indicate that MOHO has become the most widely used occupation-focused model in occupational therapy practice in the United States and internationally (Haglund, Ekbladh, Thorell, & Hallberg, 2000; Law & McColl, 1989; Lee, 2010; National Board for Certification in Occupational Therapy, 2004). An **occupation-focused model** defines an approach to therapy that focuses on a client's engagement and participation in occupations as the mechanism of change, rather than focusing specifically on remediating an impairment. In a recent nationwide random study of occupational therapists in the United States (Taylor & Lee, 2009), over 76% of therapists indicated that they used MOHO in their practice. These therapists indicated that they chose MOHO because it fit with their view of occupational therapy and reflected their clients' needs. Moreover, the vast majority of these therapists indicated that, in their experience, MOHO:

- supports occupation-focused practice,
- helps therapists prioritize clients' needs,
- provides a holistic view of clients,
- offers a client-centered approach,
- affords a strong base for generating treatment goals, and
- supplies a rationale for intervention.

These views of practitioners coincide with many of the aims that have guided the development of MOHO over the past four decades. *Kielhofner's vision for MOHO is to support practice throughout the world that is occupation focused, client centered, holistic, and evidence based and complementary to practice based on other occupational therapy models and interdisciplinary theories.* Each of these elements is discussed below.

Multinational and Multicultural

MOHO has received much attention, including criticism, elaboration, application, and empirical testing, by occupational therapists throughout the world. Attempts to apply and test MOHO in different cultures and under different national conditions have provided priceless feedback about how its theoretical arguments and technology for application can best be developed to transcend cultural differences and national boundaries. MOHO incorporates a respect for each client's individuality and cultural background, and many MOHO assessments capture a client's unique cultural perspective. Successful applications of MOHO throughout the world point to its broad relevance. For instance, MOHO-based assessments and publications are available now in more than 20 languages. Most important, however, is that members of the occupational therapy profession throughout the world are now making important contributions to the development of MOHO so that its concepts and application increasingly reflect multiple perspectives.

Practice Oriented

Every day, MOHO is widely used in hospitals, clinics, home health care settings, skilled nursing facilities, group homes, schools, and countless other settings throughout the world. When therapists use concepts from MOHO, they link them to the specific client or client group to whom they are providing services. MOHO provides a wide range of resources (assessments, case examples, intervention protocols, and programs) to aid therapists to make this link. Moreover, an important emphasis underlying the development of MOHO has been to assure that it is grounded in the real-world situations of everyday practice (Forsyth, Summerfield-Mann, & Kielhofner, 2005; Kielhofner, 2005b). Thus, this model has strongly emphasized the involvement of practitioners and consumers in research and development efforts to assure they are grounded in practice and relevant to those who receive services.

Occupation Focused

Contrary to impairment-focused models and interventions that focus on the remediation of a set of symptoms or an impairment, MOHO was the first of the contemporary models to articulate a focus on occupation. In practice, this means that the practitioner makes a deliberate effort to focus on understanding the client in light of his or her interests, daily habits, and actual performance of specific occupations. Rather than focusing solely on analyzing the client's biomechanics of movement within a medical environment or conducting a standardized cognitive assessment to determine the level of brain function, a MOHO therapist examines the client's engagement in a meaningful activity. In sum, MOHO addresses three practical concerns related to this focus:

- How is occupation motivated, organized into everyday life patterns, and performed in the context of the environment?
- What happens in the face of impairments, illness, and other factors that create occupational problems?
- How does occupational therapy enable people to engage in occupations that provide meaning and satisfaction and that support their physical and emotional well-being?

WHAT IS OCCUPATION?

According to Kielhofner (2008), MOHO was specifically developed to focus its theoretical concepts, practice application, and research efforts on the doing of occupation. **Human occupation** refers to the doing of **work**, play, or activities of daily living within a temporal, physical, and sociocultural context that characterizes much of human life. Humans are characterized by an intense need to do things (Fidler & Fidler, 1983; Nelson, 1988). Human occupation comprises three broad areas of doing: activities of daily living, play, and productivity. **Activities of daily living** are the typical life tasks required for self-care and self-maintenance, such as grooming, bathing, eating, cleaning the house, and doing laundry. **Play** refers to activities freely undertaken for their own sake; it includes exploring, pretending, celebrating, engaging in games or sports, and pursuing hobbies (Reilly, 1974). **Productivity** refers to activities (both paid and unpaid) that provide services or commodities to others, such as ideas, knowledge, help, information sharing, entertainment, utilitarian or artistic objects, and protection (Shannon, 1970). Activities such as studying, practicing, and apprenticing improve abilities for productive performance. Thus, productivity includes activities engaged in as a student, employee, volunteer, parent, serious hobbyist, and amateur.

Client Centered

In MOHO terms, being a client-centered practitioner means that the therapist observes and, when appropriate, asks the client questions that facilitate an understanding of the client's immediate needs, perspectives, and experiences within the client–therapist interaction. Even before the emergence of client-centered concepts in occupational therapy, MOHO stressed the importance of incorporating the client's perspective and desires in shaping therapy. Thus, MOHO is recognized as consistent with concepts of client-centered practice (Law, 1998). MOHO is inherently a client-centered model in two important ways. First, it focuses the therapist on the client's uniqueness and provides concepts that allow the therapist to more deeply appreciate the client's perspective and situation. MOHO-based practice requires a client–therapist relationship in which the therapist must understand, respect, and support his or her client's values, sense of capacity and efficacy, roles, habits, performance experience, and personal environment. Second, since MOHO conceptualizes the client's own doing, thinking, and feeling as the central dynamic of therapy, the client's choice, action, and experience must be central to the therapy process.

In addition, MOHO has been influenced by many of the ideas emerging from disabilities studies (Albrecht, Seelman, & Bury, 2001; Kielhofner, 2005a; Longmore, 1995; Oliver, 1994; Scotch, 1988; Shapiro, 1994) that argue that theory needs to be informed more fully by the perspectives of those with disabilities. MOHO has always been consistent with the idea of informing theory and practice with client's viewpoints. However, in the last decade, a special effort has been made to have the model resonate with the voices of disabled persons and emphasize the experience of disability. Also in concert with the disability studies theme that disability occurs because of a misfit between person and environment, MOHO pays close attention to the environment as both an enabler of and a barrier to occupation.

Holistic

MOHO seeks to explain how occupation is motivated, patterned, and performed within social and physical environments. By offering explanations of such diverse phenomena, MOHO provides a broad and integrative view of human occupation. Holistic is another word to describe this integrative approach to understanding clients. For example, two of the phenomena addressed in MOHO, motivation and performance, are not typically considered together in the same theoretical framework. That is, occupational therapy theories that concentrate on physical performance have generally attended to the bodily components (brain and musculoskeletal system) involved in physical doing, while motives have been seen as part of a separate, mental domain.

There is growing recognition of the importance of considering body and mind together in explaining phenomena (Trombly, 1995a, 1995b). After all, motivation for a task can influence the extent of physical effort directed to that task (Riccio, Nelson, & Bush, 1990), while physical impairments can weigh down the desire to do things (Toombs, 1992). MOHO concepts seek to avoid dividing humans into separate physical and mental components. Rather, body and mind are viewed as integrated aspects of the total human being.

Evidence Based

Being evidence based refers to the research that has been conducted to successfully demonstrate the validity, positive impact, and relevance of MOHO and its individual concepts to occupational therapy practice. MOHO is supported by a substantial body of research generated over the past three decades, and new research is developing at a rapid pace. To date, over 100 studies of MOHO have been published in English. Collectively, these studies have:

- supported the validity of the concepts offered in the model,
- confirmed the reliability and validity of MOHO assessments, and
- documented the process and outcomes of interventions based on MOHO.

Therapists who wish to use an evidence-based model can find substantial empirical support for MOHO, as discussed in Chapter 26.

Designed to Complement Other Models and Theories

MOHO was developed at a time when most models in occupational therapy were impairment focused and when the importance of occupation was being rediscovered (Kielhofner, 2004). The intention of the model was to fill a gap that existed in occupational therapy knowledge and to complement the focus on impairment with an understanding of the client's motivation and lifestyle as well as the environmental context. The model was always intended to be used alongside other occupational therapy models as well as interdisciplinary concepts. It is recognized that MOHO rarely addresses all the problems faced by a client, requiring the therapists to actively use other models and concepts. Most therapists who use MOHO do use it in combination with other models such as the biomechanical, sensory integration, and motor control models, to name a few. The latter models provide a focus on performance components not provided in MOHO. Thus, use of these models in combination allows a more comprehensive approach to meeting client needs.

CASE EXAMPLE: TEST YOUR KNOWLEDGE

Since the time he broke his leg on a bicycle in first grade, Ben, a 12-year-old boy from Toronto, has always had a desire to become a health care provider. Anything related to medicine interests him, from learning about the prescription medications that his mother takes for her gastroesophageal reflux disease to offering to splint the wrist of a classmate who just sprained it playing ball. Unfortunately, Ben's performance in school, coupled with his social skills, has not been strong suits for him. He has been living with a learning

disability, a diagnosis of attention deficit disorder, and sensory-processing difficulties ever since he can remember. Ben is always on the go. He loves hands-on activities, including being outdoors, and his teachers describe him as being in perpetual motion. On a typical day at school, he may forget to bring his gym shorts from home, get scolded by his teacher for talking in class, get pushed into a locker by a classmate for saying something inappropriate, and miss the bus home because he is consumed with watching the eighth graders conduct their science projects.

Ben regularly consults two occupational therapists: one at school and one on an outpatient basis. The two therapists differ drastically and disagree in terms of their approach to Ben's difficulties. The school-based occupational therapist utilizes a treatment approach rooted in principles of behavioral modification to address his social and behavioral difficulties. She uses specialized computer games to provide him with remedial opportunities in the areas of math and language arts. Although he is cooperative with this therapist, he rarely shows enjoyment or appreciation and appears to be going through the motions of therapy rather than being fully engaged in it. His outpatient therapist, on the other hand, utilizes an approach that combines principles from sensory integration theory and MOHO. Firstly, she supports Ben's need to be in constant motion by encouraging his engagement in sports that involve intense body movement, both during and after school hours. To this effect, she has recommended to Ben's parents that he take horseback riding lessons on weekends. Additionally, the therapist has recommended to Ben's teachers that they focus any homework assignments that he has on topics that somehow relate to a health care situation. The school administrator has also been encouraged to provide Ben with two gym periods (as opposed to the usual one gym period) and a few smaller, additional break periods during which he is allowed to visit and watch the science teacher teaching other classes. The therapist has also recommended to Ben's parents that they take him to as many museums and age-appropriate public lectures and venues that have anything to do with science and health care. She also recommends that Ben volunteer at a skilled nursing facility as he transitions into high school, to provide him with early experience within a health care environment.

FOLLOW-UP QUESTIONS

Use the preceding case example to answer the following questions.

1. Which of the two occupational therapists is using an impairment-focused approach? Which one is using an occupation-focused approach?
2. What are the recommendations that are made by the MOHO-based (outpatient) therapist that support Ben's interests in health care and science?
3. How does the MOHO-based occupational therapist utilize elements of the physical environment to support Ben's interests and respond to his need for constant movement?
4. What are the recommendations that are made by the MOHO-based therapist?
5. What are the pros and cons of each of the two intervention approaches (impairment focused versus MOHO)?
6. If you were Ben, which of the two intervention approaches would you prefer? Why?

Approaching This Book

This book relies on case studies from actual practice situations as well as some fictionalized, case-composite examples from the editor's practice experience to provide a hands-on overview of contemporary MOHO theory, practice application, and research. To the greatest extent possible, the voice and content of Dr. Gary Kielhofner's original contributions are preserved. In addition, the voices of the many other contributors who provided case material used in prior editions of this text have been retained and simply updated. This book is divided into four sections. The first section covers MOHO theory. Part II covers such topics as therapeutic reasoning, assessments, and planning and documenting therapy. Part III illustrates the application of MOHO in therapy by providing a series of in-depth case examples. Part IV contains resources for the use of MOHO in practice and research.

In addition to the former and new contributing authors in this edition, an effort has been made to retain the unheralded voices of Kielhofner's colleagues from around the world who helped him conceptualize MOHO, those of persons who have told their stories of living with disabilities, and those of therapists who have created practical means of applying MOHO.

Each chapter begins by defining expected learning outcomes and by presenting one or more case examples illustrating how use of a MOHO-based intervention improved occupational therapy outcomes for a client.

These cases are labeled "MOHO Problem-Solver" cases. Toward the end of each chapter, a final case example is provided to assess the applied learning of the relevant concepts covered in the chapter. Finally, the retention of basic concepts in each chapter is tested through a series of brief quiz questions.

Chapter 1 Quiz Questions

1. In two sentences or less, define the model of human occupation.
2. Name and describe the seven elements of Kielhofner's vision for advancing occupational therapy through the model of human occupation. List the seven elements of the model of human occupation that characterize its vision for advancing occupational therapy practice.
3. To what extent is the model of human occupation used in practice?
4. Define human occupation.

thePoint® For additional resources and exercises, visit http://thePoint.lww.com

Key Terms

Activities of daily living: The typical life tasks required for self-care and self-maintenance, such as grooming, bathing, eating, cleaning the house, and doing laundry.

Environment: One of the four elements that comprise MOHO. The environment refers to both physical and social aspects of the context within which a person performs a given occupation. Ideally, the physical and social elements of the environment serve to facilitate a person's engagement in occupation.

Habituation: One of the four elements that comprise MOHO. Habituation describes the emergence of a pattern of occupation over time. This pattern forms repeated habits and public and private roles.

Human occupation: The doing of work, play, or activities of daily living within a temporal, physical, and sociocultural context that characterizes much of human life.

Model of human occupation: An evidence-based conceptual practice model that explains how people adapt to disabilities and other conditions that create occupational problems and rediscover satisfying and meaningful ways to live their lives. Specifically, the model explains how occupations are motivated, patterned, and performed within an environmental context.

Occupation-focused model: Defines an approach to therapy that focuses on a client's engagement and participation in occupations as the mechanism of change, rather than focusing specifically on remediating an impairment.

Performance capacity: One of the four elements that comprise MOHO. Performance capacity describes a person's own experience and perception of the ability to perform an occupation as well as others' perceptions of that person's experience and perception of that ability.

Play: Activities undertaken for their own sake.

Productivity: Activities (both paid and unpaid) that provide services or commodities to others, such as ideas, knowledge, help, information sharing, entertainment, utilitarian or artistic objects, and protection.

Volition: One of the four elements that comprise MOHO. Volition describes how a person is motivated to perform a given occupation.

REFERENCES

Albrecht, G. L., Seelman, K. D., & Bury, M. (2001). *Handbook of disability studies*. Thousand Oaks, CA: SAGE.

Fidler, G., & Fidler, J. (1983). Doing and becoming: The occupational therapy experience. In G. Kielhofner (Ed.), *Health through occupation: Theory and practice in occupational therapy*. Philadelphia, PA: F. A. Davis.

Forsyth, K., Summerfield-Mann, L., & Kielhofner, G. (2005). A scholarship of practice: Making occupation-focused, theory-driven, evidence-based practice a reality. *British Journal of Occupational Therapy, 68*, 261–268.

Haglund, L., Ekbladh, E., Thorell, L.-H., & Hallberg, I. R. (2000). Practice models in Swedish psychiatric occupational therapy. *Scandinavian Journal of Occupational Therapy, 7*, 107–113.

Kielhofner, G. (1980a). A model of human occupation, Part 2: Ontogenesis from the perspective of temporal adaptation. *American Journal of Occupational Therapy, 34*, 657–663.

Kielhofner, G. (1980b). A model of human occupation, Part 3: Benign and vicious cycles. *American Journal of Occupational Therapy, 34,* 731–737.

Kielhofner, G. (2004). The model of human occupation. In G. Kielhofner (Ed.), *Conceptual foundations of occupational therapy* (3rd ed., pp. 147–161). Philadelphia, PA: F. A. Davis.

Kielhofner, G. (2005a). Rethinking disability and what to do about it: Disability studies and its implications for occupational therapy. *American Journal of Occupational Therapy, 59,* 487–496.

Kielhofner, G. (2005b). A scholarship of practice: Creating discourse between theory, research and practice. *Occupational Therapy in Health Care, 19,* 7–17.

Kielhofner, G. (2008). *Model of human occupation: Theory and application* (4th ed.). Baltimore, MD: Lippincott Williams & Wilkins.

Kielhofner, G., & Burke, J. (1980). A model of human occupation, Part 1: Conceptual framework and content. *American Journal of Occupational Therapy, 34,* 572–581.

Kielhofner, G., Burke, J., & Heard, I. C. (1980). A model of human occupation, Part 4: Assessment and intervention. *American Journal of Occupational Therapy, 34,* 777–788.

Law, M. C. (1998). *Client-centered occupational therapy.* Thorofare, NJ: Slack.

Law, M., & McColl, M. A. (1989). Knowledge and use of theory among occupational therapists: A Canadian survey. *Canadian Journal of Occupational Therapy, 56*(4), 198–204.

Lee, J. (2010). Achieving best practice: A review of evidence linked to occupation-focused practice models. *Occupational Therapy in Health Care, 24,* 206–222.

Longmore, P. K. (1995, September/October). The second phase: From disability rights to disability culture. *The Disability Rag & Resource,* pp. 4–11.

Mosey, A. C. (1992). *Applied scientific inquiry in the health professions: An epistemological orientation.* Rockville, MD: The American Occupational Therapy Association.

National Board for Certification in Occupational Therapy. (2004, Spring). A practice analysis study of entry-level occupational therapist registered and certified occupational therapy assistant practice. *Occupation, Participation and Health, 24*(Suppl. 1), S3–S31.

Nelson, D. (1988). Occupation: Form and performance. *American Journal of Occupational Therapy, 38,* 777–788.

Oliver, M. (1994). The social model in context. In *Understanding disability: From theory to practice.* London, United Kingdom: Macmillan.

Reilly, M. (1974). *Play as exploratory learning.* Beverly Hills, CA: SAGE.

Riccio, C. M., Nelson, D. L., & Bush, M. A. (1990). Adding purpose to the repetitive exercise of elderly women. *American Journal of Occupational Therapy, 44,* 714–719.

Rogers, J. (1983). The study of human occupation. In G. Kielhofner (Ed.), *Health through occupation: Theory and practice in occupational therapy.* Philadelphia, PA: F. A. Davis.

Scotch, R. (1988). Disability as a basis for a social movement: Advocacy and the politics of definition. *Journal of Social Issues, 44*(1), 159–172.

Shannon, P. (1970). The work-play model: A basis for occupational therapy programming. *American Journal of Occupational Therapy, 24,* 215–218.

Shapiro, J. (1994). *No pity: People with disabilities forging a new civil rights movement.* New York, NY: Times Books.

Taylor, R. R., Lee, S. W., Kielhofner, G. W., & Ketkar, M. (2009). Therapeutic use of self: A nationwide survey of practitioners' experience and attitudes. *The American Journal of Occupational Therapy, 63,* 198–207.

Toombs, K. (1992). *The meaning of illness: A phenomenological account of the different perspectives of physician and patient.* Boston, MA: Kluwer Academic Publishers.

Trombly, C. (1995a). Occupation: Purposefulness and meaningfulness as therapeutic mechanisms. *American Journal of Occupational Therapy, 49,* 960–972.

Trombly, C. (1995b). *Occupational therapy for physical dysfunction* (4th ed.). Philadelphia, PA: F. A. Davis.

The Person-Specific Concepts of Human Occupation

Takashi Yamada, Renée R. Taylor, and Gary Kielhofner (posthumous)

CHAPTER 2

EXPECTED LEARNING OUTCOMES

Upon completion of this chapter, readers will be able to:

1. Describe the basic concepts of the model of human occupation (MOHO): volition, habituation, performance capacity, and environment.
2. Understand the elements that form volition.
3. Recall the way in which habits and roles interact to form habituation.
4. Explain the two perspectives from which a client experiences performance capacity.
5. Understand the ways in which the environment can facilitate or limit action, as well as the way in which the person can influence the environment.

The Basic Concepts of Human Occupation

Clients differ in how they are motivated toward and choose to do things, in their patterns of everyday life, and in their individual capacities. In order to have a common way to understand all of their circumstances, concepts that explain how they select, organize, and undertake their occupations are needed. Within the model of human occupation (MOHO), humans are conceptualized as being made up of three interrelated components:

- Volition
- Habituation
- Performance capacity

Volition refers to the motivation for occupation. Habituation refers to the process by which occupation is organized into patterns or routines. Performance capacity refers to the physical and mental abilities that underlie skilled occupational performance. Although the following sections discuss these components separately, it is important to keep in mind that they are three different aspects of the total person.

Within MOHO, consideration of any aspect of the person (volition, habituation, and performance) always includes how the environment is influencing the person's motivation, pattern, and performance. The environment is a constant influence on occupation, and persons' occupational circumstances cannot be appreciated without an understanding of their environments.

Volition

MOHO Problem-Solver: School-Based Therapy

Arata, the son of a well-known professional soccer player, is a fifth grader who lives just outside of Tokyo. He attends the same school as his two siblings, both of whom have a reputation among faculty and other students for being exceptional at academics. By contrast, Arata has always had difficulties with academics and has also struggled with paying attention in class. At the beginning of the school year, he did poorly on his last homework assignment, which added to his feelings of ineffectiveness as a student. He does not want to let his parents down because he knows how much they value doing well in school, but he increasingly dreads going to school. Arata recently started succumbing to all of the pressures of being a student by ignoring some of his homework assignments. Concerned about Arata's increasing difficulty in school, his mother began forcing him to study during the evening time when he usually plays soccer, the only athletic activity at which Arata excels and enjoys.

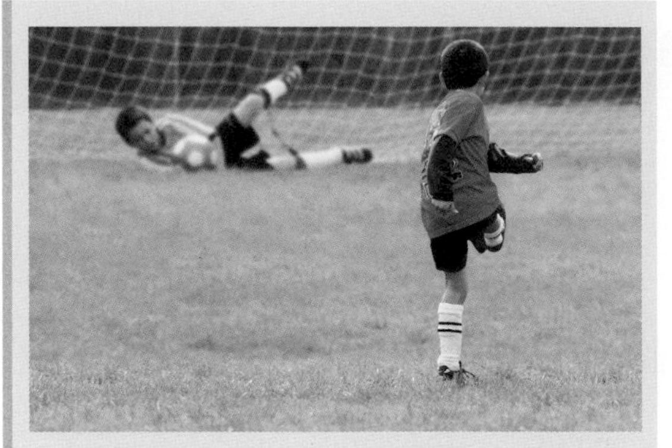
Arata performing a valued soccer activity

The decision by Arata's parents not to allow him to play after school led to increased behavioral problems and a complete refusal to engage in any homework or studying. Arata began sitting idly in front of his computer and was unresponsive in class at school. As a result of his failing grades, an individualized educational plan was created for Arata, which included regular observations and appointments with an occupational therapist in the school setting.

The therapist began her observation by focusing upon what interested Arata during school when he was not paying attention in class. The first thing she noticed was that, unbeknownst to his teacher, he often brought torn-out pages from the sports sections of newspapers and soccer magazines to school. He hid them under his computer or within the pages of his textbooks and then lured his classmates into conversations about the pictures, often bragging about his abilities. He would inform his classmates how he always scores goals and finds value in teaching soccer techniques to the younger children in the neighborhood.

Having observed Arata's interests, sense of ability, and values around being a leader among his siblings in soccer, the therapist then consulted with Arata's teacher and parents. Together, they developed an approach to remotivating Arata to engage in school work. This approach involved building relevant content involving soccer statistics and famous soccer players into his math problems and reading assignments. During one-on-one occupational therapy sessions, the therapist would encourage Arata to bring in new pictures of these interests and they would spend time searching on the Internet for relevant news articles, events, and competitions. At the same time, his parents were encouraged to allow Arata to play with his siblings and friends after school, on the condition that he received a positive evaluation for having paid attention in class.

People possess a complex nervous system, which gives them an intense and pervasive need to act (Berlyne, 1960; Florey, 1969; McClelland, 1961; Reilly, 1962; Shibutani, 1968; Smith, 1969; White, 1959). Moreover, people have bodies capable of action. Last, people have an awareness of their potential for doing things (DeCharms, 1968). Together, these factors result in a need for action that is the underlying motive for occupation. Other motives are sometimes involved in an occupation (Nelson, 1988). For example, financial rewards may partly motivate work. Daily living tasks are partly in the service of basic drives such as hunger, and recreational activities such as dating have a sexual dimension. Nonetheless, the desire for action manifests itself throughout occupation and is its dominant motive.

VOLITIONAL THOUGHTS AND FEELINGS

In addition to the need or desire to act, each person has distinct feelings and thoughts about doing things that are essential to volition. These thoughts and feelings are responses to the questions: Am I good at this? Is this worth doing? Do I like this? Thus, volitional thoughts and feelings are about the following:

- Personal capacity and effectiveness
- Importance or worth attached to what one does
- Enjoyment or satisfaction one experiences in doing things

Thus, while humans are all energized by a universal drive toward action, they want to do those things that they value, feel competent to do, and find satisfying.

PERSONAL CAUSATION, VALUES, AND INTERESTS

In MOHO, these volitional thoughts and feelings are referred to as personal causation, values, and interests (Fig. 2-1). **Personal causation** refers to one's sense of capacity and effectiveness. **Values** refer to what one finds important and meaningful to do. **Interests** refer to what one finds enjoyable or satisfying to do. In everyday life, personal causation, values, and interests are interwoven. For example, Arata's volition can be seen in the values he has internalized about the importance of school performance and his

Thoughts and feelings about self as an actor in one's world
Personal causation
Sense of competence and effectiveness
Values
What's important and meaningful to do?
Interests
What's enjoyable and satisfying to do?

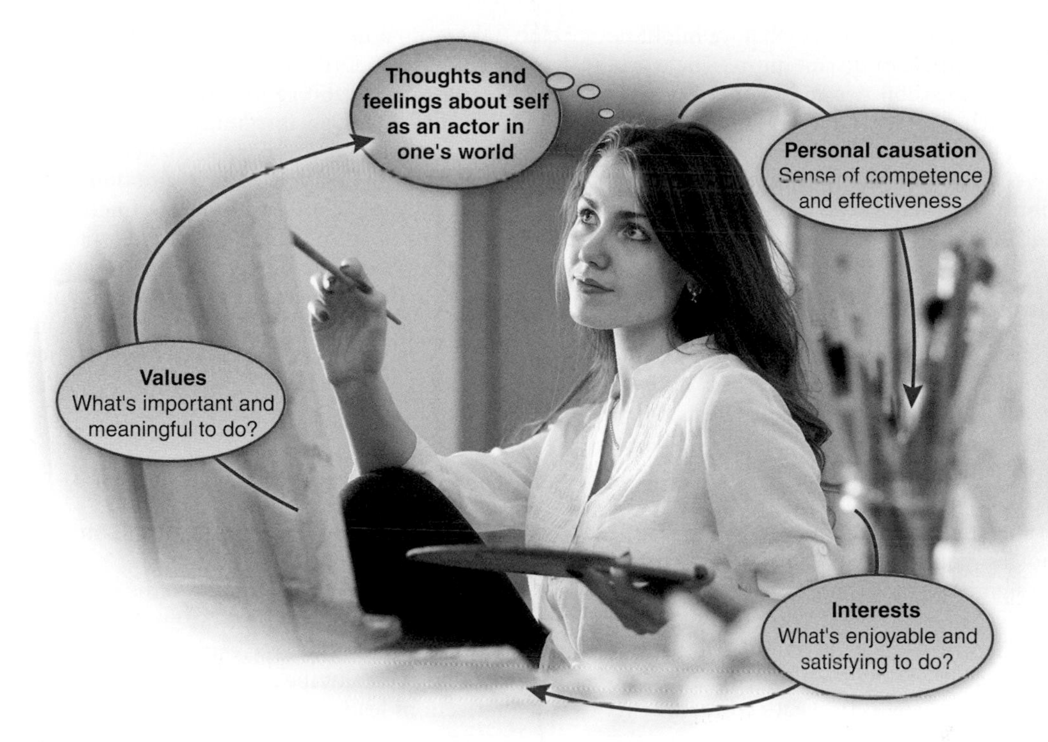

FIGURE 2-1 The Content of Volitional Thoughts and Feelings.

sense of feeling ineffective in doing well in school. His volition is reflected in a wide range of thoughts and feelings he has about the things he has done, is doing, or might do.

VOLITIONAL PROCESSES

Volition is an ongoing process. That is, volitional thoughts and feelings occur over time as people experience, interpret, anticipate, and choose occupations.

Experience

Whenever we do something, a whole range of experiences are possible. We may, for example, feel pleasure, anxiety, comfort, challenge, or boredom. Moreover, we may have thoughts of self-doubt or confidence. We may proceed deliberately with solid convictions about why we are doing what we are doing or hesitantly worrying that our actions are futile or meaningless. **Experience** refers, then, to the immediate thoughts and feelings that emerge in the midst of and in response to performance. These would include, for instance, the joy Arata feels when playing soccer or the anxiety he experiences when facing his homework.

Interpretation

Of course, we not only experience what we do, but also reflect on and interpret that experience. A person may do this in a variety of ways. For example, Arata feels badly when his parents see his negative report card and recalls the incident to consider whether he should have behaved differently in school. Later, he asks his mother whether she thinks he has improved doing his homework. Whenever people reflect on or discuss with others how they performed, what it was like to do something, and whether it is worth doing, they are engaged in the volitional process of interpretation. **Interpretation** is thus defined as recalling and reflecting on performance in terms of its significance for oneself and one's world.

Anticipation

The world presents us with immediate and future possibilities for action. Whether we pay attention to them and how we react to the opportunities and expectations for action is also part of the volitional process. For example, Arata walks into a classroom and dreads an upcoming exam. He peers out the window to see if friends have been let out of class yet.

Anticipation always considers what we might be doing in the immediate or distant future. The world presents us with possibilities and expectations for action, but which ones we notice and how we think and feel about them is influenced by what we like and feel competent and obligated to do. Consequently, **anticipation** is defined as the process of noticing and reacting to potentials or expectations for action.

Activity and Occupational Choices

Our daily lives are influenced by what we choose to do next, later on, and tomorrow. These **activity choices** are defined as short-term, deliberate decisions to enter and exit occupational activities. Examples of activity choices include deciding to go for a morning walk, have lunch with a friend later in the day, and clean one's apartment this Saturday morning. While activity choices require only brief deliberation, they determine a significant amount of what we actually do.

Individuals also make larger choices concerning occupations that will become an extended or permanent part of their lives. These occupational choices (Heard, 1977; Matsutsuyu, 1971) are commitments to enter into a course of action or to sustain regular performance over time. They include taking on a new role, establishing a new activity as part of one's permanent routine, and undertaking a project. Examples of occupational choices are starting a job, joining a club, taking up a new hobby, and deciding to tend a summer garden. Ordinarily, occupational choices require some deliberation and may involve information gathering, reflection, imagining possibilities, and considering alternatives. Occupational choices also involve commitment since they require doing over time. **Occupational choices** are thus defined as deliberate commitments to enter an occupational role, acquire a new habit, or undertake a personal project.

Together, activity choices and occupational choices influence, to a large extent, what kinds of occupational performance make up our daily lives. These choices are the function of volition. They reflect our personal causation, our interests, and our values.

SUMMARY AND DEFINITION OF VOLITION

The cycle of experience, interpretation, anticipation, and choice is an integrated process. As shown in Figure 2-2, each process flows into the next. One chooses action, the doing of which stimulates experience. One recalls and reflects on experience to interpret what was done. Finally, the meanings generated from such reflections lead to the next choices.

Thus we can say that **volition** *is a pattern of thoughts and feelings about oneself as an actor in one's world which occur as one anticipates, chooses, experiences, and interprets what one does. Volitional thoughts and feelings include personal causation, values, and interests.*

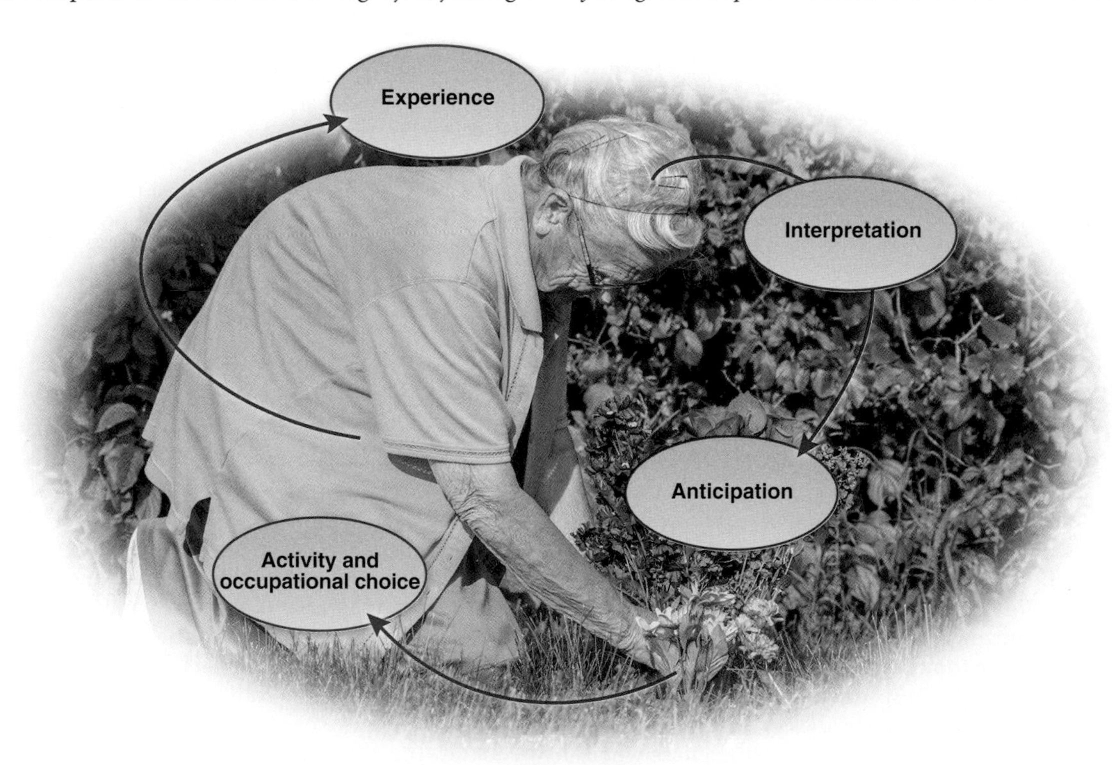

FIGURE 2-2 Volitional Processes. The World Around Us, Our Habitat, Has a Certain Stability; We, in Return, Also Have a Tendency to Act in Consistent, Patterned Ways.

Through the cycle of anticipating, choosing, experiencing, and interpreting, volition tends to perpetuate itself. For example, once we experience ourselves as competent in an occupation, we will tend to anticipate that occupation with positive feelings and choose to do it again. Volition is also an unfolding process in which changes take place. As we develop and age, and as we encounter new environments with new opportunities and demands for action, we may find new pleasures, lose old interests, discover new capabilities, or find that we are no longer so adept at a particular activity. There are elements of both continuity and change in values, interests, and personal causation over the life span.

Habituation

MOHO Problem-Solver: Adult

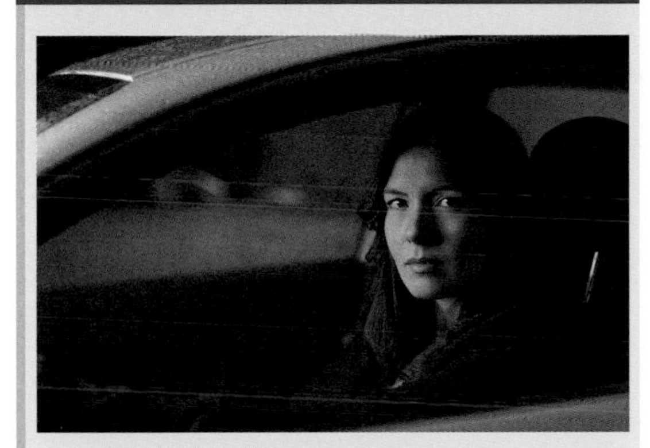

Marie behind the wheel

Marie is a middle-aged woman who worked as a delivery driver for a local florist during the day and an Uber car driver in the evenings to support her aging mother, who was unable to support herself on her own due to severe mental illness. On her way home from work, Marie experienced a mild-to-moderate traumatic brain injury resulting from a car accident. During her hospital stay, she talked with her therapist about wanting to resume her jobs as a driver upon discharge. However, a simulated driving test revealed that it may not be possible for her to return to driving full-time right away due to concentration difficulties, easy fatigability, dizziness, and headaches, which were interfering with her ability to sustain attention during the test. Additionally, a mild hand tremor interfered with her manipulation of small knobs in the car and muscle atrophy and a lack of endurance resulting from the inactivity and decreased activity levels during her hospital stay were contributing to her poor posture during the simulation.

Overall, Marie is feeling badly about herself since she has been receiving negative feedback about her driving ability. As a consequence she does not see much value in trying to drive, and she decides not to continue with occupational therapy as an outpatient. When she shares her discouragement and lack of attendance with her physician's office during a follow-up phone call, the nurse recommends consultation with a new therapist. Marie agrees to a brief, initial consultation with the new therapist.

The therapist began by interviewing Marie about her daily habits and roles before the accident, her present roles, and the roles she desire for the future. While Marie was able to identify several roles in the past, her only present role was one of caregiver for her mentally ill mother. However, she expressed a continued desire to return to her worker role as a driver in the future. Currently, Marie's daily routine involved waking up, taking her vitamins, showering, and calling her mother to make sure her mother has taken her morning medications. Marie then watches daytime television until lunchtime, at which time she walks to the corner store to get a sandwich and to pick up any groceries that she needs. In the late afternoon, Marie goes across the street to her mother's house to have dinner with her mother. She then returns home, watches evening television or a movie, and goes to bed.

Before the accident, driving had been the one occupation in addition to caretaking her mother that provided Marie with a sense of self-efficacy and value. Marie expressed to the therapist that she was keen to return to driving, yet terrified that she would be unable to do it. By this time, it had been nearly 2 months since discharge, when Marie had failed the driving simulation test. Because Marie's symptoms of headaches, dizziness, and fatigue had lessened over time, the therapist decided to explore anew Marie's interest in driving and ability to drive. The therapist began by driving Marie to the flower shop where she was working before the accident, and having Marie ride along as a passenger while the therapist simulated a half-day flower delivery route.

As the therapist was driving, she asked Marie to direct her to the best of her ability. Marie demonstrated that she was highly familiar with the routes she used to take when delivering flowers and was able to remember the directions and roads within the neighborhood immediately surrounding the flower shop without any assistance from a map or navigational device. The context of being in a car and being in a familiar neighborhood provided Marie with the confidence she needed, and so she exerted extra effort to focus and concentrate on the addresses and the route. Marie was less confident about her former worker role as an Uber driver owing to the broader driving territory and the lack of a regular daily route. However, she agreed to continue with the recommended visits from the occupational therapist, and, together, they developed renewed habit patterns to support Marie's growing ability to reengage in one of her valued worker roles as a floral delivery driver.

Much of what we do belongs to a taken-for-granted round of daily life. Most of us repeat the same familiar weekday morning scenario of getting up, grooming, and heading to work or school. On the way, we walk, ride, or drive the same route or take the same train, subway, or bus without having to consciously think about what we are doing. Once arrived, we set about doing tasks we previously have done multiple times, undertaking them in much the same way as before. We encounter others, saying and doing the same types of things with them that we have done in the past. We do these things unreflectively, and doing them feels familiar, locating us in our ordinary, taken-for-granted life. Moreover, by engaging in certain routine behaviors, we reaffirm ourselves as having a certain identity. These aspects of routine daily life unfold automatically.

The term, habituation, refers to this semi-autonomous patterning of behavior in concert with our familiar temporal, physical, and social habitats as shown in Figure 2-3. Habituation allows us to recognize and respond to temporal cues and time frames (e.g., the recurring pattern of weeks), to our familiar physical worlds (e.g., the physical layout of our home, workplace, school, and neighborhood), and to the social customs

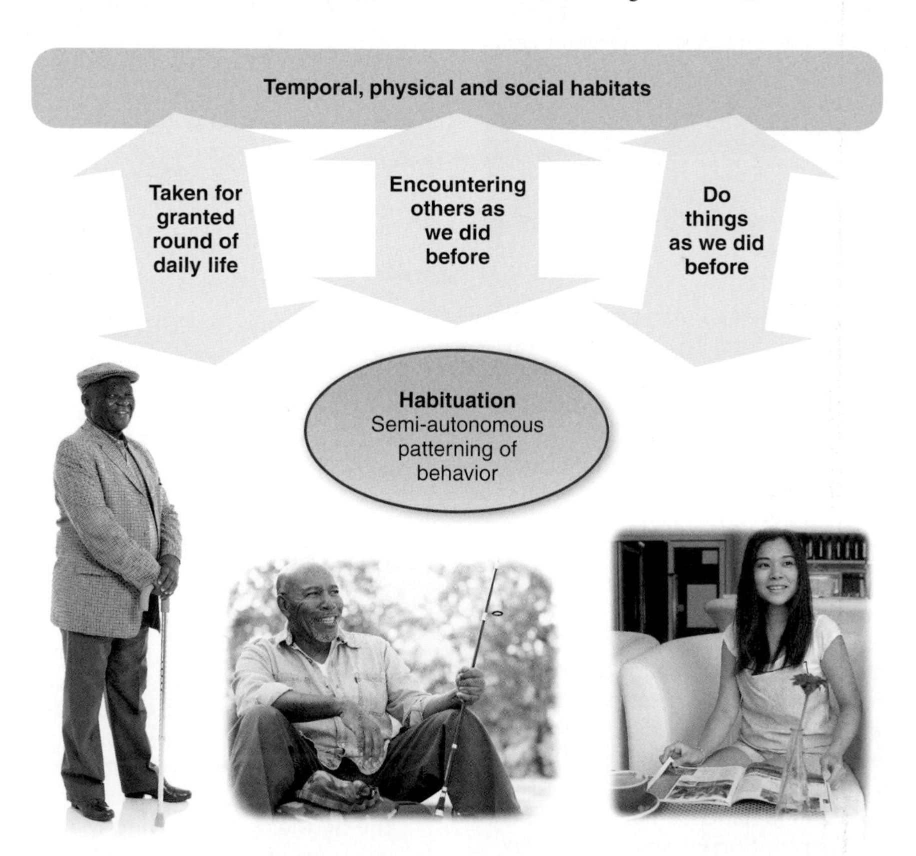

FIGURE 2-3 Habituation Shapes Interaction with Our Habitats. All Persons Who Have Objectively Describable Abilities and Limitations of Ability Also Have Corresponding Experiences of Those Abilities or Limitations.

and the patterns that make up our own culture. The world around us, our habitat, has a certain stability; we, in return, also have a habituated tendency to act in consistent, patterned ways. That we do so is a function of habits and roles.

HABITS

Habits preserve ways of doing things that we have internalized through repeated performance. We generate habits by consistently doing the same thing in the same context. What once required attention and concentration eventually becomes automatic. Thus, **habits** are defined as acquired tendencies to respond and perform in certain consistent ways in familiar environments or situations. Consequently, for habits to exist,

- we must repeat action sufficiently to establish the pattern;
- consistent environmental circumstances must be present.

Much of what we do in the course of a day or week is guided by habits. Our daily routine, our manner of going about anything we do, and the peculiar ways we always do a given task, all reflect our habits. Marie's morning call to her mother to ensure she has taken her morning medications and Arata's regular practicing of soccer techniques are both examples of habits.

INTERNALIZED ROLES

Our patterns of action also reflect roles that we have internalized. That is, we identify with and behave in ways that we have learned to associate with a particular social status or identity. For example, when people act as spouses, parents, workers, or students, they exhibit patterns of behavior that reflect those socially identified statuses. Moreover, their behavior will tend to be along the lines of what others expect them to do as part of that role.

Through a process of socialization, people acquire those roles that derive from a social status. Socialization involves interacting over time with explicit and implicit definitions and expectations for the role. As a result, one internalizes a sense of self, attitudes and behaviors that correspond to the social definition, and expectations of the role. Other roles are self-defined and shaped by the interrelated and ongoing nature of a set of tasks for which we feel responsibility. Such roles arise out of personal circumstances or necessity. They are established as one engages in a pattern of related actions and assumes an identity connected to them.

Given these considerations, the **internalized role** can be defined as incorporation of a socially and/or personally defined status and a related cluster of attitudes and behaviors. People ordinarily have several roles that occupy routine times and spaces. For example, people generally are in the worker role during the workweek and in the workplace. On the other hand, they are mostly in the role of a spouse or parent at home and outside work hours. Having a complement of roles gives one rhythm and change between different identities and modes of doing. We can see how roles play out in the lives of Arata, who struggles to meet the demands of a student, and Marie, who seeks to reenact her role as a worker.

SUMMARY AND DEFINITION OF HABITUATION

Habituation comes about as a consequence of repeating patterns of behavior under certain temporal, physical, and sociocultural contexts (Bruner, 1973; Koestler, 1969). As we interact over and over again with the various characteristics of these contexts (e.g., physical arrangement, temporal patterns, social attitudes and expectations, behaviors of others), we internalize patterns of attitude and action.

A pervasive influence on habituation is the environment. As noted earlier, habituation is a way we have learned to be within our habitats. Be it the physical arrangement of the world or the social patterns and norms that surround us, the features of our environments shape us to develop certain habituated ways of doing things.

Habituation is defined as an internalized readiness to exhibit consistent patterns of behavior guided by our habits and roles and fitted to the characteristics of routine temporal, physical, and social environments. As shown in Figure 2-4, habituation shapes what we take to be ordinary and mundane in our lives. It is responsible for our daily routine of behavior; our usual way of going about doing things; the various routes we take in going about our homes, neighborhoods, and larger community; and our patterns of involvement with others.

Performance Capacity

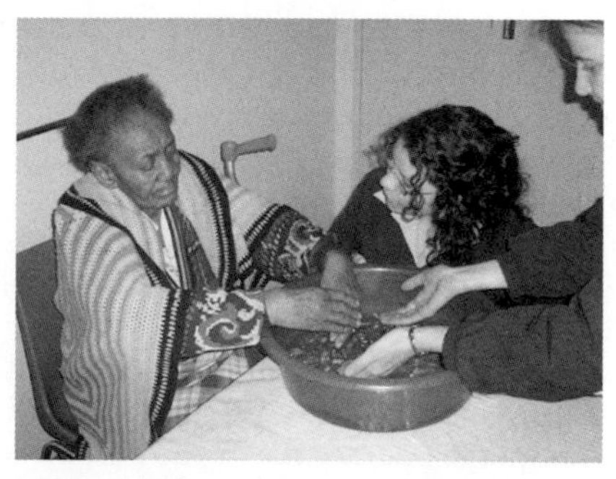

Lydia interacts with physical therapy students during a therapy session

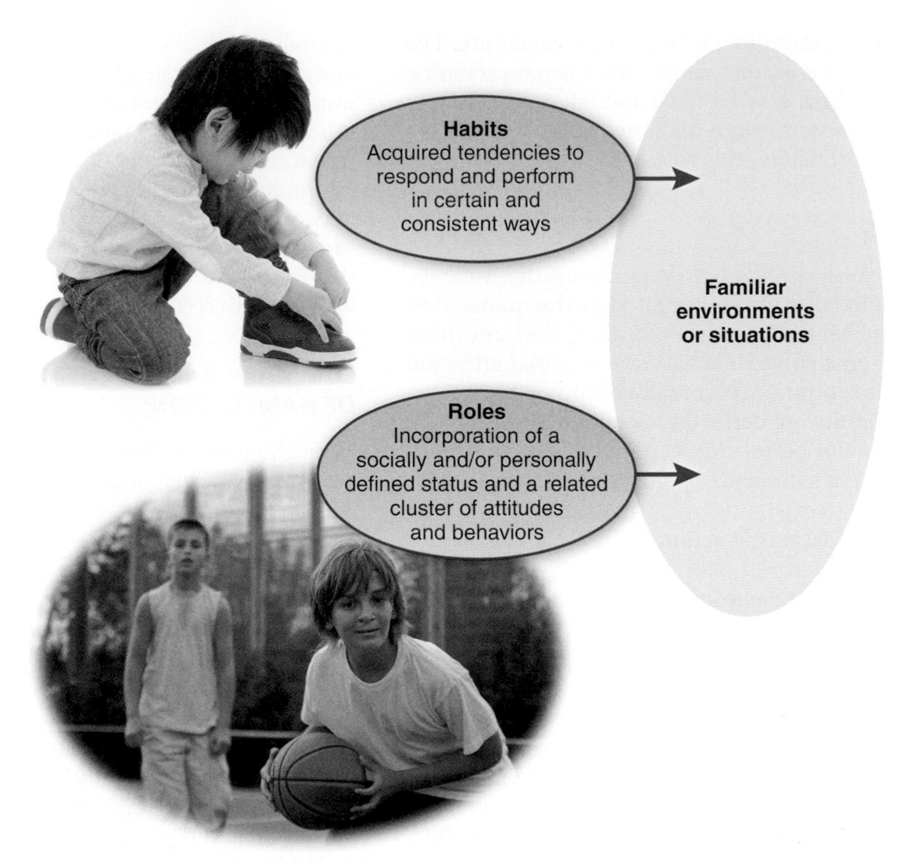

FIGURE 2-4 Habituation: Habits and Roles Influencing Behavior in Familiar Environments and Situations.

CASE EXAMPLE: OLDER ADULT IN DEMENTIA CARE

Lydia is 83-year-old Sesotho resident of the dementia care unit in Bloemfontein, South Africa. She loves young people as she raised six children of her own. She views any younger person as if he or she were her own child, offering food or assistance. Most people humor her or gently decline her offers, to which Lydia always responds, "How will I ever get you to grow up?" Lydia's caring nature and strong religious beliefs makes her a favorite among the unit staff. She willingly engages in any of the occupational therapy groups offered in the unit. She is friendly and kind to all and often sits by herself and softly sings hymns. Although she is seldom reality oriented, she loves to pray for others. She attempts to communicate in Sotho, Xhosa, Afrikaans, and/or English, depending on the language preference of the person with whom she is interacting.

The capacity to do things depends on

- musculoskeletal, neurologic, cardiopulmonary, and other bodily systems that are used when acting on the world; and
- mental or cognitive abilities such as memory and planning.

Arata's cognitive capacity is affected by his difficulty maintaining attention. Marie's and Lydia's cognition are impaired, each in different ways. As we saw, the performance capacity of each of these individuals affects their occupation.

Theory and practice in occupational therapy have always recognized the importance of these underlying components for competent performance. Notably, other models (e.g., biomechanical, cognitive-perceptual, sensory integration, motor control) provide specific explanations of physical and mental components and their contribution to performance (Bundy, Lane, & Murray, 2002; Katz, 1992; Mathiowetz & Haugen, 1994; Trombly, 1995). Because other models address performance capacity, therapists use these models as a means to understanding and addressing specific problems of performance capacity.

Within MOHO, performance capacity is approached from a different but complementary viewpoint that emphasizes subjective experience and its role in shaping how people do things. In occupational therapy and related fields, people's performance and difficulty in performing is approached objectively. For example, consideration may be given to understanding losses or disturbances of ordinary movement capacity, sensory abilities such as sight or hearing, or cognitive capacities such as memory or judgment. Various objective ways of describing, categorizing, and measuring these impairments have been developed. All objectively describable abilities and limitations of ability are experienced by the people who have them. Attention to the nature of these experiences and how they shape performance can complement and enhance the understanding we have from the objective approach to performance capacity.

Therefore, within MOHO, the concept of **performance capacity** is defined as the ability for doing things provided by the status of underlying objective physical and mental components, and corresponding subjective experience. As shown in Figure 2-5, this definition calls attention to the objective approach to capacity, which is the focus of other models, and to the subjective, experiential focus on capacity that we emphasize.

In discussing the experiential aspect of performance capacity, we employ a concept referred to as the lived body. This concept derives from the work of philosophers who argue that the body must be understood as a site of experience (Merleau-Ponty, 1945/1962). This concept also offers new ways of understanding both how we are able to perform and how disease or impairment is experienced and affects performance.

The Environment

CASE EXAMPLE: COMMUNITY-DWELLING ADULT

Carlos is a 26-year-old that lives in Mexico. As a child he was diagnosed as developmentally delayed. He is independent in his personal care, but is unable to cross the streets or manage money by himself. He enjoys music, but otherwise has few interests or pastimes. He wants to work like other young men and attends a sheltered workshop two times a week where he packages products. In the workshop, he has trouble with new tasks that involve following directions and does not get along well with his supervisor. Carlos feels frustrated that he is not able to control more aspects of his life and do things that others his age are able to do.

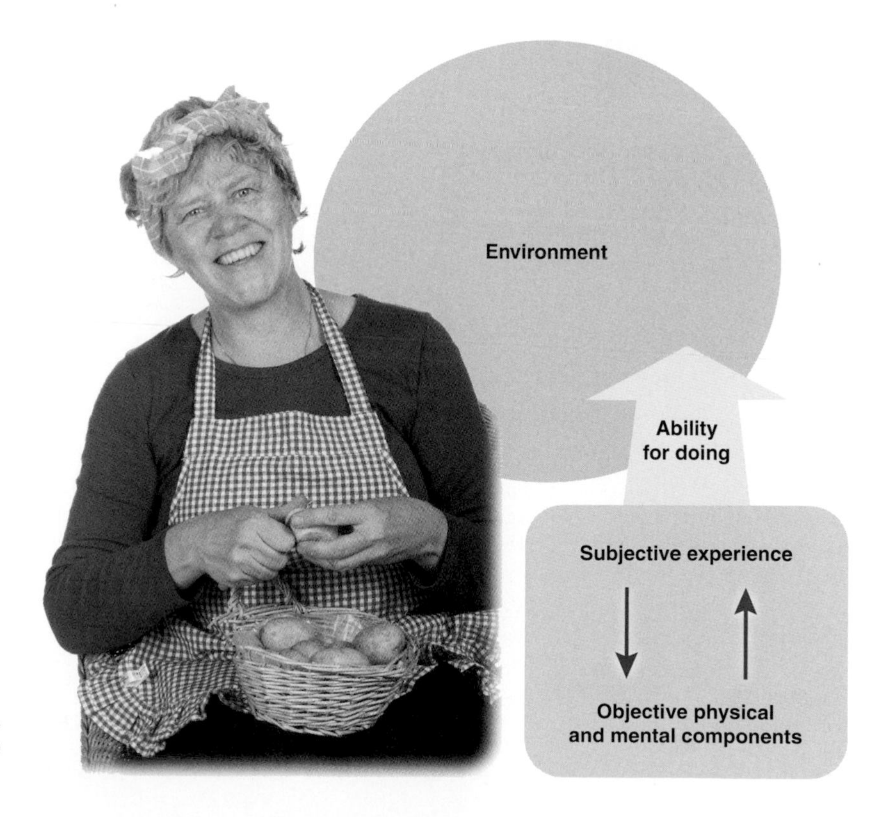

FIGURE 2-5 Objective and Subjective Components of Performance Capacity

All occupations occur in a complex multilayered environment. Occupation is always located in, influenced, and given meaning by its physical and sociocultural context. Thus the environment includes the spaces humans occupy, the objects they use, the people with whom they interact, and the possibilities and meanings for doing that exist in the human collective of which they are a part. Each environment offers potential opportunities and resources, demands, and constraints. How the characteristics of a given environment interact with each person's values, interests, personal causation, roles, habits, and performance capacities will determine what influence the environment has for that person. The opportunity, support, demand, and constraint that the physical and social aspects of the environment have on a particular individual will be referred to as **environmental impact**. Importantly, this impact can be to enable or to disable the individual. The environment is often the critical dimension that either supports or interferes with an individual's occupation. Arata's school environment presents expectations he finds difficult to meet. Marie has mixed opportunities and challenges in her work environment (i.e., her driving route for flower delivery versus her role as an Uber driver). Lydia has necessary supports that allow her to function at her level and be safe despite her dementia.

Conclusion

At the beginning of this chapter, it was indicated that volition, habituation, and performance capacity are integrated parts of each person. As shown in Figure 2-6,

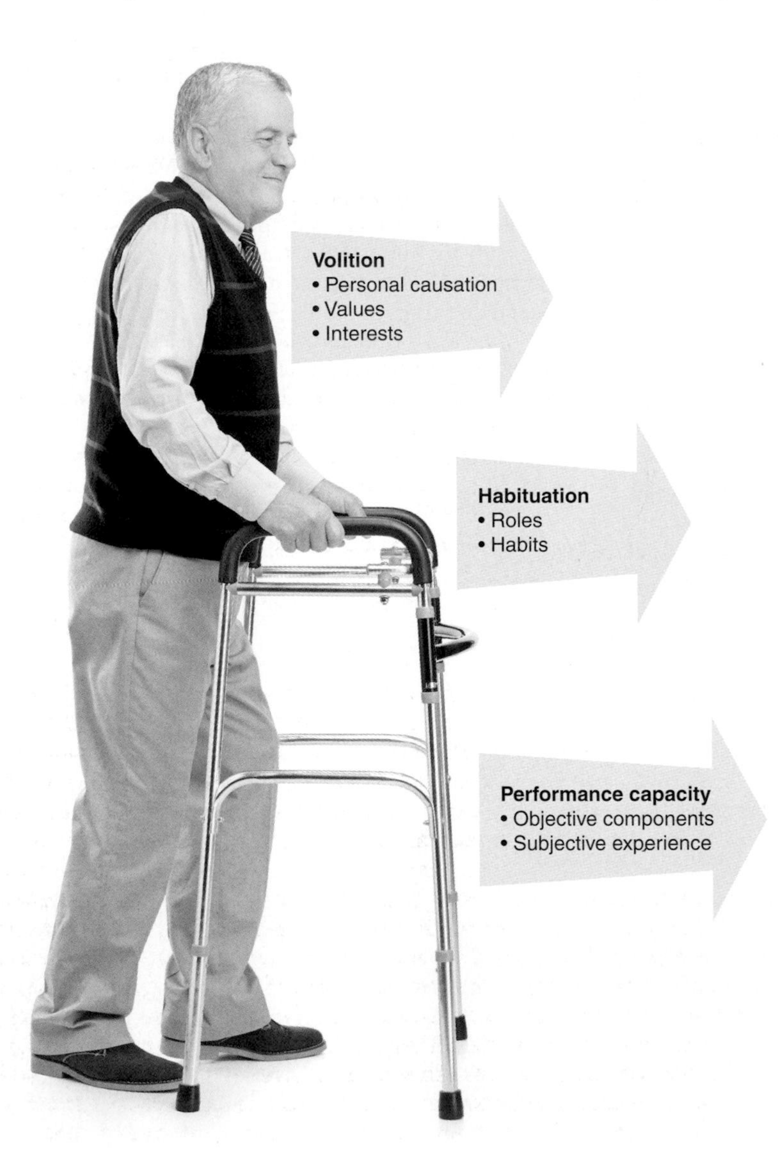

FIGURE 2-6 Integration of Volition, Habituation, and Performance Capacity into the Whole Person.

they operate seamlessly, forming a coherent whole. Volition, habituation, and performance capacity each contribute different but complementary functions to what we do and how we experience our doing. We cannot fully understand the occupation of people like Arata, Marie, Carlos, and Lydia without reference to all three contributing factors and without reference to the environment. Taking this broader view recognizes the complexity inherent in human occupation.

CASE EXAMPLE TO TEST YOUR KNOWLEDGE: ADULT NEURO-REHABILITATION

Hatsu is a 70-year-old woman with right-side paralysis resulting from a subarachnoid hemorrhage 2 years ago. She entered a long-term rehabilitation unit in Japan after receiving acute care services in a nearby hospital for a 1-year period. Before onset, she worked as a hair stylist until she was 35 years old, and then as a food-preparer, and then most recently as a house cleaner. Before the hemorrhage, she was living on the third floor of a housing complex with her eldest son who is her primary caregiver.

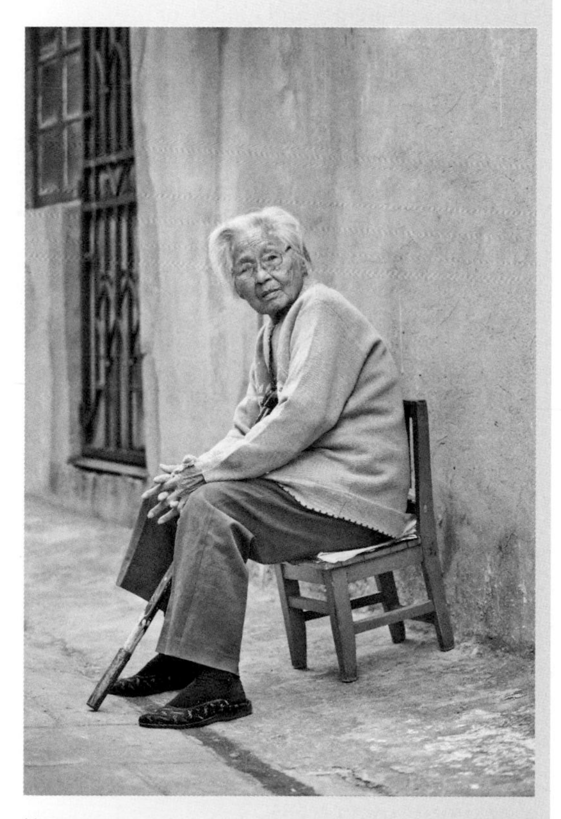

Hatsu

Hatsu's paralysis in her upper and lower limbs was mild. She followed through on the crutch-walking exercises recommended by the physiotherapist. One year had passed since the time she entered the rehabilitation unit, and Hatsu hoped for an at-home return. However, her progress with respect to the exercises assigned to her had reached a point of diminishing returns. She and her physiotherapist both believed she had reached maximal performance capacity.

As a consequence, Hatsu's eldest daughter has refused a joint-living situation due to child care. Hatsu's eldest son has been postponing the joint-living situation due to being too busy at work to provide the level of care that would be needed. He reported that he would be willing to reconsider his position if Hatsu was able to achieve independence in toileting. Thus, Hatsu's social environment outside of the rehabilitation unit was not conducive to a return home. As a result of having performed a typical checklist that was used by the original therapist on the unit (the Neuropsychiatric Interest Check List), the previous therapist was unable to identify any of Hatsu's strong interests and her progress remained stagnant for a period of time.

Recognizing the stagnation, Hatsu's son consulted her physician, and together they requested an occupational therapy consultation. Having a foundation in MOHO, Hatsu's new occupational therapist approached the relationship by attempting to understand her interests and to promote a return to home by emphasizing activities that supported those interests. The therapist decided to reassess Hatsu's interests using a version of the Interest Checklist translated for Japanese elders (ICJEV) (Nakamura-Thomas & Yamada, 2011). The ICJEV focuses on the elicitation of a client's interests, which is a component of volition within the MOHO. In this treatment scenario, the ICJEV was used in combination with other assessments to tailor a MOHO-oriented treatment program that involved transition from a neurorehabilitation unit to the home setting.

On the MOHO-based Interest Checklist, three items of cleaning and washing, listening to songs and taking care of one's physical appearance (i.e., clothing, hairstyle, and makeup) were rated as being of strong interest. Additionally, four items were rated as being of casual interest: taking a walk, visiting acquaintances, food preparation, and shopping. Hatsu reported that, because she had always worked, she had not developed any leisure activities until now. She mostly performed cleaning and washing and other housekeeping duties on her days off. The interest in maintaining her physical appearance, such as keeping up with her hairstyle, seemed to be connected with her having been a hair stylist in the past. Through this exercise, the therapist came to understand Hatsu's interests and suggested that she might begin the treatment process by practicing housekeeping activities such as cleaning, washing, and preparing foods.

The therapist also administered the Japanese translation of the Role Checklist and learned that Hatsu wanted to take on four roles in the future: caregiver, home maintainer, friend, and family member. It made sense that Hatsu valued the worker role, and that home maintainer fit very well into that value.

The therapist negotiated with Hatsu and together they set a long-term goal of returning home. However, there was a concern that, once Hatsu returned home, her eldest son would be working in the daytime. The therapist anticipated that Hatsu would be staying there alone. Thus, Hatsu would not be able to rely upon the support that would come from her immediate social environment. Based upon this information, the therapist and Hatsu reexamined her identified interests in terms of what she may start to work on at home after discharge. They decided on the following short-term goals: (a) "Hatsu will explore housework, and, at each outpatient visit, Hatsu will report on her experiences doing one housework task." (b) "Hatsu will identify one activity that she enjoys and make a habit doing this." The existing approach to occupational therapy assumed that these activities would fall within the domain of housework exercises such as "tableware transportation while walking with the crutch," "washing-up," and "washing and drying clothing" in reference to results of the Interest Checklist. The therapist talked with Hatsu about activities she might be able to enjoy other than housework and they also decided to work on quilting and crafts. Hatsu attended therapy twice a week for approximately 3 months and Hatsu's motivation to engage in various occupations of meaning became higher with time.

In parallel to this development, Hatsu's ambulatory exercise and the exercise of going up and down stairs recommended by the physical therapist advanced smoothly, and her walking became independent. The success in going up and down the stairs was enabled by monitoring, and Hatsu began to feel more comfortable navigating the stairs. Also, the occupational therapist had the daughter and the son observe the state of the exercise and planned their understanding of Hatsu's performance capacity according to MOHO. That is, the therapist educated the son and the daughter about the importance of considering both Hatsu's perceived experience of performance as well as the objective evaluation of performance. As a result, the eldest son consented to living together with his mother, and the long-term goal of the at-home return became a short-term objective.

Before discharge, the therapist conducted a home visit and performed home modifications. The modifications enabled Hatsu's physical environment to support her performance. This occurred over a period of 3 months and a final evaluation was conducted toward the end of therapy. After 6 months, Hatsu returned home and had improved in terms of her mobility, psychological well-being, and quality of life.

Questions to Encourage Critical Thinking and Discussion

- Using MOHO concepts, describe Hatsu's limitations before encountering her new occupational therapist.
- What strengths did Hatsu's new occupational therapist discover in terms of her volition, habituation, performance capacity, and environment? Describe these strengths in detail.
- What was the most informative assessment that was used in this example? Explain your answer.
- Applying your understanding of MOHO concepts, were there any other components of the model you would have recommended that the new occupational therapist focus on with Hatsu?

Chapter 2 Review Questions

1. List the four basic concepts that form MOHO.
2. Describe the three elements that form the concept of volition.
3. What role does volition play in approaching treatment using MOHO?
4. How do habits and roles interact to form habituation?

5. What are the two perspectives from which performance capacity may be described? Why is it important to describe performance capacity from these two perspectives?
6. Explain the ways in which the environment can facilitate or limit action, as well as the way in which a client can influence the environment.

HOMEWORK ASSIGNMENT

Think of a client or person you know who is having difficulty moving forward in his or her life. Describe these difficulties using MOHO concepts.

thePoint® For additional resources and exercises, visit http://thePoint.lww.com

Key Terms

Anticipation: Noticing and reacting to potentials or expectations for action.

Activity choices: Short-term, deliberate decisions to enter and exit occupational activities.

Experience: Refers, then, to the immediate thoughts and feelings that emerge in the midst of and in response to performance.

Habits: Acquired tendencies to respond and perform in certain consistent ways in familiar environments or situations.

Habituation: Internalized readiness to exhibit consistent patterns of behavior guided by our habits and roles and fitted to the characteristics of routine temporal, physical, and social environments.

Environmental impact: The opportunity, support, demand, and constraint that the physical and social aspects of the environment have on a particular individual.

Interests: What one finds enjoyable or satisfying to do.

Internalized role: Incorporation of a socially and/or personally defined status and a related cluster of attitudes and behaviors.

Interpretation: Recalling and reflecting on performance in terms of its significance for oneself and one's world.

Occupational choices: Deliberate commitments to enter an occupational role, acquire a new habit, or undertake a personal project.

Performance capacity: Ability for doing things provided by the status of underlying objective physical and mental components and corresponding subjective experience.

Personal causation: Sense of capacity and effectiveness.

Values: What one finds important and meaningful to do.

Volition: Pattern of thoughts and feelings about oneself as an actor in one's world which occur as one anticipates, chooses, experiences, and interprets what one does.

REFERENCES

Berlyne, D. E. (1960). *Conflict, arousal, and curiosity*. New York, NY: McGraw-Hill.

Bruner, J. (1973). Organization of early skilled action. *Child Development, 44*, 1–11.

Bundy, A. C., Lane, S. J., & Murray, E. A. (2002). *Sensory integration: Theory and practice* (2nd ed.). Philadelphia, PA: F. A. Davis.

DeCharms, R. E. (1968). *Personal causation: The internal affective determinants of behaviors*. New York, NY: Academic Press.

Florey, L. L. (1969). Intrinsic motivation: The dynamics of occupational therapy theory. *American Journal of Occupational Therapy, 23*, 319–322.

Heard, C. (1977). Occupational role acquisition: A perspective on the chronically disabled. *American Journal of Occupational Therapy, 41*, 243–247.

Katz, N. (1992). *Cognitive rehabilitation: Models for intervention in occupational therapy*. Boston, MA: Andover Medical Publishers.

Koestler, A. (1969). Beyond atomism and holism: The concept of the holon. In A. Koestler & J. R. Smythies (Eds.), *Beyond reductionism*. Boston, MA: Beacon Press.

Mathiowetz, V., & Haugen, J. B. (1994). Motor behavior research: Implications for therapeutic approaches to central nervous system dysfunction. *American Journal of Occupational Therapy, 48*, 733–745.

Matsutsuyu, J. (1971). Occupational behavior: A perspective on work and play. *American Journal of Occupational Therapy, 25*, 291–294.

McClelland, D. (1961). *The achieving society*. New York, NY: Free Press.

Merleau-Ponty, M. (1962). *Phenomenology of perception* (C. Smith, Trans.). London, United Kingdom: Routledge & Kegan Paul. (Original work published 1945)

Nakamura-Thomas, H., & Yamada, T. (2011). A factor analytic study of the Japanese Interest Checklist for the Elderly. *British Journal of Occupational Therapy, 74*(2), 86–91.

Nelson, D. (1988). Occupation: Form and performance. *American Journal of Occupational Therapy, 34*, 777–788.

Reilly, M. (1962). Occupational therapy can be one of the great ideas of 20th century medicine. *American Journal of Occupational Therapy, 16*, 1–9.

Shibutani, T. (1968). A cybernetic approach to motivation. In W. Buckley (Ed.), *Modern systems research for the behavioral scientist*. Chicago, IL: Aldine.

Smith, M. B. (1969). *Social psychology and human values*. Chicago, IL: Aldine.

Trombly, C. (1995). Occupation: Purposefulness and meaningfulness as therapeutic mechanisms. *American Journal of Occupational Therapy, 49*, 960–972.

White, R. W. (1959). Excerpts from motivation reconsidered: The concept of competence. *Psychological Review, 66*, 126–134.

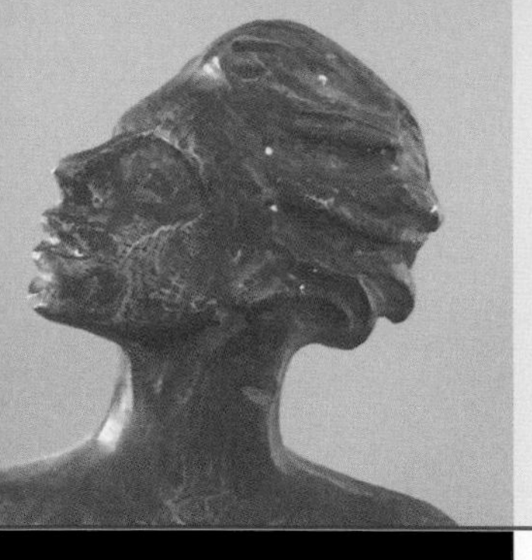

The Interaction between the Person and the Environment

Jane C. O'Brien and Gary Kielhofner (posthumous)

CHAPTER 3

EXPECTED LEARNING OUTCOMES

Upon completion of this chapter, readers will be able to:

1. Describe how volition, habituation, and performance capacity are integrated together and relate to one's environment.
2. Explain how the model of human occupation (MOHO) can be used in the process of applying dynamic systems theory to occupational therapy practice.
3. Understand MOHO theoretical principles derived from systems theory that explain the dynamics of occupation.
4. Delineate how MOHO principles inform occupational therapy practice and facilitate change.
5. Define concepts of occupational shift and resiliency as applied to occupational therapy practice.
6. Illustrate how to use MOHO to solve clinical problems regarding the dynamics of occupation.

An essential feature of occupational therapy practice models is the model's explanation of the role of **occupation** in clients' lives. The model of human occupation (MOHO) makes occupation central to the model and operationalizes factors that contribute to a person's choice for occupations, feelings, and actions for occupation. Occupation refers to the everyday things that people do and is considered to be those things that provide a person with meaning and identity (American Occupational Therapy Association [AOTA], 2014; Boyt Schell, Gillen, & Scaffa, 2014). MOHO is concerned with how people participate in daily occupations to achieve a sense of competence and identity, and explains how occupations are chosen, patterned, and performed (Kielhofner, 2008). Furthermore, MOHO describes the interactions and dynamic nature of occupation as influenced by volition, habituation, performance capacity, and the environment. Students and practitioners are urged to use MOHO assessments to help them understand the concepts contributing to occupational performance.

Engagement in occupation throughout one's life is a dynamic process. MOHO explains the process and allows practitioners to analyze occupation through definitions of concepts to facilitate and support change. Extensive practice research using MOHO throughout the life span provides practitioners with examples on which to base intervention (Kahlin & Haglund, 2009; Melton, Forsyth, & Freeth, 2010; Misko, Nelson, & Duggan, 2015; O'Brien et al., 2010; Wimpenny, Forsyth, Jones, Matheson, & Colley, 2010; Yamada, Kawamata, Kobayashi, Kielhofner, & Taylor, 2010).

This chapter explains how volition, habituation, and performance capacity are integrated and relate to one's environment. The author introduces current systems theory, including concepts such as heterarchy and emergence, and describes principles that explain the dynamics of occupation, based on MOHO theory. Concepts of change are examined, including occupational shift, resiliency, occupational competency, and occupational identity. The author uses case examples throughout to illustrate the use of MOHO in occupational therapy practice and facilitate critical thinking.

Systems Theory

Systems theory refers to a large and changing body of literature that has evolved over the last half century. MOHO was originally based on concepts of open systems and *general systems* theory (Koestler, 1969; von Bertalanffy, 1968a, 1968b). As these original systems ideas were expanded and revised to more recent dynamic systems theory (Thelen, 2005; Thelen & Smith, 2006; Thelen & Ulrich, 1991), the use of systems concepts in MOHO evolved.

Current dynamic systems theory (Thelen, 2005; Thelen & Smith, 2006) proposes that action is performed on the basis of an interaction between multiple systems. Dynamic systems theory describes how biological systems self-organize and move through fluctuations of continuity and change, particularly nonlinear forms of change (Thelen & Smith, 2006). Thus, movement is not just a matter of a person's range of motion, muscle strength, endurance, and coordination, but it is also influenced by one's desires, motivations, belief in ability, habits, routines, and the environment.

Dynamic systems theorists hypothesize that people prefer to remain in the status quo or same pattern of behavior (Thelen & Smith, 2006). In order to facilitate change, they must experience a **perturbation,** which refers to a shift or disturbance. The perturbation causes a sense of discomfort and signifies the need for a change. Perturbations can be external (e.g., loss of job) or internal (e.g., sense of discomfort). Occupational therapists often meet clients who have experienced perturbations or changes in their patterns. Therapists help clients develop new patterns of performance considering the numerous factors that influence occupational performance.

Many variables influence occupation, including motor, neurological, musculoskeletal, cognitive, emotional, and the task, objects, and environment. Humans are sensitive to environments and have the capacity to respond (Keenan, 2010). In addition, human behaviors and thoughts are reformed by processes and feedback, becoming more ordered and complex over time as multiple systems join together (Thelen, 2005).

Therapists who apply dynamic systems to occupational therapy practice examine the multitude of factors that influence occupational performance. This requires a complex view of human occupation and consideration of the dynamic nature of the factors influencing humans. MOHO provides occupational therapy practitioners with a structure for organizing one's thinking and information regarding multiple systems. MOHO stipulates an occupation-based, client-centered philosophy that can be used with any client population. Therapists using MOHO as their model of practice examine multiple factors that influence behaviors to inform evaluation, intervention, and outcomes measurement. This allows practitioners to use one model for clients of all ages and abilities. Understanding occupation through MOHO allows practitioners to integrate complex theory regarding dynamic systems and apply it to occupational therapy practice. The following case shows how MOHO supports application of theory and dynamic systems concepts into practice.

MOHO Problem-Solver: Pediatrics

Karen is an occupational therapist who recently graduated and is working in an outpatient clinic at a large hospital. She works with children of all ages and abilities. She interviews parents using a variety of evaluation tools but does not have a uniform system. She acknowledges that she misses key information and only collects data related to developmental milestones or motor skills. As she begins to develop the intervention plan, she realizes she does not have the "complete story." For example, although she knows the child has difficulty dressing due to increased muscle tone on the right side due to cerebral palsy, she does not know who dresses the child or the child's routines and habits. She does not know whether the child wants to dress, or how the child feels about his performance. As she mentions dressing to the family, they seem underwhelmed by this plan. Karen realizes her evaluation did not provide a clear view of the child or family's goals. She seeks assistance from her direct supervisor.

Karen's supervisor asks questions to get a better picture. Specifically, she wants to know:

- What is a typical day like for the child?
- What is the environment like? Is it accessible?
- What is the social environment?
- Where does the child go to school?
- What resources are available?
- What resources may be available?
- What are the child's goals? Wants and likes?
- What are the family's goals?
- What are the child's strengths? Weaknesses?
- How does the child view his abilities?
- What are the child's routines?
- Does the child have siblings? Who are his friends?

As Karen contemplates these questions, she realizes her current developmental assessment tools provide her with a small piece of the puzzle. How can she gather the information she needs (in a short period of time)? How can she organize the information to make sense of all the variables influencing occupational performance? She decides to use MOHO as her model of practice. Specifically, she relies on the SCOPE (Bowyer et al., 2008) to organize her initial evaluation. This evaluation provides data for measuring outcomes and allows her to organize the interview so that she receives a thorough picture of the child and family for intervention purposes. It does not take her any longer to complete, and makes developing meaningful goals much easier. Karen finds that she is able to establish a rapport with the child and family more easily with this tool. She can use MOHO with all of her clients. Notably, team members are impressed with the thoroughness of her new reports and meaningfulness of her goals. This model also works well with a variety of intervention approaches (e.g., motor control, biomechanical, rehabilitation). Karen is pleased that MOHO offers a variety of assessments specific to pediatric clients. As she uses the assessments, she understands the complexities of human occupation more clearly.

Reflect on the following questions:

- Categorize each question from the supervisor according to the core aspects of MOHO.
- Develop a list of questions for each core aspect of MOHO.

Principles Guiding Process

MOHO identifies personal factors as volition, habituation, and performance capacity, and defines environmental factors as elements of social, institutional, and physical space (Kielhofner, 2008). Volition refers to the client's values, interests, and personal causation. Habituation refers to habits, routines, and roles, whereas performance capacity includes skills defined as actions that make up occupational engagement and include motor skills, process skills, and communication and interaction skills. The physical environment is made up of objects and space, whereas tasks, social groups, and cultural/sociopolitical surroundings make up the social environment. Institutional space refers to the political or institutional environment (or culture) (e.g., school, university, hospital). The following principles guide the MOHO process of understanding the complexity of human occupation:

1. Occupational actions, thoughts, and emotions arise out of the dynamic interaction of volition, habituation, performance capacity, and environmental context.
2. Change in any aspect of volition, habituation, performance capacity, and/or the environment can result in change in the thoughts, feelings, and doing that make up one's occupation.
3. Volition, habituation, and performance capacity are maintained and changed through what one does and what one thinks and feels about doing.
4. A particular pattern of volition, habituation, and performance capacity will be maintained so long as the underlying thoughts, feelings, and actions are consistently repeated in a supporting environment.
5. *Change requires that novel thoughts, feelings, and actions are sufficiently repeated in a consistent environment to coalesce into a new organized pattern.*

DYNAMIC INTERACTION

Occupational actions, thoughts, and emotions arise out of the dynamic interaction of volition, habituation, performance capacity, and environmental context.

To understand why and how people engage in a variety of occupations, one must consider the unique interactions possible. A person's actions, thoughts regarding their actions, and emotions toward occupational performance and engagement are the result of the dynamic interaction of volition (values, beliefs, and interests), habituation (habits and roles), and performance capacity (skills and abilities) within a given environment (that supports or hinders the occupation). People reflect and have emotions regarding engagement in occupations. For example, a teen may feel pleased with volunteering at a pet shelter (volition); aware of his ability to complete high-quality homework responses (performance capacity); and satisfied that, once again, he has made it to school on time (habituation). All these thoughts regarding a person's actions shape the behavior for the next time and strengthen the motivation to engage in meaningful occupations. Feeling positive about volunteer work, a homework assignment, or arriving at school on time reinforces the behaviors so that the teen attempts to repeat them. The environment and person cooperate in producing occupation.

People's actions are also influenced by their interests (part of volition) that develop over time. In early childhood, children explore the environment and seek out those activities that are pleasurable. As toddlers age, they repeat activities that are rewarding and fun or that bring them praise. They may be exposed to family activities (e.g., music, religious observances, meals) to which they attach meaning. While teens begin to establish their own identity, they experience new occupations and attach emotion and meaning to those things. They may determine that they have a specific affinity for activities or talent (such as drawing, writing, singing) and decide to develop or pursue this further. Adults have established volitional patterns for occupations. For example, one adult may enjoy indoor word search games and find patterns of occupation that require cognitive skills. Another adult may enjoy physical activity outside in a variety of challenging areas. The experiences over one's lifetime affect the thoughts and emotions attached to occupational actions and may determine the client's pattern of behaviors. Volitional patterns may require adjustments over time. For example, illness or injury may interfere with established patterns, requiring that people develop new interests and volitional patterns.

MOHO provides a structure to understand each person's problems and strengths and how these are related to a unique pattern of motivation, habits, performance capacity, skills, and/or the environment. The major concepts of MOHO underpin all stages of the process (Maciver et al., 2015). This process considers a person's habituation (habits and roles), which refers to the repetitive pattern of what people do. As people take on new roles, they complete actions related to the role, which may alter previously established occupations. For example, the demands of a new job may limit leisure time pursuits. Routines, roles, and habits provide the pattern of behaviors necessary for occupational engagement. It gives people a structure that serves as a foundation for work, education, and leisure. Waking up, taking a shower, grooming, getting dressed, eating breakfast, and driving to work are familiar patterns that provide a sense of structure to one's day. These familiar reactions may be taken for granted until a person experiences a disruption. For example, clients in the hospital report that they miss the "everyday things," such as brushing one's teeth or taking a morning shower. Since MOHO provides an understanding of the dynamic interactions of routines, roles, and habits, occupational therapists can assist clients in new ways of completing "everyday things."

Performance capacity refers to one's skills and abilities for a given occupation. A person may find that his abilities are not sufficient as the demands increase for a specific skill. This leads to changes in occupations and may affect one's volition and habituation. It may require different environmental supports. As one engages in routines successfully, one experiences a sense of efficacy (belief in one's skills) and positive emotions that reinforce participation. As people perform their daily activities and participate in an array of social roles, they develop **occupational competence**. With time and practice, individuals develop the ability to perform occupations with skill and ease, referred to as occupational competence.

The following case example illustrates the dynamic interaction of volition, habituation, performance capacity, and environment leading to occupational shift.

CASE EXAMPLE: YOUNG ADULTHOOD

Marlene is a 20-year-old college student who has always been energized by music. As she states, it is her "passion." She seeks out opportunities to spend leisure time at concerts, studies music at school, and learns to play a variety of instruments. Marlene enters a college where she can pursue her love of music; the environment is supportive of her passion. In one of her courses, she completes an internship at a local school, teaching music. This new opportunity allows her to engage in activity related to music in a different way. Marlene realizes that she loves teaching others piano and that she has many skills to be an effective teacher (belief in efficacy of skill). She enjoys the interactions with the children and the daily routine of teaching. She is proud of her students' accomplishments and is energized by the newly found role. She decides to seek out a degree in teaching music, while continuing to explore other avenues in the music industry.

Marlene's actions changed as she reflected on the thoughts and emotions that arose while doing and in consideration of the other aspects of her life (environment). As people evolve, habits, routines, volition, and performance capacity develop in different ways, leading to a variety of occupational choices, termed **occupational shift**. Occupational shift refers to changes in occupations as a result of the interactions between volition, habituation, and performance capacity within a given environment. In Marlene's case, she changed her occupation when reflecting upon her newly found performance capacity and volition for teaching. She was able to continue her passion and abilities in music by slightly changing her occupation.

The complex interactive process allows people to develop routines that promote occupational performance. The following case example sets the stage for understanding occupation.

Understanding Occupation

CASE EXAMPLE: ADULT OUTPATIENT

A highly organized process unfolds as people go about their everyday occupations.

Consider, for example, Rigo doing his morning routine of getting washed up, groomed, and dressed. After getting out of bed, he puts on some coffee, takes medications for rheumatoid arthritis, performs stretching exercises, takes a shower and

shaves, and then dons his work clothes. During much of this time, Rigo is thinking about an upcoming fishing trip that he is taking on the weekend with his best friend, Carlos. During his drive to the construction site where he is foreman of a plumbing crew, he plans how the crew will finish up the job. As he pulls into the construction site, he calls Carlos to remind him to stop by the bait and tackle shop after work to buy fishing supplies.

- **Describe the aspects of volition, habituation, and performance capacity illustrated in this case.**
- **How does the environment influence Rigo's occupational performance?**

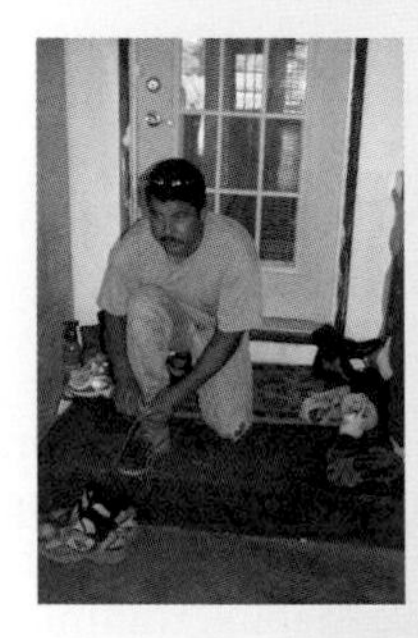

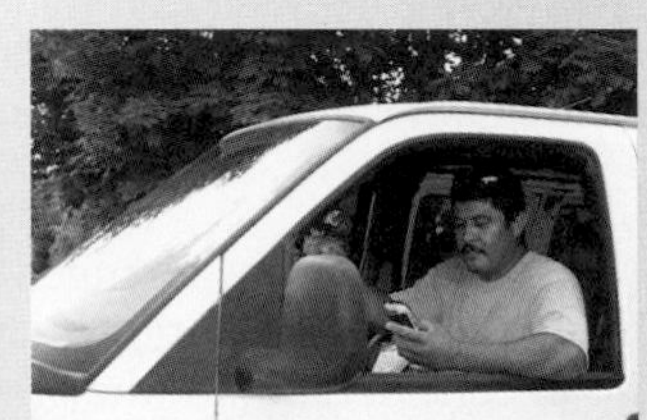

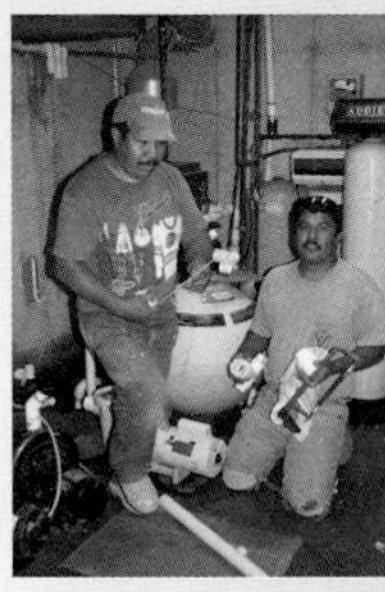

Rigo tying shoes, talking on the phone, working

This short scenario illustrates several aspects of volition, habituation, and performance capacity. For instance, Rigo's habits guide his morning routine and free him to engage in volitional anticipation of the upcoming fishing trip. Similarly, while his habit of driving to work unfolds, his awareness of the responsibilities of his foreman role stimulates him to plan the activities of the work crew. During all this time, Rigo's physical and mental capacities are being called upon as he engages in tying his shoes, watching the traffic as he drives, and planning an errand after work. As this small slice of Rigo's occupational life illustrates, occupation always involves an ongoing interplay of volition, habituation, performance capacity, and the environmental context. This interplay reflects two important systems concepts, heterarchy and emergence.

Heterarchy is the principle according to which aspects of a person and that person's environment are linked together into a dynamic whole (Capra, 1997; Clarke, 1997; Thelen & Ulrich, 1991; Turvey, 1990). In a heterarchy, each component contributes something to a total dynamic. For instance, as shown in Figure 3-1, Rigo's habits for going about his morning routine provide a tendency to manifest a sequence of behaviors. Rigo's performance capacity (i.e., problem-solving, strength, endurance) make possible certain abilities that are called upon when habitual self-care unfolds. Rigo's interests (i.e., his love of fishing) and his values (i.e., doing a good job) are also at play. Each of these elements contributes something to the total dynamic of the morning routine.

Importantly, the environment is central to these dynamics (Clarke, 1997). For example, his activities of daily living involve and are shaped by the objects and spaces that make up his home. Moreover, while Rigo's memory may provide him with rough instructions for driving to the construction site, he must rely on the physical environment to give him cues about when to speed up, slow down, or stop; how to steer on the road; and when to turn at an intersection.

The concepts of heterarchy and emergence can be used to generate a comprehensive and dynamic understanding of occupation. In contrast, hierarchy provides a more "top-down" approach and refers to a sequential approach whereby each level leads to the next. For example, using heterarchical concepts to understand what kind of occupational task a person will choose, we must consider that it is a function of the interaction of the following factors:

- The kind of things a person feels effective in doing;
- What the person likes to do;
- What the person finds valuable or meaningful to do; and
- What opportunities or expectations are present in the environment for doing things.

For example, whether a person will be motivated and choose to enter the worker role will be influenced by:

- The extent to which the person feels capable of doing work based on past experiences;
- Whether and what kinds of work tasks the person has enjoyed doing in the past;
- How important work, and other factors either positively or negatively associated with work, is to this person;
- What kinds of jobs are available to the person and whether they match the felt capacity, interests, and values of the person;
- What other factors in the environment are affected by working (e.g., the availability of disability income or medical insurance); and

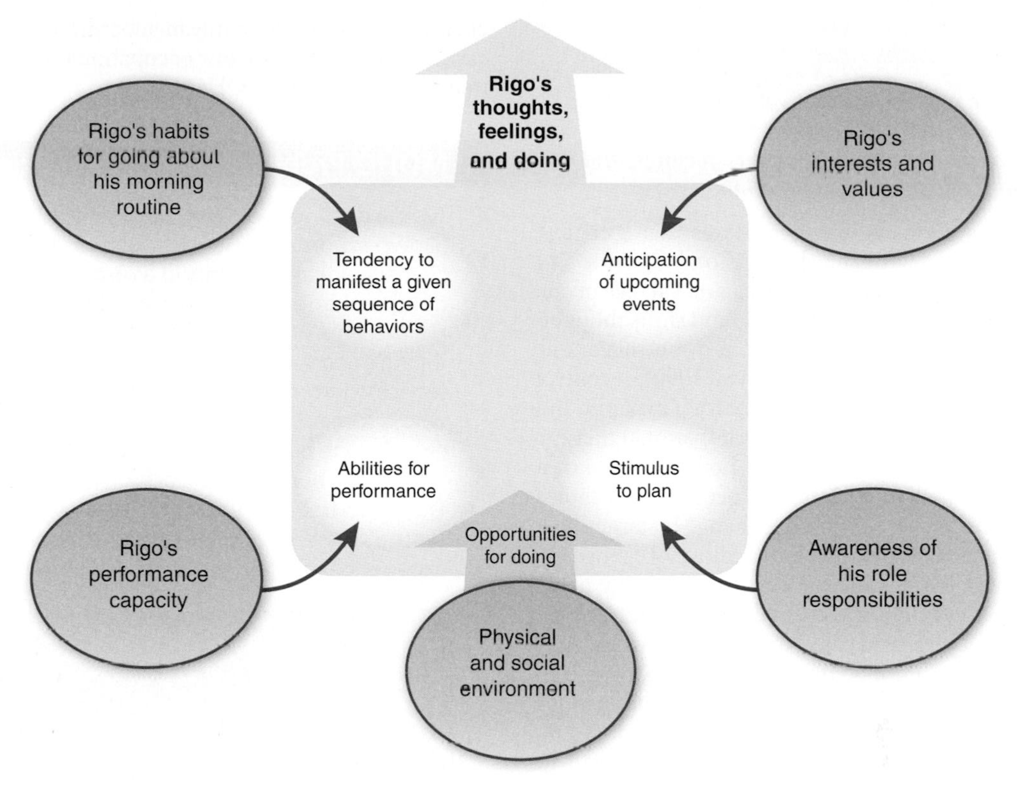

FIGURE 3-1 An Illustration of Heterarchical Contributions of Volition, Habituation, Performance Capacity, and Environment to an Occupation.

- The extent to which others in the environment expect and want the person to work.

In the same way, the quality of a person's performance in doing the task will be influenced by the interaction of:

- The underlying capacity the person has for the performance;
- The complexity and demands of the task itself; and
- The kinds of objects present in the environment for engaging in the task.

For example, whether and how a child with severe motor problems can use a computer depends on:

- How the child's impairments affect fine motor movements;
- Whether adapted keyboards or other adapted interfaces are available and appropriate; and
- Whether the child has developed the habit of using these adaptive objects.

Every instance of human occupation reflects a unique configuration of such elements that together determine what a person chooses to do, how that person performs, and what is the outcome of the performance. Occupational therapy practitioners examine this configuration to determine how to intervene.

What Rigo does, thinks, and feels *emerges* out of the collective conditions created by the interaction of personal and environmental elements. **Emergence** is the principle that complex actions, thoughts, and feelings spontaneously arise out of the interactions of several components (Clarke 1997; Haken, 1987; Kelso & Tuller, 1984). As shown in Figure 3-1, Rigo's thoughts, emotions, and actions in the morning routine emerge from the dynamic interaction of his volition, habituation, performance capacity, and environment.

This means that no single causal factor can ever account fully for emergent behavior, thought, or feeling. Furthermore, volition, habituation, performance capacity, and the environment do not always make synergistic contributions. For example:

- Anxiety from a lack of belief in capacity can interfere with performance even when a person has the necessary underlying capacities;
- Old habits can resist new volitional choices; and
- The pull of values can keep one going despite pain and fatigue.

In these and other circumstances, values, interests, personal causation, role, habits, performance capacity, and the environment may produce a complex dynamic in which some factors support and others constrain a particular behavior, emotion, or thought. It is always the summation of their total contributions to the dynamic whole that results in the outcome.

Change

Change in any aspect of volition, habituation, performance capacity, and/or the environment can result in a change in the thoughts, feelings, and doing that make up one's occupation.

Another systems concept indicates that a critical change in one factor can shift the total dynamic and result in a different emergent behavior. Change in one factor that creates a new dynamic and shifts thought, emotion, and/or action is known as a control parameter (Thelen & Ulrich, 1991; Turvey, 1990). A control parameter sufficiently changes the total dynamic and something different emerges. Occupational therapy (OT) practitioners understand how a change in a control parameter may influence occupational choice and performance. Facilitating change by targeting a control parameter may lead to additional changes in the system. For instance, if Rigo had a flare-up of his arthritic condition, if a storm damaged or destroyed his house, if his friend called to say a family emergency meant he could not go on the fishing trip, or if Rigo lost his job, then his actions, thoughts, and feelings during the morning routine would be quite different.

Resiliency refers to the ability to respond to changes and adapt or recover from some defined event (Abelenda & Helfrich, 2003; Carmichael, 2015). It is the ability to withstand adverse environmental conditions involving multiple dimensions, such as hardships or challenges across the life span (Abelenda & Helfrich, 2003; Greene, 2014). Resiliency is based on a variety of factors that allow persons to problem-solve, change behaviors, and recreate meaning. Abelenda and Helfrich (2003) summarized that families who have loved ones with mental illness had three basic needs: (1) information about the nature, course, treatment, and prognosis of the mental illness; (2) skills for coping with consequences (e.g., problem-solving, managing symptoms, dealing with conflict and stress, and possessing motivation); and (3) support for themselves. Families and individuals engage in a process of change that permits occupational adaptation. **Occupational adaptation** refers to making needed changes to continue to engage in one's chosen activities, or developing new activities. People respond to changes throughout one's life. For example, a gardener who has difficulty kneeling as she ages, plants items so she can stand; a child completes more difficult puzzles as he grows up; an adult changes habits to adjust to the occupational requirements for caring for a family. Individuals who possess traits of resiliency make necessary adjustments so they may continue to engage in those occupations that they find meaningful and that give them a sense of identity (Greene, 2014). The perturbation (or impetus for change) may be internal (emotional, change in feelings or thoughts) or external (decreased skill, environmental change, family member). The following case example illustrates how occupational adaptation may be explained in MOHO terms.

MOHO Problem-Solver: Pediatrics

Tyrone is a 3-year-old boy who has Trisomy 21 (Down syndrome). He lives with his brother (7 years old) and parents in a rural neighborhood and attends a day care 5 days a week. He receives occupational therapy, physical therapy, and speech therapy early intervention services. Tyrone plays well with his brother, who is somewhat "bossy" with Tyrone. However, Tyrone plays aimlessly at preschool, not knowing whom to approach or what to do. The adults frequently end up playing with him. Tyrone's parents are concerned that he will experience difficulty at preschool in the Fall.

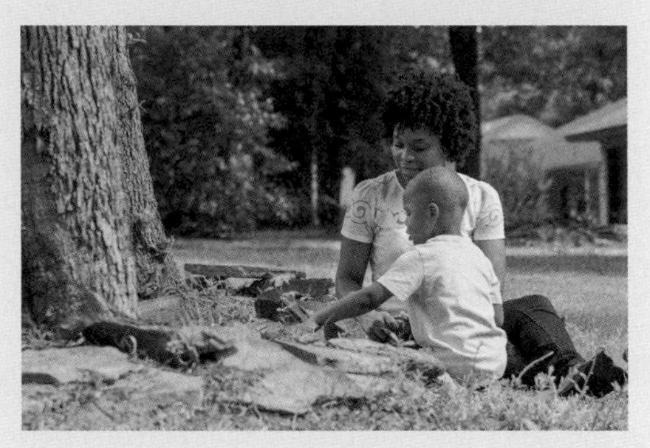

Child with Down syndrome playing

The occupational therapist (Kim) working with Tyrone has been focusing on developing his ability to use his hands (for fine motor skills for school), feed himself, and exhibit improved posture for play. While they have made some progress, the parents are very concerned about his ability to "fit in" at school and have asked for a more comprehensive intervention plan.

Critical questions:

- How would MOHO help Kim frame evaluation and intervention to comprehensively address Tyrone and his family's concerns?
- What are the occupational challenges that Tyrone will face in preschool?
- How can therapy help Tyrone adapt his occupational performance?
- What is the role of the environment?
- What MOHO assessments may provide Kim with additional information?

Kim reviewed Tyrone's information and completed the SCOPE (Bowyer et al., 2008) through observation and parental interview. She interviewed the parents to better determine their concerns. As Tyrone is young, Kim ascertained his interests and preferences by engaging him in a variety of activities where he got to choose between two things. She summarized the findings, presented in what follows, and developed an intervention plan to focus on the transition to preschool.

Volition

Tyrone enjoys playing with older children or adults who provide him with more direction. He likes playing with trucks and running (to find hidden objects) but has difficulty following two-step directions. Tyrone watches other children playing and shows interests in their games, but disrupts others' play when he tries to engage. His parents are concerned that Tyrone will not fit in at preschool.

Habituation

Tyrone has a typical morning routine. He assists with dressing, feeds himself with set up (but is messy), and continues to have "accidents" with toileting. Tyrone washes his hands upon request. He has an established nap and bedtime routine. Tyrone typically plays with his brother on weekends and after day care. He stays close to adults at day care.

Performance Capacity

Tyrone has low muscle tone throughout, open mouth posture, and typical features of Down syndrome. He had cardiac complications at birth, but it was repaired. Tyrone exhibits global developmental delays. He communicates his needs verbally (but articulation is delayed). Tyrone followed one-step verbal directions and made eye contact with adults frequently. Tyrone smiled frequently during the observation and asked for help. At times Tyrone asked for help before trying, but after encouragement, he was able to accomplish the task.

Environment

Tyrone attends a well-equipped day care center. He will be attending preschool in the Fall at a local school with 15 children in his classroom with an experienced teacher. Tyrone's home is in a rural neighborhood. He has a wide range of toys and a large backyard that is child friendly. He has his own computer and child-sized chairs for eating and coloring. He spends time with his older brother, who tells Tyrone what to do.

Assessment

Tyrone is comfortable playing with his older brother (who is clear about what Tyrone should do). Tyrone will need to learn to enter the play of other children and engage with others for preschool. He exhibits global developmental delays but has a supportive environment.

Plan

Tyrone will learn to follow two-step directions as necessary for preschool. The OT practitioner incorporated his love of trucks and running into therapeutic activity, whereby he must (1) run to the tree and pick up the truck and (2) return the truck to the "truck stop." Kim changed the game to introduce novelty to the activities. Kim also encouraged his brother to allow Tyrone to be the "boss" for a play activity each day. Kim worked with Tyrone to role-play some examples of games he could lead. This helped Tyrone develop a sense of competence and feelings of self-efficacy. It allowed Tyrone to practice social skills needed for preschool (while also reinforcing developmental gross and fine motor play skills). Kim encouraged adults to play with Tyrone and another child, modeling play behaviors and supporting Tyrone's need to learn to play with others in a nonintrusive way. As Tyrone gained skills to enter play groups, Kim encouraged the parents to establish a play date at the home so Tyrone could be in charge, develop confidence, and make friends before entering preschool. They visited the preschool playground so Tyrone was comfortable in this new environment.

In summary, using MOHO provided a well-rounded evaluation and intervention plan for Tyrone. The intervention assisted Tyrone in occupational adaptation so that he could more easily transfer skills to preschool. It included the parent's goals, considered the child's habits and routines, and was an occupation-based client-centered plan. By building on Tyrone's strengths (volition for play), Kim afforded him with habits and routines that supported occupational competence for preschool.

Thinking and Doing

Volition, habituation, and performance capacity are maintained and changed through what one does and what one thinks and feels about doing.

Human beings are highly organized systems that are maintained by underlying, physiological, mental, affective, and behavioral processes (Brent, 1978; Sameroff, 1983). Humans become what they do, think, and feel about doing. People change and develop over time depending on their ongoing occupations. Consequently, from the time we enter this world, we set about doing things. Within the first weeks of life, we have begun a course of occupation that has already established some performance capacity, given us a rudimentary sense of ourselves and of the world around us, and created a basic daily routine. From then on, we persist in a process of doing that continually shapes and reshapes ourselves (Capra, 1997; Wolf, 1987).

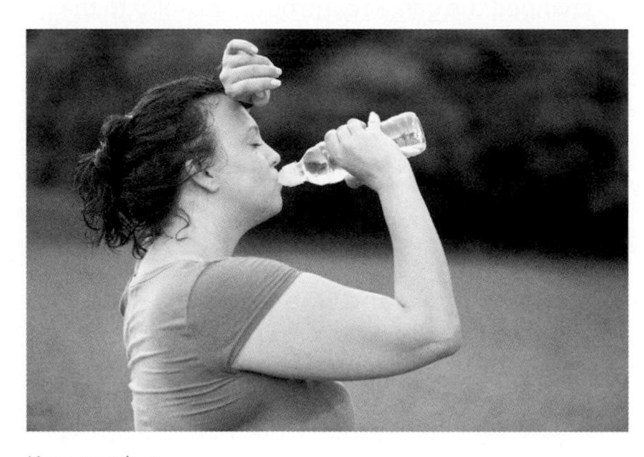

Kara running

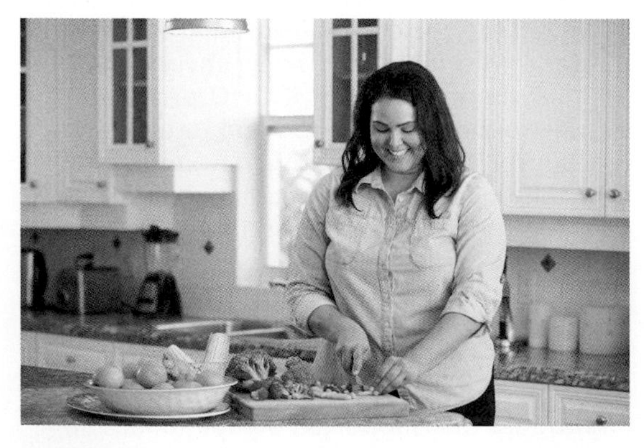

Kara making a nutritious meal

People thus shape themselves through their occupations. Consider, for instance, what happened to Kara's volition, habituation, and performance capacity when she took up running. Repeated running reshaped her existing physical, psychological, and social structures involved. Her aerobic capacity increased, the muscles she used to run gained strength, the image of herself as capable of running was enhanced, and her public identity as a runner was affirmed when she swapped stories and tips about running with others, shopped for running clothes, joined a friend for a regular run after work, and participated in organized races.

When Kara took up and repeated running and related behaviors, her actions and the associated thoughts and feelings rearranged her personal causation, role, and performance capacity into that of a runner. She became what she did. Moreover, as long as she sustains these occupations, the corresponding organization is maintained. However, if Kara were to abandon the behavior for long enough, her aerobic capacity would diminish, her muscles would weaken, and her confidence for running and her runner role identity would wane. As this illustrates, we can also unbecome what we cease to do.

To consider how this process continues to unfold throughout life, we need to answer two questions. How do we maintain our organized patterns? How do we change? The remainder of this chapter attempts to provide some basic answers to these questions.

MAINTAINING OCCUPATIONAL PATTERNS

A particular pattern of volition, habituation, and performance capacity will be maintained so long as the underlying thoughts, feelings, and actions are consistently repeated in a supporting environment.

Thinking and feeling about what we are doing is a natural ongoing process that includes experience over doing and reflecting on our performance, which, in turn, creates the foundation for our future (Nygren, Sandlund, Bernspang, & Fisher, 2013). People exhibit certain constancy in who they are and what they do over time. Individuals develop an **occupational identity** as they maintain and repeat a pattern of engagement. Occupational identity pertains to the idea that we each develop a sense of who we are and wish to become as an occupational being based on our own accumulated and reflected life experiences (Kielhofner, 2008; Nygren et al., 2013). Maintaining these organized patterns of emotion, thought, choice, and behavior involves the following elements:

- Our existing volition, habituation, and performance capacity (which we previously generated through our doing) provide certain resources, limitations, and tendencies for emoting, thinking, and behaving.

- We encounter consistent environmental conditions, seek them out, or create them.
- Given the interaction of internal resources, limitations, and tendencies with consistent environmental conditions, we repeat what we have done before, sustaining an organized pattern of behaving and of the thoughts and feelings that accompany behavior.

Importantly, this organized pattern represents a way of operating with its own internal coherence that resists change. Once we have a way of feeling, thinking, and behaving, we tend to behave so as to preserve it. For example, a study of women with chronic pain revealed distinct patterns of doing, thinking, and feeling (Keponen & Kielhofner, 2006). For instance, one group of women saw themselves as moving on. They emphasized recognizing the limitations imposed by their chronic pain and making decisions about what occupations were important to them to do, asking others to understand and assist them to live their lives as positively as possible, and having plans for the future. Another group saw themselves as fighting. They tried to hide their pain from others and gave priority to doing the things they felt obligated to do, often sacrificing their own interests and life satisfaction. These women found it impossible to imagine the future. Women in both these groups saw their way of living with chronic pain as the only option. They persisted in behavior that reinforced their thoughts and feelings. As the example illustrates, each individual "actively constructs his or her view of self" (Gergen & Gergen, 1983, p. 255). Once a person's volition, habituation, or performance capacity has become organized in a particular way, it tends to stay that way. Nonetheless, change does occur and occupational therapists can facilitate change. The next section considers how change occurs.

NEW ORGANIZED PATTERNS: OCCUPATIONAL SHIFT

■ ***Change requires that novel thoughts, feelings, and actions are sufficiently repeated in a consistent environment to coalesce into a new organized pattern.*** ■

An alteration of any single internal or external component in a heterarchy can contribute something new to the total dynamic out of which new thoughts, feelings, and actions may emerge. Therefore, a shift in volition, habituation, performance capacity, or the environment can alter the overall dynamics, leading to the emergence of something new. Thus, a key element in change is some alteration (i.e., perturbation) in internal or external circumstances that results in the emergence of novel thoughts, feelings, and behaviors. Occupational shifts may occur naturally, such as changes associated with puberty. Shifts may also be imposed on people through illness, disease, or health conditions, such as a decline in performance after a stroke. It may also result from a change in a major life role, such as transitioning from soldier to civilian. A veteran who returns from war must adapt his daily activities to adjust to "civilian" life. He may need to find civilian employment and readjust his thinking. The internal and external circumstances from the changes in setting, work, and identity result in the need for an occupational shift. At first, he will find these changes difficult and will need additional thought, support, and assistance to participate. Over time and with support, he may accommodate to the changes and adjust. However, some occupational shifts require ongoing adjustments. For example, a veteran may experience posttraumatic stress disorder interfering with his feelings of security and competence.

The next requirement for change is that the novel thoughts, feelings, and behaviors must continue over time. Only by repetition do we begin to reshape ourselves. Repetition of new behaviors, thoughts, and feelings requires supportive environmental conditions. If the new pattern is repeated enough, then volition, habituation, and performance capacity will coalesce toward a new organization. Occupational therapy practitioners often facilitate change and support clients as they engage in new behaviors over time.

Ordinarily, there is a natural history of new behaviors, thoughts, and emotions, whereby volition, habituation, and performance capacity are altered incrementally together over time. Throughout this natural history of change, the elements will resonate with each other, each taking turns in contributing something new to the mix of components that spur on the ongoing changes process.

Implications for Therapy

Occupation is a complex process and the central focus of occupational therapy intervention. Understanding the complexities of occupation allows practitioners to design effective intervention for clients of all ages. In accordance with dynamic systems theory, OT practitioners consider multiple factors when working with clients to help them engage in occupation and, importantly, regain occupational identity. Occupational identify refers to how clients view themselves in terms of how they spend their time. It implies that people are what they do. People engage in those activities for which they find meaning or pleasure. They repeat patterns of behaviors that fulfill them and serve to create an identity or sense of purpose. For example, certain responsibilities are associated with specific roles (i.e., parent role requires caring for children; coworker role requires proper dress). The behaviors correlated with occupation are the result of the interactions between volition, habituation, and performance capacity within the environment.

The systems concepts discussed in this chapter have important implications for the process of occupational therapy. First, they indicate that assessment (the goal of which is to understand a person's "needs, problems, and concerns"; AOTA, 2014) requires consideration of how volition, habituation, performance capacity, and environmental factors contribute to the client's circumstance. Without assessing all these factors, one cannot fully understand a client's situation. The purpose of evaluation is to understand and consider how all the factors make up the total dynamic affecting the client's doing, thinking, and feeling. This means that the assessment process should be holistic and dynamic. To be holistic, it should, to the extent possible, consider the status of performance capacity, habits, roles, personal causation, values, interests, and environmental circumstance. To be dynamic, the occupational therapist considers how these factors interact to create the total situation of the client. No single factor is necessarily the most important to consider first in assessment. Rather, it is important to have adequate information on each to determine how it is influencing the client's occupational life. Contemporary occupational therapy has called for a top-down approach to assessment (Fisher, 1998), which begins with consideration of the person's occupation and then proceeds to consideration of the underlying performance capacity. What is being suggested here is not a top-down, but a dynamic approach to assessment that ensures all factors (volition, habituation, performance capacity, and environmental) are examined and considered simultaneously.

Most often, several factors are involved simultaneously. For example, if Rigo, whom we discussed earlier, sustained a spinal cord injury in a car accident, a new set of dynamics would emerge as shown in Figure 3-2. While the most obvious change would be a major loss of sensory and motor capacity following the spinal cord injury, a cascade of other factors would also be involved. Rigo's values and interests may no longer be consistent with what he is capable of doing. He may have lost his physically demanding job. His old friend may feel uncomfortable and become avoidant

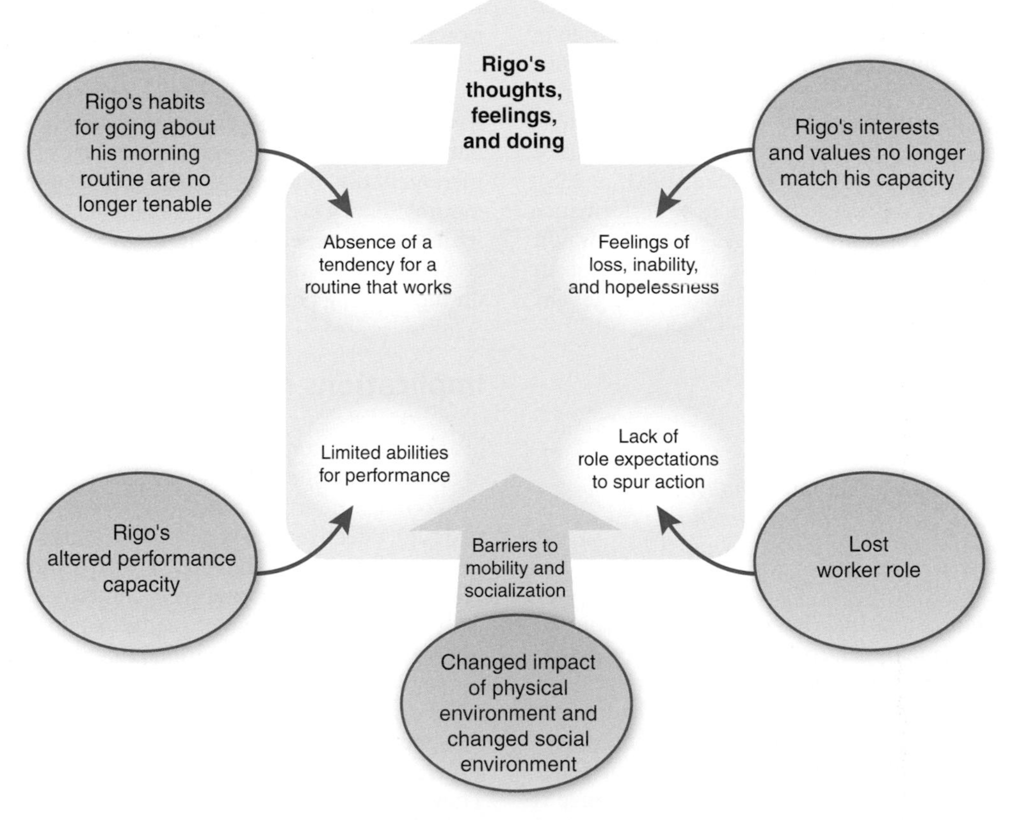

FIGURE 3-2 An Illustration of Altered Heterarchical Contributions of Volition, Habituation, Performance Capacity, and Environment Following a Traumatic Inset of a Disability.

of Rigo. The once familiar environment of his home, truck, and worksites would all be physically inaccessible to him. The habitual ways he learned to do things no longer would work in the face of his motor and sensory impairments. Without consideration of all these factors, one cannot fully understand the nature of a person's occupational problems.

Second, since many factors contribute to the emergence of occupational behaviors, thoughts, and feelings, it is important to consider multiple possibilities for addressing a client's problems and challenges to help him or her regain occupational engagement. For example, when a person experiences some limitation of capacity (e.g., mobility, strength, attention, or memory), therapy can use strategies that increase/restore capacity. However, there are also other possibilities that may be used. They include, for instance:

- Compensating for loss of one capacity by modifying habits of how necessary activities are done;
- Altering the environment to provide supports for doing; and
- Making new choices for action so that those things that can no longer be done can be replaced by an alternative activity.

Successful occupational therapy often involves a combination of strategies. Intervention planning requires an ongoing process of deciding, in collaboration with the client, what combination can best create a positive dynamic out of which positive actions, thoughts, and feelings can emerge.

Third, therapy should, to the extent possible, consider and address all the factors contributing to the client's occupational dynamic. This means that diminished performance capacity, problematic habits, lost roles, a sense of inefficacy, problems operationalizing values and interests, and environmental barriers are all potential factors to be addressed in therapy. Addressing some factors and not others can result in less than optimal outcomes of therapy. Nonetheless, it is important that the process of deciding what factors to address be client centered, meaning that those factors most important to the client should be addressed first or given the most emphasis. Therapists should, when appropriate, assist clients to understand how all relevant factors may impact their occupational lives.

Fourth, because the aim of therapy is always to achieve a new and positive pattern of occupational life, it requires sustained occupational engagement in a supportive environment. Therapy must support the client to engage in new forms of doing, thinking, and feeling that can reorganize volition, habituation, performance capacity, and the environment into a new and positive dynamic. Therapists facilitate change in a number of ways. For example, they may identify environmental resources, create opportunities for skill development, and design activities to develop coping strategies. Therapists use critical thinking to examine clients' abilities and interactions between volition, habituation, performance capacity, and the environment to design intervention. As therapists facilitate change, clients reengage in occupations or develop new occupational identities. This process is ordinarily begun during therapy and continues on beyond the period of intervention.

Conclusion

This chapter used systems concepts to explain how volition, habituation, and performance capacity are integrated together and relate to the environment. Five key principles were proposed to explain the dynamics of occupation. Finally, the chapter offered a discussion of the implications of systems concepts for therapy. These concepts and principles discussed in this chapter will be reflected and integrated throughout this text.

CASE EXAMPLE TO TEST YOUR KNOWLEDGE: PEDIATRICS

Devin is a 10-year-old boy who has difficulty in school. His teacher reports that he gets into trouble, forgets his homework, does not listen to instructions, and is irritable. The teacher says he has few friends and is behind in all classes. His parents report a cooperative boy at home who stays to himself. He has trouble getting ready for school and taking care of his chores. He plays too roughly with his sister and cousins and frequently gets hurt. He is unable to ride a bike or swim. Devin is fearful of heights and picky regarding food. He does not like to read but loves to draw and play on the computer. Devin is a very vocal child who engages in conversations easily with adults. He was referred to occupational therapy at school.

Questions to Encourage Critical Thinking and Discussion

- **Using MOHO concepts, describe Devin's limitations.**
- **What are Devin's strengths in terms of volition, habituation, performance capacity, and environment?**
- **How could you frame Devin's occupational performance challenges to help him succeed?**
- **What principle outlined in the chapter may serve to inform how a practitioner would design intervention?**
- **How would you begin this evaluation? Why?**
- **How does dynamic systems theory support your intervention?**

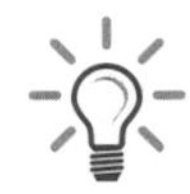

Chapter 3 Review Questions

1. Define the five principles regarding MOHO's view of occupation.
2. What is meant by heterarchy? Control parameters?
3. Compare and contrast resiliency and occupational adaptation.
4. Define contemporary dynamic systems theory.
5. What is occupational shift?
6. How do occupational therapists facilitate change?

HOMEWORK ASSIGNMENTS

1. Provide an example of an occupational shift in your life.
2. Describe an occupation in which you engage and identify how it has changed over time. Using MOHO theory, describe what prepared you for the changes.
3. Outline an occupation with which you are not familiar. Analyze the volition, habituation, performance capacity, and environmental factors.
4. List your habits and roles. How would you adapt if you lost the ability to use your dominant hand; home; or electricity for a week?
5. List MOHO principles regarding the dynamic nature of occupation and provide an example to describe how the principle is applied to practice.

thePoint® For additional resources and exercises, visit http://thePoint.lww.com

Key Terms

Control parameter: Change in a factor that creates a new dynamic and shifts thought, emotion, and/or action.

Emergence: The principle that complex actions, thoughts, and feelings spontaneously arise out of the interactions of several components.

Heterarchy: The principle according to which aspects of a person and that person's environment are linked together into a dynamic whole.

Occupation: The everyday things that people do and is considered to be those things that provide a person with meaning and identity (AOTA, 2014; Boyt Schell et al., 2014).

Occupational adaptation: Making needed changes to continue to engage in one's chosen activities, or developing new activities.

Occupational competence: The ability to perform occupations with skill and ease.

Occupational identity: The sense of who we are and wish to become as an occupational being based on our own accumulated and reflected life experiences (Kielhofner, 2008; Nygren et al., 2013).

Occupational shift: Changes in occupations or activities as people evolve and develop in different ways. Occupational shift refers to changes in occupations as a result of the interactions between volition, habituation, and performance capacity within a given environment.

Perturbation: A shift or disturbance. The perturbation causes a sense of discomfort and signifies the need for a change. Perturbations can be external (e.g., loss of job) or internal (e.g., sense of discomfort).

Resiliency: The ability to respond to changes and adapt or recover from some defined event (Abelenda & Helfrich, 2003; Carmichael, 2015). It is the ability to withstand adverse environmental conditions involving multiple dimensions, such as hardships or challenges across the life span (Abelenda & Helfrich, 2003).

REFERENCES

Abelenda, J., & Helfrich, C. (2003). Family resilience and mental illness. *Occupational Therapy in Mental Health, 19*(1), 25–39.

American Occupational Therapy Association. (2014). Occupational therapy practice framework: Domain and process (3rd ed.). *American Journal of Occupational Therapy, 68* (Suppl. 1), S1–S48.

Brent, S. B. (1978). Motivation, steady-state, and structural development. *Motivation and Emotion*, *2*, 299–332.

Bowyer, P., Kramer, J., Ploszaj, A., Ross, M., Schwartz, O., Kielhofner, G., et al. (2008). *The Short Child Occupational Profile (SCOPE)* [Version 2.2]. Chicago, IL: MOHO Clearinghouse, University of Illinois at Chicago.

Boyt Schell, B. A., Gillen, G., & Scaffa, M. (2014). Glossary. In B. A. Boyt Schell, G. Gillen, & M. Scaffa (Eds.), *Willard and Spackmans' occupational therapy* (12th ed., p. 1237). Philadelphia, PA: Wolters Kluwer Health/Lippincott Williams & Wilkins.

Capra, F. (1997). *The web of life*. London, United Kingdom: HarperCollins.

Carmichael, D. G. (2015). Incorporating resilience through adaptability and flexibility. *Civil Engineering and Environmental Systems, 32*(1–2), 31–43.

Clarke, A. (1997). *Being there: Putting brain, body and world together again*. Cambridge, MA: MIT Press.

Fisher, A. (1998). Uniting theory and practice in an occupational framework: 1998 Eleanor Clark Slagle Lecture. *American Journal of Occupational Therapy, 52*(7), 509–521.

Gergen, K. J., & Gergen, M. M. (1983). Narratives of the self. In T. R. Sarbin & K. E. Scheibe (Eds.), *Studies in social identity*. New York, NY: Praeger.

Greene, R. R. (2014). Resilience as effective functional capacity: An ecological-stress model. *Journal of Human Behavior in the Social Environment, 24*, 937–950.

Haken, H. (1987). Synergetics: An approach to self-organization. In F. E. Yates (Ed.), *Self-organizing systems: The emergence of order*. New York, NY: Plenum.

Kahlin, I., & Haglund, L. (2009). Pyschosocial strengths and challenges related to work among persons with intellectual disabilities. *Occupational Therapy in Mental Health, 25*(2), 151–164.

Keenan, E. K. (2010). Seeing the forest for the trees: Using dynamic systems theory to understand stress and coping and trauma and resilience. *Journal of Human Behavior in the Social Environment, 20*(8), 1038–1060.

Kelso, J. A. S., & Tuller, B. (1984). A dynamical basis for action systems. In M. S. Gazzaniga (Ed.), *Handbook of cognitive neuroscience*. New York, NY: Plenum.

Keponen, R. & Kielhofner, G. (2006). Occupation and meaning in the lives of women with chronic pain. *Scandinavian Journal of Occupational Therapy, 13*(4), 211–220.

Kielhofner, G. (2008). *A model of human occupation: Theory and application* (4th ed.). Baltimore, MD: Williams & Wilkins.

Koestler, A. (1969). Beyond atomism and holism: The concept of the holon. In A. Koestler & J. R. Smythies (Eds.), *Beyond reductionism*. Boston, MA: Beacon Press.

Maciver, D., Morley, M., Forsyth, K., Bertram, N., Edwards, T., Heasman, D., et al. (2015). Innovating with the model of human occupation in mental health. *Occupational Therapy in Mental Health, 31*, 144–154.

Melton, J., Forsyth, K., & Freeth, D. (2010). A practice development programme to promote the use of the model of human occupation: Contexts, influential mechanisms and levels of engagement amongst occupational therapists. *British Journal of Occupational Therapy, 73*(110), 549–558.

Misko, A. N., Nelson, D. L., & Duggan J. M. (2015). Three case studies of community occupational therapy for individuals with human immunodeficiency virus. *Occupational Therapy in Health Care, 29*(1), 11–26.

Nygren, U., Sandlund, M., Bernspang, B., & Fisher, A. G. (2013). Exploring perceptions of occupational competence among participants in Individual Placement and Support (IPS). *Scandinavian Journal of Occupational Therapy, 20*, 429–437.

O'Brien, J., Asselin, L., Fortier, K., Janzegers, R., Lagueux, B., & Silcox, C. (2010). Using therapeutic reasoning to apply the Model of Human Occupation in pediatric occupational therapy practice. *Journal of Occupational Therapy, Schools & Early Intervention, 3*, 348–365.

Sameroff, A. J. (1983). Developmental systems: Contexts and evolution. In P. H. Mussen (Ed.), *Handbook of child psychology*. New York, NY: John Wiley & Sons.

Thelen, E. (2005). Dynamic systems theory and the complexity of change. *Psychoanalytic Dialogues, 15*(2), 255–283.

Thelen, E., & Smith, L. B. (2006). Dynamic systems theories. In R. Lerner & W. Damon (Eds.), *Handbook of child psychology: Theoretical models of human development* (6th ed., pp. 258–312). New York, NY: John Wiley & Sons.

Thelen, E., & Ulrich, B. D. (1991). Hidden skills: A dynamic systems analysis of treadmill stepping during the first year. *Monographs of the Society for Research in Child Development, 56*(1), 1–98.

Turvey, M. T. (1990). Coordination. *American Psychologist, 45*, 938–953.

von Bertalanffy, L. (1968a). General system theory: A critical review. In W. Buckley (Ed.), *Modern systems research for the behavioral scientist*. Chicago, IL: Aldine.

von Bertalanffy, L. (1968b). *General systems theory*. New York, NY: George Braziller.

Wimpenny, K., Forsyth, K., Jones, C., Matheson, L., & Colley, J (2010). Implementing the model of human occupation across a mental health occupational therapy service: Communities of practice and a participatory change process. *British Journal of Occupational Therapy, 73*(11), 507–516.

Wolf, P. H. (1987). *The development of behavioral states and expression of emotion in early infancy*. Chicago, IL: University of Chicago Press.

Yamada, T., Kawamata, H., Kobayashi, N., Kielhofner, G., & Taylor, R. (2010). A randomized clinical trial of a wellness programme for healthy older people. *British Journal of Occupational Therapy, 73*(11), 540–548.

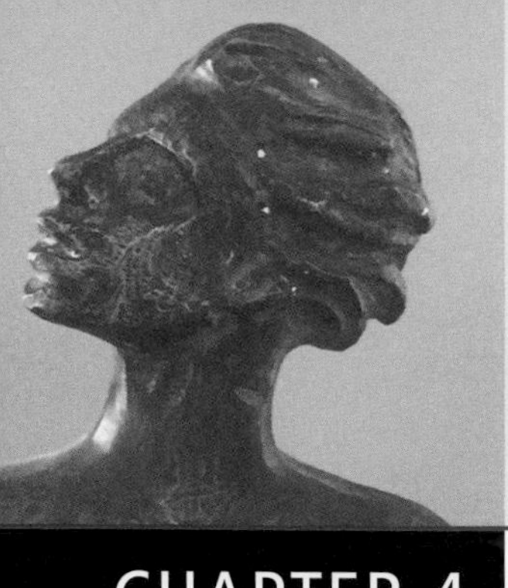

Volition

Sun Wook Lee and Gary Kielhofner (posthumous)

CHAPTER 4

EXPECTED LEARNING OUTCOMES

Upon completion of this chapter, readers will be able to:

1. Understand and state the meaning of volition.
2. Name three components of volition.
3. Describe the volitional process of a person, using an example.
4. Describe the volitional stages in relation to a client's occupational participation.
5. Identify the strengths and limitations of a client's volition to facilitate the therapy process (goals/strategies).

MOHO Problem-Solver: Pediatrics

Eight-year-old Jiyeon has a diagnosis of cerebral palsy. Like many children her age in Korea, she is very interested in playing a game, *gong-gi nolyi*, that involves five small marbles. Jiyeon also very much wants to use chopsticks since Koreans customarily use a spoon for eating rice and chopsticks for the side dishes. Because of her strong desire to play marbles and use chopsticks like other children in her culture, she is frustrated with her inabilities in these areas.

Jiyeon's occupational therapist is helping her achieve these goals. Jiyeon's fine motor skills don't allow her to play the marble game according to its usual rules (i.e., tossing one marble in the air and then grabbing a marble off the floor before catching the tossed marble). Therefore, the occupational therapist has arranged a modified version of the game that allows Jiyeon to engage in an activity of interest while developing better fine motor skills. She has responded well to this adaptation of the game. The occupational therapist also devised an activity to allow Jiyeon to work toward being able to use chopsticks. They began using wooden thongs that resemble chopsticks to pick up and move objects and later to eat side dishes. By harnessing things that Jiyeon valued and found enjoyable, the therapist was not only able to help Jiyeon increase skills, but also develop greater belief in her ability to do things

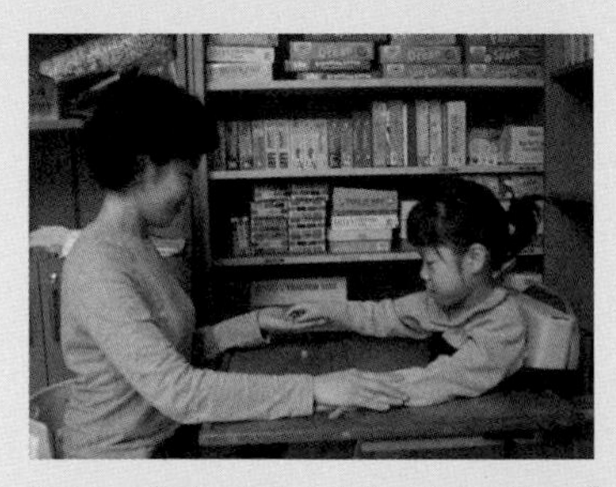

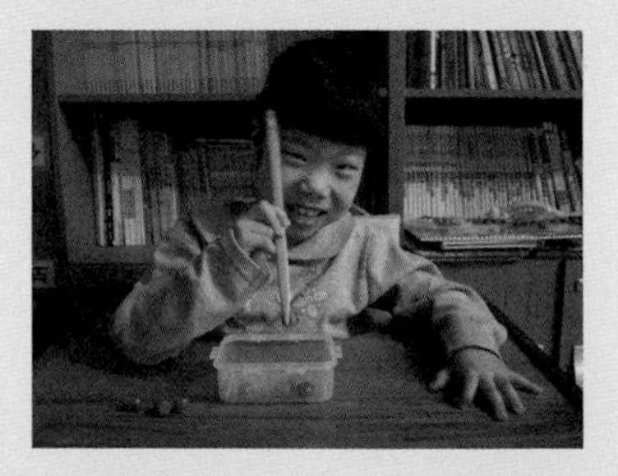

Jiyeon playing an adapted version of the Korean marble game, *gong-gi nolyi*, with her occupational therapist and using a tong to develop fine motor skills for handling chopsticks

Jiyeon's values and interests led her to choose to be involved in the tasks described above; the experience of feeling successful in doing these things may result in her reflection about how she can have more control over her life which, in the future, will shape her orientation to the world and the choices she makes.

This and the remaining scenarios in this chapter illustrate the concept of volition. They demonstrate how volition involves thoughts and feelings about what one holds important (values), what one perceives as being able to do and effective at doing (personal causation), and what one finds enjoyable (interests). They also illustrate aspects of the volitional cycle (Fig. 4-1) of anticipating, choosing, experiencing, and interpreting what one does. As this cycle is repeated, it maintains or reshapes one's values, personal causation, and interests. With each new experience and reflection, people come to think and feel about themselves and their lives in similar or in slightly different ways. Then, they anticipate possibilities for and make decisions to do things accordingly and the cycle repeats itself. The case example of Elizabeth explains how moving to a different culture represents a new experience that affects the volitional cycle.

How Does Culture Shape Volition?

Although values and personal causation are universal human concerns, how persons think and feel about personal effectiveness and assign significance to what they do will greatly depend on culture. Culture shapes what kinds of abilities are of concern, what kinds of meanings are tied to actions, what pastimes are enjoyed, and what one should strive for in life (Bruner, 1990; Gergen & Gergen, 1983, 1988; Markus, 1983). How culture shapes volitional thoughts and feelings can be appreciated by considering Elizabeth's dilemma:

CASE EXAMPLE: ADOLESCENT AT SCHOOL

Elizabeth is 14 and has just begun attending high school in a Midwestern American city. She feels a great deal of pressure from her peers to wear the latest fashions in clothes. Because of her insecurity about her own competence and being accepted by peers, she feels very compelled to fall in line with her peers' values about clothes. Because her family has less resources than many of her peers' families in the school she attends, Elizabeth often feels she cannot keep up materially with her classmates. In the past her brother loaned her some money to buy trendy clothes, but lately he has refused. Elizabeth was hoping to buy a new pair of jeans to wear to school. Feeling that she had no other way to get the resources, Elizabeth decided to just take the money and try to replace it somehow in the future. After taking her brother's money without permission, Elizabeth feels even more out of control and remorseful that she did something she knew was not honest.

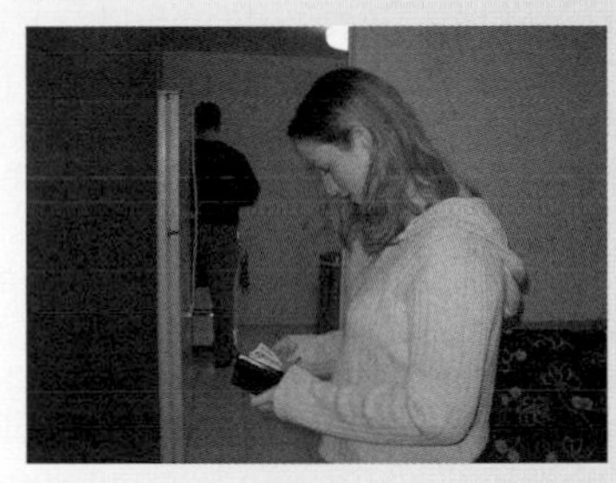

Elizabeth takes some of her brother's funds without permission in order to buy new clothes

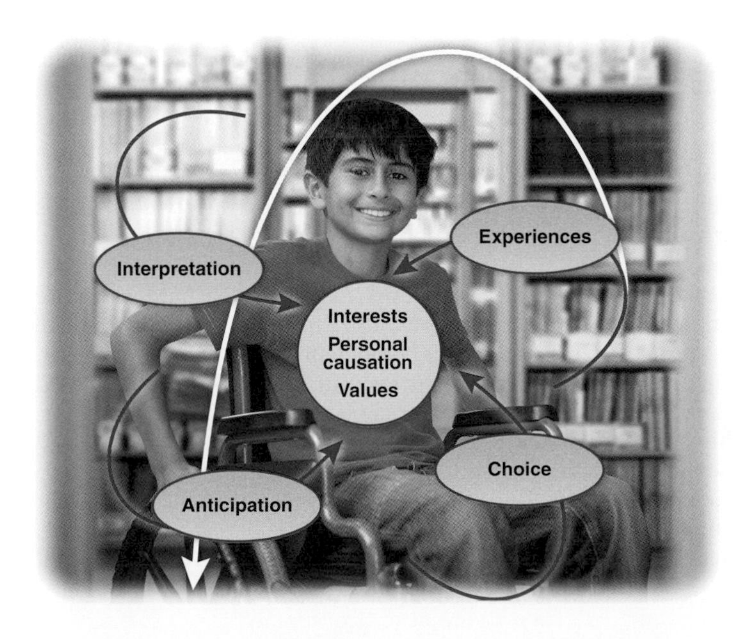

FIGURE 4-1 The Process of Volitional Change Over Time.

Elizabeth's culture emphasizes certain ways of dressing and she feels deeply obligated to conform. At the same time, she has incorporated values from her family about honesty and justice. These two sets of values clash when she finds herself trying to fit in with the values of her peers. Moreover, her cycle of anticipating, choosing, experiencing, and interpreting what she does threatens to spiral Elizabeth toward a greater and greater sense of failure and being out of control. This affects her volition in other areas of her life.

How Do Personal Circumstances and History Influence and Shape Volition?

Each person has unique volitional thoughts and feelings. Volition begins with biological propensities such as one's level of arousal, preferred sensory modes, and temperaments and impairments. These personal inclinations influence what capacities one develops, what one enjoys, and what one considers important. Additionally, as life unfolds each person accumulates a personal history of doing, experience, and reflection that shape volition. These experiences:

- afford the opportunity to learn what one can and cannot do well,
- provide occasions to discover what one enjoys doing, and
- shape what one considers important to do.

At any point in time a person's volition will reflect a unique personal history and circumstances that have shaped and continue to shape it. Let us look at Richard's situation:

CASE EXAMPLE: ADOLESCENT AT WORK

Richard is 17 years old and lives in a small English village. He very much wants to be successful like his older brother who is an officer in the military. He recently left school after not doing very well and wants to work. He has secured a job at a center that employs persons with disabilities, but he is struggling. Richard has a right-sided weakness and trouble with attention due to a neurological condition. Thus, he tires quickly and sometimes is unable to follow sequences. Because Richard wants to be seen as competent, he often pushes himself when fatigued instead of resting, which causes him to make mistakes. For the same reason, Richard will not ask for assistance when he is unsure how to complete work tasks and consequently sometimes does them incorrectly. These behaviors, although intended to make himself appear more competent, paradoxically result in Richard receiving negative feedback. This only increases Richard's sense of inefficacy on the job.

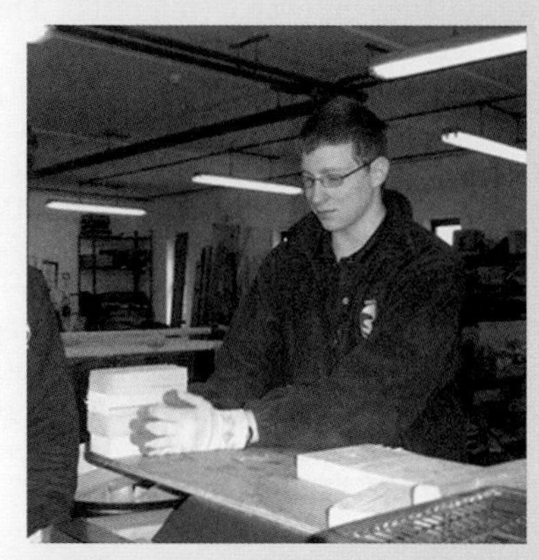

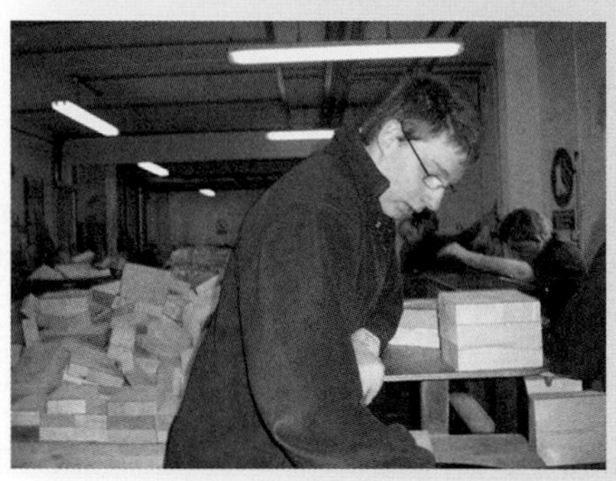

Richard at work

Richard's experiences of following a highly successful older brother, living with a neurological impairment, and his reflecting difficulties in school and recently at work all combine to form his unique sense of volition. His volition includes, among other things:

- a strong value of performing well like his brother and
- feelings of incapacity and failure

These aspects of his volition led Richard to choose to ignore his own difficulties in an effort to make himself appear competent. These choices, however, only generate further difficulties that keep him locked in a cycle of poor choices and negative experiences. When Richard's occupational therapist recognized this dynamic, she was able to help Richard learn to ask for help and support when he needed it in order to have more positive experiences at work. In time, this led Richard to accumulate positive feedback that built up his sense of efficacy at work.

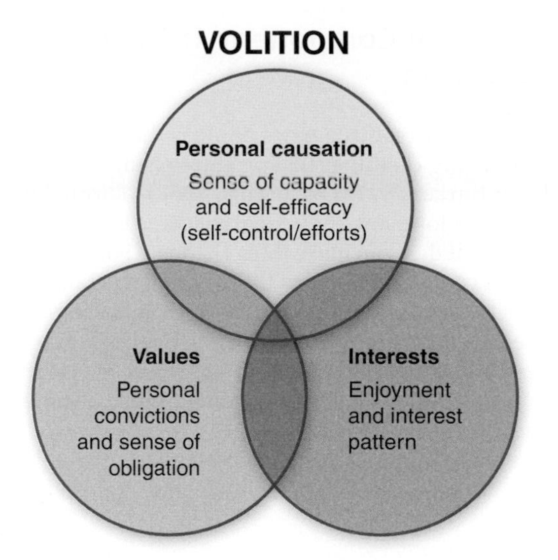

FIGURE 4-2 The Components of Volition.

Confluence of Personal Causation, Values, and Interests

Thoughts and feelings about competence, enjoyment, and value are always interwoven. People want to be competent at doing the things they value. They tend to find enjoyable those things that they do well and to dislike those that overtax them. They feel bad when they cannot do the things they care about deeply. Consequently, a person's **volition** can only be understood fully by examining the dynamic relationship among personal causation, values, and interests (Fig. 4-2). While the following sections discuss each separately, one should be mindful that personal causation, values, and interests are each aspects of a larger volitional whole.

Each of the following examples shows how occupational therapists get a sense of enacting client-centered, occupation-focused practice by examining what ways clients see their own capacities, what they value, and what they enjoy. Often, these volitional components are interwoven. Can you identify key factors of volition that the therapists utilized in each successful therapy journey?

MOHO Problem-Solver Cases: Occupational Therapists' Focus on Volition

MOHO Problem-Solver: Adult Neurorehabilitation

Peter is a 28-year-old male occupational therapist in an inpatient rehabilitation hospital located in a Metropolitan area. Today, he is nervous because of his appointment with Eva, his middle-aged client, who is scheduled for bathing. Eva had a stroke resulting from a concussion 2 weeks ago and has been sponge-bathed since then. She still has weakness along with balance issues. However, Eva desperately wants to try bathing herself. Peter thinks Eva could try bathing but he wanted to take it slowly. He has a good working relationship with Eva because of his humorous personality, but bathing can be a sensitive issue, and he is concerned about any uncomfortable events that might occur, which might jeopardize Eva's self-image, motivation for therapy, safety, and their therapeutic relationship. After instructing Eva about precautions and step-by-step methods required for bathing in her condition, Peter stepped out of the bathroom while keenly paying attention to any indication of her needing help or negative incidents during her bathing. Suddenly, Eva screamed in the shower, alarming Peter, who asked if everything was ok. Eva responded. "No. Nothing. This feels just so good! Thank you so very much, Peter, I feel like I'm a person again." Peter was relieved and assured about his decision to enact his client's interests, leading to the therapeutic journey of enabling client-centered practice.

MOHO Problem-Solver: Adult Inpatient with Spinal Cord Injury

Ellen is a new therapist in an acute rehabilitation hospital. Jin, a client referred to occupational therapy (OT), has C6 complete paralysis due to a spinal cord injury resulting from a car accident. Ellen evaluated him physically and started his ADL training. Jin was very cooperative. Jin had been a truck driver and had recently become a father. One day, he appeared gloomy and asked Ellen if he would ever be cured. Ellen could not respond, knowing that he would have permanent limitations lingering for the rest of his life. Jin said, "I am crippled. What can I do? I am like an infant." Instead of listening to his concerns, Ellen urged Jin to focus on the current therapy. From that day, Jin's motivation for therapy deteriorated. Ellen realized the strengthening, endurance, and

ADL training was crucial for Jin's occupational functioning, but her approach failed to support and nurture equally important aspects for his journey back to life—his sense of capacity and self-efficacy as a doer in the world. Ellen then put herself in Jin's shoes and saw how difficult it must have been to have worked at a masculine job and then to have suddenly become fully dependent (stating that he felt similar to an infant) while he himself was a father to a newborn. In the next OT session, she inquired of Jin how he spends much of his time in bed because of his condition and what he enjoys. He smiled. "My wife says she fell in love with my singing voice." Ellen realized she had found the spark to ignite Jin's heart for life. Jin agreed to record his lullabies for his baby as a starting point.

MOHO Problem-Solver: Adult Geriatrics

Miyan, who is a female Asian occupational therapist, met with an 80-year-old male client, Kim, who previously refused to receive OT from Miyan because she was a female therapist. The rehab team decided to encourage Kim to keep his therapist due to logistical inconveniences, and he reluctantly accepted the plan. Kim was experiencing left side paralysis and expressed high regard for self, demanding care from his daughter-in-law per his value of filial piety, saying "I am the father-in-law." In an effort to facilitate his occupational participation, Miyan instructed Kim in a modified method of dressing technique; this incident made him upset and he refused therapy. In a family meeting, Kim's daughter-in-law lamented that she worked to support her own family and was not able to meet Kim's expectation, which made her feel guilty. Miyan asked Kim's daughter-in-law what mattered the most to Kim, and she responded that he would do anything for his five-year-old grandson. Miyan then asked Kim if he would like to help with a pantomime of an injured soldier in the field, which was his grandson's preschool art day assignment. Having a fun time with his grandson, Kim said, "I am the grandfather." Following his shift in role identification that was prompted by this volitional intervention, Kim was willing to cooperate with the self-care training with the therapist.

Volitional Component 1: Personal Causation

One of the first discoveries of life is that one can be a cause (i.e., do things that produce results) (Bruner, 1973; Burke, 1977; DeCharms, 1968). Throughout early development, individuals become increasingly aware that they can make things happen. For example, infants come to realize that their movements can make objects move and create noises. This awareness that one can cause things to happen is the beginning of **personal causation** (DeCharms, 1968). Over time as one engages in a wider and wider range of action, one discovers:

- what one is capable of doing and
- what kinds of effects one's doing can produce.

TWO DIMENSIONS OF PERSONAL CAUSATION

As the previous statement indicated, personal causation involves two components: a sense of one's personal capacity and knowledge of one's self-efficacy in the world. The **sense of personal capacity** is a self-assessment of one's physical, intellectual, and social abilities (Harter, 1983, 1985; Harter & Connel, 1984). The second dimension, **self-efficacy**, refers to one's sense of effectiveness in using personal capacities to achieve desired outcomes in life (Lefcourt, 1981; Rotter, 1960). Self-efficacy is specific to different spheres of life (Connel, 1985; Fiske & Taylor, 1985; Lefcourt, 1981; Skinner, Chapman, & Baltes, 1988), that is, we feel more able to control outcomes in certain circumstances than in others.

Persons who feel capable and effective will seek out opportunities, use feedback to correct performance, and persevere to achieve goals. In contrast, individuals who feel incapable and lack a sense of efficacy will shy away from opportunity, avoid feedback, and have trouble persisting (Burke, 1977; DeCharms, 1968; Goodman, 1960). Consequently, personal causation influences how one is motivated toward doing things.

As shown in Figure 4-3, personal causation can be conceptualized as growing out of the original awareness of being a cause and developing over time—through a continuing cycle of anticipation, choice, experience, and interpretation—into the sense of personal capacity and self-efficacy. The following sections consider these two components of personal causation.

Sense of Capacity

People observe themselves through the common-sense lens of their culture, building up a store of

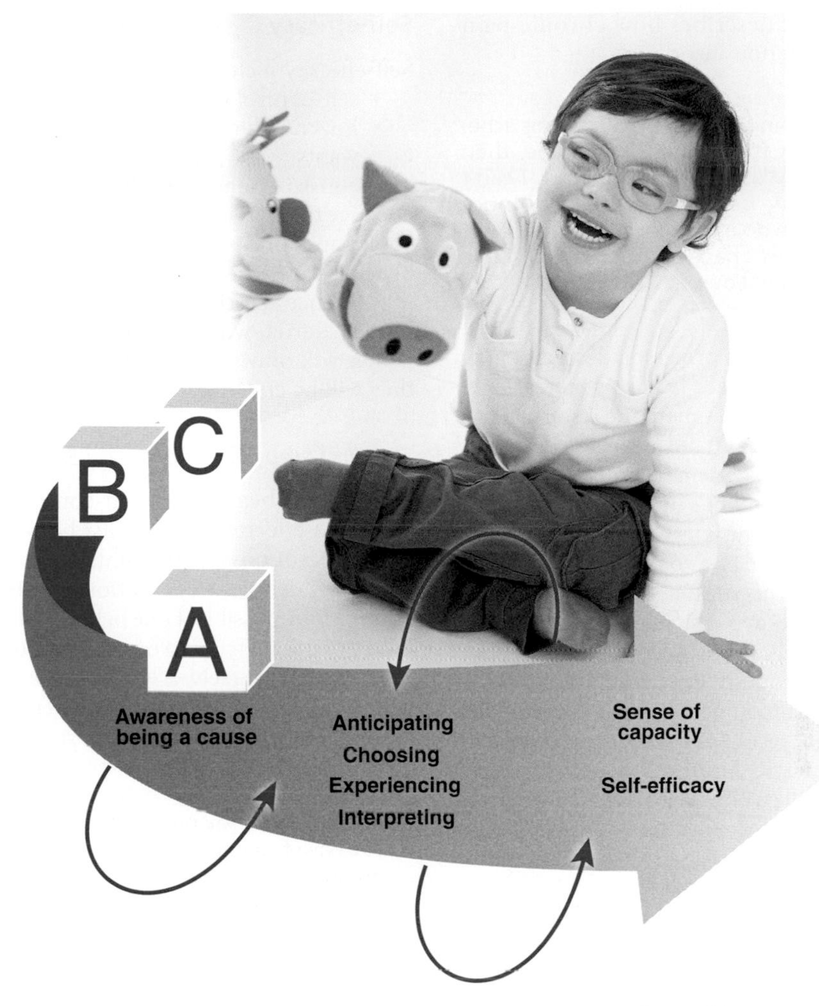

FIGURE 4-3 The Development of Personal Causation Over Time as One Encounters the World.

knowledge about what kind of capacities they have for doing the things that matter. The sense of capacity is an active awareness of one's capabilities for carrying out the life one wants to live. Moreover, as one proceeds through life, new experiences can alter one's sense of capacity.

What Happens When One's Sense of Capacity Is Challenged?

While all people must realize the limits of their capacities, having impairment uniquely challenges the view of self as capable (Molnar, 1989; Wright, 1960). As we saw at the beginning of the chapter, both Jiyeon and Richard are facing challenges to their sense of capacity related to their unique impairments. These challenges are particularly felt when the impairments limit their ability to do things that they want to do.

Pain, fatigue, and limitations of sensation, cognition, or movement can constrain people to achieve less than they desire (Werner-Beland, 1980). For example, Sienkiewicz-Mercer and Kaplan (1989, p. 64) write about their experience of cerebral palsy as being trapped in a body that "followed few directions of its mind and ignored the simple commands of speech and movement that nearly everyone takes for granted." Similarly, Deegan (1991) writes about her experience of schizophrenia and its impact on everyday tasks:

> I remember being asked to come into the kitchen to help knead some bread dough. I got up, went into the kitchen, and looked at the dough for what seemed an eternity. Then I walked back to my chair and wept. The task seemed overwhelming to me. (p. 49)

Another woman describes how chronic pain interferes with doing housework:

> Hanging the washing on the line. The arms ache. I might get about four things on the line, then it starts to ache. Washing up I can start. I can't do the saucepans, because of the scrubbing. Cooking—oh, I can do a bit of cooking, but I can't lift heavy saucepans. I have dropped them. I have burnt myself. (Ewan, Lowy, & Reid, 1991, p. 178)

Murphy (1987, p. 80), a professor, describes how his progressive paralysis made lecturing increasingly problematic as his voice "lost timbre and resonance, no longer projecting as well as it did." As these examples illustrate, incapacity is experienced as difficulty doing the things that matter in one's life.

The knowledge that one is less capable than others or than one once was can be a source of considerable emotional pain. For this reason, some persons will go out of their way to avoid situations that provide occasions for failure (Cromwell, 1963; Moss, 1958). For example, emotionally disturbed adolescents indicate feelings of incompetence and often prefer solitary tasks whose results are not judged by others (American Psychiatric Association [APA], 2000; Smyntek, 1983). Adults with developmental disabilities are often plagued with doubts about their abilities and go to great lengths to disguise their limitations (Edgerton, 1967; Kielhofner, 1983).

For example, Doris, a middle-aged woman who spent much of her childhood and young adulthood in a state hospital after being diagnosed as mentally retarded, was haunted by concerns about her capacity. She carried and often showed her [decade old] discharge papers as "proof" that she was competent (Kielhofner, 1980). When shame or fear of failure governs a person's sense of capacity there is disincentive to take risks, to learn new skills, or to make the best use of what one has. A negative sense of capacity can be even more limiting than the impairments on which it is based.

People are disposed to undertake that for which they feel capable and to avoid that which threatens them with failure. The close link between the sense of capacity and the desire to act accordingly is underscored by Murphy's (1987, p. 193) observation that, "With all bodily stimuli to movement muted and almost forgotten, one gradually loses the volition for physical activity." The sense of capacity readies one to anticipate, choose, experience, and interpret behavior. Those who see themselves to be capable are disposed to act and generate further evidence of their capacity. Those who view themselves as incapable feel compelled in the opposite direction.

Self-efficacy

Self-efficacy includes one's perception of:

- self-control and of
- how much one is able to bring about what one wants.

Through experience, people generate images of how effective they are in using their capacities and of how compliant or resistant life is to their efforts. Persons' beliefs about whether they can use their capacities to influence the course of events or circumstances in the external world are also powerful motivators. People will only put their efforts where they believe they will be effective.

The First Step of Self-efficacy: Self-control

Self-efficacy begins with self-control. To use one's capacities effectively, one must be able to shape or contain emotions and thoughts and exercise control over one's decisions and actions. A strong sense of efficacy is impossible if one believes that one is at the mercy of overwhelming emotions or uncontrollable thoughts. Conversely, a strong sense of self-control can greatly enhance how persons adapt, as illustrated in the following passage from a young woman with quadriplegia:

> The ability to say my mind is in charge here. Not this environment. Not what's happening to me—it's not in charge. What determines what I will do and how I will handle things is right here (pointing to her head), and I do have control over it. That's the important thing, that events can't shake you, physical environments can't shake you as long as you are able to say, "my mind is in control here. . . " (Patsy & Kielhofner, 1989)

Impact of Efforts on Self-efficacy

Self-efficacy also concerns whether one's efforts are sufficient to accomplish desired ends. The ability to achieve wanted outcomes in life can be challenged in a number of ways by impairments. That disease and trauma arrive uninvited and with negative consequences readily engenders feelings of being controlled by outside factors (Burish & Bradley, 1983; Trieschmann, 1989). Children who grow up with impairments learn that they cannot do what others do and are prone to develop feelings of ineffectiveness (Molnar, 1989). Such children may become unnecessarily dependent on others, because they do not see their own actions as the most effective route for achieving their desires (Wasserman, 1986). Feeling helpless is concomitant with many forms of mental illness (APA, 2000; Meissner, 1982). Persons with mental illness often lack a sense of control over life outcomes (Lovejoy, 1982; Wylie, 1979; Youkilis & Bootzin, 1979). Depression in particular is associated with the belief that one lacks control (Becker & Lesiak, 1977; Lefcourt, 1976; Leggett & Archer, 1979).

The loss of abilities significantly impacts self-efficacy. Hull (1990) gives a poignant description of how loss of sight took away personal control:

> I just sit here. The creatures emitting the noise have to engage in some activity. They have to scrape, bang, hit, club, strike surface upon surface, impact, make their vocal cords vibrate. They must take the initiative in announcing their presence to me. For my part, I have no power to explore them. I cannot penetrate them or discover them without their active cooperation. (p. 83)

Such constant reminders of one's inability to control the external world can result in feelings of powerlessness. Countering them requires extraordinary effort (Miller & Oertel, 1983; Murphy, 1987).

Dependence on medical personnel, family, or friends can exacerbate feelings of inefficacy. The patient role itself can contribute to a decreased sense of efficacy (Goffman, 1961). As persons are hospitalized and lose responsibility for their daily occupations, they may come to doubt whether they can manage their own lives. As Delaney-Naumoff (1980) notes:

> The patient feels he has lost power, direction, and goals—behaviors that characterize the mature adult in his interactions with others. Rather than feeling that he is in the center of activity, he feels pushed to the periphery. He becomes an outsider dependent upon the ministrations of others. (p. 87)

Disabled persons frequently note that the challenge of maintaining appropriate feelings of efficacy is complex and difficult. For example, Sienkiewicz-Mercer, who has cerebral palsy, describes her own struggle with self-efficacy. After the disappointments of not being able to stand and feed herself, being able to talk was the one area in which she kept up hope since it was "something that was infinitely more important to me than anything else" (Sienkiewicz-Mercer & Kaplan, 1989, p.12). Although she had to go on to deal with not being able to speak, she found her voice in her autobiography, *I Raise My Eyes to Say Yes*.

Self-efficacy can be complicated by important and consequential factors that might take away personal control in the future. For example, Thelma, who has bipolar disorder, discusses the uncertainty surrounding her disease and social welfare:

> And if I ever got a job (then) I got to pay full fee for my (subsidized) apartment . . . I don't want to be making the wrong move and then I'll be stuck with nothing, you know . . . You see, you may get (a job) and then you may get sick again, or have a relapse. You're out in the cold again trying to get back on disability. (Helfrich, Kielhofner, & Mattingly, 1994, p. 316)

As Thelma illustrates, it is difficult to have a sense of self-efficacy when illness or the vagaries of a welfare system may foil one's efforts to achieve a better life.

Disabled persons must often achieve a fine balance between necessary hope for the future and unrealistic expectations. The search for efficacy involves knowing disappointment, realizing what one cannot control, and finding and emphasizing what one is able to influence. Finding such a balanced view is not easy (Burish & Bradley, 1983).

Appraising the Self

How people judge their own capacity and efficacy is a matter of great importance and consequence. Thoughts and feelings about personal capacity and control incur strong emotions. So just how accurately can people assess themselves?

A number of factors impact self-appraisals. Cognitive limitations may impair comprehension of one's capacity. The psychological pain of acknowledging limitations and failures invites denial, avoidance, and projection (Valient, 1994). On the other hand, secondary gains related to being incapacitated (e.g., freedom from unsatisfying work conditions) may bias persons toward overestimating their limitations.

Persons who exaggerate their limitations may unnecessarily limit their actions. Those who overestimate their capacities may make choices that can lead to injury, exacerbation of symptoms, and failure in performance. The view of personal capacity and efficacy can also impact therapy. For example, Krefting (1989) discusses about a young man with a head injury that resulted in cognitive and communication deficits. He insisted that his only problem was walking and as a consequence "saw no need to compensate for his deficits" (p. 74).

Achieving an accurate view of one's capabilities and efficacy is not always easy. Persons with newly acquired impairments have not yet discovered what their capacities will be. Similarly, persons with progressive conditions or those who experience exacerbations and remissions cannot anticipate what abilities they will have in the future. In the face of a disability, personal causation is a highly individualized process of discovering how impairment may curtail or complicate the things one must and wants to do. This discovery may be ongoing as one's impairment and life change.

Volitional Component 2: Values

Over the course of development, people acquire beliefs and commitments about what is good, right, and important to do (Grossack & Gardner, 1970; Kalish & Collier, 1981; Klavins, 1972; Lee, 1971; Smith, 1969). These **values** are derived from culture that specifies what things matter, communicating how one ought to act, and what goals or aspirations are desirable (Bellah, Madsen, Sullivan, Swidler, & Tipton, 1985). These cultural messages commit people to a way of life and impart commonsense meaning to the lives they lead. Thus, values are convictions that carry with them a strong disposition to act accordingly. As shown in Figure 4-4, the process of anticipating, choosing, experiencing, and interpreting in our cultural context generates personal convictions and the sense of obligation that goes with them.

Importantly, values influence the sense of self-worth that one derives from doing certain things. Since values involve commitments to performing in culturally meaningful and sanctioned ways, one experiences a sense of belonging and appropriateness when following values (Lee, 1971). Moreover, one does not act contrary to one's values without a feeling of shame, guilt, failure, or inadequacy, as illustrated by the example of Elizabeth at the beginning of this chapter.

PERSONAL CONVICTIONS

All values are part of a coherent worldview about which people feel deeply (Bruner, 1990; Gergen & Gergen, 1988; Mitchell, 1983). These **personal convictions** are strongly held views of life that define what matters. For example, personal convictions may be organized around a fundamental religious viewpoint of right and wrong that defines what a good life is. A very different set of convictions underlie a street-smart adolescent who learns a code of gang solidarity, territoriality, and survival by aggression. While these two sets of convictions are vastly different, each represents a deeply held way of viewing the world.

SENSE OF OBLIGATION

Values bind people to action (Bruner, 1990; Fein, 1990). Because values evoke powerful emotions such as feelings of importance, security, worthiness, belonging, and purpose, they create a sense of obligation to perform in ways consistent with those values. This

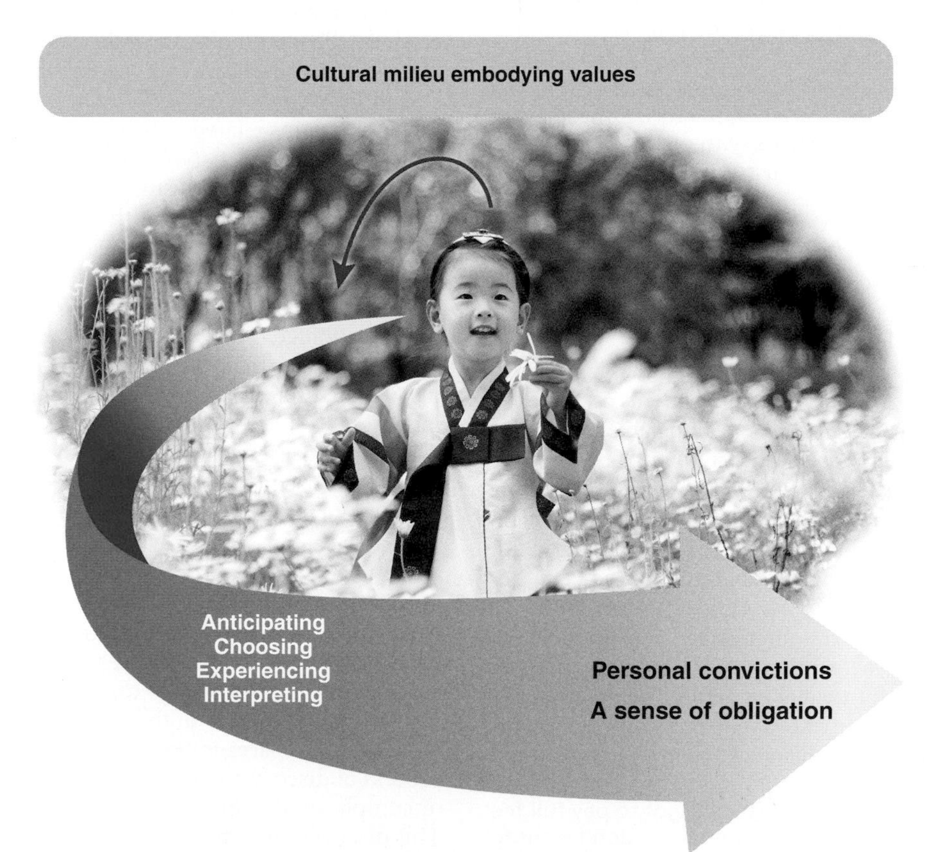

FIGURE 4-4 The Emergence of Values from Interactions with the Cultural Milieu.

sense of obligation may include such things as how time should be spent, what one should do, how one should do something, what constitutes adequate effort or outcomes, and what goals one should pursue (Cottle, 1971; Hall, 1959; Kluckholn, 1951). In sum, the **sense of obligation** is a strong emotional disposition to follow what are perceived as right ways to act.

IMPACT OF IMPAIRMENTS ON ONE'S VALUES

The interface of impairment and value is complex and multifaceted. Values shape how persons experience impairments. Values that conflict with what one is able to do can lead one to self-devaluation. Finally, experiencing an impairment may challenge one's values.

Persons with disabilities often find that their very condition is in conflict with mainstream cultural values. As Murphy (1987, pp. 116, 117) notes, "The disabled, individually and as a group, contravene all the values of youth, virility, activity, and physical beauty." Similarly, DeLoach, Wilkins, and Walker (1983, p. 14) note that the American work ethic has "tended to discredit anyone who does not or cannot work." Indeed, persons with acquired disabilities often find themselves devalued by the very standards that they have held all their lives.

A discontinuity between one's capacity and what one values can lower self-esteem (Zane & Lowenthal, 1960). For example, a woman experiencing functional limitations imposed by repetitive strain injury notes: "I got to the stage where you felt that you weren't worth anything, you were good for nothing. You couldn't do anything. What's the good of me? I can't do anything" (Ewan et al., 1991, p. 184). Loss of capacity can mean either rejecting old values or devaluing self as unable to live up to old values (Rabinowitz & Mitsos, 1964; Vash, 1981).

Values can commit one to impossible ideals (Fein, 1990). Persons with disabilities sometimes struggle futilely to achieve values inconsistent with their capacities. For example, Mike, throughout his adolescence and young adulthood, accepted his parents' vision that he would follow in the footsteps of his father, a successful surgeon. In college, he found the coursework overwhelming, failed his classes, became withdrawn and inactive, and finally required hospitalization for depression. Following this, he worked in a blue-collar position, which he enjoyed. Plagued with the idea that he was not living up to his parents' ideal, he returned to college only to experience the same pattern of failure, depression, and hospitalization. Twice more he repeated the same cycle, needing rehospitalization each time. Only after these repeated failures was he able to admit that the values he had pursued were not consistent with his abilities or his interests.

Like Mike, individuals may strive after certain values in the belief that their lives will not be fulfilled or that they will not have worth unless they somehow realize those values. In such instances, values can drive individuals toward choices that make life disappointing or difficult to bear.

Disability can radically challenge the whole view of life in which one's values are embedded. Consider, for example, persons who have made sense of their hard work as a means to a valued promotion and career development. In the face of a progressively disabling disease, their ideal of the progressive work career would no longer be viable.

As the previous example illustrates, the future as one imagined it may be partially or totally invalidated by disability. Without an image of what life will be like, it is more difficult to manage the taxing problems imposed by disability (Litman, 1972; Rogers & Figone, 1978, 1979). Without a sense of some valued future goal or state toward which one is striving, persons may question the worth of life and find themselves alienated and without a sense of purpose (Frankl, 1978; Korner, 1970; Menninger, 1962; Mitchell, 1975; Schiamberg, 1973).

Disability Values

While preexisting values can have an important impact on what a disability means to an individual, the existence of a disability can also be the critical occasion for development of new values. This is not easy since most cultures devalue disability and persons with disabilities (Longmore, 1995a, 1995b; Oliver, 1996; Scotch, 1988; Shapiro, 1994). Indeed, one of the consistent messages that persons with disabilities receive is that the part of the self which is disabled is essentially "bad" and must be balanced or overcome with the parts which are still "good" or not disabled (Gill, 1997).

Because dominant societal values tend to denigrate persons with disabilities, a growing community of disabled persons emphasizes a different valuation of disability. They identify their disability as a positive value rather than an aberration from what is good or right. A disability culture is beginning to emerge that extols ideals such as disability pride and encourages exhibiting rather than hiding one's disability (Gill, 1994, 1997).

Exposure to others who share common experiences and positive disability values is important for disabled persons (Gill, 1994, 1997). Such exposure can be hampered by the fact that people with disabilities are a diverse group and a single disability culture does not yet exist (Hahn, 1985). Until a disability culture and the values it extols become more widespread, disabled persons will continue to carry the burden of mainstream cultural values that demean them.

Values, Disability, and Choice

By rendering many of the things one used to do as impossible, impairment may force persons to examine what is most important to them. For example, Roberts (1989) recalls his own experience:

> One of my therapists insisted that I learn to feed myself. Meals took hours, and I was always exhausted. After, I realized then that I could either use my time to feed myself or have an attendant feed me, allowing me to spend the time saved to go to school. I went to school. (p. 234)

Another example is Melanie, who had arthritis. She routinely entertained her husband's business associates in their home, highly valuing her ability as a gourmet cook and expert hostess. However, after the onset of arthritis she found that her routine of shopping for products, preparing a complex meal, dressing appropriately, and then decorating the home for guests was no longer feasible. Her pain was so great by the time guests arrived that she could not enjoy the evening. Although she valued all components of the routine, she had to choose which aspects would be dropped or modified. She chose to have meals catered so that she would have the energy and relative freedom from pain to be a good hostess.

Disability can become a source of rethinking personal values and one's fundamental view of life. Wright (1960) argues that to adjust to disability persons may need to enlarge the scope of their values to incorporate behaviors for which they are still capable. In addition, persons may need to learn new values, which judge their performance given their capacities, and reject old values, which compare one's performance to that of others without disabilities. Since impairments typically invalidate some aspect of one's values, adjusting to disability almost invariably means a quest for new ways of viewing and valuing life.

One important example has been the way the disability community has critiqued the Western value of independence. They note that independence is typically thought of only in terms of functional capacity of persons to take care of themselves with insufficient attention to enabling self-determination though the exercise of free choice (Brisenden, 1986; Longmore, 1995a, 1995b; Oliver, 1993; Scheer & Luborsky, 1991). Moreover, as pointed out by Longmore (1995a), interdependence is a much more acceptable value for many disabled persons. Thus, personal choice and interdependence are proposed as values preferable to independence.

Volitional Component 3: Interest

Interests are what one finds enjoyable or satisfying to do. Thus, interests reveal themselves both as the enjoyment of doing something and as a preference for doing certain things over others (Matsutsuyu, 1969). As shown in Figure 4-5, interests reflect highly individual tastes generated from the cycle of anticipating, choosing, experiencing, and interpreting one's actions. Dreikie provides a moving example of how interests can continue to energize volition even in the midst of severe cognitive decline. She reenacts as best she can the activities that gave her enjoyment and satisfaction as a nurse (straightening out patient's beds, greeting new patients, and leading them about the ward).

ENJOYMENT

The **enjoyment** of doing things ranges from the simple satisfaction derived from small daily rituals to the intense pleasure people feel in pursuing their driving passions. The feeling of enjoyment may come from a wide range of factors. These include:

- Bodily pleasure associated with physical exertion
- Handling certain materials or objects
- Fulfillment of intellectual intrigue
- Aesthetic satisfaction from artistic production
- Fulfillment of using one's skill to face a challenge
- Creation of a pleasing product
- Fellowship with others

Attraction to any particular occupation most likely represents a confluence of several such factors. Those occupations that evoke the strongest feelings of attraction for us are generally those that evoke several sources of enjoyment. Csikszentmihalyi (1990) describes a form of ultimate enjoyment in physical, intellectual, or social occupations, which he calls flow. The experience of flow is a complete saturation of one's awareness with the positive experience of performing the activity. According to his research, flow occurs when a person's capacities are optimally challenged.

PATTERN

Since we do not experience all occupations with equal pleasure or satisfaction, we each develop a unique pattern of interests. One's **interest pattern** is the unique configuration of preferred things to do that one has accumulated from experience. In some cases, a pattern of interests will reflect an underlying theme such as athletic interest or cultural interests like theater and art. On the other hand, persons may have very diverse and seemingly unrelated preferences. Preferring certain occupations to others allows one to choose. Feeling a preference for certain activities makes it easier to select what to do. Consequently, one's pattern of interests is usually paralleled by a routine in which one's interests are at least partially indulged.

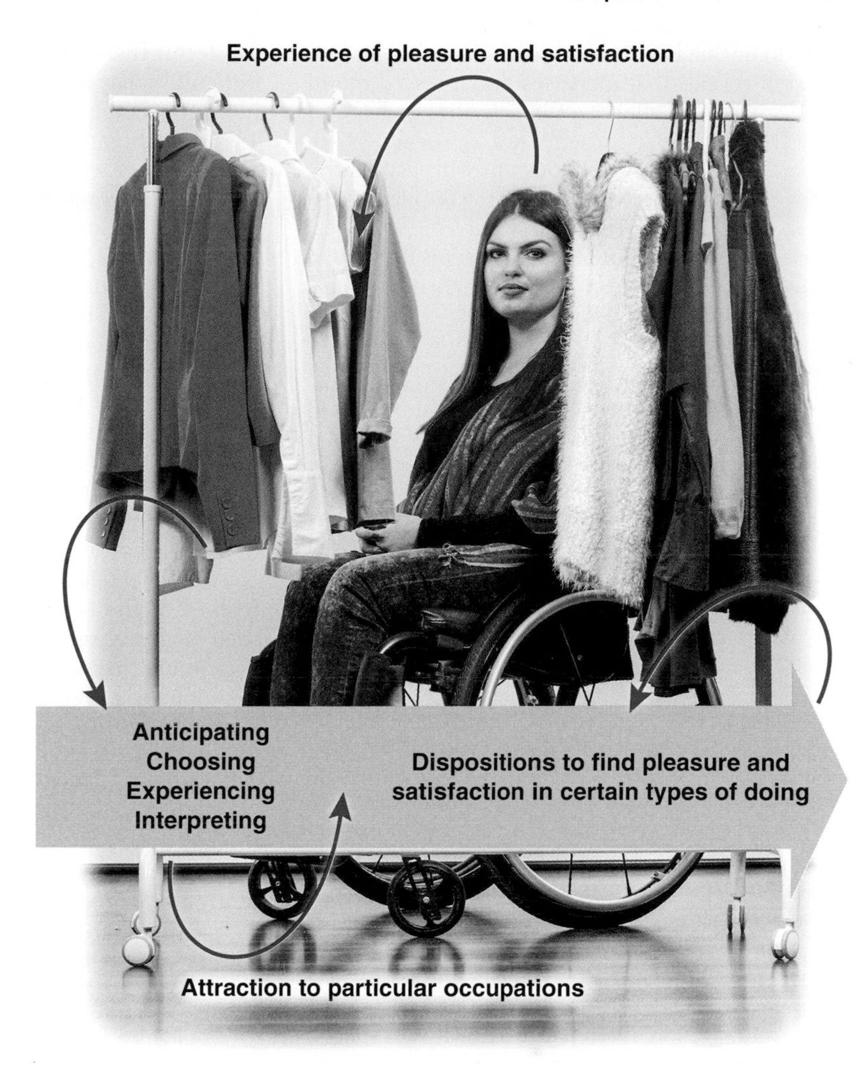

FIGURE 4-5 Interests.

IMPACT OF IMPAIRMENTS ON ONE'S INTERESTS

Although commonly overlooked, one of the most pervasive effects of impairment on occupation is its influence on the experience of satisfaction and pleasure in life. The daily pleasures, comforts, and enjoyments that enliven existence and help maintain energy and mood can be threatened or altered by disability.

Children with disabilities may have been given fewer opportunities to develop normal investment and satisfaction in occupational performance. Further, difficulties with performance and fear of being recognized as incompetent may lead a child to avoid opportunities to develop a sense of attraction to occupations.

Physical impairments and attendant fatigue, pain, and preoccupation with failure may reduce or eliminate the feeling of pleasure in occupations. Physical or procedural adaptations necessary to allow performance may negatively affect the ambiance and spirit of activities, making it difficult to experience the same sense of satisfaction as before. Many persons with acquired disabilities describe that it is no longer worth engaging in old pastimes. They are no longer enjoyable or do not warrant the additional effort required.

Further, persons may be prevented by limitations of capacity from participating in activities they previously enjoyed (Rogers & Figone, 1978; Trieschmann, 1989; Vash, 1981). For example, persons may have to give up activities involving excessive physical stress or requiring lost sensory, perceptual, or cognitive abilities.

Some psychiatric illnesses involve a loss of attraction to activities. For example, depressed persons frequently indicate few current interests even when their past interests were substantial (Neville, 1987). Many depressed persons speak about losing their enthusiasm for former interests and describe that they no longer enjoy doing things. Supporting such individual reports, research reveals that increases in depressed mood and decreases in enjoyment in activities go hand in hand (Neville, 1987; Turner, Ward, & Turner, 1979). Research also suggests that persons with psychiatric problems engage in few interests (Grob & Singer, 1974; Spivak, Siegel, Sklaver, Deuschle, & Garrett, 1982). Jack, who is psychiatrically disabled, represents the kind of limbo some people inhabit when they are neither able to establish nor be guided by interests:

> I don't have any drive. There's nothing I really feel like working for. I guess I wouldn't mind being a song-writer. But I never wrote anything worthwhile. No, I'd like to be an architect. I'd like to design bizarre houses. I'll never do it, because I'd lose interest. I'd like to do something with my life, but what I don't know. (Estroff, 1981, p. 142)

In discussing how persons with spinal cord injury may experience changes in interests, Trieschmann (1989) notes:

> Reduced access to satisfying activity can certainly lower mood, which tends to lower a person's interest in activity, which further lowers mood. Thus, a vicious circle evolves. (p. 242)

Her argument is supported by the finding that when persons increase their activities, their mood improves as well (Turner et al., 1979). Thus, it appears that the reduction in interest and attraction associated with many forms of disability may reflect a complex process in which decreased feelings of attraction, decreases in activity, and demoralization interrelate in a downward spiral.

Thus, one of the challenges presented by disability is often to find new interests or new avenues for channeling one's interests. One of my earliest client encounters was a young man who had great promise as a swimmer and diver. He had won regional and national championships and was an Olympic hopeful. He broke his neck in a diving accident and was rendered a high-level quadriplegic. Fortunately, he discovered that he was also a talented writer and speaker and was able to channel his interest in sports toward the field of sports journalism. Others do not so easily redirect their interests. Another client I knew at the same time had been an accomplished dancer in a nationally famous dance troupe. Following her spinal cord injury, she became despondent over her loss of ability. She slipped into chronic substance abuse.

WHEN INTERESTS FAIL

Persons may develop preferences that lead to problematic activity choices. For example, there is evidence to suggest that some adolescents with psychosocial difficulties may be attracted to socially unacceptable interests (Lambert, Rothschild, Atland, & Green, 1978; Werthman, 1976). As another example, adults with developmental disabilities tend to have mainly solitary and sedentary interests (Cheseldine & Jeffree, 1981; Coyne, 1980; Matthews, 1980; Mitic & Stevenson, 1981). As a consequence of their interests, these persons made choices to do things that isolated themselves, led to chronic physical inactivity, or got them into trouble.

Other research has found that persons with alcoholism are less likely to pursue their stated interests (Scaffa, 1982). Some persons appear to substitute the pleasure induced by substance abuse for the enjoyment of doing things. Others feel they cannot enjoy themselves without the assistance of drugs or alcohol.

A prospective study of more than 3000 aircraft workers found that those who hardly ever enjoyed their job tasks were 2.5 times more likely to report a back injury than subjects who almost always enjoyed their job tasks (Bigos et al., 1991). Whereas there is some reason to suspect that many workers today may feel disaffected from their work (Kielhofner, 1993), this may be particularly true when one has a disability. For example, Alice, who has a psychiatric disability, notes:

> I hate my job. I just hate it. It takes the mind of a seven-year-old to work there. It's boring. My supervisor is like a slave driver. I tried so many Civil Service jobs you wouldn't believe it. Sometimes two to three job interviews a week. But no one would hire me. No one. They never did tell me why. I bet I'll be stuck at Goodwill forever . . . (Estroff, 1981, p. 136)

Since work is a fact of life for so many adults, the degree of interest persons find in their work is no small issue.

INTEREST AS INSPIRATION

Interests can infuse life with meaning and energy, as illustrated in a story told by Christi Brown in his autobiography, *My Left Foot*. Brown, severely disabled with cerebral palsy, explains that as a 10-year-old boy he became depressed and despondent. With a set of watercolors bartered from his brother, he learned to paint with his foot. He explains:

> I didn't know it then, but I had found a way to be happy. Slowly I begin to lose my early depression. I had a feeling of pure joy while I painted, a feeling I had never experienced before which

seemed almost to lift me above myself. (Brown, 1990, p. 57)

Brown's characterization of painting as a way to be happy underscores an important point about interests. The process of finding pleasure and satisfaction in doing things is a central component of adapting in occupational life. The contentment we find in doing things gives us positive emotional experiences. Even more importantly, we must find some enthusiasm for doing particular things that urges us to action and gives us something to which we can look forward. Interest gives life much of its appeal. Inspiration can be a more effective motivator than fear.

Volitional Processes

The previous sections examined personal causation, values, and interests independently. As noted at the outset of this chapter, these three elements are woven together in the thoughts and feelings we have about our actions and our world. Moreover, it was noted at the beginning of this chapter that volition is a dynamic process involving a cycle of anticipation, making choices, experience while doing, and subsequent evaluation or interpretation. This last section examines the dynamic process of volition. In doing so, it considers how personal causation, values, and interests are part of a coherent pattern of thoughts and feelings unfolding in everyday life.

ANTICIPATION

People's interests, values, and personal causation influence how they anticipate action—that is, what they notice and search out in the world and what they feel and think about prospects for doing things. People tend to be unaware of that in which they have no volitional investment. Conversely, they notice what corresponds to their competence, interests, and commitments. What is out there in the world for anyone is very much a function of volition. For example, Dreikie notices those things on the dementia ward that reflect opportunities for her to enact the nurse-like behaviors that give her satisfaction.

MAKING CHOICES

People's choices for action shape their everyday doing and influence the course of their lives. These choices involve complex contributions from all components of volition. Thus choices are shaped by one's interests, personal causation, and values. Activity choices shape the immediate future. They involve decisions to begin or terminate activities as well as how to go about them. Thus they commence, shape, and terminate what one does. Occupational choices (i.e., decisions to begin or end roles, alter a habit pattern, or undertake a personal project) occur much less frequently than activity choices, but they have a much more far-reaching impact on our lives. In fact, what most characterizes an occupational choice is that it changes something fundamental about one's life. Consequently, most occupational choices are made over a period of deliberation as one considers what they mean for one's life. The onset of an acquired disability is often an occasion for occupational choice. When a disability interferes with role performance, requires extra time to do things, or makes old habits or projects no longer viable, people must make a series of different occupational choices to find a new pattern of behavior. The success of such choices will have a great deal to do with how well a person adapts to the circumstance of having a disability. Richard's desire to enter a worker role and Jiyeon's efforts to learn the tasks that her peers do are both examples of importance of this process of choice-making.

EXPERIENCE

Volition also influences how we experience what we do. When we engage in occupations our volition determines which ones we find more or less enjoyable or valuable. It also determines the extent of confidence or anxiety we feel. Volition leads each of us to experience action in our own unique way.

CASE EXAMPLE: GERIATRICS ADULT WITH ALZHEIMER'S DEMENTIA

Driekie is a 72-year-old resident of a specialized care unit in South Africa. She is the seventh member of her family to be diagnosed with Alzheimer's disease. Driekie is a trained nurse and spent a substantial amount of her working years in a local hospital when she lived in Zambia with her family. Her caring nature is still evident as she is very preoccupied with many of the residents on the ward who are bedridden. Under supervision of staff she spends a lot of time fidgeting with these residents' bedclothes, as she tugs and pulls at them apparently in an effort to "straighten her patients' beds." Despite lacking verbal communication she welcomes all newcomers on the ward by approaching them and speaking incoherently. She also likes to take fellow residents by the hand and lead them up and down the ward hall. Finally,

one of Driekie's favorite occupations is to explore the ward's multisensory garden.

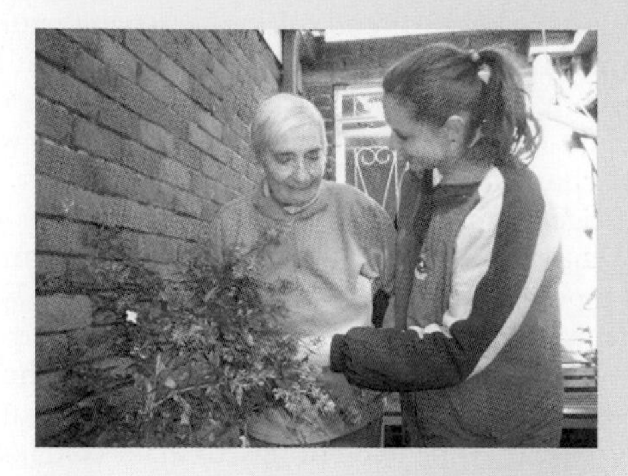

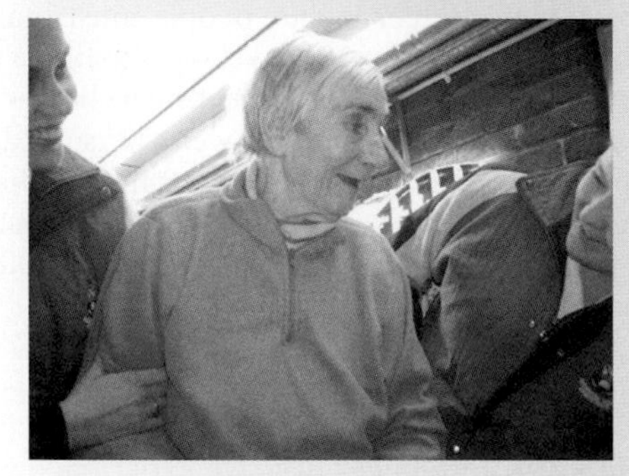

Driekie interacting with OT students and exploring the multisensory garden

Our experience in performing is closely linked to our quality of life. After all, how we experience the things we do—be it enjoyment, boredom, fulfillment, angst, triumph, or disappointment—determines much of what we get out of life. Finding harmony between our volition and what we actually get to do in the course of daily life contributes to life satisfaction.

For instance, the fact that Driekie's environment allows her to continue to do occupations that satisfy her allows her to achieve a measure of life satisfaction despite her severe impairment.

Finally, experience is also a critical dimension of therapy. The therapeutic transformation that comes from doing things depends on what we experience in the midst of performance. Research has shown that volition is an important determinant of how therapy is experienced and a critical factor in whether clients benefit from therapy (Barrett, Beer, & Kielhofner, 1999; Helfrich & Kielhofner, 1994; Kielhofner & Barrett, 1998).

INTERPRETATION

Volition influences how we interpret our actions. Our personal causation, values, and interests have an important influence on the significance we assign to what we have done. For example, Richard's commitment to achieving a productive life like his brother will influence how he makes sense of everyday experiences on the job. Elizabeth's feelings of insecurity and inefficacy around her peers influences the way she views her interpersonal performance. As these examples show, volition provides the framework by which people make sense of their actions.

Summary

Volition has a pervasive influence on occupational life. It shapes how people see the world and the opportunities and challenges it presents. It guides the activity and occupational choices that together determine much of what we do. It determines the experience of doing. It shapes how people make sense of what they have done, including effectiveness in achieving desired ends and success in realizing important values. To a large extent, how people experience life and how they regard themselves and their world has to do with volition.

CASE EXAMPLE TO TEST YOUR KNOWLEDGE: GOAL-SETTING FOR A PALLIATIVE CARE CLIENT

An OT was asked to work with an 81-year-old Asian man, who had been diagnosed with pancreatic cancer 3 days prior. Family members inquired about palliative care for him, and the internal medicine team referred the family to a palliative care program. The OT—a member of the palliative care team—visited the patient and his family for an evaluation. A preliminary phone call with family members indicated that they were in shock. The OT was asked about the best way to inform the client about the diagnosis, as well as about designing an individualized palliative care program for him. At the time that the OT introduced herself to the client and began her informal interviews, the client was still hospitalized, but his cognition level was high. However, there were a few obstacles the OT needed to address: First, the family informed her that the client was very sensitive, with a lifelong anxiety history concerning his health status. Second, he had a degenerative hearing disability. While respecting the family's wishes to find the gentlest way to inform the client about his health status, the OT wanted to involve him in a goal-setting process for his remaining days.

Question to Encourage Critical Thinking and Discussion: How can we identify the client's volition? What questions should be asked and how should one observe and gather information about his interests, values, and personal causation?

Discussion: The OT provided structured questions to help the client identify his life goals. The following is a conversation between the client and the OT about creating a timeline of goals:

OT: What would you like to do if you were to live another 10 years?

Client: Then I would finish my writing.

OT: *What would you like to do if you were to live for another 5 years?*

Client: *Then I would still finish my writing.*

OT: *What would you like to do if you were to live for another 1 year?*

Client: *Well, Then I would finish my writing as much as I could.*

OT: *What would you like to do, if you were to live for another 1 hour?*

Client: Then, I would pray for the Lord's Son to come and take me.

Through the structured and unstructured interview with the client and the family members, the OT was able to identify what mattered the most, what the client was interested in, and what could make the client feel in control and capable, given the circumstances. The OT and the client collaborated to summarize a bucket list for 1 year as follows:

1. To finish writing a book
2. To be a proper son, visiting his parents' tombstone with his own family members
3. To be a father, meeting his children and grandchildren, eating a Chinese meal together

Things to check on to understand the volition of my client:

- If my client is willing to do something, does that always mean she/he has a high volition?
- When does my client's volition become problematic?
- In what circumstances should I encourage my client to become aware of her/his volition?

Chapter 4 Review Questions

1. Define the three elements of volition.
2. Using an example, explain how these three elements interact to motivate an individual to engage in an occupation.
3. Provide an example of the occupational behavior of a person with a lower level of volition—someone in the exploratory stage of volition.
4. Provide an example of the occupational behavior of a person with a moderate level of volition—someone in the competency stage.
5. Provide an example of the occupational behavior of a person with a high level of volition—someone in the achievement stage.

HOMEWORK ASSIGNMENTS

Complete a self-analysis of your own volition and that of someone close to you. For each analysis, answer the following questions:

1. Describe three of this person's primary interests.
2. Explain this person's sense of personal causation, particularly as it relates to his or her primary interests.
3. Describe this person's values. How are they aligned with his or her interests and personal causation? If they are not well aligned, please explain why not.
4. Characterize this person in terms of his or her stage of volition.

SELF-REFLECTION EXERCISE

Fill in the blanks with a list of your occupations.	What volitional concept can you find?
"I like to_______________________________."	Interest
"To do_________________________ is important to me."	Value
"I can _________________________ but not _________________________, and I'm not sure whether I can_______________________________."	Sense of Capacity
"I feel like I'm out of control. No matter what I do, nothing will change."	Self-efficacy
"___________makes me want to do more in my life and I can't wait to _______________."	Volitional Process

thePoint® For additional resources and exercises, visit http://thePoint.lww.com

Key Terms

Enjoyment: The feeling of pleasure or satisfaction that comes from doing things.

Interest pattern: The unique configuration of preferred things to do that one has accumulated from experience.

Interests: What one finds enjoyable or satisfying to do.

Personal causation: One's sense of competence and effectiveness.

Personal convictions: Views of life that define what matters.

Self-efficacy: Thoughts and feelings concerning perceived effectiveness in using personal abilities to achieve desired outcomes in life.

Sense of obligation: Strong emotional dispositions to follow what are perceived as right ways to act.

Sense of personal capacity: Self-assessment of one's physical, intellectual, and social abilities.

Values: What one finds important and meaningful to do.

Volition: Pattern of thoughts and feelings about oneself as an actor in one's world, which occur as one anticipates, chooses, experiences, and interprets what one does.

REFERENCES

American Psychiatric Association. (2000). *Diagnostic and statistical manual of mental disorders* (4th ed., Text Revision). Washington, DC: Author.

Barrett, L., Beer, D., & Kielhofner, G. (1999). The importance of volitional narrative in treatment: An ethnographic case study in a work program. *Work, 12,* 79–92.

Becker, E. W., & Lesiak, W. J. (1977). Feelings of hostility and personal control as related to depression. *Journal of Clinical Psychology, 33,* 654–657.

Bellah, R., Madsen, R., Sullivan, W., Swidler, A., & Tipton, S. (1985). *Habits of the heart.* Berkeley: University of California Press.

Bigos, S. J., Battie, M. C., Spengler, M. D., Fisher, L. D., Fordyce, W. E., Hansson, T. H., et al. (1991). A prospective study of work perceptions and psychosocial factors affecting the report of back injury. *Spine, 16,* 1–6.

Brisenden, S. (1986). Independent living and the medical model of disability. *Disability, Handicap, and Society, 1,* 173–178.

Brown, C. (1990). *My left foot.* London, United Kingdom: Minerva.

Bruner, J. (1973). Organization of early skilled action. *Child Development, 44,* 1–11.

Bruner, J. (1990). *Acts of meaning.* Cambridge, MA: Harvard University Press.

Burish, T. G., & Bradley, L. A. (1983). *Coping with chronic disease: Research and applications.* New York, NY: Academic Press.

Burke, J. P. (1977). A clinical perspective on motivation: Pawn versus origin. *American Journal of Occupational Therapy, 31,* 254–258.

Cheseldine, S., & Jeffree, D. (1981). Mentally handicapped adolescents: Their use of leisure time. *Journal of Mental Health Deficiency Research, 25,* 49–59.

Connel, J. P. (1985). A new multidimensional measure of children's perceptions of control. *Child Development, 56,* 1018–1041.

Cottle, T. J. (1971). *Time's children: Impressions of youth.* Boston, MA: Little, Brown & Co.

Coyne, P. (1980). Developing social skills in the developmentally disabled adolescent and young adult: A recreation and social/sexual approach. *Journal of Leisure, 7,* 70–76.

Cromwell, R. L. (1963). A social learning approach to mental retardation. In N. R. Ellis (Ed.), *Handbook of mental deficiency.* New York, NY: McGraw-Hill.

Csikszentmihalyi, M. (1990). *Flow: The psychology of optimal experience.* New York, NY: Harper & Row.

DeCharms, R. E. (1968). *Personal causation: The internal affective determinants of behaviors.* New York, NY: Academic Press.

Deegan, P. (1991). Recovery: The lived experience of rehabilitation. In R. P. Marinelli & A. E. Dell Orto (Eds.), *The psychological and social impact of disability* (3rd ed.). New York, NY: Springer-Verlag.

Delaney-Naumoff, M. (1980). Loss of heart. In J. A. Werner-Beland (Ed.), *Grief responses to long-term illness and disability.* Reston, VA: Reston Publishing.

DeLoach, C. P., Wilkins, R. D., & Walker, G. W. (1983). *Independent living: Philosophy, process, and services*. Baltimore, MD: University Park Press.

Edgerton, R. B. (1967). *The cloak of competence: Stigma in the lives of the mentally retarded*. Berkeley, CA: University of California Press.

Estroff, S. E. (1981). *Making it crazy*. Berkeley: University of California Press.

Ewan, C., Lowy, E., & Reid, J. (1991). 'Falling out of culture': The effects of repetition strain injury on sufferers' roles and identity. *Sociology of Health and Illness, 13*, 168–192.

Fein, M. L. (1990). *Role change: A resocialization perspective*. New York, NY: Praeger.

Fiske, S., & Taylor, S. E. (1985). *Social cognition*. New York, NY: Random House.

Frankl, V. E. (1978). *The unheard cry for meaning*. New York, NY: Touchstone Books.

Gergen, K. J., & Gergen, M. M. (1983). Narratives of the self. In T. R. Sarbin & K. E. Scheibe (Eds.), *Studies in social identity*. New York, NY: Praeger.

Gergen, K. J., & Gergen, M. M. (1988). Narrative and the self as relationship. In L. Berkowitz (Ed.), *Advances in experimental social psychology* (pp. 17–56). San Diego, CA: Academic Press.

Gill, C. (1994). A bicultural framework for understanding disability. *The Family Psychologist, Fall*, 13–16.

Gill, C. (1997). Four types of integration in disability identity development. *Journal of Vocational Rehabilitation, 9*, 39–46.

Goffman, E. (1961). *Asylums*. New York, NY: Doubleday.

Goodman, P. (1960). *Growing up absurd*. New York, NY: Vintage Books.

Grob, M., & Singer, J. (1974). *Adolescent patients in transition: Impact and outcome of psychiatric hospitalization*. New York, NY: Behavioral Publications.

Grossack, M., & Gardner, H. (1970). *Man and men: Social psychology as social science*. Scranton, PA: International Textbook.

Hahn, H. (1985). Disability policy and the problem of discrimination. *American Behavioral Scientist, 28*, 293–318.

Hall, E. T. (1959). *The silent language*. Greenwich, CT: Fawcett Publications.

Harter, S. (1983). The development of the self-system. In M. Hetherington (Ed.), *Handbook of child psychology: Social and personality development* (Vol. 4). New York, NY: John Wiley & Sons.

Harter, S. (1985). Competence as a dimension of self-evaluation: Toward a comprehensive model of self-worth. In R. L. Leahy (Ed.), *The development of the self*. Orlando, FL: Academic Press.

Harter, S., & Connel, J. P. (1984). A model of relationships among children's academic achievement and self-perceptions of competence, control, and motivation. In J. Nicholls (Ed.), *The development of achievement motivation*. Greenwich, CT: JAI.

Helfrich, C., & Kielhofner, G. (1994). Volitional narratives and the meaning of therapy. *American Journal of Occupational Therapy, 48*, 318–326.

Helfrich, C., Kielhofner, G., & Mattingly, C. (1994). Volition as narrative: Understanding motivation in chronic illness. *American Journal of Occupational Therapy, 48*, 311–317.

Hull, J. M. (1990). *Touching the rock: An experience of blindness*. New York, NY: Vintage Books.

Kalish, R. A., & Collier, K. W. (1981). *Exploring human values*. Monterey, CA: Brooks/Cole.

Kielhofner, G. (1980). *Evaluating deinstitutionalization: An ethnographic study of social policy* (Unpublished doctoral dissertation). University of California, Los Angeles, CA.

Kielhofner, G. (1983). "Teaching" retarded adults: Paradoxical effects of a pedagogical enterprise. *Urban Life, 12*, 307–326.

Kielhofner, G. (1993). Functional assessment: Toward a dialectical view of person-environment relations. *American Journal of Occupational Therapy, 47*, 248–251.

Kielhofner, G., & Barrett, L. (1998). Meaning and misunderstanding in occupational forms: A study of therapeutic goal-setting. *American Journal of Occupational Therapy, 52*, 345–353.

Klavins, R. (1972). Work-play behavior: Cultural influences. *American Journal of Occupational Therapy, 26*, 176–179.

Kluckholn, C. (1951). Values and value orientations in the theory of action: An exploration in definition and classification. In T. Parsons & E. Shils (Eds.), *Toward a general theory of action*. Cambridge, MA: Harvard University Press.

Korner, I. (1970). Hope as a method of coping. *Journal of Consulting and Clinical Psychology, 34*, 134–139.

Krefting, L. (1989). Reintegration into the community after head injury: The results of an ethnographic study. *Occupational Therapy Journal of Research, 9*, 67–83.

Lambert, B. G., Rothschild, B. F., Atland, R., & Green, L. B. (1978). *Adolescence: Transition from childhood to maturity* (2nd ed.). Monterey, CA: Brooks/Cole.

Lee, D. (1971). Culture and the experience of value. In A. H. Maslow (Ed.), *Neural knowledge in human values*. Chicago, IL: Henry Regnery.

Lefcourt, H. (1981). *Research with the locus of control construct* (Vol. 1: Assessment and methods). New York, NY: Academic Press.

Lefcourt, H. M. (1976). *Locus of control: Current trends in theory and research*. Hillsdale, NJ: Erlbaum.

Leggett, J., & Archer, R. P. (1979). Locus of control and depression among psychiatric patients. *Psychology Report, 45*, 835–838.

Litman, T. J. (1972). Physical rehabilitation: A social-psychological approach. In E. G. Jaco (Ed.), *Patients, physicians and illness: A sourcebook in behavioral science and health* (2nd ed.). New York, NY: Free Press.

Longmore, P. K. (1995a). Medical decision making and people with disabilities: A clash of cultures. *Journal of Law, Medicine & Ethics, 23*, 82–87.

Longmore, P. K. (1995b, September/October). The second phase: From disability rights to disability culture. *The Disability Rag & Resource*, pp. 4–11.

Lovejoy, M. (1982). Expectations and the recovery process. *Schizophrenia Bulletin, 8*, 605–609.

Markus, H. (1983). Self knowledge: An expanded view. *Journal of Personality, 51*, 543–562.

Matsutsuyu, J. (1969). The interest checklist. *American Journal of Occupational Therapy, 23*, 323–328.

Matthews, P. R. (1980). Why the mentally retarded do not participate in certain types of recreational activities. *Therapeutic Recreation Journal, 14*, 44–50.

Meissner, W. W. (1982). Notes on the potential differentiation of borderline conditions. *Psychoanalytic Review, 70*, 179–209.

Menninger, K. (1962). Hope. In S. Doniger (Ed.), *The nature of man in theological and psychological perspective*. New York, NY: Harper Brothers.

Miller, J. F., & Oertel, C. B. (1983). Powerlessness in the elderly: Preventing hopelessness. In J. F. Miller (Ed.), *Coping with chronic illness: Overcoming powerlessness*. Philadelphia, PA: F. A. Davis.

Mitchell, A. (1983). *The nine American lifestyles*. New York, NY: Macmillan.

Mitchell, J. J. (1975). *The adolescent predicament*. Toronto, ON: Holt, Rinehart & Winston.

Mitic, T. D., & Stevenson, C. L. (1981). Mentally retarded people as a resource to the recreationist in planning for integrated community recreation. *Journal of Leisure Research, 8*, 30–34.

Molnar, G. E. (1989). The influence of psychosocial factors on personality development and emotional health in children with cerebral palsy and spina bifida. In B. W. Heller, L. M. Flohr, & L. S. Zegans (Eds.), *Psychosocial interventions with physically disabled persons*. New Brunswick, NJ: Rutgers University Press.

Moss, J. W. (1958). *Failure-avoiding and stress-striving behavior in mentally retarded and normal children*. Ann Arbor, MI: University Microfilms.

Murphy, R. (1987). *The body silent*. New York, NY: WW Norton.

Neville, A. M. (1987). *The relationship of locus of control, future time perspective and interest to productivity among individuals with varying degrees of depression* (Unpublished doctoral dissertation). New York University, New York.

Oliver, M. (1993). Disability and dependency: A creation of industrial societies. In J. Swain, V. Finkelstein, S. French, & M. Oliver (Eds.), *Disablingbarriers—Enabling environment* (pp. 49–60). London, United Kingdom: SAGE.

Oliver, M. (1996). The social model in context. In *Understanding disability from theory to practice* (pp. 30–42). New York, NY: St. Martin's Press.

Patsy, D., & Kielhofner, G. (1989). *An exploratory study of psychosocial adaptation to spinal cord injury*. Unpublished manuscript.

Rabinowitz, H. S., & Mitsos, S. B. (1964). Rehabilitation as planned social change: A conceptual framework. *Journal of Health and Social Behavior, 5*, 2–13.

Roberts, E. V. (1989). A history of the independent living movement: A founder's perspective. In B. W. Heller, L. M. Flohr, & L. S. Zegans (Eds.), *Psychosocial interventions with physically disabled persons*. New Brunswick, NJ: Rutgers University Press.

Rogers, J. C., & Figone, J. J. (1978). The avocational pursuits of rehabilitants with traumatic quadriplegia. *American Journal of Occupational Therapy, 32*, 571–576.

Rogers, J. C., & Figone, J. J. (1979). Psychosocial parameters in treating the person with quadriplegia. *American Journal of Occupational Therapy, 33*, 432–439.

Rotter, J. B. (1960). Generalized expectancies for internal versus external control of reinforcement. *Psychological Monographs: General Applications, 80*, 1–28.

Scaffa, M. (1982). *Temporal adaptation and alcoholism* (Unpublished master's thesis). Virginia Commonwealth University, Richmond.

Scheer, J., & Luborsky, M. L. (1991). Post-polio sequelae: The cultural context of poliobiographies. *Orthopedics, 14*, 1173–1181.

Schiamberg, L. B. (1973). *Adolescent alienation*. Columbus, OH: Merrill.

Scotch, R. (1988). Disability as a basis for a social movement: Advocacy and the politics of definition. *Journal of Social Issues, 44*(1), 159–172.

Shapiro, J. (1994). *No pity: People with disabilities forging a new civil rights movement*. New York, NY: Times Books.

Sienkiewicz-Mercer, R., & Kaplan, S. B. (1989). *I raise my eyes to say yes*. New York, NY: Avon Books.

Skinner, E. A., Chapman, M., & Baltes, P. B. (1988). Control, means-end, and agency beliefs: A new conceptualization and its measurement during childhood. *Journal of Personality and Social Psychology, 54*, 117–133.

Smith, M. B. (1969). *Social psychology and human values*. Chicago, IL: Aldine.

Smyntek, L. E. (1983). *A comparison of occupationally functional and dysfunctional adolescents* (Unpublished master's project). Virginia Commonwealth University, Richmond.

Spivak, G., Siegel, J., Sklaver, D., Deuschle, L., & Garrett, L. (1982). The long-term patient in the community: Life-style patterns and treatment implications. *Hospital Community Psychiatry, 33*, 291–295.

Trieschmann, R. B. (1989). Psychosocial adjustment to spinal cord injury. In B. W. Heller, L. M. Flohr, & L. S. Zegans (Eds.), *Psychosocial interventions with physically disabled persons*. New Brunswick, NJ: Rutgers University Press.

Turner, R. W., Ward, M. F., & Turner, D. J. (1979). Behavioral treatment for depression: An evaluation of therapeutic components. *Journal of Clinical Psychology, 35*, 166–175.

Valient, G. E. (1994). Ego mechanisms of defense and personality psychopathology. *Journal of Abnormal Psychology, 103*, 44–50.

Vash, C. L. (1981). *The psychology of disability*. New York, NY: Springer-Verlag.

Wasserman, G. A. (1986). Affective expression in normal and physically handicapped infants. Situational and developmental effects. *Journal of the American Academy of Child and Adolescent Psychiatry, 25*, 393–399.

Werner-Beland, J. A. (Ed.). (1980). *Grief responses to long-term illness and disability*. Reston, VA: Reston Publishing.

Werthman, C. (1976). The function of sociological definitions in the development of the gang boy's career. In R. Giallombardo (Ed.), *Juvenile delinquency: A book of readings* (3rd ed.). New York, NY: John Wiley & Sons.

Wright, B. A. (1960). *Physical disability: A psychological approach*. New York, NY: Harper & Row.

Wylie, R. (1979). *The self-concept: Theory and research* (2nd ed.). Lincoln, NE: University of Nebraska Press.

Youkilis, H., & Bootzin, R. (1979). The relationship between adjustment and perceived locus of control in female psychiatric in-patients. *Journal of Genetic Psychology, 135*, 297–299.

Zane, M. D., & Lowenthal, M. (1960). Motivation in rehabilitation of the physically handicapped. *Archive of Physical Medicine and Rehabilitation, 41*, 400–407.

Habituation: Patterns of Daily Occupation

Sun Wook Lee and Gary Kielhofner (posthumous)

CHAPTER 5

EXPECTED LEARNING OUTCOMES

Upon completion of this chapter, readers will be able to:

1. Understand and state the meaning of habituation.
2. Name two components of habituation.
3. Identify and describe the dynamics of one's roles and habits given certain circumstances. Provide an example.
4. Describe the impact of one's habituation in relation to the client's occupational participation.
5. Find the strength/challenges of habituation in order to facilitate the therapy process (goals/strategies).

The way in which one goes about everyday life can affect one's success and satisfaction. Chapter 1 proposed that the organization of routine life is a function of habituation. **Habituation** is an internalized readiness to exhibit consistent patterns of behavior guided by our habits and roles and fitted to the characteristics of routine temporal, physical, and social environments. As shown in Figure 5-1, habituation allows persons to cooperate with their environments in order to do the routine actions that make up everyday life.

In the following cases, Michael is struggling with finding a routine way to manage his homework. Chung-Haw is seeking to enrich his life with a new role as a serious tennis player. Mr. Chen has decided to alter his daily and weekly routine in order to have more balance between work and family and leisure pursuits.

MOHO Problem-Solver Cases

MOHO Problem-Solver Case #1: School-Based Therapy

Michael, a primary school student with attention-deficit hyperactivity disorder, struggles with organization of his schoolwork. Despite a folder with numerous pockets provided by his therapist, Michael has developed a habit of placing all of his papers in the same pocket. This only results in him having problems finding the items and getting them out in a timely manner. He has become quite frustrated with the folder solution his therapist provided for his difficulty in keeping his homework assignments and other papers organized.

Recognizing that her approach was not working, the therapist revised her approach by offering new folders of different types and sizes, and by encouraging him to put iconic stickers onto each of his folders, each of which reflects a specific, imaginary role or character. When it was time for science class, Michael assumed the role of a medical doctor, and his papers were placed in a folder that looked like a patient's medical chart, complete with a red cross on the front of a white background. When it was time for reading, Michael became a bookworm, and stored his reading materials in a folder with a large worm sticker on it—the worm wearing glasses and appearing interested in a book he was reading. Imaging himself in the roles of each of these different characters as he changed subjects motivated Michael to compartmentalize and appropriately organize the subjects and materials in his mind, making it less likely that he would lose his materials and homework assignments.

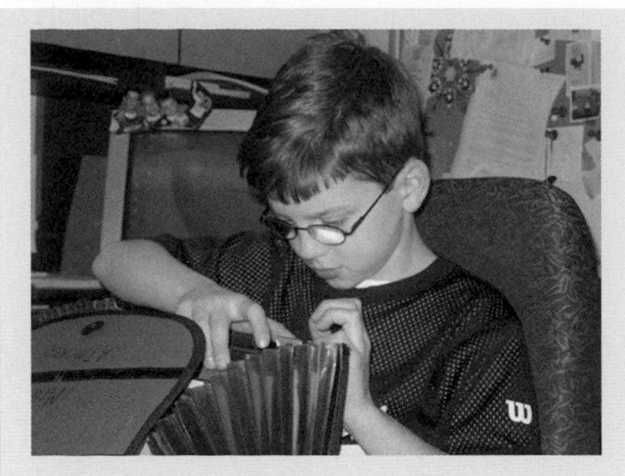

Michael looking in backpack

MOHO Problem-Solver Case #2: Adult Outpatient Balancing Roles

Chun-Haw is a 32-year-old first-year medical student in Taiwan. He sees his role as a medical student as being vital to his future, both as a way of contributing to humanity and as a lifelong, gainful occupation. However, his true passion involves his role as a tennis player. Chun-Haw has given up a lot for his passion, delaying his education in order to support his tennis habit. He has gone through several intensive training courses and constantly focuses on increasing his tennis skills. This role has become increasingly important to him lately, because he has recently received a diagnosis of rheumatoid arthritis and is receiving occupational therapy in order to learn self-management approaches. Recognizing the limits of his own body, Chun-Haw realizes that he will not be able to play tennis forever, and he very much wants to elevate the level of competition in which he engages. Additionally, he experiences a great deal of pleasure and satisfaction from it and has incorporated tennis playing as a significant part of his identity. When talking about his tennis playing, Chung-Haw also notes that he sees it as beneficial to his physical and psychological health since it improves his cardiopulmonary function and reduces the stress associated with his strenuous studies. Moreover, playing tennis has been a major way that Chung-Haw interacts with peers and built friendships.

Together, he and his occupational therapist have come up with a plan that allows him to engage in his much-loved role as a tennis player while at the same time putting some of his educational goals into perspective. Although he has the talent and ability to become a physician, ultimately, Chun-Haw decides that a career as a physical therapist is a better fit for his daily routine. Transferring relevant credits from medical school, Chun-Haw enters a blended online/classroom program as a part-time physical therapy student. The online component allows him to complete his studies around a flexible schedule, and the part-time nature of his enrollment allows him to pace himself so that he does not become overwhelmed by academic stress and a chronic sense of overcommitment.

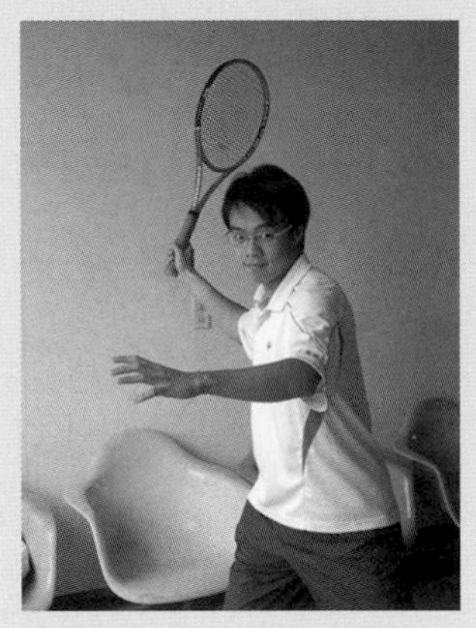

Chen-Haw playing tennis

MOHO Problem-Solver Case #3: Adult Outpatient Reassessing and Reprioritizing

Mr. Chen is a successful professional who has been able to provide a comfortable life for his family in Taiwan. In the past, Mr. Chen found it challenging to balance the multiple demands associated with being a husband, father, and son, while working in a high-pressured job. After experiencing the loss of his spouse and suffering a heart attack just weeks later, he was referred to occupational therapy with the goal of reassessing his life and priorities. Now he is working to maintain more balance and satisfaction from his involvement in his family roles and from his leisure lifestyle. He has decided to have more modest life goals, be satisfied with what he does accomplish, earn less income, and have more time for family, rest, and leisure. One aspect of his changed lifestyle is that Mr. Chen has taken up golf, which he does regularly with his son. As a consequence of changes he made in his life, Mr. Chen has experienced a new sense of achievement and pleasure.

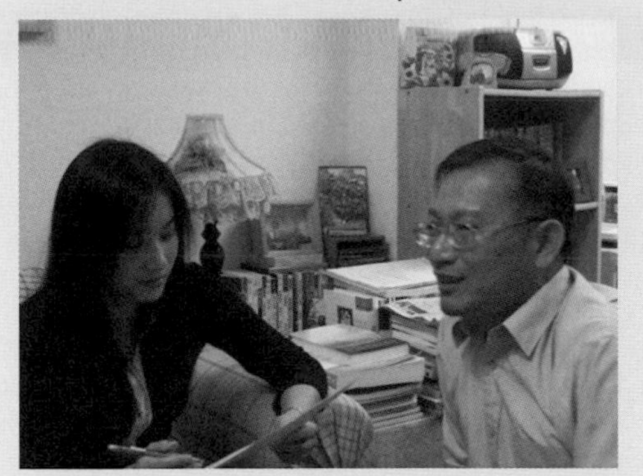

Mr. Chen with therapist

Interdependency of Habituation and Habitat

The regularity in our habituated behavior depends on the reliability of our habitats. A degree of sameness in the physical environment provides a stable arena for performance. The recurring temporal patterns—such as day and night, workweek and weekend—provide a stable structure within which routines unfold. Similarly, the social order has sufficient stability to furnish us known situations for which we have ways of responding. Because of the regularity of our environments, we are mostly grounded in the familiar, not having to calculate our moves consciously. As Young (1988, p. 79) notes, habituated performances are "generated and locked into place by recurrences."

Habituation involves the internalization of action-oriented representations that, in the words of Clarke (1997, p. 49), "simultaneously describe aspects of the world and prescribe possible actions."

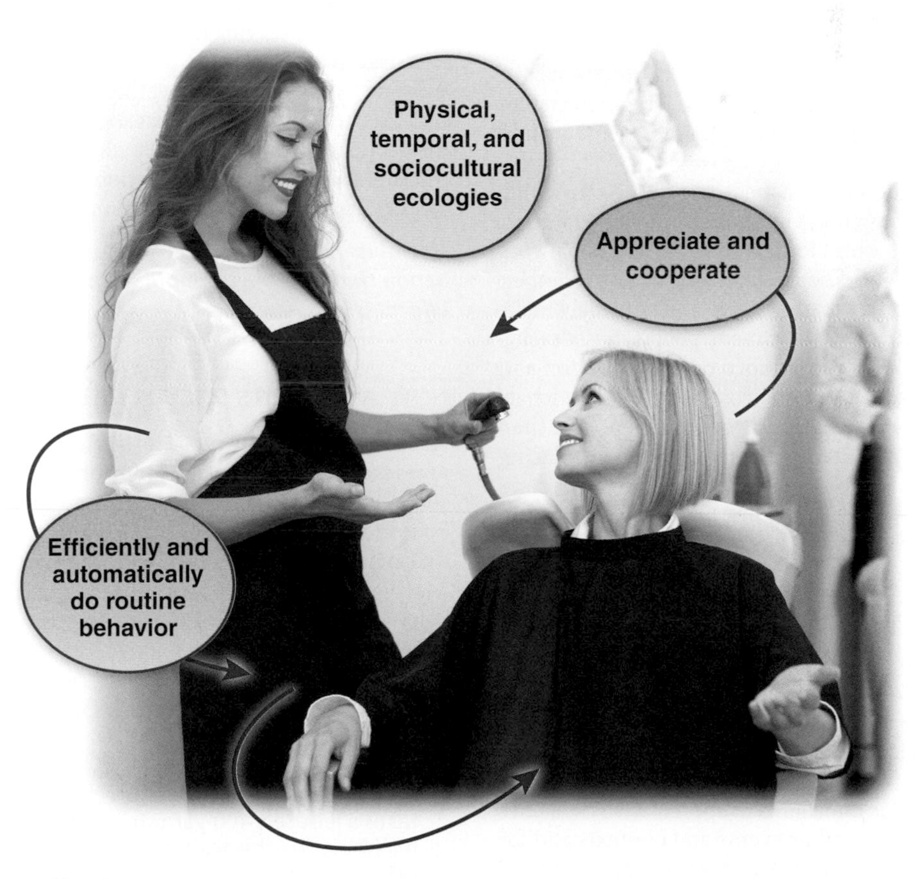

FIGURE 5-1 Habituation.

When we repeat behavior in a constant context, we learn to attend to aspects of the environment that will help sculpt the action that is part of any habit or role.

Habituation Component 1: Habits

Habits can be defined as acquired tendencies to automatically respond and perform in certain, consistent ways in familiar environments or situations. Habits regulate behavior by providing a regulated manner of dealing with environmental contingencies (Camic, 1986; Dewey, 1922). Habits guide behavior in the way that grammar organizes language or rules regulate a game (Koestler, 1969; Young, 1988). Bourdieu (1977) underscores that learning a habit is to acquire a set of rules for how to simultaneously appreciate and act in the world. Appreciating the environment means that we automatically locate ourselves in the midst of familiar environmental features, apprehending their action implications for a habitual behavior we are doing. For example, in the routine of getting dressed, people automatically recognize which piece of clothing goes where and which pieces of clothing need to be donned before others. We attend to and comprehend our environments in terms of their implications for our routine doing. Therefore, a large component of any habitual action will be strategies for incorporating the things, people, and events around us into what we do.

This is exactly the aspect of habit with which Michael is struggling. He has been provided folders that would allow him to separate different homework assignments and keep related materials together. However, in order to effectively and routinely make use of objects in the environment, people must develop personal habits that capitalize on their volition and on the features of the environment. Until Michael is able to attach meaning to the folders and then practice and acquire a new set of rules for placing materials in the appropriate folders in an orderly and systematic fashion, it will not provide a solution to his homework woes.

We incorporate features of the environment into how we go about doing habitual things.

So long as we experience the world as familiar, habits operate smoothly and without need of attention. It is the unfamiliar (i.e., that for which we do not have internalized rules) that extricates us from our habitual way of doing things. Consequently, habits operate as internalized, appreciative capacities for recognizing familiar events and contexts and for guiding action. Habits give us a way to appreciate and construct action appropriate to what is going on in the world around us.

HOW DO HABITS BRING ABOUT EFFECTIVENESS AND EFFICIENCY TO OUR LIVES?

Habits preserve a way we have learned to do something from earlier performance in a given environment. Habits will incorporate ways of doing things that have a certain value within the environment in which they are performed. This does not mean that all habits are effective in every way. Matthew's habit of dumping his papers into one section of the folder may serve some purpose such as avoiding the challenging process of sorting them out, but it does not help him be more organized in his approach to homework. Adaptive habits allow persons to compete routine activities in a consistent and effective manner (Camic, 1986).

Habits hold together the patterns of ordinary action that give life its familiar character. Young (1988) argues that habits serve as a kind of self-perpetuating flywheel conserving patterns of action. Once launched, habits provide a momentum that allows action to unfold on its own. This frees up conscious attention for other purposes (James, 1950). Habits can also allow two or more behaviors to occur simultaneously. While one is performing habituated behaviors (e.g., getting dressed in the morning, driving home after work), it is possible to engage in other thoughts and behaviors (e.g., making a phone call, planning a meeting, or listening to the radio). Therefore, habits decrease the effort required for occupational performance not only by reducing the amount of conscious attention required, but also freeing up persons for other simultaneous activity.

Habits hold together the patterns of ordinary action that give life its familiar and relatively effortless character.

HOW ARE HABITS SOCIALLY RELEVANT?

Habits also serve a purpose for society. Young (1988) notes that habits shared by a group of people constitute social customs. Thus, by acquiring habits humans become carriers and messengers of the customs that make up the way of life of a particular group. Moreover, in a social group one person's habitual behavior may be part of the environmental context necessary for another's habits. For example, Rowles (1991) provided the following description of a group of elderly men engaging in the habit of gathering at the post office:

> Every morning, shortly before 10:00 a.m., Walter takes a leisurely 400-yard stroll down the hill from his house to the trailer that serves as the post office to "pick up the mail." He traces exactly the same path each day. Several male age peers from different locations within Colton embark on

> the same trip at about the same time . . . picking up the mail provides a rationale for an informal gathering of the elderly men of the community at the bench outside the Colton Store, which is located adjacent to the post office. The men generally linger throughout the morning. They watch the passing traffic, converse with patrons of the store, and discuss events of the day. Then, around lunchtime, the group disperses and Walter finds his way home again. (p. 268)

Walter's habit of getting the mail and meeting with other older residents illustrates how habits guide us to take advantage of, and be in harmony with, others' behavior (Cardwell, 1971).

Our typical behaviors are to a large extent those recognized, expected, and depended on by others in the environment. For example, the habits of punctuality and industriousness reflect typical expectations of Western society. One is to be at work, meetings, and appointments at scheduled times and to focus on the task at hand during periods so designated. A person who is not punctual or attentive to work tasks will not be in synchrony with such an environment. Consequently, habits also allow a person to be integrated into the smooth functioning of society. This point is illustrated by Mr. Chen's alternation of his routine which allowed him to come into more harmonious relationship with his family. Whereas his previous habits of working kept him away from leisure activities with family members, his new routine allowed more contact with family.

THREE INFLUENCES OF HABITS IN DAILY OCCUPATIONS

The influence of habits on everyday behavior is pervasive (Camic, 1986). What we do, when we do it, and how we go about it reflect our habits. As shown in Figure 5-2, we can recognize three influences of habits:

- Habits impact how routine activity is performed;
- Habits regulate how time is typically used;
- Habits generate styles of behavior that characterize a range of occupational performances.

Habits of Occupational Performance

Each person has his or her own way of performing routine activities such as grooming and dressing,

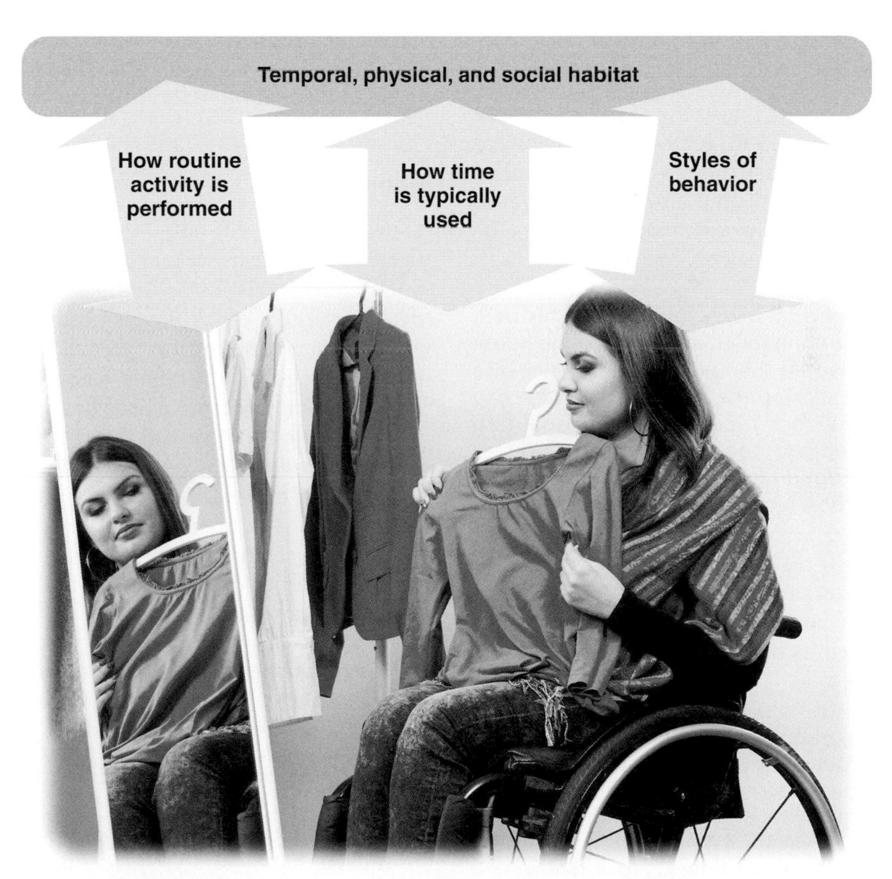

FIGURE 5-2 Influences of Habits on Occupation.

making the bed, preparing morning coffee, taking out the dog, paying bills, and going to work or school. Habits may fit with our ideas about proper etiquette or form. They may reflect the way a parent or mentor taught us. They may simply emanate from what is simplest and most efficient. Whatever the reasons, people tend to be firmly entrenched in their particular ways of doing familiar activities.

Seamon (1980) noted that habits ordinarily involve a sequence of physical movements. He refers to them as body ballets, noting that they are "a set of integrated behaviors which sustain a particular task or aim" (p. 157). Habitual ways of performing ordinary activities organize actions together to accomplish a goal under routine conditions. Dewey (1922, p. 24) referred to such daily habits as "passive tools waiting to be called into action." Indeed, our habits are tools of a sort that we call upon to get done what we do in ordinary life. Although the habitual ways of doing almost everything we do go largely unnoticed, getting through the day without them would be unbearably cumbersome.

Although the habitual ways of doing almost everything we do go largely unnoticed, getting through the day without them would be unbearably cumbersome.

Habits of Routine

The influence of habits is also found in our routine use of time. Seamon (1980) refers to such habits as time–space routines since they are ordinarily linked not only to what time it is but also to where we are or how we are moving through space. He offers the following description of such a routine:

> He would be up at seven-thirty, make his bed, perform his morning toilet, and be out of his house by eight. He would then walk to the corner cafe up the street, pick up the newspaper (which *had* to be the *New York Times*), order his usual fare (one scrambled egg, toast, and coffee), and stay there until around nine when he would walk to his nearby office. (p. 158)

Each of us will recognize similar routine use of time that characterizes our everyday patterns.

Chapin (1968) points out that our routines include not only daily habits but habits within a variety of temporal cycles:

> . . . cooking, eating and washing dishes during the twenty-four hour period of a day; the work, school, shopping, recreation or socializing routine during a seven day week; visiting out-of-town relatives and family vacation or other holiday outing routines during a year's time . . . (p. 13)

Consequently, routines may be linked to a variety of cycles. Some cycles are tied to the kind of work one does. For example, teachers have changing routines across the school term and farmers' routines depend on the seasons and the weather.

Routines do provide a degree of structure and predictability to life. In a longitudinal study of retirement, one of the greatest challenges for older persons was to find a new routine after working (Jonsson, Josephsson, & Kielhofner, 2001). While no 2 days are exactly the same, most persons have and can identify a routine that is typical for a given day of the week. In industrialized societies persons generally have patterns that characterize schooldays and workdays as well as alternate patterns that characterize days off from work or school. The degree of consistency in a routine depends on one's environment. Some environments demand a fixed routine such as the grade school or factory schedule that requires persons to show up, do certain tasks, take lunch and breaks, and terminate the day at specific times. Other environments require a more flexible pattern of action.

Habits of routine help locate us effectively within the stream of time. They enable us to be where we should be and get done what we should be doing over the course of daily, weekly, and other life cycles. To a very large extent, our everyday lives are defined and shaped by these cyclical routines. They create the overall pattern by which we go about our various occupations.

Habits of Style

Dewey (1922, p. 20) noted that one's habits were reflected in a typical "style of . . . being-in-the-world." Such characteristics as being big-picture versus detail-oriented, quick versus plodding, or prompt versus procrastinating are examples of styles of performance regulated by habits. Habits of style are also found in our interpersonal behavior. Whether we tend to be quiet or talkative, direct or evasive, trusting or cautious, and formal or informal are examples of social habits of style.

Habits of style are manifest across a whole range of activities. That is, we tend to bring our personal styles to the performance of all that we do. Camic (1986) defines such habits as:

> The durable and generalized disposition that suffuses a person's action throughout an entire domain of life or, in the extreme instance, throughout all of life—in which case the term comes to mean the whole manner, turn, cast, or mold of the personality. (p. 1045)

Indeed, habits of style give a unique and stable character to performance.

HOW ARE HABITS FORMED AND CHANGED?

Children come into the world without internal regulators of patterned behavior save, perhaps, certain biorhythms. Soon, however, they are integrated into the rhythms, routines, and customs that make up the physical, social, and temporal world. Children first acquire routines through parental guidance and support. These are routines of day and night with the attending patterns of sleeping, waking, eating, bathing, and so on. Over the course of development, as routines, customs, and ways of doing things are reexperienced, the child incorporates complex habit patterns.

A number of these patterns remain somewhat stable throughout life, such as sleeping and eating patterns. Others change with the attainment of developmental stages such as entering the student or worker roles. Interestingly, each new environmental context has its own regular rhythms that encourage individuals to internalize a pattern of action like that of others in the social system. Eventually, a number of rhythms may interweave, such as the rhythms and patterns of home life and those of school or work life.

All habits serve to preserve patterns of action, so they are naturally resistant to change. Whenever we make alterations in our schedules or environments, we encounter the tenacity of old habits. We show up at old appointed times or we visit the wrong cabinet or office for some time after we have relocated where we keep things or where we work.

Habits resist change since they are based on our most fundamental certainties about how the world is constructed (Berger & Luckman, 1966). Habits presuppose a particular order in the physical, temporal, and social world. When habits and their background assumptions are disrupted or altered, a feeling of disorientation or unreality follows. For example, when our sleep patterns are disrupted or altered, we can find ourselves waking up without the usual sense of being firmly anchored in the temporal world (i.e., thinking it is dawn when it is really dusk). A similar feeling of disorientation can occur when we are in the midst of a familiar task and lose our place (e.g., suddenly realizing we do not recognize where we are on the road when driving to a familiar destination). In such cases, we are shocked into sudden consciousness with no clear footing in what is ordinarily a familiar and taken-for-granted world.

WHAT HAPPENS TO HABITS WHEN DISABILITY OCCURS?

Habits organize our use of underlying performance capacity so that we can perform within our environment. The fit of our habits to our performance capacity and to our environment will determine how effective we are in our everyday routines. Habits play an especially important role when persons face the challenges of a disability. As the following discussions show, habits may either contribute to a disability or they may effectively compensate for underlying impairments.

Dysfunctional Habits

We intuitively know that the wrong habits can negatively affect us. All of us have possessed habits we would rather have been without. Sometimes, however, dysfunctional habits become more than a nuisance. They become a serious liability threatening one's welfare (Kielhofner, Barris, & Watts, 1982).

Acquired impairments can lead to an erosion of habits that further exacerbate the consequences of these functional limitations. For example, persons facing depression may be unable to pursue their routines because of limited motivation and energy (American Psychiatric Association, 2000). Over time, this can lead to an erosion of habits that contributes to inactivity (Melges, 1982). When this happens and the person loses previously effective and satisfying routines, mood and energy can be further degraded. In such cases, the disruption of habits becomes part of a downward spiral. Impairments negatively affect habits and their disruption further exacerbates the symptoms and/or consequences of the underlying condition.

Another habit problem associated with disability is that persons may learn dysfunctional habits due to their environments. For example, the inactivity imposed by hospitalization can contribute to the loss of habits. Unfortunately, opportunities for persons to practice old or new habits are often not provided during rehabilitation (Shillam, Beeman, & Loshin, 1983). Many persons with more severe emotional and cognitive impairments are placed in institutional environments. In such settings the routines can result in residents learning habits of passivity and inactivity that do not serve them well in the institution or later when they are placed in the larger community (Borell, Gustausson, Sandman, & Kielhofner, 1994; Kielhofner, 1979, 1981, 1983).

Impact of Impairments on Habits

When capacities are diminished, previously established habits can be severely disrupted. One may be forced to develop new habits for many or most aspects of everyday life. Alterations in a person's functional status can totally disrupt the effectiveness of an existing habit. Zola (1982) illustrates this in his description of trying to complete his morning routine from the new viewpoint of a wheelchair:

> Washing up was a mess. Though the sink was low enough, I nevertheless managed to soak myself thoroughly. In retrospect, I should not have worn anything. Ordinarily when washing my face, chest, and arms, I would lean over the sink, and any excess water from my splashing would drip into it. My body angle in a wheelchair was different. I could not extend over the sink very far without tipping. Thus, much of the water dripped down my neck onto me. Splashing with water was out, and the use of a damp washcloth, what I once called a "sponge bath." (p. 64)

When impairments are more pronounced so are the complications of everyday routines. When persons have to make extensive use of adaptive equipment or require assistance from other persons, entirely new routines must be acquired. Sometimes, new habits related to the management of the disability are required. For example, people may need to learn new habits for bowel and bladder care, for joint protection and energy conservation, or for following complicated medication regimens. Remissions and exacerbations, or progressive decreases in physical functioning, can make acquiring these necessary new habits difficult.

Disabled persons whose abilities are variable may need to develop extremely flexible habits. For example, persons with unpredictable impairments must be ready to capitalize on those times when things are better such as the following gentleman with Parkinson's disease:

> I cram in to the periods when I'm flexible all the things I would have liked to have done the rest of the day . . . One day I may be nine-tenths of the day free, although that's very rare, and another much less. There's nothing I can do about it. (Pinder, 1988, p. 79)

On the other hand, steadily progressive impairments may mean that habits are to an extent replaced with conscious strategies. For example, Murphy (1987) explains how his progressive paralysis meant that everyday routines had to be calculated. As he notes, the routine of transferring from wheelchair to toilet required him to strategize how to get up, "choosing . . . supports with care, calculating the number of steps it would take to reach [the toilet]" (p. 76). When habits cannot automatically regulate what one does, additional effort and concentration are required, taking away the ease and efficiency that ordinarily accompany everyday routines.

When habits cannot automatically regulate what one does, additional effort and concentration are required, taking away the ease and efficiency that ordinarily accompany everyday routines.

Disruption of Space and Time

The onset of a severe impairment can radically alter the spatial and temporal dimensions of routine performance. For example, the spinal cord–injured person must learn to organize behavior around the constraints of where one can go in a wheelchair and how long it will take (Paap, 1972). With the onset of a disability, the entire relationship of persons with their environments may change in dramatic ways, resulting in the need for new habits. In this regard Hull (1990) notes:

> On the whole, my experience has been that, if I have a bad habit, it . . . is naturally corrected . . . In other words, blindness itself imposes an iron law upon the user of the white cane. Lampposts, curbs, and stairways are the best teachers. (p. 15)

In a similar fashion, wheelchairs or other devices to assist walking require their users to choose not simply the closest route to a destination, but rather the route with friendly ramps, curbs, and surfaces. The habits that accommodate a new disability must not only deal with altered performance capacity, but must also grapple with a physical world whose implications for action are radically changed. Additionally, people can become more vulnerable to external contingencies such as bad weather or crowded public places.

Time also becomes a different matter. When their impairments require additional time to conduct routine tasks, persons must develop daily routines that involve doing fewer things. Such temporal challenges can be further constrained by the necessity of adding new self-care habits to the daily routine.

How Can Habits Be Reconstructed?

As the previous discussions illustrate, the task of organizing daily life in the face of disability means reconstructing one's habits. Accommodations and trade-offs must take place. Some activities may need to be eliminated. New ways of doing things must be discovered and learned. Finally, one may have to delegate some tasks to family members or an attendant to have time for other more valued activities.

As Williams (1984) notes:

> If the disabled individual is to move toward "mere" impairment, eventually alternative ways of accomplishing the tasks of everyday life will be committed to memory and habit, engrained

> in relationships with a new world which is once again "had." (p. 110)

The path to these new habits involves leaving behind a once familiar world that has been invalidated by disability. As Merleau-Ponty (1945/1962) notes:

> It is precisely when my customary world arouses in me habitual intentions that I can no longer, if I have lost a limb, be effectively drawn into it: the utilizable objects, precisely in so far as they present themselves as utilizable, appeal to a hand I no longer have. (p. 82)

Only by reencountering the world with one's altered condition can a new relationship to the world emerge and once again become familiar and taken for granted. DeLoach and Greer (1981) describe this transformation in the following way:

> A person begins to learn new ways of doing what she did before—and ways of accomplishing, as well, some brand-new things. These new, different ways are, at first, awkward, stress-producing, and frustrating . . . little by little, a person gets accustomed to a new modus operandi. What at first was awkward, painful, or embarrassing becomes just a regular part of living, incorporated into one's routine. After such habituation, the person begins to concentrate more on participation in life now rather than on what used to be or what might have been. (p. 251)

As they indicate, the transformation of habits is a necessary pathway through which persons find their way back to the participation in everyday activities of daily living, work, and leisure.

Habituation Component 2: Internalized Roles

Routine action is influenced by the fact that each of us belongs to and acts in social systems. Much of what we do is done as a spouse, parent, worker, student, and so on. Having internalized such roles, we act in ways that reflect our role status (Fein, 1990). Internalizing the role means taking on an identity, an outlook, and actions that belong to the role. Consequently, an **internalized role** is the incorporation of a socially and/or personally defined status and a related cluster of attitudes and actions. Chun-Haw's involvement in the leisure role of playing tennis is an example of this process of internalizing a role. He sees himself as and has acquired equipment and clothes that signify he is a tennis player. He has sought out training to improve his game. He interacts with others who share this role and is working toward involvement in formal competitions that will allow him to publicly enact the role in new contexts.

Internalizing a role involves gaining a sense of one's relationships to others and of expected behaviors. As Sarbin and Scheibe (1983, p. 8) note, effective action depends on the "correct placements of self in the world of occurrences." Consequently, internalized roles give us the necessary social bearings to act effectively.

ROLE IDENTIFICATION

We see ourselves as students, workers, parents, and so on because we recognize ourselves as occupying certain statuses or positions and also because we experience ourselves acting as someone who holds these roles. As Sarbin and Scheibe (1983, p. 7) note, "a person's identity at any time is a function of his or her validated social positions." We identify with our roles in part because we see ourselves reflected in the attitudes and actions of others toward us. Consequently, role identity is generated when others recognize and respond to us as occupying a particular status. Who we are is intertwined with the roles we inhabit (Cardwell, 1971; Ruddock, 1976; Schein, 1971; Turner, 1962).

Identifying with any role means internalizing elements of what society attributes to the role along with one's personal interpretation of that role (Fein, 1990). For example, one person may develop a student role identity that stresses being an intellectual. For such a person being a student may resonate with the volitional sense of having intellectual capacity, interests, and values. Another student, whose interest and values lie elsewhere, may view the student role as only instrumental to gaining a credential. Both inhabit the student role, but the ways in which they internalize it, identify with it, and enact its expectations will differ significantly.

Whatever way we come to think of and experience ourselves in a role becomes part of our self-understanding. To an extent, we see ourselves and judge our actions in terms of our own perception of the roles we inhabit. As Miller (1983) argues, personal identity reflects our awareness of all our various roles. Integrating one's various roles into a personal identity involves assigning centrality or importance to some roles over others. This process is dynamic and changes over time as different roles assume different places in our lives or demand extra effort or attention (Hall, Stevens, & Meleis, 1992). Mr. Chen is an examples of someone who has redefined his worker, leisure, and family roles.

However, not all roles have a clearly defined social status. Some roles are more informal. Some arise out of personal circumstances (Rosow, 1976). One example of an informal role without a clear social status is that of caregiver for a disabled spouse or parent (Schumacher, 1995). Such roles that do not correspond to a formal social status have more ambiguous meanings and expectations attached to them. Consequently, internalization of such roles requires more improvisation. Persons are often left to impart their definition on the role and to find social partners who will recognize and validate the role. This is one of the reasons that support groups are so popular. They often provide persons access to others who, like themselves, occupy a role that is not well defined. In such groups persons find validation for their role and sort out what are reasonable expectations for the role.

People know how to act in a given role because of an internalized script that guides how they perceive themselves and their role partners (Fein, 1990; Miller, 1983; Mancuso & Sarbin, 1983). The script allows one to tacitly appreciate how one should proceed. For example, how we perform a greeting is guided by the role relationship we have with another. Depending on whether a pair is parent and child, worker and boss, student and teacher, or two close friends, the greeting may take on quite different forms.

■ ***When we know our role relationship to others, we recognize both how they see and should act toward us and what should be our attitudes and actions toward them.*** ■

INFLUENCES OF ROLES ON OCCUPATION

As shown in Figure 5-3, roles organize action in three main ways. First, they influence the manner and content of our actions. Moving from one role to another is often demarcated by such changes as how we dress, our manner of speech, and our way of relating to others. Second, each role carries with it a range of actions that make up that role. Consequently, roles shape what kinds of things we do. For example, a student is expected to attend class, take notes, ask questions, read articles or books, complete assignments, study, and take exams. The actions expected for a role are clearly defined by some social groups.

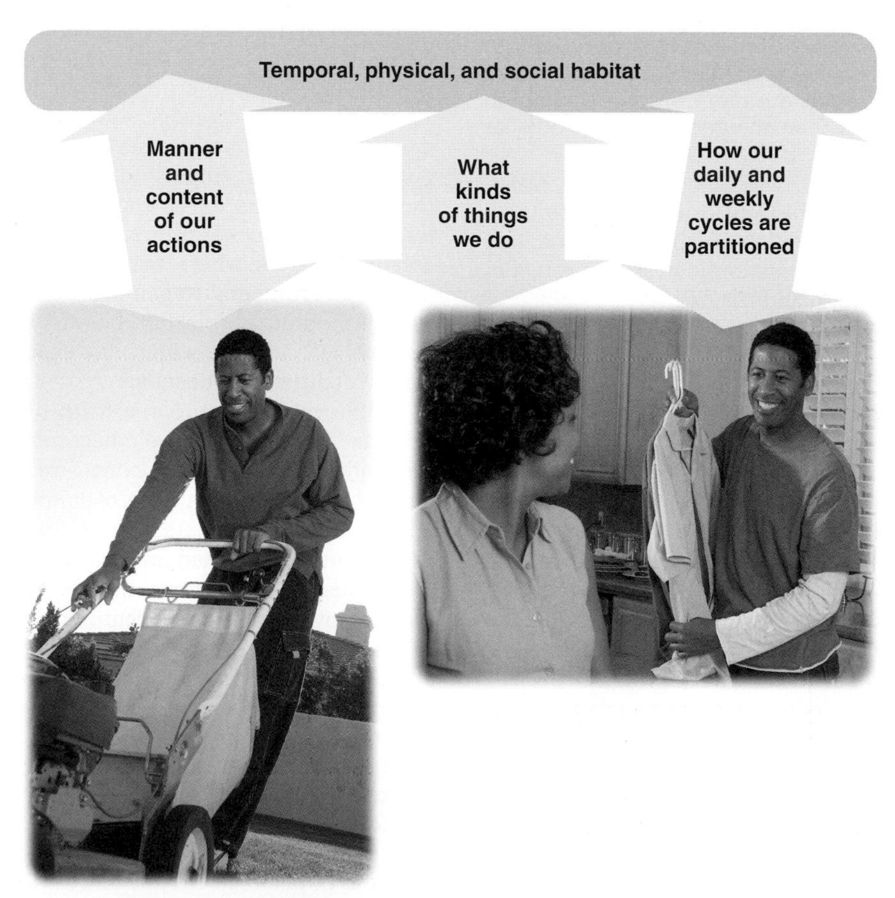

FIGURE 5-3 Influences of Roles on Occupation.

In other situations, persons must negotiate or define for themselves what actions make up the role.

Third, roles partition our daily and weekly cycles into times when we inhabit certain roles. The course of each day ordinarily involves a succession of roles and overlapping roles. Any parent who has attempted to talk on the phone with a coworker while holding a fussy baby and watching food on the stove will immediately appreciate how roles can overlap. Across our days, weeks, and lives, roles are social spaces that we enter, enact, and exit.

■ *Across our days, weeks, and lives, roles are social spaces that we enter, enact, and exit.* ■

SOCIALIZATION AND ROLE CHANGE

Beginning in childhood, we perceive others to fill positions that everyone takes for granted. The people who occupy such positions as mothers, teachers, and baby-sitters tend to behave in predictable ways. As time goes on, we discover that we too have been assigned roles. We learn that we are expected to act in certain ways because of the roles we occupy (Grossack & Gardner, 1970; Katz & Kahn, 1966; Turner, 1962).

The process of communicating role expectations is referred to as socialization (Brim & Wheeler, 1966). For example, as children develop, expectations of being a family member are communicated.

These expectations involve where and how to play, conformity to family routines, and the responsibilities for self-care and chores. These expectations for performance as a family member are generally more informal than the role expectations that come later in life. Thus, role socialization generally involves a developmental progression from informal to formal roles. This role progression parallels the child's growing ability to internalize role scripts and to use them as guides for action. Later in development, socialization may be much more formal, including education, practicing or apprenticing in the role, credentialing, and supervision. For many roles society goes to great lengths to socialize and regulate those who fill the role.

Persons being socialized into a new role typically negotiate their role in a give-and-take process (Heard, 1977; Schein, 1971). Each person fulfills a role uniquely but is also bound by how others are affected. An individual who enacts a role in ways that negatively affect others invites their invectives to conform to the role's expectations.

Socialization is an ongoing process because roles change throughout life. Society expects and structures role transitions at various life stages such as entering and exiting the student role, beginning work, and retiring. Persons also choose to enter and leave roles. Finally, role change is sometimes thrust on people by circumstances.

Role change is complex, involving alterations of one's identity, one's relationship to others, the tasks one is expected to perform, and how one's lifestyle is organized. An example of the complexity of role change is the experience of family members when aging parents require children to take care of them. This circumstance entails:

> A clear reversal of roles as the older generation loses power, and the authority to make the most personal kinds of decisions gravitates into the hands of their children . . . Roles need to be thoroughly redefined, often in the face of stiff resistance and understandable resentment. (Hage & Powers, 1992, p. 118)

Thus, while role change is part and parcel of human development, it is often the occasion for significant reorganization within individuals and their social systems.

IMPACT OF DISABILITY ON ROLES

Disabled persons may be barred from, have difficulty performing, or lack opportunities to learn or enter occupational roles. In addition, having a disability can assign one to unwanted, marginal roles. Consequently, living with a disability poses a number of challenges for occupying roles.

Role Performance Difficulties Associated with Disability

Disability often presents itself as a problem with role performance. For example, a common factor that leads persons with mental illness or substance abuse problems to enter mental health care is a failure in school or work roles (Black, 1976; Mechanic, 1980). Adolescents with mental illness have more problems in academic, leisure, and work roles than their peers (Barris, Dickie, & Baron, 1988; Barris et al., 1986; Holzman & Grinker, 1974; Offer, Ostrov, & Howard, 1981).

Problems with role behavior may occur when one has not internalized appropriate role scripts and, therefore, one does not meet the expectations of the social group. By virtue of having a disability, people may have fewer experiences in which to acquire role scripts (Smith, 1972; Versluys, 1983). For example, persons with cognitive impairments are often denied access to opportunities to learn adult roles (Guskin, 1963; Kielhofner, 1983; Wolfensberger, 1975). In such cases, limitations of capacity are magnified by the lack of learning experiences.

Limitations of physical capacity may disrupt or terminate role performance. In other cases, a person can retain a role only by making major modifications in how the role is enacted. For example, a person who acquires a disability may continue as a worker but needs to engage in a new type of work. In many instances, this can mean moving to a lesser-paying job.

A disability may create problems of role performance such as being unable to discharge the role in ways consistent with one's own or others' expectations for the role. For example, persons whose impairments are not visible to others may be viewed by friends, family, or coworkers as malingering (Schiffer, Rudick, & Herndon, 1983). In other cases the conflict may be between one's own view of the role and how one is able to perform. For example, one gentleman who has multiple sclerosis notes of his family roles: "I feel left out of discipline over the children because I am static in an armchair and cannot even phone the school. I had lost the ability to be a real father and husband" (Robinson, 1988, p. 60). Hull (1990) similarly describes how being blind has robbed him of the ability to supervise and to participate in play with his children, eroding and constricting what kind of father he can be. Such shifts in the identity and function of ongoing roles can be sources of conflict and self-devaluation.

Role strain may occur when a person cannot meet the multiple obligations or aspirations represented in several roles (Beutell & Greenhaus, 1983; Coser, 1974; Gerson, 1976; Gray, 1972). Impairments may require persons to exert more time and energy toward maintaining such major life roles as work or homemaking, requiring them to relinquish other roles (Hallet, Zasler, Maurer, & Cash, 1994). Overall, persons with disabilities tend to occupy fewer roles than their nondisabled counterparts (Dickerson & Oakely, 1995; Ebb, Coster, & Duncombe, 1989).

Social Barriers to Roles

Although impairments may contribute to difficulties in role performance, one of the most significant obstacles for persons with disabilities is social barriers (Hahn, 1985, 1988). For many people, the presence of a visible disability creates immediate difficulties of access to ordinary roles. Beginning in childhood, persons with disabilities may be discouraged or prevented from exploring, learning, and occupying roles. Such persons may be chronically frustrated as they are unable to attain a series of roles (Kielhofner, 1979, 1981). Social barriers to roles range from subtle attitudinal barriers that make social access difficult, to social policies whose consequence is to make roles inaccessible to persons with disabilities.

Sometimes barriers to roles are evident when people refuse to admit persons with disabilities into various social groups. One of the most dramatic examples is the area of work. Despite legislation in most industrialized countries that assures some equal access to the marketplace, persons with disabilities still have a harder time finding employment (Erikson, 1973; Trieschmann, 1989). In the United States less than one-third of severely disabled persons of working age work (Hale, Hayghe, & McNeil, 1998; Louis Harris and Associates, 1998; Trupin, Sebesta, Yelin, & LaPlante, 1997). Barriers to work include discrimination in the workplace and public policy that often penalizes persons financially or in terms of health benefits if they seek employment (Brandt & Pope, 1997; National Council on Disability, 1996).

What Are the Consequences of Role Loss and Rolelessness?

Research suggests that involvement in too few roles is even more likely to be detrimental to psychosocial well-being than having too many role demands (Marks, 1977; Seiber, 1974; Spreitzer, Snyder, & Larson, 1979). Without sufficient roles one lacks identity, purpose, and structure in everyday life. For example, unemployment has been linked to suicide, depression, stress-related physical health problems, child abuse, and increased substance abuse (Borrero, 1980; Briar, 1980).

A loss of identity and self-esteem may occur as persons take on roles they believe to be less important or as they lose roles (Thomas, 1966; Werner-Beland, 1980). For example, Krefting (1989) notes:

> Most head-injured people remember parts of their old selves and recognize that the old self is gone. But they have nothing upon which to build a new self-identity. This is largely a result of lack of opportunity to fill legitimate roles in society. If an individual's personhood is not acknowledged by others, it is difficult for him or her to develop a sense of self-identity. (p. 76)

This view is echoed throughout accounts that persons with disabilities have given of themselves. There is a substantial cost to personal identity when persons no longer are recognized as the fathers, mothers, spouses, students, workers, caretakers, or friends that they used to be.

■ ***There is a substantial cost to personal identity when persons no longer are recognized as the fathers, mothers, spouses, students, workers, caretakers, or friends that they used to be.*** ■

Sick and Disabled Roles

Disability may not only remove or bar people from occupational roles, but may also relegate them to sick and deviant roles (Bogdan & Taylor, 1989; Parsons, 1953; Werner-Beland, 1980). When a person is ill and incapacitated, normal role expectations are typically suspended and the person is relegated to the sick role and expected to do what is necessary to get well (McKeen, 1992; Parsons, 1953). The sick role and its expectations for passivity and compliance can be problematic for persons with a long-term illness or disability.

A case in point is Bill who was diagnosed with sarcoma that required him to leave his job as a mechanic in order to undergo a regimen of surgery and chemotherapy over 3 years. Bill became accustomed to the sick role, in which others made decisions about the care that dominated his life. His identity as a cancer patient overshadowed other aspects of his identity. His interactions with others and his daily routine centered on his patient role. At the end of 3 years, Bill was left with an able body but found it overwhelming to consider reentry into work and other adult roles.

The reactions of others can cast a person in a disabled role (Asch, 1998; Toombs, 1987; Werner-Beland, 1980). For example, others may unnecessarily lower their expectations, become overly protective or helpful, or consider the person to be disabled beyond his or her actual limitations. For example, Zola (1982) discusses how using a wheelchair transformed his social interactions:

> As soon as I sat in the wheelchair I was no longer seen as a person who could fend for himself. Although Metz has known me well for nine months, and had never before done anything physical for me without asking, now he took over without permission. Suddenly, in his eyes, I was no longer able to carry things, reach for objects, or even push myself around. Though I was perfectly capable of doing all these things, I was being wheeled around, and things were being brought to me—all without my asking. Most frightening was my own compliance, my alienation from myself and from the process. (p. 52)

As he suggests, the identity of being disabled can, of itself, trigger new expectations and behaviors. This dramatic transformation validated the sensibleness of Zola's earlier attempts to avoid being cast into the role of a disabled person:

> I had separated myself early from the physically handicapped by refusing to attend a special residential school. Later, I had simply never socialized with anyone who had a chronic disease or physical handicap. I too had been seeking to gain a different identity through my associations. (Zola, 1982, p. 75)

Distancing oneself from the disabled role is understandable in light of social reactions to disability. However, by doing so people with disabilities are less likely to develop a positive identity as a disabled person or to engage in social and political action that might ameliorate social prejudice toward disability (Gill, 1997).

Conclusion

This chapter explained how occupation is patterned by habituation. The habits and internalized roles that make up habituation plant people in the familiar territory of everyday life ready to interact with our physical, temporal, and social ecology. When habituation is challenged by impairments and/or environmental circumstances, people can lose a great deal of what has given life familiarity, consistency, and relative ease. One of the major tasks of living with disability is to reconstruct habits and roles.

CASE EXAMPLES TO TEST YOUR KNOWLEDGE

CASE #1: A Mother's Difficulty with Her Role

Maria is a 24-year-old mother who has been referred to occupational therapy for chronic fatigue syndrome and depression. She states: "I think this flu will go away in a few days this time. Could it? Sore throat, repetitive body aches penetrating every inch of my body, endless sleep . . . I sleep a lot with no proper refreshed feelings afterwards. My 3-year-old girl crawls up to my bed. I suddenly think of work to do. My boss's face dawns on me. I remember I have not cooked for her for days; the laundry must be piled up. I can't remember how long it has been since I have done it. Still, I don't like her to come to me. Gosh, I don't like it! What kind of mom am I?! I must like to spend time with her, to read story books, and to play Legos . . . She needs me . . . but my physical state simply cannot handle her energy. Her smiling face is now in front of my nose. I can see the image of my own face reflected in her eyes. I feel like I'm looking down a well. Small fingers drag my 10 ton-heavy, yet ironically, weary arm. Her dad came along and becomes my savior saying, "Shhh. Momma is tired." Disappointed, two big eyes finally faded away. I hear a door slam sound showering over my closed eyes. Tears drip onto the pillow. I feel like my life is a ball of tangled iron thread, which I can find no way to untangle."

CASE #2: A Young Adult with a Shopping Habit

"Through the bus window, pretty shops in the street come into my sight. I have a few minutes

to stop by those before I go to work. I step down from the bus. I shop around. It's already twelve o'clock. I have no appointment today . . ." Susie thinks to herself. Shame creeps into her thinking. She ignores that feeling. It's been 6 months since she last shopped like this. It seemed like naïve and even understandable behavior at first, after she lost her child. Susie is an outpatient bipolar disorder client who immigrated upon marriage. Recently, her close friends moved out to other states. Being an introvert, she doesn't have anyone to talk with. Even if there is someone, she doesn't want to talk, so as not to bother other people. Her husband is verbally abusive and doesn't pay her the proper attention she craves. Her clothes-purchasing addiction, fueled by denigrating comments about her body by her husband, is severely cutting into her time these days. Shopping is the only way to temporarily avoid her pain. She works at a school and used to be a very conscientious worker. She used to almost always finish things in advance. These days, she cannot make the deadlines and it pains her, eroding her self-esteem as a successful worker, yet she can't stop her urge to go to the shopping mall and take in the pleasant scent of beautiful outfits and to find something new, which might help her forget about her child and her marriage.

Both stories exemplify how one's habituation, composed of roles and habits in a close relationship with environment (physical and social), performance capacities, and volition (one's sense of capacities, self-efficacy, what one values, and her/his interest) are constantly shaped by, and evolve with, life events.

Question to Encourage Critical Thinking And Discussion: Can you identify each client's roles And habits? What should we know in order to identify if a client's habituation has been influenced by abrupt injury and/or chronic symptoms?

Discussion: Occupational therapists who worked with these two women identified their habituation dynamic as heading in a downward spiral, unaligned with and unassimilated with their valued roles in varying social and physical environments. A sudden event that triggers temporary illness—as indicated in Susie's story—versus a lifelong battle has distinctive features, yet the commonality between these cases is a disruption of the client's habituation, and the impact of the disruption on life of the client and the lives of the people around the client. In both cases, the therapist needed to sit with the client and validate her feelings, with great empathy skills. Once the clients were openly able to discuss their true feelings, the therapists worked with them to establish self-awareness of time use, habits of avoidance of their feelings, and self-defeating tendencies. Below is the dialogue between the therapist and the client with chronic fatigue syndrome:

Client: I wish . . . I don't know what's wrong with me. I mean I know life is unfair but I am struggling.

OT: [Sighing . . . looking into the client's eyes, striving to feel how she would feel now.]

Client: I feel like there is nothing I can do for my baby. I'm just so sick and these will get worse only.

OT: You feel you can't do anything.

Client: Yes. I'm a terrible mother.

OT: Has your child ever said or indicated that to you?

Client: No. She hasn't. She is too young to say anything. I just know I can do better, if I were not sick like this.

OT: That maybe true, but we do the best we can.

Client: [. . .]

OT: What does she like?

Client: My daughter? Oh, she loves flowers. Her favorite storybook is a flower book.

OT: Do you like flowers, too?

Client: Somewhat. Once, I wanted to learn about flower arrangements.

OT: You did?! Do you think you and your daughter can do a flower arrangement together?

Client: Maybe . . . but I don't know if I would be able to afford the time.

OT: How about doing a small project between us first. That'll be a fun experience for me, too. Would you help me to learn about it?

Receiving feedback from the therapist, the clients began to develop new insights, acknowledging their striving and efforts to do the best they could and not feeling ashamed by focusing on "what should have been done" and "what could have been done." Therapists advised the clients to identify interests that could be fulfilled within the limits of their performance capacity. For example, the therapist helped the client with chronic fatigue syndrome to negotiate with her three-year-old daughter to participate in physical activities with her dad and to play pretend with the client, which required minimal physical energy and was enjoyable for both. The client then negotiated with her husband to help minimize her house chores. With Susie, the therapist advised her to get involved with a local church group that could support her during the difficult time after the loss of her child. Volunteering with children and subsequently occupying her time instead of wandering the streets shopping was advised. Continuous empathy with encouragement gradually helped both women feel in control of their feelings. They found true enjoyment without shame or guilt, participating in occupations that supported their roles, and in turn, their habits marked an upward spiral of habituation.

Things to check on in order to understand the habituation of my client:

- If my client has established roles and routines, does that mean necessarily she/he has a strong habituation?
- When does habituation become problematic?
- How could I help my client want to change/maintain/alter her/his habits and roles?

Chapter 5 Review Questions

1. What are the two elements of habituation?
2. How do these two elements interact with the environment and shape an individual's occupational engagement pattern? Provide an example.
3. Give an example of the occupational behavior of a person with negative life patterns—someone with conflicting roles and habits. How could these patterns be reduced, if not eliminated?
4. Provide an example of the occupational behavior of a person with positive life patterns. How could these be reinforced?

HOMEWORK ASSIGNMENTS

Complete a self-analysis of your own habituation, as well as the habituation of someone close to you. For each analysis, respond to the following:

1. Describe three of your own and three of this person's primary roles.
2. Explain your and this person's roles and habits, particularly as they relate to his or her primary volition (personal causation, values, and interests), performance capacities, and environment.
3. Describe your and this person's habits. How are they aligned with roles? If they are not well-aligned, please explain. How can these habits be maintained, changed, substituted, and/or eliminated?
4. Characterize your and this person's life in terms of his or her pattern of occupation.

SELF-REFLECTION EXERCISE

Fill in the blanks with a list of your occupations.	What habitational concept can you find?
I spent most of my day: ____________________.	Habit
I consider myself to be ____________________.	Roles
For me, _______ is the most important role I have in my life.	Roles
I wish I could change my life so that ______________.	Habituation
Spending time ___________ makes me feel like I'm doing an ok job as a _________(role[s]).	Habituation

thePoint® For additional resources and exercises, visit http://thePoint.lww.com

Key Terms

Habits: Acquired tendencies to automatically respond and perform in certain, consistent ways in familiar environments or situations.

Habituation: An internalized readiness to exhibit consistent patterns of behavior guided by our habits and roles and fitted to the characteristics of routine temporal, physical, and social environments.

Internalized role: The incorporation of a socially and/or personally defined status and a related cluster of attitudes and actions.

REFERENCES

American Psychiatric Association. (2000). *Diagnostic and statistical manual of mental disorders* (4th ed., Text Revision). Washington, DC: Author.

Asch, A. (1998). Distracted by disability: The "difference" of disability in the medical setting. *Cambridge Quarterly of Healthcare Ethics, 7,* 77–87.

Barris, R., Dickie, V., & Baron, K. (1988). A comparison of psychiatric patients and normal subjects based on the model of human occupation. *Occupational Therapy Journal of Research, 8,* 3–37.

Barris, R., Kielhofner, G., Burch, R. M., Gelinas, I., Klement, M., & Schultz, B. (1986). Occupational function and dysfunction in three groups of adolescents. *Occupational Therapy Journal of Research, 6,* 301–317.

Berger, P. L., & Luckman, T. (1966). *The social construction of reality.* New York, NY: Doubleday/Anchor.

Beutell, N. J., & Greenhaus, J. H. (1983). Integration of home and nonhome roles: Women's conflict and coping behavior. *Journal of Applied Psychology, 68,* 43–48.

Black, M. (1976). The occupational career. *American Journal of Occupational Therapy, 30,* 225–228.

Bogdan, R., & Taylor, S. J. (1989). The social construction of humanness: Relationships with severely disabled people. *Social Problems, 36,* 135–148.

Borell, L., Gustausson, A., Sandman, P., & Kielhofner, G. (1994). Occupational programming in a day hospital for patients with dementia. *Occupational Therapy Journal of Research, 14,* 219–238.

Borrero, I. M. (1980). Psychological and emotional impact of unemployment. *Journal of Sociology and Social Welfare, 7,* 916–934.

Bourdieu, P. (1977). *Outline of a theory of practice* (R. Nice, Trans.). London, United Kingdom: Cambridge University Press.

Brandt, E. N., & Pope, A. M. (Eds.). (1997). *Enabling America: Assessing the role of rehabilitation science and engineering.* Washington, DC: National Academy Press.

Briar, K. H. (1980). Helping the unemployed client. *Journal of Sociology and Social Welfare, 7,* 895–906.

Brim, O. J., & Wheeler, S. (1966). *Socialization after childhood: Two essays.* New York, NY: John Wiley & Sons.

Camic, C. (1986). The matter of habit. *American Journal of Sociology, 91,* 1039–1087.

Cardwell, J. D. (1971). *Social psychology: A symbolic interaction perspective.* Philadelphia, PA: F. A. Davis.

Chapin, F. S. (1968). Activity systems and urban structure: A working schema. *Journal of the American Institute of Planners, 34,* 11–18.

Clarke, A. (1997). *Being there: Putting brain, body and world together again.* Cambridge, MA: MIT Press.

Coser, L. (1974). *Greedy institutions.* New York, NY: Free Press.

DeLoach, C. P., & Greer, B. G. (1981). *Adjustment to severe physical disability: A metamorphosis.* New York, NY: McGraw-Hill.

Dewey, J. (1922). *Human nature and conduct.* New York, NY: Henry Holt & Company.

Dickerson, A. E., & Oakely, F. (1995). Comparing the roles of community-living persons and patient populations. *American Journal of Occupational Therapy, 49,* 221–228.

Ebb, E. W., Coster, W., & Duncombe, L. (1989). Comparison of normal and psychosocially dysfunctional male adolescents. *Occupational Therapy in Mental Health, 9,* 53–74.

Erikson, K. T. (1973). Notes on the sociology of deviance. In H. S. Becker (Ed.), *The other side: Perspectives on deviance.* New York, NY: Free Press.

Fein, M. L. (1990). *Role change: A resocialization perspective.* New York, NY: Praeger.

Gerson, E. M. (1976). On "quality of life." *American Sociological Review, 41,* 793–806.

Gill, C. J. (1997). Four types of integration in disability identity development. *Journal of Vocational Rehabilitation, 9,* 39–46.

Gray, M. (1972). Effects of hospitalization on work-play behavior. *American Journal of Occupational Therapy, 26,* 180–185.

Grossack, M., & Gardner, H. (1970). *Man and men: Social psychology as social science.* Scranton, PA: International Textbook.

Guskin, S. L. (1963). Social psychologies of mental deficiency. In N. R. Ellis (Ed.), *Handbook of mental deficiency.* New York, NY: McGraw-Hill.

Hage, G., & Powers, C. H. (1992). *Post-Industrial lives: Roles & relationships in the 21st Century.* Newbury Park, NJ: SAGE.

Hahn, H. (1985). Disability policy and the problem of discrimination. *American Behavioral Scientist, 28,* 293–318.

Hahn, H. (1988). Toward a politics of disability: Definitions, disciplines and policies. *Social Science Journal, 22,* 87–105.

Hale, T. W., Hayghe, H. W., & McNeil, J. M. (1998). Persons with disabilities: Labor market activities, 1994. *Monthly Labor Review, 121*(9), 3–12.

Hall, J. M., Stevens, P. E., & Meleis, A. I. (1992). Developing the construct of role integration: A narrative analysis of women clerical workers' daily lives. *Research in Nursing & Health, 15,* 447–457.

Hallet, J., Zasler, N., Maurer, P., & Cash, S. (1994). Role change after traumatic brain injury in adults. *American Journal of Occupational Therapy, 48,* 241–246.

Heard, C. (1977). Occupational role acquisition: A perspective on the chronically disabled. *American Journal of Occupational Therapy, 41,* 243–247.

Holzman, P., & Grinker, R. (1974). Schizophrenia in adolescence. *Journal of Youth and Adolescence, 3,* 267–279.

Hull, J. M. (1990). *Touching the rock: An experience of blindness.* New York, NY: Vintage Books.

James, W. (1950). *The principles of psychology.* New York, NY: Dover.

Jonsson, H., Josephsson, S., & Kielhofner, G. (2001). Narratives and experience in an occupational transition: A longitudinal study of the retirement process. *American Journal of Occupational Therapy, 55,* 424–432.

Katz, D., & Kahn, R. L. (1966). *The social psychology of organizations.* New York, NY: John Wiley & Sons.

Kielhofner, G. (1979). The temporal dimension in the lives of retarded adults. *American Journal of Occupational Therapy, 33,* 161–168.

Kielhofner, G. (1981). An ethnographic study of deinstitutionalized adults: Their community settings and daily life experiences. *Occupational Therapy Journal of Research, 1,* 125–141.

Kielhofner, G. (1983). "Teaching" retarded adults: Paradoxical effects of a pedagogical enterprise. *Urban Life, 12,* 307–326.

Kielhofner, G., Barris, R., & Watts, J. (1982). Habits and habit dysfunction: A clinical perspective for psychosocial occupational therapy. *Occupational Therapy Mental Health, 2,* 1–22.

Koestler, A. (1969). Beyond atomism and holism: The concept of the holon. In A. Koestler & J. R. Smythies (Eds.), *Beyond reductionism.* Boston, MA: Beacon Press.

Krefting, L. (1989). Reintegration into the community after head injury: The results of an ethnographic study. *Occupational Therapy Journal of Research, 9*, 67–83.
Louis Harris and Associates. (1998). *Highlights of the N.O.D/Harris 1998 Survey of Americans with Disabilities*. Washington, DC: National Organization on Disability.
Mancuso, J. C., & Sarbin, T. R. (1983). The self-narrative in the enactment of roles. In T. R. Sarbin & K. E. Scheibe (Eds.), *Studies in social identity*. New York, NY: Praeger.
Marks, S. R. (1977). Multiple roles and role strain: Some notes on human energy, time, and commitment. *American Sociological Review, 42*, 921–936.
Mechanic, D. (1980). *Mental health and social policy* (2nd ed.). Englewood Cliffs, NJ: Prentice-Hall.
Melges, F. T. (1982). *Time and inner future: A temporal approach to psychiatric disorders*. New York, NY: John Wiley & Sons.
Merleau-Ponty, M. (1962). *Phenomenology of perception* (C. Smith, Trans., Original work published 1945). London, United Kingdom: Routledge & Kegan Paul.
McKeen, D. G. (1992, July/August). Such a good little patient. *The Disability Rag & Resource*, p. 43.
Miller, D. R. (1983). Self, symptom and social control. In T. R. Sarbin & K. E. Scheibe (Eds.), *Studies in social identity*. New York, NY: Praeger.
Murphy, R. F. (1987). *The body silent*. New York, NY: WW Norton.
National Council on Disability. (1996). *Achieving independence: The challenge for the 21st century*. Washington, DC: Author.
Offer, D., Ostrov, E., & Howard, K. (1981). *The adolescent: A psychological self-report*. New York, NY: Basic Books.
Paap, W. R. (1972). The social reconstruction of reality: The rehabilitation of paraplegics and quadriplegics. *Dissertation Abstracts International, 33*, 45-A. (University Microfilms No. 72-19, 234)
Parsons, T. (1953). Illness and the role of the physician: A sociological perspective. In C. Kluckhohn, H. Murray, & O. Schneider (Eds.), *Personality in nature, society, and culture* (2nd ed.). New York, NY: Alfred A. Knopf.
Pinder, R. (1988). Striking balances: Living with Parkinson's disease. In R. Anderson & M. Bury (Eds.), *Living with chronic illness: The experience of patients and their families*. London, United Kingdom: Unwin Hyman.
Robinson, I. (1988). Reconstructing lives: Negotiating the meaning of multiple sclerosis. In R. Anderson & M. Bury (Eds.), *Living with chronic illness: The experience of patients and their families*. London, United Kingdom: Unwin Hyman.
Rosow, I. (1976). Status and role change through the life span. In R. H. Binstock & E. Shanas (Eds.), *Handbook of Aging and the Social Sciences*. New York, NY: Van Nostrand Reinhold.
Rowles, G. D. (1991). Beyond performance: Being in place as a component of occupational therapy. *American Journal of Occupational Therapy, 45*, 265–272.
Ruddock, R. (1976). *Roles and relationships*. London, United Kingdom: Routledge & Kegan Paul.
Sarbin, T. R., & Scheibe, K. E. (1983). A model of social identity. In T. R. Sarbin & K. E. Scheibe (Eds.), *Studies in social identity*. New York, NY: Praeger.
Schein, E. H. (1971). The individual, the organization, and the career: A conceptual scheme. *Journal of Applied Behavioral Science, 7*, 401–426.
Schiffer, R. B., Rudick, R. A., & Herndon, R. M. (1983). Psychologic aspects of multiple sclerosis. *New York State Journal of Medicine, 3*, 312–316.
Schumacher, K. L. (1995). Family caregiver role acquisition: Role-making through situated interaction. *Scholarly Inquiry for Nursing Practice: An International Journal, 9*, 211–226.
Seamon, D. (1980). Body-subject, time-space routines, and place-ballets. In A. Buttimer & D. Seamon (Eds.), *The human experience of space and place*. London, United Kingdom: Croom Helm.
Seiber, S. D. (1974). Toward a theory of role accumulation. *American Sociological Review, 39*, 567–578.
Shillam, L. L., Beeman, C., & Loshin, P. (1983). Effect of occupational therapy intervention on bathing independence of disabled persons. *American Journal of Occupational Therapy, 37*, 744–748.
Smith, C. A. (1972). Body image changes after myocardial infarction. *The Nursing Clinics of North America, 7*, 663–668.
Spreitzer, E., Snyder, E. E., & Larson, D. L. (1979). Multiple roles and psychological well-being. *Social Focus, 12*, 141–148.
Thomas, E. J. (1966). Problems of disability from the perspective of role theory. *Journal of Health and Human Behavior, 7*, 2–14.
Toombs, S. K. (1987). The meaning of illness: A phenomenologi cal approach to the patient-physician relationship. *Journal of Medicine & Philosophy, 12*(3), 219–240.
Trieschmann, R. B. (1989). Psychosocial adjustment to spinal cord injury. In B. W. Heller, L. M. Flohr, & L. S. Zegans (Eds.), *Psychosocial interventions with physically disabled persons*. New Brunswick, NJ: Rutgers University Press.
Trupin, L. D., Sebesta, S., Yelin, E., & LaPlante, M. P. (1997). Trends in labor force participation among persons with disabilities, 1993-94. *Disability Statistics Report, 10*, 1–39.
Turner, R. (1962). Role-taking, process versus conformity. In M. Rose (Ed.), *Human behavior and social processes*. Boston, MA: Houghton Mifflin.
Versluys, H. P. (1983). Psychosocial adjustment to physical disability. In C. A. Trombly (Ed.), *Occupational therapy for physical dysfunction* (2nd ed.). Baltimore, MD: Lippincott Williams & Wilkins.
Werner-Beland, J. A. (Ed.). (1980). *Grief responses to long-term illness and disability*. Reston, VA: Reston Publishing.
Williams, R. S. (1984). Ability, disability and rehabilitation: A phenomenological description. *Journal of Medicine and Philosophy, 9*, 93–112.
Wolfensberger, W. (1975). *The origin and nature of our institutional models*. Syracuse, NY: Human Policy Press.
Young, M. (1988). *The metronomic society: Natural rhythms and human timetables*. Cambridge, MA: Harvard University Press.
Zola, I. K. (1982). *Missing pieces: A chronicle of living with a disability*. Philadelphia, PA: Temple University Press.

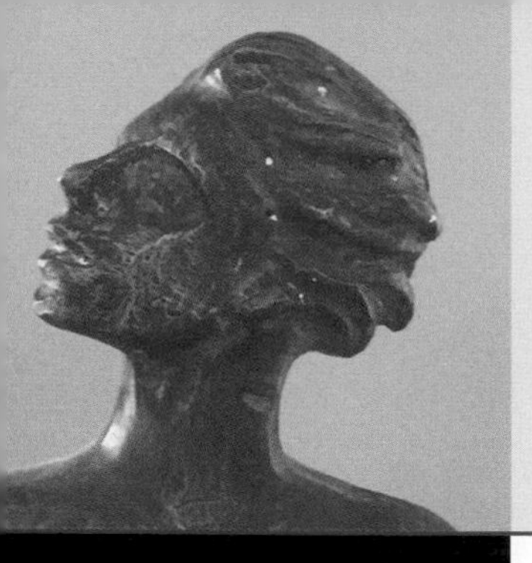

Performance Capacity and the Lived Body

Kerstin Tham, Anette Erikson, Mandana Fallaphour, Renée R. Taylor, and Gary Kielhofner (posthumous)

CHAPTER 6

EXPECTED LEARNING OUTCOMES

Upon completion of this chapter, readers will be able to:

1. Differentiate between the objective and subjective aspects of performance capacity.
2. Understand and define the lived body.
3. Provide examples of mind–body dualism in the model of human occupation (MOHO).
4. Describe the embodied mind and explain how knowing is situated within the body.
5. Explain why subjective experience is important to performance, particularly as it is applied to disabled persons.

MOHO Problem-Solver Case

Until intensive chemotherapy, a bilateral mastectomy, and radiation for stage-three breast cancer left her with severe fatigue and chemotherapy-associated peripheral neuropathy, Linda had worked as a United Parcel Service delivery driver. In the evenings and on weekends, Linda was an intensely competitive bowler and enjoyed spending time with her grandchildren. She was a member of a local women's bowling league and had been looking forward to another undefeated season. As an outpatient, Linda participated actively in all aspects of rehabilitation. The rehabilitation consisted of postsurgical upper extremity range-of-motion exercises prescribed by an occupational therapist, and of walking and cycling prescribed by a physical therapist, to rebuild her balance and endurance.

After the prescribed period of rehabilitation, results from multiple range-of-motion, motor, balance, and endurance assessments conducted by her therapists indicated that she had regained her range of motion and was exercising to the greatest degree that her fatigue and pain levels would allow. Discontinuation of outpatient therapy was recommended, and Linda was encouraged to perform the daily exercises at home. When she asked about bowling, her treatment team gave a noncommittal response, maintaining that she could "try it when she was ready" but that it would probably be difficult and painful to hold and throw the ball because of the lingering postsurgical pain, muscle atrophy, and neuropathy she was experiencing. Having learned that her rehabilitation had reached a point of diminishing returns, Linda feared that she would not improve, and expressed a feeling that she would never be able to bowl again. As a result, she developed a reactive major depressive episode.

Uncomfortable terminating therapy with Linda and knowing she was in a depressive state, the occupational therapist decided to refer her to a colleague specializing in the psychosocial aspects of cancer rehabilitation. Relying upon MOHO as his conceptual foundation for practice, the new occupational therapist, Nick, began by interviewing Linda and asking her a series of questions about the occupations in her daily life before the cancer. He specifically asked about activities that gave her the greatest sense of joy and competence. In addition to activities associated with her former job role, the topic of bowling came up as the top leisure priority. Nick then asked Linda what she thought about the news and recommendations from the treatment team, and she confessed that they were probably right about her not being able to carry and throw the ball without experiencing severe pain.

She then added, "But they never gave me a chance to say that I wanted to try it now, anyway, or at least work toward doing it again one day." She added that she has been simulating throwing a bowling ball throughout her rehabilitation, and that she feels her strength and range are improving. She articulated: "When I grab an inflatable ball and try swinging my arm, I feel excruciation and ecstasy at the same time. My arm becomes bionic and free. Like a warrior, I accept the pain as part of my mission, and my arm takes me past the pain and to a place of strength. Planning to bowl again and pretending I was bowling is what has kept me going all of these months."

At that point, Nick posed the question whether she wanted to first try a videogame-based bowling simulation or whether she wanted to begin by working at it in an actual bowling alley. Linda responded with the latter choice, stating that she knew that she would not be able to get her arm back or up, and that she knew that even the lightest ball was going to be too heavy and very painful, but that she wanted to do it anyway. She said, "I want to at least smell the familiar smells, see the familiar sites, and get the ball to roll halfway down the gutter. . . I want to buy a wig, I want my friends to see that I am back, and I want to feel like a person again." Together Nick and Linda began the painful process of conditioning her arms to be able to lift them over her head enough to put on a wig. They then planned a party at the bowling alley that would reunite her with the friends in her league. Lastly, they began a second process of throwing balls down the gutter at the local bowling alley when no one was around. Linda's depression had improved significantly as she continued to work toward her goal.

In summary, asking about Linda's lived experience of simulated bowling during her period of rehabilitation, rather than focusing on her actual ability and assessment findings, turned out to be the key to getting her slowly back into the actual sport of bowling, subsequently freeing her from her depression.

Performance Capacity

The multitude of things people do requires them to sense and interpret the world, move their bodies in space, manipulate objects, plan actions, and communicate and interact with others. Even the most ordinary occupation reflects the complex and exquisite organization of the human capacity to perform. As noted in Chapter 2, **performance capacity** is the ability to do things provided by the status of underlying objective physical and mental components and corresponding subjective experience (Fig. 6-1). This definition highlights that capacity involves both objective and subjective aspects.

Objective Components of Performance Capacity

Performance depends on musculoskeletal, neurological, cardiopulmonary, and other body systems. The capacity to perform also depends on cognitive abilities such as memory. When people do things, they exercise these capacities.

Other conceptual practice models in occupational therapy provide detailed explanations of specific performance capacities. These models address such phenomena as the biomechanics of movement, motor control processes, organization of sensory information, and perceptual and cognitive processes (Fisher, Murray, & Bundy, 1991; Katz, 2005; Trombly, 1995). Collectively, these models address performance capacity by objective study of physical (e.g., muscle, bone, nerve, brain) and psychological (e.g., memory, perception, cognition) phenomena. These models explain performance as a function of the status of objective performance capacities. Objective description invokes a language that names, classifies, and measures systems that appraise capacity by systematically observing performance. For example, we can speak about joint range of motion measured in degrees of movement or cognition measured by test scores.

This objective approach is typically coupled with an effort to explain problems of function in terms of disturbances to underlying structures and functions. For instance, limitations of movement might be attributed to loss of muscle strength and damage to joints. Similarly, limitations in problem-solving might be attributed to disturbances of attention following brain damage. Such depictions of impairments are important and helpful because the objective understanding of their nature can provide useful cues to how they might be remediated or their negative consequences minimized.

Subjective Approach to Performance Capacity

Objectively describable abilities and limitations of ability are also experienced by those who have them.

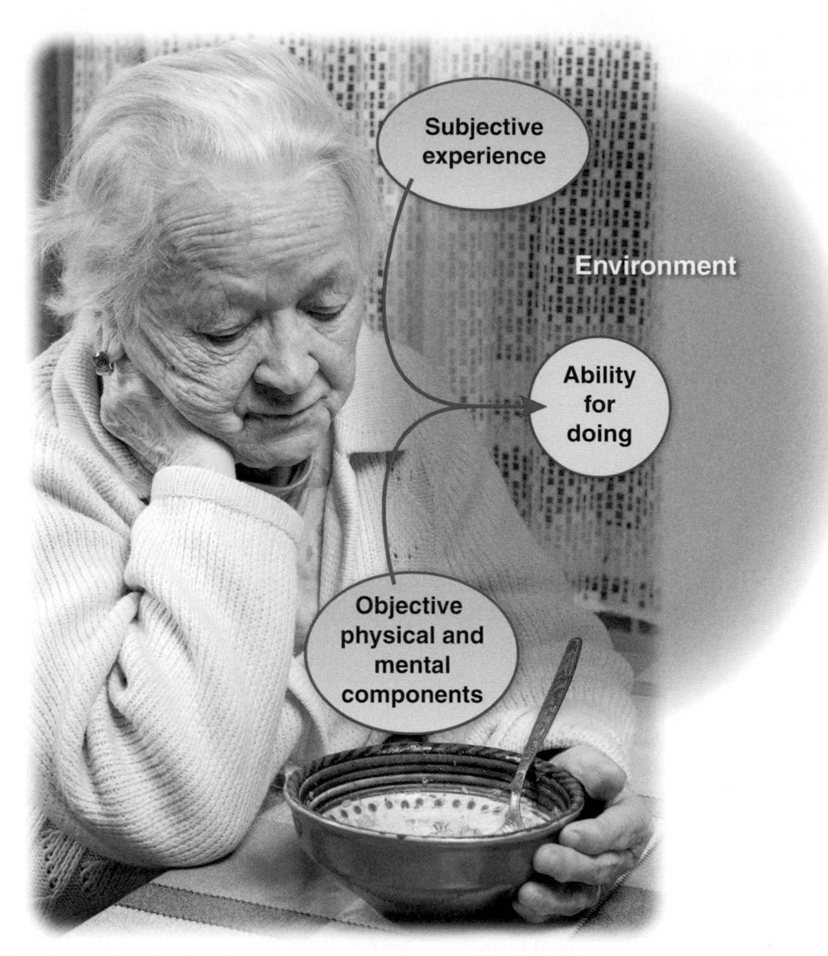

FIGURE 6-1 Objective and Subjective Components of Performance Capacity.

However, the objective approach generally views these experiences as only consequences of the real problem that must be appraised from an outsider's detached viewpoint. Even when therapists using this approach ask people about their subjective experience, they do so with an eye toward building an objective picture of performance capacity.

Nonetheless, subjective experience also shapes how people perform (Kielhofner, 1995). Paying careful attention to subjective experience in its own right can reveal a great deal about performance capacity and limitations of performance. It can also reveal important information about how to undertake therapy.

Focusing on the subjective aspect of performance capacity is complementary to the traditional objective approach. As shown in Figure 6-2, the objective approach provides a view of performance capacity from the outside, whereas the additional approach offered in this chapter provides a view of performance capacity from the inside. Both the observer's objective perspective and the performer's subjective experience have something to tell us about performance capacity. Neither perspective fully accounts for the other. Both the objective and the subjective are bound together in any instance of performance, and both contribute to the performance. For example, in moving one arm to reach out for something, there is the question of both how it feels to perform the movement and how the arm actually moves in space. Both tell something about what is involved in reaching. The objective approach provides a picture of how muscle contractions generate forces across joints producing degrees of extension and rotation that carry the arm through the trajectory of movement for reaching. The subjective experience will tell another story. This chapter is mainly about the nature of that story.

The Lived Body

The concept of the lived body ultimately emanates from the work of the philosopher Merleau-Ponty (1945/1962), based in phenomenology and the concept of life-world (Husserl, 1970). Merleau-Ponty further

Objective perspective:
View from the outside
Subjective perspective:
View from the inside
Performance

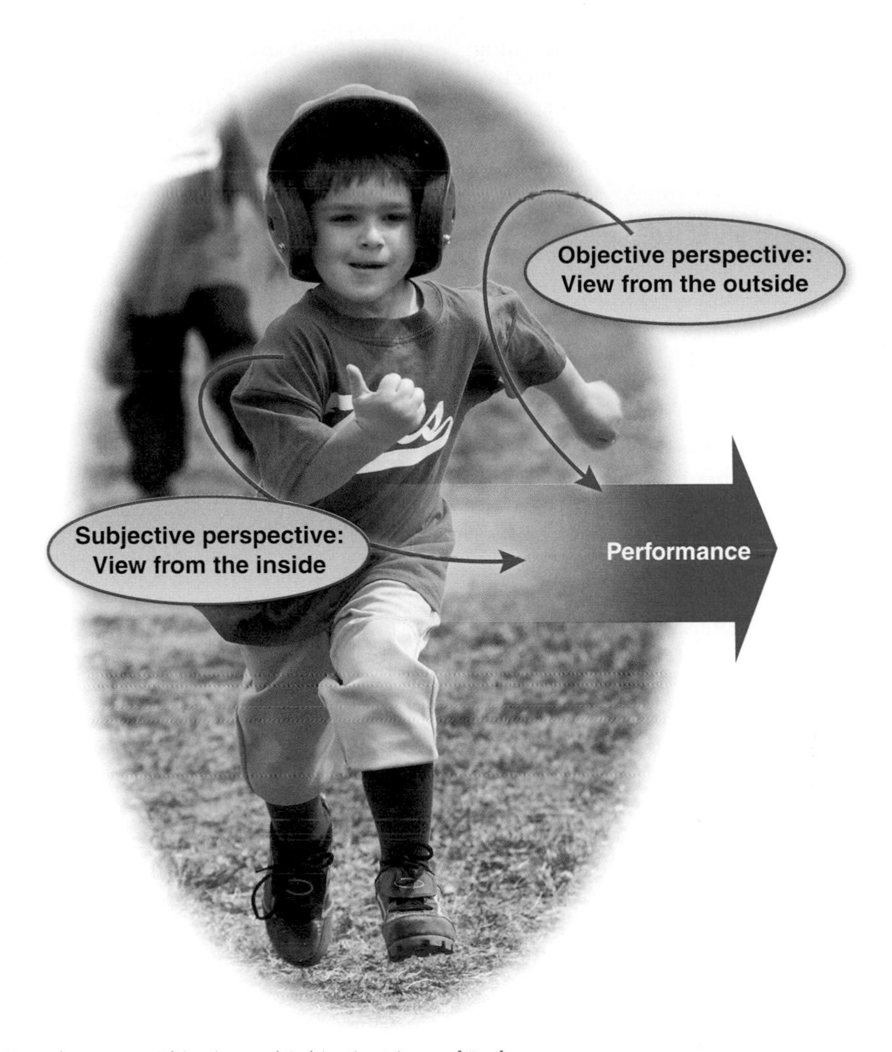

FIGURE 6-2 Complementary Objective and Subjective Views of Performance.

developed a view of human performance that paid careful attention to the nature of experience. He used experience as a central concept in explaining how performance was possible. Unlike the objective approach that describes performance from a detached, objective perspective, he emphasized a phenomenological approach that considered subjective experience as fundamental to understanding human perception, cognition, and action.

Using this phenomenological approach, Leder (1990, p. 1) employed the term "lived body" to emphasize how we experience, that is, live through our bodies. He describes the lived body as follows:

> Human experience is incarnated. I receive the surrounding world through my eyes, my ears, my hands . . . My legs carry me toward a desired goal seen across the distance. My hands reach out to take up tools . . . My actions are motivated by emotions, needs, desires, that well up from a corporeal self. Relations with others are based upon our mutuality of gaze and touch, our speech, our resonances of feeling and perspective. (p. 1)

Following Leder's (1990) utilization, we employ the concept of the **lived body** to refer to the experience of being and knowing the world through a particular body. The concept of the lived body applies both to human embodiment in general and to unique specific forms of embodiment associated with disability.

The lived body concept underscores two fundamental ideas. First, mind and body are seen not as separate phenomena, but as part of a single, unitary entity—namely, the lived body. Second, subjective experience of performance is not simply an artifact of performing. Rather, it is fundamental to how we perform. That is, in doing things and learning how to do things, we call on not only the objective components that make up performance capacity, but also the experience of exercising our capacities. The following sections discuss these two aspects of the lived body.

MIND–BODY UNITY

The tendency to view body and mind as separate entities has been a dominant force in Western science and culture. It began with the philosopher Descartes, who observed that the body is an object like other objects in the physical world and, therefore, subject to the same causal laws (Leder, 1984). According to his classic and influential argument, the workings of the human body should be understood through the same objective methods with which other objects in the physical world can be investigated and understood. The other side of Descartes' philosophical argument was that the mind was immaterial and thus operated according to different, abstract principles. Hence, Cartesian dualism proclaimed that the body and mind represented completely separate realms and that understanding them required radically different approaches.

To cease regarding the body and mind as two separate entities and, instead, see them as dual aspects of a single entity is not easy. Dualism is deeply ingrained in our way of thinking. Nonetheless, we can begin to understand mind–body unity by paying attention to both how the body is experienced and how the mind is embodied.

Bodily Experience

We can experience our own bodies as objects in the way Descartes identified. For example, we can look at our hands just as we gaze at other things in the world. In such looking, our experience is directed to our hands (Leder, 1990). However, this is neither the only nor the dominant way in which we experience our hands. Rather, we routinely experience from our hands to that which is outside ourselves.

When we reach into a purse for coins, grasp a door handle, pull on our socks, pat our dog, wave to our friends, or caress our loved ones, we are attending and acting to the world and from our hands. In those instances, our hands are subjects not objects. Our hands are, in these instances, our point of view for reaching, grasping, pulling, patting, waving, and caressing.

Thus, the fundamental difference between experiencing our bodies as objects and as subject goes as follows: When I experience some part of my body as an object in the world, I am attending to that body part and am distinguishing between my body and myself. When I am attending to the world from my body, there is no distinction between self and body. As Sartre (1970) noted, one does not just have one's body, one is one's body.

Leder (1990) describes this phenomenon in the following way. He notes that when we are doing things, our bodies disappear to us. Our experience is directed to that part of the world with which we are interacting, and our bodies recede, vanishing from our awareness. Moreover, our bodies are that from which our attention and action are focused on what is outside us. Thus, in the course of our daily occupational lives, our bodies are invisible viewpoints from which we experience and act upon the world. We experience our bodies "as an attitude directed towards a certain existing or possible task" (Merleau-Ponty, 1945/1962, p. 100).

Because of this experience, it can seem that the body is not really a part of conscious experience. For example, when we are reading a book we experience it as a mental activity, unaware that we are holding it with our hands, and seeing it with our eyes. It is the body that is doing the reading.

In everyday life, the body is the taken-for-granted place from which we exist and from which we attend to and act on the world. We may become aware of our bodies as objects when we perceive fatigue or pain and, therefore, attend to the tired or aching limb. For the most part, however, doing things requires that we attend from our bodies to what we are doing.

Because our bodies are in use much of the time, our experience of our bodies is grounded in doing things. Consequently, we each experience our body as the self that is always taking in the world around us and doing things in that world. Moreover, we experience our body not as "a collection of adjacent organs, but as a synergic system, all the functions of which are exercised and linked together in the general action of being in the world . . ." (Merleau-Ponty, 1945/1962, p. 234). For example, when we are walking outside and viewing the scenery, we have no separate awareness of the movements of legs and arms in walking or the orientation of our head and eyes in attending to the things around us. When we raise our hands above our eyes to shade the sun, it is simply part of looking, not a separate act by a separate part of the body. We experience all the parts of the body as a unified whole engaged in the action of walking and looking. Moreover, most of our experience of our bodies is the awareness we have of doing things as a body. We can imagine a walk outside, but it is only a facsimile (and a poor one at that) of feeling the sun on our brow and the ground at our feet, of apprehending the world in the midst of moving around within it. We are most aware when we are bodies in the midst of action.

When we consider the body in this way, we cannot readily separate it from what we call mind. Further, we can see that awareness is not something belonging to a separate mind and imposed on the body. Rather, the body is an intimate part of how we are aware.

Embodied Mind

Whatever else we might attribute to mind, it consists of knowing about things and knowing how to do things. Descartes posited knowledge as what distinguished the mind from the body. However, knowing is seated in the body. Importantly, we do not mean simply that knowledge is stored or processed biochemically in the brain. Rather, we mean that the whole of the body is the way we apprehend and thus know about how to do things. The body is the existential medium of knowing.

Knowing Things

What we know about the world around us begins with our bodies looking at, touching, and probing the world (Merleau-Ponty, 1945/1962). Abstract properties we attribute to various objects in the world echo how our bodies experience those objects. For example:

> How do I know that the ball is spherical, solid, and leathery? My moving, throwing and pressing hands reveal these properties . . . [that] do not exist solely in the ball and not at all in my hands. It is only when my hands touch the ball that these properties are revealed to me. (Engelbrecht, 1968, p. 12)

Sartre (1970, p. 231) elaborates this notion in the following example of how bodily action gives us an experience of the world:

> We never have any sensation of our effort . . . We perceive the resistance of things. What I perceive when I want to lift this glass to my mouth is not my effort but the heaviness of the glass.

When we do things, we generate bodily experiences of the world that we come to interpret as properties of that world. Nevertheless, the world we know is always on the other end of something we are doing with our bodies. Perception is not simply the registration and evaluation of sense data, but rather an active taking hold of the world. When we perceive objects and their characteristics, the foundation of our knowing them always has to do with how our bodies encounter and engage them. Once again, we are speaking here not of the objective ways sensory data are taken in by sensory organs and networked through the central nervous system. Instead, we are referring to the body as a way of generating experience in response to its own questions that are posed as forms of acting toward and in the world. What the mind asks of the world and the answers that make up the mind's accumulated knowledge are asked, in large measure, through bodily action.

Even abstract knowledge grows out of bodily experiences. For example, only by using our bodies to do things—touching, grasping, lifting, shoving, observing, and listening to the world—do we have access to experiences that give meaning to concepts of distance, direction, temporality, clarity, resistance, resilience, and obscurity (Leder, 1990; Merleau-Ponty, 1945/1962; Sudnow, 1979). Thought itself builds on what our bodies do and experience. As Sudnow (1979) argues:

> When I sit before the piano keyboard, I am directly aligned to its center . . . I sit down and there I am, as exactly middled as before the dinner plate, the steering wheel, the bathroom faucets—before whatever action moves out from the center. Dividing in half all the body's ways, is part of the calculus, topography, trigonometry, and algebra that my body does . . . Mathematics is perhaps the purest form of human thought, not because its pictures struggle toward a perfect concept of nature, but because its pictures have their origin in the ways of the body . . . (p. 79)

The structure and content of mental operations are always based on the body's way of comprehending the world. As Leder (1990, p. 7) notes, abstract cognition "may sublimate but never fully escapes its inherence in a perceiving, active body."

Knowing How to Do Things

When typing or playing the piano, one's fingers instinctively know where to go for the right letter or note (Sudnow, 1979). For example, the most efficient strategy for locating the computer key "H" on a computer keyboard is to begin to type a word beginning with that letter. Without consciously thinking about its location, the right index finger will begin to move to the right center of the keyboard where "H" is located. What is also notable in this and other instances of bodily knowing is that the body instinctively knows which part of itself should perform any action.

Our bodies readily perform all manner of things that we cannot readily describe how to do. Imagine doing any ordinary action such as a dance step, a swim stroke, whistling a tune, or tying a shoe. Describing the action only gives us a vague trace of what it is. We must typically watch our bodies do things to notice exactly what we are doing. Compare thinking about how to tie a shoe with actually tying the shoe, and one can readily see how much the knowing is in the body.

SUBJECTIVE EXPERIENCE AND PERFORMANCE

As noted previously, every action we perform is objectively describable. It can be divided into so much flexion, extension, or rotation at joints. It can be described in terms of the trajectory, speed, and the efficiency with which movement is accomplished.

Such bodily action is known differently from within. When we reach for a cup of coffee, open a door, walk to the bus, or operate a car, we do not objectively know or do the movements involved. Instead, we are inside the movements and experience them from that vantage point. Consequently, when we use our bodies to do things, we aim for the subjective experience of doing them. Indeed, we cannot fully attend to the objective features of our performance without disrupting it in some way. For example, if we concentrate too much on how to move our hands in tying our shoes, we will interrupt our performance.

When learning to do something, we may at first aim for the objective movements. For example, when learning to hold silverware or chopsticks, we first attend to how they are placed in the hand and how the fingers should be positioned. But learning to do something means that we must grasp the experience—to learn how it feels. Most of us will also recall that when learning to ride a bicycle, roller skate, ski, or any other skilled form of doing, we began with a sense of what was objectively involved and ended up learning what the right movement felt like. Once we have grasped the feeling of how it is to do something, repeating the performance is altogether different. After that feeling is achieved, we no longer pay attention to the objective aspects of doing the action. Rather, we focus on the experience and use it as our guide to performing. As Sudnow (1978) describes it:

> . . . when one first gets the knack of a complex skill . . . the hang of it has been glimpsed . . . the experience is tasted. All prior ways of being seem thoroughly lacking, and the new way is encountered with a "this is it" feeling, almost as a revelation. (p. 83)

Being inside any performance allows us to assess it in a uniquely subjective way (Clark, 1993). When we are about to reach somewhere or step somewhere, we appraise the kind of getting there that the distance entails. In moving our bodies, we do not estimate distances as so much objective distance to be traversed, but rather as so much traveling to do. We aim toward the experience of a performance, not to the objective features of performance. Consequently, learning to perform involves finding the right experience, and performance involves aiming for that experience.

THE LIVED BODY IN PERSPECTIVE

Although a great deal of objective knowledge about performance capacity has been generated, the subjective experience of performance has been largely neglected. The previous section highlighted the subjective experience of the lived body. The discussion covered two important themes. First, physical and mental aspects of performance do not represent separate realms. Both moving one's body to accomplish a task and planning the steps in the task are functions of a lived body that is at once both physical and mental. Second, the nature of subjective experience and its role in performance were examined. It was argued that experience is not simply an artifact or consequence of doing, but rather that experience is central to how we manage to perform. To learn any performance, we must find the experience of it—how it feels. To do any performance, we are guided not by the objective features of what is involved, but by how it feels to do it. Understanding both performance and limitations of performance requires attention to these features of the lived body.

Disability and the Lived Body

Although there is little systematic study of the embodied experience of disability, a number of writers who have disabilities have offered important insights into their experiences. Toombs (1992), who has multiple sclerosis, reminds us that there is a particular experience that goes with a disability. It is often radically different from experience in a nondisabled state. She notes, for example, that with a physical impairment:

> My attention is focused on my hand as hand. I must observe how it is that my fingers grasp the handle of the cup and I am conscious of my hand's unaccustomed ineffectiveness as an instrument of my action. In illness the body intrudes itself into experience. (Toombs, 1992, p. 71)

Zasetsky describes the challenges of trying to write following his traumatic brain injury:

> I didn't have enough of a vocabulary or mind left to write well . . . I'd spend ages hunting for the right words. I had to remember and turn up words that were are at least fairly similar or close enough to what I wanted to say. But after I'd put together these second choices, I still wasn't able to start writing until I figured out how to compose a sentence. (Luria, 1972, pp. 78, 79)

Others write about how the world is transformed. For example, Sechehaye (1968) describes her experience of schizophrenia as transforming the world into a place where there:

> Reigned an implacable light, blinding, leaving no place for shadow; an immense place without boundary, limitless, flat; a mineral, lunar country, cold as the wastes of the North Pole. In this stretching emptiness, all is unchangeable, immobile, congealed, crystallized. Objects are strange trappings, placed here and there, geometric cubes without meaning. (p. 44)

Similarly, Williams (1994) describes how her experiences as a child with autism placed her in an extraordinary world:

> I discovered the air was full of spots. If you looked into nothingness, there were spots. People would walk by, obstructing my magical view of nothingness. I'd move past them. (p. 3)

Others have written about the alteration of experiences that comes with medical treatments. For example, Jamison (1995) describes living with the consequences of taking lithium necessary to control her manic-depressive illness. In addition to feeling "less lively, less energetic, less high spirited" (p. 92), she also found that some of her ability to read was impaired:

> . . . I had to read the same lines repeatedly and take copious notes before I could comprehend the meaning. Even so, what I read often disappeared from my mind like snow on a hot pavement. (p. 95)

Such testimonies from persons who experience various impairments offer important windows into the experience of limitations or alterations of capacity. Systematic descriptions of the experience of impairments and the course of change over time also have the potential to offer us new ways of understanding and intervening. In what follows, we examine this potential more closely.

UNDERSTANDING TRANSFORMATIONS IN THE LIVED BODY

Collectively, we have undertaken three studies that have examined the experience of the lived body among persons with disabilities. Each focuses on:

- Nature of the experience
- Contribution of experience to disability
- Evolution of experience over time
- Role of experience in changes in performance capacity.

The following sections briefly describe the findings from the three studies. Following this are a discussion of their implications for better understanding the nature of experience in disability and how experience can be used in the therapeutic process.

Example I: Recapturing Half of Self and the World

Brain damage often significantly alters experience. One of the more dramatic alterations is unilateral neglect following cerebrovascular accident. Objectively, persons with unilateral neglect are unable to orient their attention toward the left hemispace and are often unaware of the left half of their body (Bisiach & Vallar, 1988).

A study of four Swedish women with unilateral neglect (Tham, Borell, & Gustavsson, 2000) described the unfolding of lived body experiences as these women lost and then slowly began to recapture half of themselves and their worlds. Many are oblivious to their neglect (McGlynn & Schacter, 1989; Tham et al., 2000). The following are highlights of their discoveries.

Initially, the left half of the women's worlds did not exist for them. They lived and acted only in the remaining right half of the world, with no sense that the left half of the world had disappeared. Rather, they experienced their half-world as complete.

Only with time, as the women began to perform previously familiar tasks, did they begin to sense something vaguely unfamiliar. Their bodies, and their perceptions of space and time, felt oddly different.

As they encountered the left half of the body, it didn't feel as though it belonged to them. Each woman's arm and leg simply didn't seem like part of the self. They felt instead like objects apart from the self. One woman reported that she had to trace her left arm with her right hand to the shoulder in order to realize that it was really attached to her. Another woman, referring to her hand placed on the table in front of her, said her fingers seemed to her like five sausages just lying there. All four women spoke about the left side of the body in the third person, characterizing it as estranged and cold. One woman lamented that her left hand "wants to reject people. It is not generous. It will just give chilliness."

In this way, as the women first became aware of their left halves, they did not experience them as an encounter with part of the self. Rather, they saw the left half as something alien, not belonging to themselves.

As these women began to move about and do things, they also found that they were disoriented to space. They repeatedly found that they did not know where they were, and could not orient themselves in space. Moreover, both people and objects could suddenly disappear or appear. For example, one woman recalled how "When I had dinner, I suddenly didn't know where my husband went. He just disappeared."

They also found that they could no longer rely on previously automatic ways of doing things. While they were still unaware of their neglect at this point, they could discern its consequences. They found these consequences of neglect confusing and could not fathom why they had problems in performing certain tasks. They could not link their problems of performance to their neglect since it did not yet exist for them.

Over time, they began to recognize familiar problems in performance, though they still did not comprehend that they were missing half the world. Bumping into things with their wheelchairs was a common problem. While they couldn't perceive what was happening on their left side, they could perceive certain features of the collision, such as the crashing sound and the sudden stopping of the wheelchair.

As such neglect-related experiences accumulated, they began to reflect upon them, searching for explanations for these difficulties. At first, their explanations were still not grounded in their neglect. For instance, they attributed their inability to find objects to unfamiliarity of the rehabilitation environment, expecting to find it much easier to locate objects at home. At this point, they could not consciously use any strategies to compensate for their neglect since they were unaware of their unawareness of the left half of the surrounding world.

As they regained movement in their left side, the sense of that side as belonging to the self began to return. Because improvements in mobility occurred first in the legs, the four women first felt that their left legs mostly belonged to them, although alienation of the left arm persisted.

Despite its continued estrangement, they began to feel a responsibility to the arm. One woman described the experience like this:

> I have to accept it, because it is sitting here on my body. All the time when I am doing something I have to think of it, and to bring it with me. It is like I am carrying a baby all the time, a baby you can't leave on a table and then go your way. You have to bring it with you. You can't forget your hand because everything can go wrong if you do that. Instead, you bring your baby and it is the same with your hand, you can't ignore the hand, because you have it, and in the future you will need it.

While the women began to own responsibility for the left arm, they still did not own it as a part of themselves. This was highlighted by the fact that they could lose the left side of the body, as one woman noted:

> Always when I am going to bed I think that I need a pillow for my arm and if the arm is not lying there, I get scared to death. I think something is wrong because I must always have my arm with me. If I don't have that, it will become swollen. If I can't find my arm, I use the alarm to call someone and ask, 'can you find my bad arm?' And, of course, they always can.

At this point, before they could actually use it, the left hand began to reemerge as a point of view for doing things. As one woman described:

> Suddenly I forget that I can't use my left hand, especially when I am eating. For example if I find some crumbs at the table, beside my plate, I want to clean them up and to put them together. So I try to put the crumbs in my left hand, even if I know that I can't use it.

Such regaining of intentionality in the neglected side was also reflected in their beginning efforts to incorporate the left body parts in their daily life.

Next, they began to comprehend that they were missing the left half of the environment. The understanding was objective, however, and they still did not have any direct experience of this limitation. Importantly, this realization came about as others (therapists, nurses, family members, aides) told them about their neglect, explained how problems were related to neglect, or demonstrated that there were objects to the left by coaching them to search there. Thus, for these women, neglect was first understood as an objective fact, related to them by others.

Armed with this objective knowledge of their neglect and its consequences, they wanted to improve their ability to find objects and to orient to the left half of the environment. The four women gradually became more and more able to use conscious strategies to perform better by compensating for their unilateral neglect.

There appeared to emerge for each woman a kind of existential pull from the left, when objects located there were part of an occupation in which they were engaged or when circumstances on their left needed their attention. For example, one woman, while working in the kitchen, suddenly saw the toaster on her left side when she noticed that its electrical cord was hanging over the sink. She noted, "I could see the electrical cord to the left because I know it is unsafe to have it over the sink. The electricity can short, and that is dangerous."

They could also more readily locate objects that they knew should be present. For example, one woman described searching for lotion and toothpaste in her dressing case:

> I look and I look. At first I can't see the things but I know that they should be there. Then I move my

eyes and I turn my head so I really can see everything because I know that the things should be there.

Increasingly, the women developed a way of reasoning that considered how things should be so that they could compare it with what they perceived. This proved effective in overcoming some problems posed by the neglect. For example, one woman noted:

Sometimes when I am eating I think, but God, didn't I get the fish? They told us that we should be served fish today. But of course, it is placed on the left side of the plate, I think. So, I begin to search to the left, and then I can see it.

Sometimes, they were able to anticipate problems that would occur because of the neglect and use a strategy to avoid them. For example, one woman surveyed and memorized any new environment before she began to move around with the wheelchair. She could use her mental map to avoid crashing into objects that she would not see once she was moving along.

Five months after their strokes, the four women had accumulated substantial experience using such conscious compensatory strategies. Their understanding and awareness of their neglect became deeper, and their compensatory strategies became habitual.

Thus, although they still did not naturally have access to the left half of the world, they were aware that it existed outside of their immediate experience. They began to spontaneously remember to access this world. They used a number of strategies for gaining access to what was present or going on in the left half of the world. They would, for instance, use sounds that came from the left. They would search to the left by reaching and feeling for things. Finally they could actively visually search to the left. As one woman put it:

Look to the left, look to the left, I tell myself, and then when I look to the left, I can find the thing that I am looking for.

In the end, the left half of the world existed for them, but not in the same way that it did before their cerebrovascular accidents. It was not an immediate presence like the rest of the world. It was a hidden place that had consequences for action, where things resided unseen. Through special efforts, objects in the left half of the world could be found and their arrangement, although unseen, could be imagined. Thus, they regained the lost half of the world in pragmatic terms, although it was forever lost to them in immediate experience.

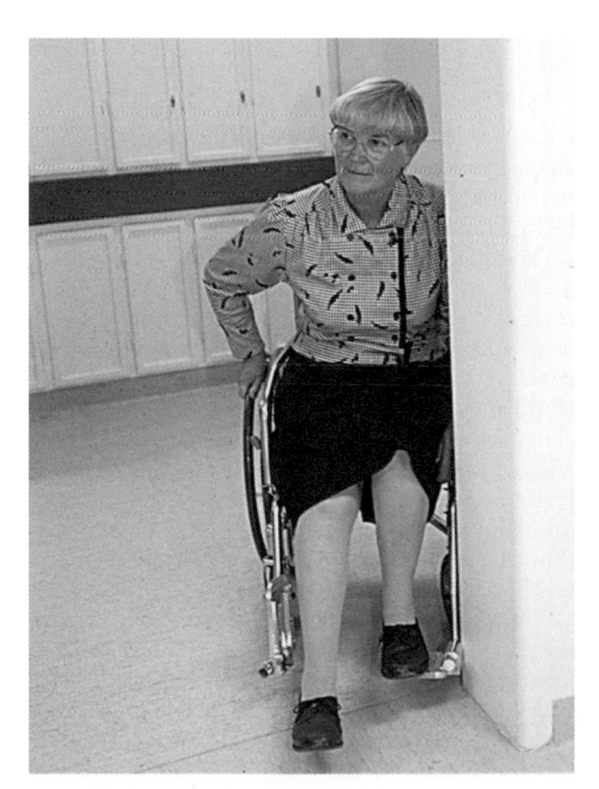

Woman living in "half-world"

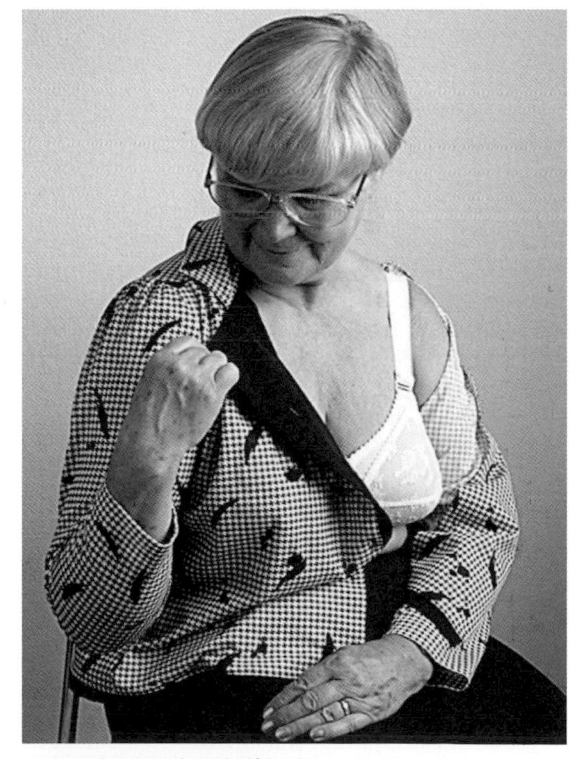

Woman living with a "half-body"

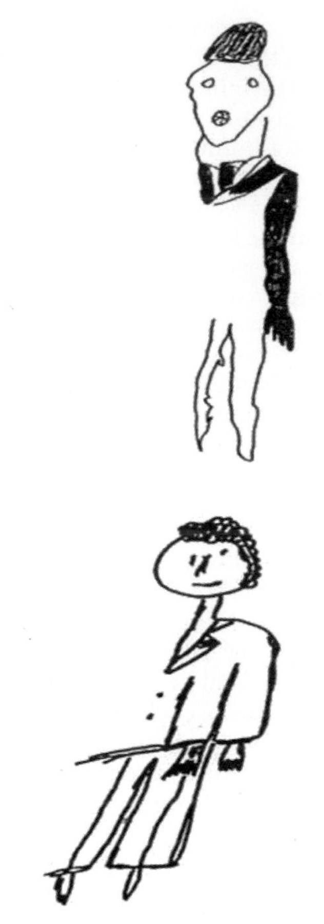

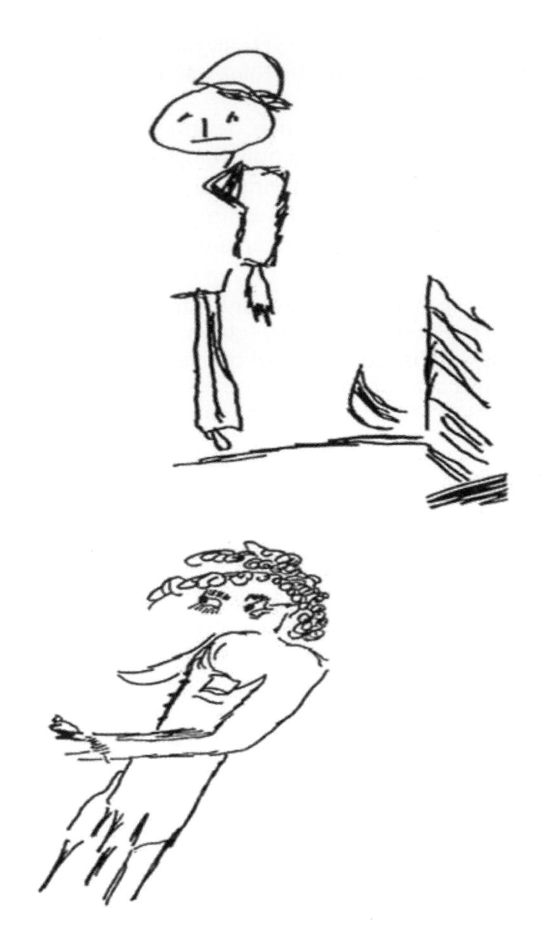

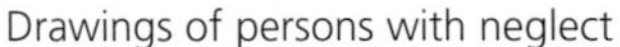

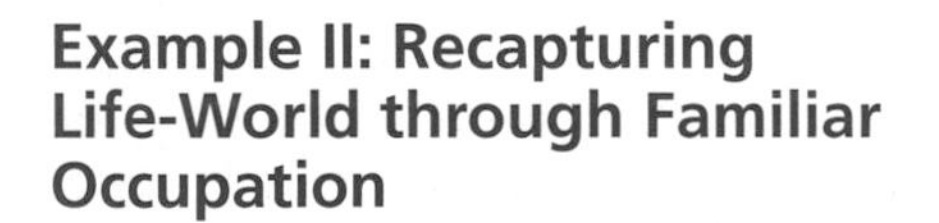

Drawings of persons with neglect

Example II: Recapturing Life-World through Familiar Occupation

When people are confronted with major life-altering events such as brain injury and memory impairment, their experiences with the life-world change to a world that may be difficult to understand (Erikson, Karlsson, Borell, & Tham, 2007). The evolution of experiences over time for persons with memory impairment is described in a phenomenological study (Erikson et al., 2007) with the objective of identifying what characterized the lived experience of memory impairment in daily occupations during the first year after acquired brain injury. After the brain injury, the life-world changed from a taken-for-granted world to a chaotic world that was difficult to understand; the world had changed from familiar to unfamiliar. The routine performance of daily activities and the habit patterns had broken down, so it was mostly the familiar activities that were already integrated in the "habit-body" that enabled coherent doings in everyday life during the year (Fig. 6-1). The findings contribute to an understanding of how to use familiar and meaningful occupations as a therapeutic medium in the rehabilitation of clients with memory impairment following acquired brain injury.

Immediately after the brain injury, the participants described a chaotic life-world; the world had changed from familiar to unfamiliar. This "new" world was described as confusing and frightening, which contributed to feelings of chaos. It was a fragmented world also experienced in the performance of daily activities; as one of the participants described a situation in which she was washing up: "My head doesn't really work; when I put away the dishes, I normally do it automatically without thinking, but I have to think. I get stuck in my thoughts. It's strange, isn't it? It is horrible; it doesn't fit with who I am."

During the first year after injury, especially initially, the participants were *struggling for coherent doing in new contexts.* When the participants were confronted with the challenge of mastering new activities that were not integrated into their habit-body, the individual's coherence in doing was disrupted. This meant that they needed to reflect on each step of what they did, which contrasts with the ease of the life-world we normally take for granted (Husserl, 1970). As one of the participants, who had weaving as a hobby, described the struggle for her initially to recapture her weaving skills: "When I've counted the threads, I don't remember how many threads I should have had. I constantly have to go back and check again." The automaticity in doing had broken down.

When confronted by unfamiliar situations, the coherence in doing was disrupted. Mastering unfamiliar situations necessitated the learning of new activities or the incorporation of new information that could be used in an activity in different contexts. For example, as one of the participants described, the demands at work or the learning of new activities or procedures were too difficult to handle; it was such a challenge that it caused a headache after a short time at work. *Unplanned events also disrupted coherence in doing;* for example, phone calls disrupted concentration and focus during performance, as some of the participants described that they could not remember where in the performance process they were (e.g., when cooking or baking) and that they needed to develop strategies in order to be able to handle these situations.

It gradually emerged during the year that *demanding activities restrained automaticity* in doing. It was particularly difficult to achieve automaticity in activities that were especially demanding on cognitive capacity, including both new activities and activities internalized in the previous habit pattern, for example, control of time, reading the newspaper, times or dates.

To be able to create a structure to establish new habits in new contexts, conscious strategies were needed. One example was a participant who transferred some responsibility to the physical environment by reducing his world in his home to a more limited physical area. He placed objects on the kitchen table, centrally located in his home and significant to activities at home and to the rehabilitation clinic. This strategy gave him a structure for his memory and also control in his daily life.

During the year of rehabilitation, the participants *achieved new habits. By performing familiar activities* integrated in the participants' previous habit patterns in everyday life, it was easier to achieve *automaticity in doing* after the brain injury. Also, re-creation of inner pictures from the past helped the participants re-create their habit patterns; for example, to find a certain place. They acquired in different ways experiences that made them recognize the world, which gave them a link to their former lives. The individual's habit-body was brought back to life, and performance ran smoothly without being disrupted by conscious thinking. In well-known contexts in which they had formerly internalized habit patterns, such as the home environment, it was easier to rely on their habit-body. As one participant described, "At home I think it is going quite well actually. There I am in an environment where it is easier to remember, it is an environment that I am used to. But with this room [at the hospital] I am totally unfamiliar. There are so many new impressions." Familiar activities that were more physical in nature, such as vacuuming, also facilitated automaticity in contrast to activities demanding cognitive capacity. By using former internalized habits as strategy, automaticity in doing was achieved. As one of the participants said, he did not need to use a recipe when he cooked paste with meat sauce. On the other hand, when performing an activity where new facts had to be learned, he explained that he needed to "drill" the activity. "If I am going to do something new, I must read the recipe several times. If he had the opportunity, he chose dishes that were internalized in his habit-body, or, as he said, "in my spinal cord." Another participant, who was used to cooking for his children, also explained the significance of the habit-body to automaticity in doing by saying, "I have been cooking for my children in the past, so all that is still there, now I just do the old dishes that I remember."

As the rehabilitation proceeded, the individuals were gradually confronted with more activities that they became more familiar with and felt more secure about performing.

It was obvious during the year that *internalization of new habits relied on old habits.* Even at the end of the year of rehabilitation, it was apparently mostly the specific activities previously internalized into their habit pattern that participants could perform in a coherent flow without consciously thinking. These activities were performed more as a routine and had become a part of the new habit pattern. This may be exemplified by one participant who felt the different steps in household activities were initially challenging but were now a matter of routine. His body was now taken for granted, and he was no longer aware of it while performing activities. "The housework is not a problem anymore; I am vacuuming and washing the dishes. I do it so quickly; it goes smoothly and easily." As soon as the activities were internalized in the participant's habit pattern, he no longer suffered from stress caused by things such as whether he forgot to turn off the stove. Another example of how an activity could be performed in a coherent flow without conscious thinking came from the participant whose hobby was weaving. Initially, it was a challenge and a struggle for her to recapture the weaving skills, but by the end of the rehabilitation process, she stated that during heddling her fingers could work in a coherent flow without being disrupted by her thinking. The performance now emanating from her body could easily manage the heddling without guidance from her mind.

The participants underwent a reality adjustment during the year. Even if their competence after injury gradually increased during the year, they described an uncertain future horizon. By performing daily activities over the year, participants gradually discovered the consequences of their brain injury to their activities, which led to a reality adjustment and still, 1 year after stroke, created feelings of uncertainty toward their own abilities and their future.

Example III: "I Am Not Living My Life"

A recent phenomenological study (Fallahpour, Jonsson, Joghataei, Nasrabadi, & Tham, 2013) focusing on the lived experience of participation in everyday occupations after stroke in Tehran, Iran, found that individuals after their stroke were profoundly disrupted in their participation, leading them to experience disability and an enormous change in their everyday life. The results stress the nature of experience and its contribution to disability and changes over time.

The meaning structure of the phenomenon of participation in everyday occupations is presented in Figure 6-2, which illustrates their disability experience expressed as "I am not living my life". The first characteristic, "I cannot do activities as before," expressed change in their "doing" and interacted with the second characteristic, "I am not the same person—discovery of a different self," which expressed a changed experience of being in the world physically and socially. The third characteristic, "I am not living my life," was expressed as a result of changes in participants' "doing" and "self," and the interactions between the first two characteristics.

I CANNOT DO ACTIVITIES AS BEFORE

The participants described a tremendous change in doing and how their everyday life was characterized by "not being able to do" the way they did before stroke. Participants described their experiences over time and compared themselves in their "doing" before and after stroke, which was perceived differently. They described their "doing" as a continuum from "doing nothing alone" to "doing something" to "can make it happen but differently." They described their experience as going from being capable to being incapable; as one related:

> I did everything at home. If there were any problems with the plumbing, or anything else at home, I fixed them. I renovated different parts at home if it was needed as that was my job, but now I can't do anything.

Three subcharacteristics were identified for this characteristic:

Losing Former Everyday Routines

The participants experienced a painful loss of their former daily routines and a shift to an undesired and unpleasant new routine. One participant experienced her former pleasant everyday occupation, morning walk, being replaced by daily physical therapy exercise as an unpleasant daily torture, which she experienced as a mandatory stressful new routine. She described how painful it had been for her to start the day after her stroke, because mornings reminded her of her former enjoyable occupation to start the day.

Two participants described their new daily routine as a temporary situation and hoped to perform their former routines in the future. Other participants reported this change as an obvious permanent "loss" that created a significant gap in their lives, and experienced their routines being replaced by a new daily routine as meaningless.

Losing Being a Subject Capable of Acting and Deciding

Participants stressed the importance of being a subject in order to experience engagement and satisfaction instead of being an object. As they experienced, to be a subject meant not only to act but also to make their own choices and to be the center of their own worlds. They described their change after stroke in terms of loss of being a subject in different ways. Some participants experienced a total loss and being treated like objects. A few experienced that others respected their integrity and viewed them as subjects making their own decisions in everyday life.

This loss was clearly described by a male participant who perceived himself as being "a piece of meat present there," like a passive object and unable to be an active subject to do different daily tasks. The participants experienced satisfaction when they were active subjects; they described how the sense of being a subject could be preserved despite not doing the activities by themselves. Two participants described, for instance, that they could do activities only by getting help from their partners. Although similar to the first example where help came from others, neither of these participants described themselves as being passive objects, despite being severely dependent. Instead, they experienced themselves as subjects who did daily activities together with their partners with their constant and supportive accompaniment.

They experienced, instead, that two subjects could do daily tasks together, perceiving a living interaction and understanding between the two subjects, an intersubjectivity.

The participants experienced it as also important to be able to make choices to perceive themselves as active subjects. One participant described how, after her stroke, she had lost the ability to make her own decision about inviting people to her place and, instead, was dependent on her two formal caregivers, and that this loss made her feel disabled.

Losing Former Roles and Authority in the Family

Participants experienced a dramatic change in their valued life roles that influenced the way they viewed themselves in the family. This experience was different in two genders. Female participants perceived their main role as that of taking care of the family through various responsibilities (e.g., home management activities, and control over family relationships), whereas male participants described their main valued life role as that of a productive person who worked full time before stroke and the transition to not being able to work. This experience of loss created a significant gap in their life and influenced their position in the family. One male participant described how not being able to do his different tasks made him experience himself as a dependent disabled person who consequently lost his authority and former role as highest in the family hierarchy, from being somebody who was productive and head of the family to being a dependent consumer.

I AM NOT THE SAME PERSON—DISCOVERY OF A DIFFERENT SELF

Participants also described significant changes in their bodies, abilities, and engagement in different areas of everyday life. They experienced a different "body" and "self" reflected in their new ways of "engaging in different activities." They sadly experienced a big change discovered by continuously comparing their unfamiliar different "present self" with their familiar active "former self."

A Senseless Body—Affected Side as an Object

The participants experienced their bodies as different, disabled, and unfamiliar after stroke. With their new discovered body, they also experienced their bodies as differently connected to the world. The participants experienced their bodies in the beginning after their stroke as lacking sensory perception senseless. They described their affected side as a separate object that they had no control over, like a senseless object restricting them in doing tasks. They described their bodies as being present physically, but not present to do, move, or act, and experienced it as a senseless passive body like an object on the bed, not a physical and emotional subject.

Discovering "Who They Are" through "What They Do"

The participants described a dramatic change between their self-images based on what they did before stroke and current images based on what they could do after stroke. They experienced these changes differently—from a total loss of their former "self" in some participants to a "changed self" in some others, depending on what they could do. Those who had experienced a total loss of "doing" described a total loss of their former "self"—the one that they had known throughout their life—their familiar "self" that "doesn't exist anymore." The greater their gaps in "doing," the greater they experienced the difference compared with the present-former self. The participants expressed their strong desire to get back to their familiar former self as an ideal self.

Discovering a Different Self in Communication with Others

The participants also experienced themselves differently in connection to other people, and, more importantly, the way others in general and the family, in particular, treated or viewed them was important in creating this new image of their new self. The way the participants perceived this discovery in relation to others varied. Some of them perceived themselves as being an object depending on how the family behaved. For instance, one participant experienced that nobody listened to her pain. She felt scared of her painful everyday physical exercises and of not getting the support she needed and being treated like a child. Another participant described how others did not view her the same way as before. This led her to discover her different "self" when communicating with others.

I AM NOT LIVING MY LIFE

Participants experienced their current situation after stroke as not living their life, which was related to "what they could not do after stroke" and "their discovery of a different self." These two aspects interacted with each other and made individuals experience "not living their life." One participant described her life as being difficult to deal with:

> . . . I talked to my friends on the phone; I also met my friends in their homes, and they also came to my place to visit me. I do not live my life. I feel sad since I've not been living my life . . . (she cries). . . .My husband has bought a new oven, and a dishwasher, I have never used them. My caregivers always use them. I can never use them. What does this mean? (She cries desperately) . . . I am not living, I have no life, not at all . . . this is my life. What life is this? I am never living my life . . . .

The participants described their present changed lives as stressful, challenging, and dissatisfying to deal with. They experienced restrictions in their social interactions owing to dissatisfaction with their current life. They tended to avoid socializing to decrease the stress, to control their lives, to keep their former image in others' eyes, to stay close and connected to their former familiar self. They have therefore moved toward social isolation in this new current undesired black "life" after stroke.

Discussion

The three studies just presented systematically examined the lived body experience. These studies illuminated both the nature of disability experience and the role of experience in how persons managed to overcome or adapt to their impairments. The third example also illustrates the disability experience when the environment is not supportive or enriching and how it may influence the lived experiences and occupational adaptation after stroke.

DISABILITY EXPERIENCE

Disability always represents a particular way of being embodied. This is an altered way of existing that thrusts itself on the person with a disability. Hence, persons with disabilities must live the reality of their embodiment. Moreover, they are challenged to adapt to their experiences. Any change in capacity must often be in terms of those experiences. As Csordas (1994) reminds us, people with disabilities must take up an existential position in the world that reflects their particular embodiment.

There appear to be some phenomena that are more general to the disability experience and others that are specific to a type of impairment. Still others are unique to the individual. For example, all the subjects in the studies we examined experienced some form of alienation from their bodies or parts of their bodies. Both Murphy (1987) and Sachs (1993) have also described the experience of disability as including alienation from one's own body.

Although alienation involves the common feature of not experiencing the body or some part of the body as belonging to the self, the particular experience of alienation varies. For the women with neglect, there was at one stage disbelief that their left side was attached to the rest of them. For the persons with memory impairment in the second example, it was easier to rely on their habit-body in well-known contexts in which they had formerly internalized habit patterns such as the home environment, which also facilitated automaticity in occupational performance in contrast to activities demanding cognitive capacity. In the third example, persons experiencing that they were not living their lives anymore after the stroke expressed how their body was experienced as different and unfamiliar and as a senseless object and that they as persons often were treated as objects by others.

Despite these differences, all the persons needed to find ways of coming to terms with this alienation. The three examples suggest that the persons needed to discover their new bodies and ability by having experiences from doing familiar occupations of significance for the individual. Familiar activities seemed to be of particular importance for persons with cognitive impairments as in the first and second examples. The third example shows that the persons did not get those enriched experiences in everyday life, which seemed to make it more difficult for them to get access to their lived body or connection to their world. In the first example, the women who had neglect regained the sense of acting from their left side and in the second example the persons with memory impairments acquired experiences that made them recognize the body and world, which gave them a link to their former habit-body, memory, and lives. These findings suggest that coming to terms with bodily alienation may be an important task in regaining capacity and access to the world for a range of persons with disabilities.

Understanding disability in terms of subjective experience is important because it often explains aspects of a person's functional capacity not accounted for in objective approaches. Understanding the experiences of persons with cognitive impairments like the persons living in a half-world in example one or living with memory impairment in example two can be challenging. However, this understanding is needed, in therapy, to meet the individuals in their unique life-worlds in order to enable transformation in experience contributing to change in the therapeutic process. The second example illustrates how important it is to understand the subjective experience of struggling for coherent doing in new contexts. Consequently, we see that how people perform not only reflects the objective status of performance components, but also emanates from how they experience themselves and their worlds. Altered experience alters performance.

IMPORTANCE OF EXPERIENCE FOR TRANSFORMING CAPACITY

Each of the three cases presented could be described from an objective view of the body and mind. For example, the difficulties in mastering new situations and contexts can be seen as attributable to the persons' changes in the brain structure, leading to memory impairments; the women's acquisition of ways to deal with world-neglect can be described in terms of neglect syndrome including lack of awareness; and the difficulties among the persons in the case examples can be seen as attributable to inability to organize their daily tasks. These objective descriptions are certainly valid and important for understanding what happens to such persons as their impairments change over time. However, as the studies clearly illustrate, these descriptions would only partly explain how change took place.

In all three studies, it was through the realm of experience that effective strategies of change were discovered. The actual events and human actions that resulted in change were a function of experience. Each of these persons had to use their experience as a way of solving their own problems and challenges, and other people played an important role in enabling experiences contributing to change. For example, the women with neglect had to come to know a new reality in which their practical world consisted not just of what they could perceive, but also of something outside perception; and the persons with memory impairment had to connect to their former habit-body to solve problems in their new situation in everyday life after stroke. Learning to exist effectively in such a world meant that they had to come to a way of understanding their new experiences. Both these examples indicate how transformation in performance capacity depends on a transformation in experience.

Conclusion

This chapter offered a subjective approach to understanding performance capacity that is complementary to the usual objective approach. The concept of the lived body derived from phenomenology offers a unique way of conceptualizing subjective experience and its role in performance. Through careful attention to this subjective experience, we have a way to better understand performance capacity.

CASE EXAMPLE: TO TEST YOUR KNOWLEDGE: A WOMAN WITH A SENSORY PROCESSING DISORDER

During a standard intake interview, an occupational therapist asked Katie, a 46-year-old music professor with a mild sensory processing disorder, about her goal for therapy. She replied, "I have always wanted a thicker skin in life, literally and physically . . . When I look at people, I see expressions in their faces and small bodily movements that others do not seem to see. When I hear sounds, they are either painfully noxious or sublime. When I try on a shirt, it feels either like sand paper or like silk. . . I just wish I did not live in a world of extremes." For these reasons, I am fragmented. If I am not at work, I avoid people, places, and things that I know will make me uncomfortable and exhausted. As a result, my daily reality is either narrow and empty or incredibly stressful. I go to work, teach my students, show up at faculty meetings, and compose music at home. This is my world. The world becomes more stable when I am performing my music. Only at this time do I feel whole."

Questions to Encourage Critical Thinking and Discussion

- **How would an occupational therapist describe the objective aspects of Katie's performance capacity?**
- **How might an occupational therapist describe the subjective aspects of Katie's performance capacity?**
- **How might an occupational therapist use Katie's subjective experience to transform her performance capacity?**

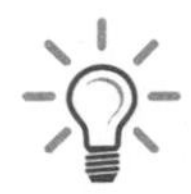

Chapter 6 Review Questions

1. Provide an example of bodily knowing.
2. From a client's perspective, which aspects of performance capacity are more important to understand—objective aspects or subjective aspects? Explain your answer.
3. Define the lived body.
4. Why is it important to understand disability in terms of a client's subjective experience?
5. Explain how a person's experience of disability changes over time.

thePoint® For additional resources and exercises, visit http://thePoint.lww.com

Key Terms

Lived body: The experience of being and knowing the world through a particular body.

Performance capacity: Ability to do things provided by the status of underlying objective physical and mental components and corresponding subjective experience.

REFERENCES

Bisiach, E., & Vallar, G. (1988). Hemi neglect in humans. In F. Boller & J. Grafman (Eds.), *Handbook of neuropsychology*. Amsterdam, The Netherlands: Elsevier.

Clark, F. (1993). Occupation embedded in a real life: Interweaving occupational science and occupational therapy. *American Journal of Occupational Therapy, 47*, 1067–1078.

Csordas, T. (Ed.). (1994). *Embodiment and experience: The existential ground of culture and self.* New York, NY: Cambridge University Press.

Engelbrecht, F. (1968). *The phenomenology of the human body*. Sovenga, South Africa: University College of the North.

Erikson, A., Karlsson, G., Borell, L., & Tham, K. (2007). The lived experience of memory impairment in daily occupation after acquired brain injury. *OTJR: Occupation, Participation, and Health, 27*, 84–94.

Fallahpour, M., Jonsson, H., Joghataei, M. T., Nasrabadi, A. N., & Tham, K. (2013). "I am not living my life": Lived experience of participation in everyday occupations after stroke in Tehran. *Journal of Rehabilitation Medicine, 45*(6), 528–534. doi:10.2340/16501977-1143

Fisher, A., Murray, E., & Bundy, A. (1991). *Sensory integration theory and practice.* Philadelphia, PA: F. A. Davis.

Husserl, E. (1970). *The crisis of European sciences and transcendental phenomenology.* Evanston, IL: North Western University Press.

Hutson, J. (1998). *Qualitative study of the experience of an injured worker* (Master's Thesis, Department of Occupational Therapy, University of Illinois at Chicago).

Jamison, K. R. (1995). *An unquiet mind: A memoir of moods and madness.* New York, NY: Vintage Books.

Katz, N. (2005). *Cognition and occupation across the life span.* Rockville, MD: AOTA Press.

Kielhofner, G. (1995). A meditation on the use of hands. *Scandinavian Journal of Occupational Therapy, 2*, 153–166.

Leder, D. (1984). Medicine's paradigm of embodiment. *Journal of Medical Philosophy, 9*, 29–43.

Leder, D. (1990). *The absent body*. Chicago, IL: University of Chicago Press.

Luria, A. R. (1972). *The man with a shattered world: The history of a brain wound.* New York, NY: Basic Books.

McGlynn, S. M., & Schacter, D. L. (1989). Unawareness of deficits in neuropsychological syndromes. *Journal of Clinical Experimental Neuropsychology, 11*, 143–205.

Merleau-Ponty, M. (1962). *Phenomenology of perception* (C. Smith, Trans.). London, United Kingdom: Routledge & Kegan Paul. (Original work published 1945)

Murphy, R. (1987). *The body silent.* New York, NY: Henry Holt & Company.

Sachs, O. (1993). *A leg to stand on.* New York, NY: Harper Collins.

Sartre, J. P. (1970). The body. In S. F. Spricher (Ed.), *The philosophy of the body: Reflections on Cartesian dualism.* Chicago, IL: Quadrangle Books.

Sechehaye, M. (1968). *Autobiography of a schizophrenic girl: The true story of Renee* (G. Rubin-Rabson, Trans.). New York, NY: Grune & Stratton.

Sudnow, D. (1978). *Ways of the hand: The organization of improvised conduct.* Cambridge, MA: Harvard University Press.

Sudnow, D. (1979). *Talk's body: A meditation between two keyboards.* New York, NY: Knopf.

Tham, K., Borell, L., & Gustavsson, A. (2000). The discovery of disability: A phenomenological study of unilateral neglect. *American Journal of Occupational Therapy, 54*, 398–406.

Toombs, K. (1992). *The meaning of illness: A phenomenological account of the different perspectives of physician and patient.* Boston, MA: Kluwer Academic.

Trombly, C. A. (1995). Occupation: Purposefulness and meaningfulness as therapeutic mechanisms: 1995 Eleanor Clarke Slagle Lecture. *The American Journal of Occupational Therapy, 49*(10), 960–972.

Williams, D. (1994). *Nobody nowhere: The extraordinary autobiography of an autistic.* New York, NY: Avon Books.

The Environment and Human Occupation

Gail Fisher, Sue Parkinson, and Lena Haglund

CHAPTER 7

EXPECTED LEARNING OUTCOMES

Upon completion of this chapter, readers will be able to:

1. Explain how the environment influences occupational participation.
2. Define each dimension and level of the environment.
3. Identify examples of opportunities and resources as well as demands and constraints in a client's immediate environment.
4. Provide examples of a variety of components and qualities in the physical, social, and occupational environment that impact participation.
5. Describe how the environmentally focused model of human occupation (MOHO) assessments are used in practice, using case studies.
6. Illustrate how occupational therapists can support the creation of environments that enable occupational performance and participation.

MOHO Problem-Solver: Reshaping Expectations in the Work Environment

Susanne is a 25-year-old woman who was treated in the outpatient mental health unit at the local hospital for a bipolar diagnosis. When she came to the hospital she was extremely talkative about where to live, quickly alternating her plans from apartment to house to moving away. She was arguing with her parents loudly regarding money and she had not slept during the last 5 days. She had met a new boyfriend last night and wanted to go away with him and get married.

Susanne was on sick leave from her job and was concerned that she might not be able to keep her job due to her recent behavioral issues at work. She had been working in management in a bank and she loved her worker *role*. She was stationed at the front desk of a bank; she was the person all new customers at the bank met. The therapist collected the initial information and did the first evaluation of Susanne's work situation. Susanne reported that some easy work scenarios she could manage by herself; other more complicated circumstances she forwarded to another staff member. She reported that the customers stand in a line to make an inquiry, and that when the line gets too long she gets anxious and begins to rush, making more mistakes and leading her to make inappropriate comments.

After 1 month of treatment in an integrative program that included occupational therapy, she felt that she was not making much progress. While she enjoyed the social skills training and self-management skills she was learning, she did not feel as though they would adequately translate to real life. This feeling was intensified by her medication, which reportedly made her feel "like someone without a personality." Feeling restless, she contacted her supervisor to indicate that she wanted to go back to work. The supervisor and her treatment team both expressed some reservations about her restarting her job. Nonetheless, she was permitted to return. Within a week, she was written up for making a sarcastic comment to a customer.

Susanne reentered treatment, and her occupational therapist decided to draw upon model of human occupation (MOHO) to develop a better, more empathetic understanding of her experience, and to examine the demands and constraints within Susanne's different environmental contexts. Together, Susanne and the occupational therapist identified that she needed to increase her ability to choose and do tasks that were well matched to her capacity to promote a sense of personal causation (*self-efficacy*) and return to work. She needed to find time in her daily routines that allowed her to rest and attend her therapy sessions. Additionally, modifications within her *social environment* were needed. She needed to accept her vulnerabilities, communicate more effectively with her supervisor, and ask for help from her friends and colleagues at work when she becomes overwhelmed.

After working on these issues through a series of interviews about her occupational history, Susanne informed her therapist that she felt ready to return to work. The occupational therapist recommended that Susanne undergo a formal evaluation of her ability to return to the job prior to making a decision. The supervisor would need to be involved in this evaluation. Initially, the supervisor expressed concerns, wondering if the bank job was the best option for Susanne. She expressed some hesitancy to have Susanne continue to work there, citing that she becomes easily overwhelmed when there is a long line of customers waiting to see her. Reluctantly, however, she agreed.

The therapist chose to conduct the *Work Environment Impact Scale (WEIS)* (Moore-Corner, Kielhofner, & Olson, 1998) interview. The WEIS allows a client and therapist to identify environmental characteristics that facilitate successful employment experiences. Factors that inhibit worker performance and satisfaction and which may require accommodation are also addressed in order to maximize the "fit" of the worker and their skills to the job environment. It is a semistructured interview and rating scale designed to assist the therapist to gather information on how individuals with physical or psychosocial disabilities experience and perceive their work environments. Typical candidates for this assessment are persons who are experiencing difficulty on the job, and persons whose work is interrupted by an injury or episode of illness. The 17 items reflect the social and physical environment, supports, temporal demands, objects used, and daily job functions.

In this case, the aim of doing the WEIS was to find out how the work environment influenced Susanne, help Susanne to increase her knowledge of how her disease influenced her work situation, and identify strategies to support her performance capacity. After the WEIS interview and follow-up discussion, they agreed on four recommendations involving the work environment:

- Educate Susanne's coworkers about her bipolar condition. Susanne needs to explain her vulnerabilities and ask them to help her to recognize early symptoms and call them to her attention before problems occur.
- The supervisor needs to have an identified administrator to contact if she sees Susanne experiencing difficulty with job tasks or interpersonal interactions.
- The workplace should allow flexible work hours to allow Susanne to leave 30 minutes early on Fridays to continue treatment.
- The occupational therapist will suggest to the bank to use a numbered ticket system for the customers, rather than a line. Susanne will be given a number each day that represents the tipping point. This tipping point number will be used to signal the supervisor that Suzanne needs more support. This will decrease the stress of seeing a long line and will still allow the supervisor to monitor how many customers are waiting.

Susanne was able to return to work with these supports, on a trial basis. After 1 month and continued treatment using other MOHO-based interventions, her need for the supports at work began to lessen and she did not require extra supervision.

There is a growing appreciation of the fact that the environment can facilitate or limit participation in everyday occupations. Occupational therapists' focus on the environment has increased dramatically since the 1990s (Law, 2015). The environment is recognized as a critical factor influencing participation in the International Classification of Functioning, Disability and Health (World Health Organization, 2001) as well as the American Occupational Therapy Association Practice Framework (American Occupational Therapy Association, 2014). It plays a major role in supporting optimal functioning and participation in education, employment, leisure, and all aspects of community living for people with disabilities (Magasi, Hammel, Heinemann, Whiteneck, & Bogner, 2009).

The environment can also be a barrier that restricts participation and creates disparities if aspects of it do not meet the person's needs and desires (Magasi et al., 2015). As such, the environment is key to the process of change, being inextricably linked with personal performance to the point of being inseparable. This dynamic relationship between the environment and the person is reciprocal, as the environment influences the person but is also potentially influenced and modified by the person (Bronfenbrenner, 1992). Individuals will seek out certain types of environments and seek to change their environments to meet their needs and preferences, when provided with the opportunity to do so.

For example, a woman can choose to decorate her immediate environment, her living area, to reflect her values and culture, invite supportive friends over to create a positive social environment, and include favorite music that lifts her mood.

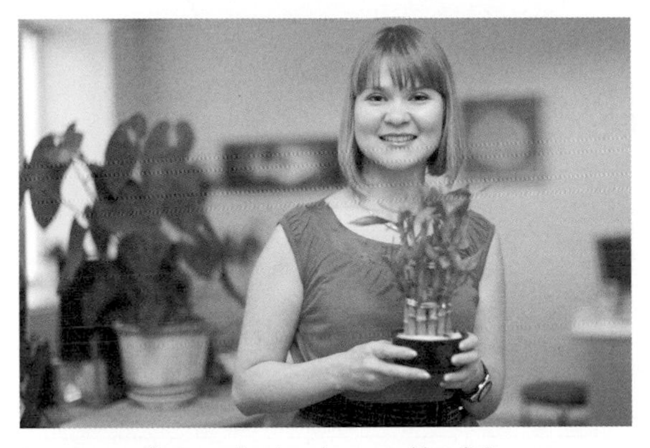

A woman reflects on having decorated her living room

A man with limited use of his hands can convince his neighborhood library to add voice recognition software on their computers so that he can produce documents without using a keyboard, creating a local or community-level support.

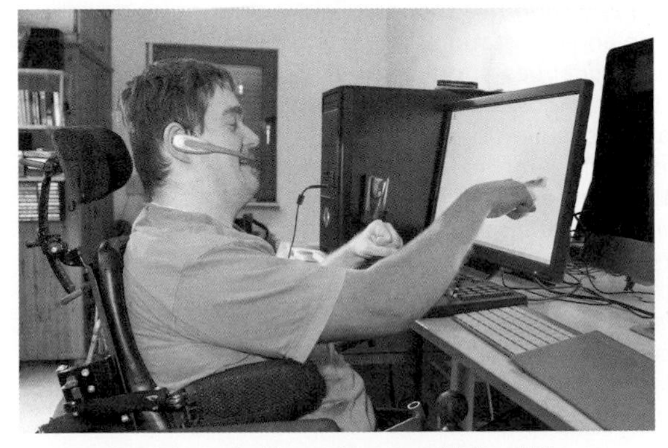

Man uses voice recognition software at his local library

At the global level, disability rights groups can advocate for a change in government policies to provide more funding for job retraining after a work injury.

The role of occupational therapy practitioners using the MOHO can include facilitating the creation of environments that support personal causation and are well matched to the person's values, interests, roles, habits, performance capacity, skills, participation, and ultimately occupational adaptation. Indeed, the environment can be viewed as "the most important tool that occupational therapists have" (de las Heras, Llerena, & Kielhofner, 2003, p. 10). Using a comprehensive analysis of environmental components and qualities, the occupational therapist can evaluate the impact of the environment on the person's occupational performance and participation, recommend modification of the environment, support implementation of recommended environmental changes, and reevaluate the modified environment's impact on the person.

Dimensions of the Environment

The **environment** can be defined as the particular physical, social, occupational, economic, political, and cultural components of one's contexts that impact upon the motivation, organization, and performance of occupation (Kielhofner, 2008). According to this conceptualization, we can envision the environment (Fig. 7-1) as including three dimensions: physical, social, and occupational. At the same time, economic, political, and cultural factors and social attitudes also exert an influence on occupational life, along with geographical and ecological aspects. Most people operate in a variety of contexts (e.g., home, school, workplace, therapy facility, and neighborhood). It is within these contexts that people encounter different physical **spaces**, objects, relationships, interactions, occupations, and activities, as well as expectations and opportunities for doing things, all within a cultural context that is unique to the individual.

The physical, social, and occupational environmental dimensions exist at three levels: in immediate contexts such as home, work, and school; local contexts such as neighborhood and community; and global societal contexts. The dimensions interact with the person and with each other, across all levels, as depicted by the two-way arrows between the person and the environmental contexts and the arrows linking the environmental dimensions and contexts. The dimensions are briefly described below and further detailed in Table 7-1.

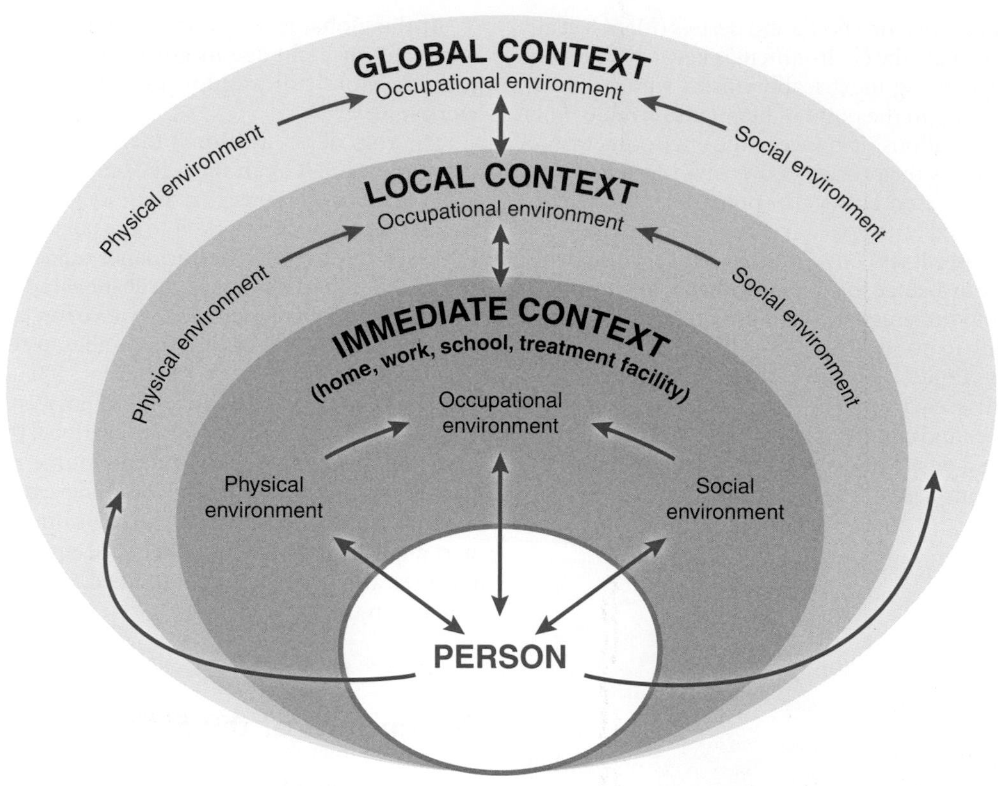

FIGURE 7-1 Interactions between the Person and the Physical, Social, and Occupational Environment across Three Contexts.

Table 7-1 Examples of Environmental Components and Qualities

Physical Environment—Space and Objects	
Environmental Components	***Environmental Qualities***
Space • architecture, streets, sidewalks • buildings (e.g., homes, workplaces, schools, shops, leisure and social spaces, health care facilities) • rooms and amenities (e.g., interior rooms, hallways) • outdoor spaces (e.g., gardens, parks, walking/biking paths) • woodland, beaches, countryside *Objects* • tools, equipment, materials, supplies for work, school, personal and domestic activities • clothing, furniture, possessions • assistive technology and devices for communication and self-care • vehicles, public transportation	*Accessibility and safety of space*—ease of getting around safely: distance, layout, barriers, hazards, universal design elements, surfaces, bathroom, entrances, stairs, lighting, impact of local geography *Adequacy of space*—match between space and person: amount of space, type and purpose of space, flexibility, design aspects *Choices of space*—options of where to live, work, go to school, shop, and go outdoors; what spaces and rooms to access and use *Visual and cognitive supports*—signage, cues for navigation and orientation, facilitating exploration *Sensory qualities*—noises, smells, visual impact, temperature and local climate conditions, air quality, tactile and movement opportunities *Overall appearance*—introduction of personal and culturally meaningful elements, warm/cold décor *Availability of objects*—availability of assistive technology and devices, ease of access: cost, storage, positioning *Adequacy of objects*—match between objects and occupations: work, study, homemaking, and leisure interests; match with person's capabilities, variety of objects

Table 7-1 Examples of Environmental Components and Qualities (continued)

Social environment—Relationships and Interactions	
Environmental Components	***Environmental Qualities***
Relationships • family—spouse/partner, children, siblings, extended family • roommates, fellow residents • social networks—friends, neighbors, faith groups • work colleagues, supervisors, clients, fellow students, fellow therapy service recipients • health care professionals, caregivers, advisers, teachers, peer coaches/advisors • community members, wider society • safety officers, shop owners, elected officials *Interactions* • verbal, nonverbal communication, pictures • physical and cognitive support and facilitation	*Availability of people and relationships*—opportunities for accessing people and developing desired relationships, personal care assistance available *Emotional support*—respect, validation, acceptance, empathy, collaboration, understanding, trust, cultural sensitivity *Empowerment*—encouragement for goal achievement, self-expression, choice, self-advocacy, and autonomy if desired *Physical and cognitive facilitation*—assistance at the right level and using the best mode: coaching, moving and handling, collaborative problem-solving, prompts, cognitive cues *Form of interaction*—in person, written messages, telephone contact, e-mail, text message, Internet contact *Adequacy of communication*—communication at desired cognitive level, volume, and speed; in preferred language, with cultural sensitivity; access to needed information; supports for decision-making and problem-solving: advice, strategies, photos, factual information *Community and broader societal attitudes and services*—supportive attitudes and practices, social support services available, presence of discrimination or stigma and strategies to avoid it or address it

Occupational Environment—Occupations, Activities, and Overarching Context	
Environmental Components	***Environmental Qualities***
Occupations/Activities • self-care/personal activities • domestic activities, home maintenance, gardening • care-giving activities • paid work, volunteering, study • leisure, play, relaxation, exercise, sleep • instrumental activities—travel, financial management • using computer and electronic communication devices • participation in organizations, community, religious observance • health care and therapy participation *Overarching context* • cultural values and practices • economic and political influence	*Occupation and activity choices*—match with capabilities: level of physical, cognitive, social, and emotional challenge *Appeal of occupations and activities*—level of attraction: status, variety, value, interest, enjoyment, familiarity/novelty, rewards *Supports available*—adaptations, positioning, transportation systems, health care and therapy services, safety concerns addressed *Participation*—opportunities for decision-making, involvement, new learning, self-expression, role development, exploration of interests *Time elements*—match with person's needs and expectations: duration, pace, balance with other demands *Structure*—predictability, flexibility, frequency, continuity over time *Flexibility*—opportunity for adaptation, able to do it the way you want *Sustainability*—environmental considerations that protect the natural world *Cultural aspects*—reflecting cultural preferences and rituals *Funding and policies*—government and economic support for participation in desired occupations and activities, adequate resources available to initiate and sustain occupations

PHYSICAL ENVIRONMENT

- Spaces within which people do things, both natural and built space
- Objects that people use when doing things, including assistive technology and devices
- Physical and cognitive accessibility, safety, sensory qualities, and availability of space and objects

SOCIAL ENVIRONMENT

- Availability of people and relationships, including family, friends, neighbors, roommates, work colleagues, caregivers, and community members
- Quality of interactions, including the physical, verbal, cognitive, and emotional support provided
- Community and societal attitudes and practices

OCCUPATIONAL ENVIRONMENT

- Presence of occupations and activities that reflect the person's interests, roles, capacity, and cultural preferences
- Qualities of occupations and activities, such as timing, structure, flexibility, continuity, sustainability, and cultural relevance
- Funding and policies that influence what occupations and activities are available, expected, or required by the context

Dynamics of the Environment–Person Interaction

According to MOHO, aspects of the environment influence each other and act together to influence the person. As one aspect of this dynamic system changes, the other aspects inevitably change, in minute or significant ways.

ENVIRONMENTAL OPPORTUNITIES AND RESOURCES

The environment provides a wide range of opportunities and resources that enable choosing and doing things. For example, a natural resource such as a lake or forest may afford opportunities to enjoy the view, to photograph the scene, or to go hiking or swimming. The environment may also provide resources to sustain our motivation. For instance, family members and friends may offer emotional support and reassurance to sustain effort toward a goal. In contrast, when opportunities and resources are not available, it may have an adverse effect. For example, some retirees who no longer have the expectations of the work environment find it more difficult to maintain their motivation for doing things (Jonsson, Josephsson, & Kielhofner, 2000).

Although the environment provides opportunities and resources that may facilitate performance, it is important to note that what seems to be an opportunity may also have negative consequences for the person. Complex technology may prove to be overwhelming for some people, too much choice may lead to indecision, and opportunities for promotion at work may be viewed with apprehension. Therefore, a match between the opportunities and the resources that are available and the desires of the individual is the critical determinant of whether the resource provided is truly a support.

A central term that can assist our understanding of how the environment influences human occupation is *enabling*. All elements of the physical, social, and occupational environment can enable occupation in immediate, local, and global contexts if the client experiences them as positive.

- Objects in the physical environment of the home that are well matched to the person's capabilities can enable independence. For example, a coffeemaker with enlarged digits can enable an older person with impaired vision to make his/her own coffee. The availability of similar products is enhanced when objects that incorporate universal design principles are readily available in ordinary stores.
- A supportive social environment can enable occupation at different levels. For a boy with an autism spectrum disorder, having friends at school that share his interests leads to opportunities to get together on the weekend to enjoy activities together. This boy's caring older brother can provide coaching and encouragement to his younger brother to enable full participation in weekend community events.
- The occupational environment can be evaluated and modified to enable maximal occupational participation. A work setting that is flexible can provide opportunities for a young worker with an intellectual disability to adjust the order of completing tasks to match challenging tasks to his/her most productive time of the day. This supportive work environment enables the worker to be more economically self-sufficient, which may allow him/her to enjoy the occupation of going out to eat with a coworker to celebrate their birthday.
- The three dimensions of the environment—physical, social, and occupational—coexist, and each may provide options to enable maximal participation. For example, following a stroke, a person may have difficulty driving to the store weekly to buy groceries, an essential occupation. If his neighborhood has an accessible small store

that is close by, he/she may be able to walk there with a shopping cart at a slow pace and make the trip twice a week instead of once a week to lessen the load. Or, he/she can ask his/her neighbor to provide social support by giving him/her a ride to the store when they goes shopping. Alternatively, the local community can provide a special van or car to take him/her to and from the store. The provision of social or physical resources, or adjusting the pace or frequency of the activity, enables the stroke survivor to choose an alternative strategy to complete the desired occupation of grocery shopping.

ENVIRONMENTAL DEMANDS AND CONSTRAINTS

Environments may place limits on or strongly direct action (Law, 1991; Lawton, 1980). Such features of the physical environment as fences, walls, steps, walkways, and doorways constrain where one can go or how much effort it takes. Others' expectations, laws and regulations, job requirements, and social norms can affect people's actions, patterns of activity, and even motivation, whether for better or for worse.

Environments encourage particular behaviors and discourage or disallow others. For example, in an airport the counters and agents, roped areas, security checkpoints and guards, posted rules and announcements, gates, and lines of passengers influence and, in part, dictate the sequence of things we do. Standing in line, obtaining a boarding pass, checking luggage, passing security, going to the gate, and boarding the plane are all done according to environmental demands. Such boundaries may limit our freedom, but they also provide safety and security.

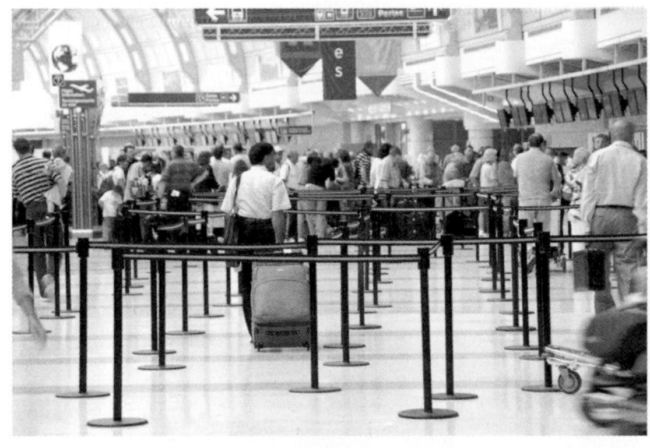

The resource and constraints afforded by an airport security line

Environmental demands and constraints also influence the development of habits and roles. For example, a school's physical arrangement and rules and requirements, combined with teachers, peers, and others' perceptions of the student role, all funnel and shape the attitudes and actions that come to make up each student's role. A teacher who rearranges the desks in groupings throughout the classroom promotes student interaction and cooperative learning during morning lessons.

By shaping habits and roles, the demands and constraints of an environment can also negatively affect motives and action. In particular, many service environments have been noted to have adverse effects on their occupants. For example, rules, organized events, and concerns of staff in a day hospital for persons with dementia were found to stifle clients' attempts to engage in spontaneous behaviors and encouraged passivity and inactivity (Borell, Gustavsson, Sandman, & Kielhofner, 1994). People with Alzheimer's disease living in special long-term care units that were more institutional and less homelike tended to have more psychotic symptoms and aggressive behaviors (Zeisel et al., 2003).

Demands and constraints that are present in the physical, social, and occupational environment can also have a positive effect.

- An individual with dementia often benefits from being in familiar surroundings that are not overstimulating. In addition, the care facility limits access to objects that may present a safety risk. These practices constrain the physical environment to promote safety and well-being.
- Likewise, the social environment makes demands on a person, by requesting behaviors and demanding social norms. The attitudes and expectations of others are pivotal. An individual who is unemployed may stop looking for work unless their friends and family, and the wider society continue to expect their participation.
- Finally, the occupational environment has constraints and demands that may enhance or inhibit performance. For example, the challenges of keeping up with the pace of a more advanced exercise class may result in a young person experiencing a greater feeling of achievement.

IMPACT OF THE ENVIRONMENT

It is important to note the difference between features of an environment and its actual influence on specific persons. As Gitlin and Corcoran (2005) noted, the environment "may evoke varying degrees of influence on daily performance depending on factors such as a person's level of cognitive and physical competency, the person's appraisals of role and environmental demands, and the characteristics of ongoing interactions or transactions that transpire within the environment." **Environmental impact** refers to the opportunity, support, demand, and constraint that the environment has on a particular individual. Whether and how environmental opportunities, resources, constraints, and demands are noticed or felt depends on each person's current values, interests, personal causation, roles, habits, and performance capacities. For example, environments that challenge a person's capacities tend to evoke involvement, attentiveness, and maximal performance (Csikszentmihalyi, 1990; Lawton & Nahemow, 1973). On the other hand, when environments demand performance well below capacity, they can evoke boredom and disinterest. When demands are too far beyond capacity, they can make a person feel anxious, overwhelmed, or hopeless. Since persons have different capacities and beliefs in their own abilities, the same environment may engage and excite one person, bore another, and overwhelm a third.

The social model of disability recognizes that participation restrictions occur when the environmental factors create barriers and limit possibilities (Oliver, 1990). Qualitative research with 201 people with primarily physical disabilities provides real-life examples of how different environmental factors influence everyday participation in both positive and negative ways (Hammel et al., 2015). Positive outcomes include more choice and control, the ability to manage everyday life, and increased community access; negative or disabling outcomes include social isolation, segregation, and discrimination, with economic factors playing a major role (Hammel et al., 2015). Each person with a disability or health condition experiences environmental features differently, depending on their functional needs in mobility, cognitive, sensory, communication, or social domains (Hammel et al., 2015). This points to the importance of considering multiple factors when assessing environmental impact (Magasi et al., 2015). However, the priority should be to assess aspects of the environment that can be changed or that are expected to affect outcomes (Heinemann et al., 2015). Efforts are underway to develop environmental measures that will allow self-assessment of environmental demands by people with disabilities (Hammel et al., 2015; Heinemann et al., 2015), furthering understanding of the impact of the environment on participation across levels.

Levels of Environmental Influence

Bronfenbrenner's well-known work on social ecological theory describes four systems that affect the individual, from the immediate environment to the macrosystem, with cultural aspects cutting across all systems (Bronfenbrenner, 1993). Extensive qualitative

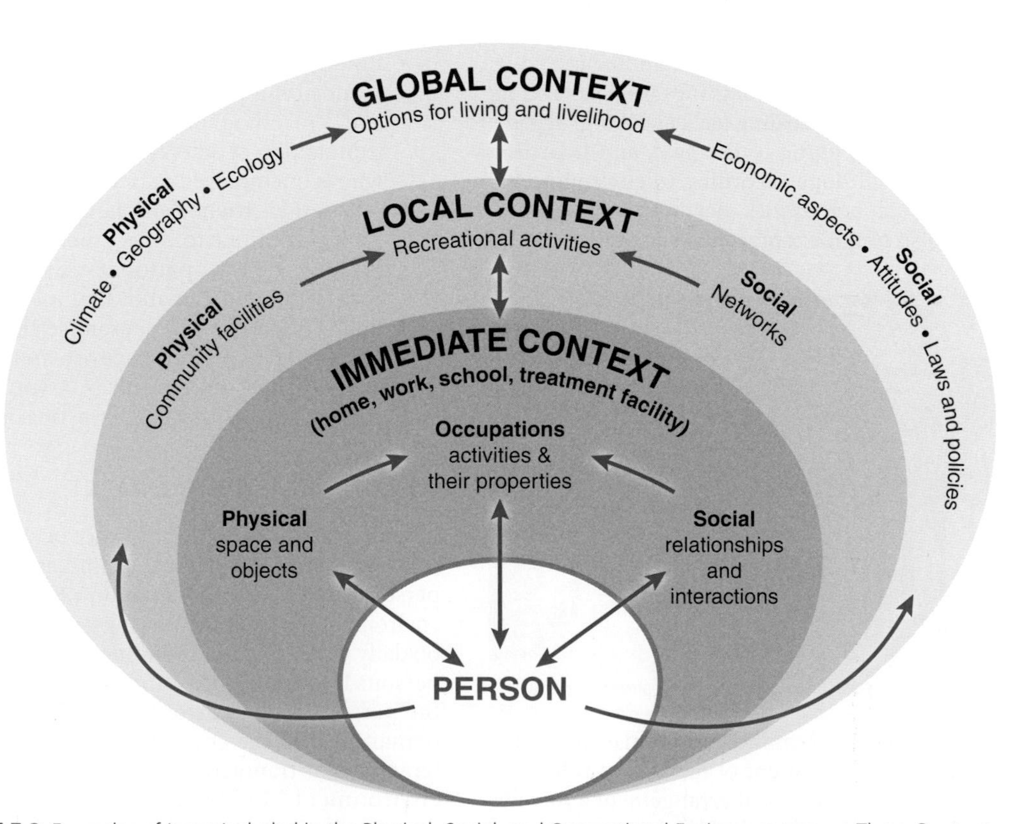

FIGURE 7-2 Examples of Items Included in the Physical, Social, and Occupational Environment across Three Contexts.

research indicates that environmental factors are experienced by people with disabilities at individual, community, and societal levels (Hammel et al., 2015).

The conceptualization of each person as interacting with multiple levels of the environment is useful to assist occupational therapy practitioners in considering relevant environmental aspects that are affecting the person. Therefore, the levels of *immediate, local, and global context* will be used to illustrate the environmental constructs and how they influence individuals and their participation in society.

- Immediate context includes home, work, school, and treatment facility/program
- Local includes community, neighborhood, and school campus
- Global includes economic and political aspects, social attitudes, laws and policies and systems of care, as well as aspects of climate and geography

The three dimensions of the environment—physical, social, and occupational—exist within each level. Figure 7-2 shows the same levels of environmental influence as depicted in Figure 7-1, but with greater detail and examples.

Cultural aspects, while not specifically named in Figure 7-2, are present at every level and are embedded in the physical and social environment of the home, workplace, community, and society (Altman & Chemers, 1980). **Culture** is historically defined as the beliefs and perceptions, values and norms, customs and behaviors that are shared by a group or society and are passed from one generation to the next through both formal and informal education (Altman & Chemers, 1980; Brake, 1980; Ogbu, 1981; Rapoport, 1980). It is important to consider if an environment is respectful and inclusive of an individual's cultural background and practices, whether at home, work, school, or in the community.

Similarly, accessibility and universal design features of the physical environment are relevant to consider at all levels. Universal design attempts to ensure access to spaces and objects by designing them to be barrier free, ensuring physical, cognitive, sensory, and linguistic access by all types of users (Law, 2015).

CASE EXAMPLE: SOCIAL JUSTICE TO ENABLE PARTICIPATION IN A SCHOOL SETTING

Lucy, aged 15 and in her second year of high school, was feeling invisible. While she had spinal muscular atrophy, a progressive neuromuscular condition that required her to use a wheelchair for mobility, she had above average intelligence and wanted to have a successful high school experience so she could be admitted to the college of her choice. Her occupational therapist in her first year of high school had helped her with some wheelchair modifications and adaptive devices for writing, which were helpful, but she did not address Lucy's frustration with the school's lack of attention to her needs. Her new occupational therapist was very familiar with the MOHO and chose to complete a *School Setting Interview* (SSI; Hemmingsson, Egilson, Hoffman, & Kielhofner, 2005) to highlight Lucy's priorities and environmental constraints.

The SSI is a student-centered interview assessment focusing on the school environment of students with disabilities. The SSI examines the level of student–environment fit of students from approximately 7 years of age and older and assists in planning target occupational therapy interventions in school. The assessment includes 16 items (and questions) concerning everyday school activities for which students may need adjustments and support to be able to participate. Each item is scored using a four-step rating scale ranging from *perfect fit* (when students do not need any adjustments at all) to *unfit* when the student lacks adjustments in school although the student has participation restrictions. The SSI is applicable for students with motor, cognitive, and psychosocial limitations and takes about 30 to 40 minutes to complete.

Lucy noted a lack of fit to her needs in the following areas: getting assistance, accessing the school, interacting with staff, and participating in practical activities during breaks. There was not an accessible bathroom on the third floor where most of her classes were held, no private space for her breathing treatments, a lack of fire safety options for students in wheelchairs, and a stage in the gym that was used for award ceremonies was not accessible to wheelchair users. Lucy felt stigmatized and frustrated by the lack of respect and social support. The school environment displayed limited compliance with policies that guaranteed her right to an equal education. The therapist recognized that Lucy's environment was characterized by constraints in *accessibility* and *adequacy of space*, availability of key objects such as a ramp, *emotional support*, supportive *attitudes*, and *adaptations*.

The occupational therapist worked with Lucy to investigate community resources to address these inequities. They found a local agency, *Equip for Equality*, that helped people with disabilities who felt their rights were being violated. The agency agreed to consult with Lucy and prepare her to address her complaints by educating her

on her legal rights. They assisted in drafting a letter to the school principal outlining her concerns and requested remediation, which included creating an additional accessible bathroom on the third floor, providing the nurse's office for her breathing treatments, implementing a fire rescue plan, and installing a ramp or lift for the stage. The occupational therapist coached Lucy in preparing for a meeting with the principal by role-playing how she could state her assessment of the problems and her requests for meeting her medical and safety needs so she could fully engage in her *occupational role* of being a student.

With the occupational therapist's support, Lucy was able to give examples of her limited occupational functioning and suggested remediation plans, and stated her plan to contact *Equip for Equality's* attorneys if the school did not comply with the school system law that guaranteed her the right to an equal education. The principal agreed to make the requested changes, which took 6 months to fully implement. Lucy was able to begin her third year of high school at a higher level of independence in a more supportive environment, thanks to her occupational therapist using the MOHO to focus on the constraints affecting her occupational role in the context of the school environment, rather than only addressing discrete physical limitations.

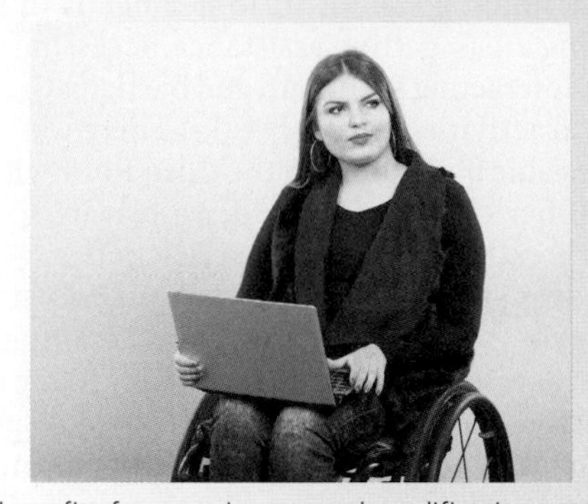

Lucy benefits from environmental modifications at school

Environmental Components: Assessment and Intervention

The varied components of the environment can impact a person's volition, roles and habits, skills and occupational participation. People participate in multiple environments, such as school, home, and community organizations. The differing resources and demands across the environments create both challenges and opportunities for the therapist to consider.

It is useful to consider different components of each environmental dimension—*physical, social, and occupational*—to evaluate how the environment is impacting the person, how the person is affecting the environment, how the components influence each other, and whether environmentally focused intervention is needed and can be implemented. Several MOHO assessments of the immediate work, home, and school environment have been developed to guide recommendations. Chapters 17 and 18 include detailed examples on how these assessments are implemented and used in practice. Furthermore, many of the other MOHO assessments include observation and description of environmental factors that can guide identification of the optimal environment as well as challenges and supports.

In addition to these MOHO assessments, a systematic description of environmental elements can assist therapists to use their observation and analysis skills to recognize the strengths, opportunities, and resources in the environment as well as the challenges, constraints, and demands, and how they affect the person. The knowledge gained will aid therapeutic reasoning and guide the intervention plan. Table 7-1 provides a MOHO-based taxonomy for environmental components and qualities that may impact the client's volition, habituation, performance, or participation. Not all of the elements are relevant to every client's situation, and the therapist determines what to focus on based on what is important to the client and context, as well as observation or report of problem areas. The left column of Table 7-1 includes examples of physical, social, and occupational environmental elements for the occupational therapist to consider when evaluating and modifying the environmental context within a MOHO framework. The right column includes the qualities of those environmental components that are possible areas for assessment and intervention to support personal causation, roles, habits, skills, and participation. Each component includes examples relevant to immediate, local, and global contexts.

While depicted as three separate elements, the components may affect each other. For example, the type of occupations and activities that are offered in a long-term treatment facility will be affected by the social environment and how knowledgeable the staff are about the residents' interests and preferences. Likewise, the willingness of the residents to participate in activities may affect their relationship with the staff. This complex interplay of factors within the three components is part of the overall environmental context and will challenge the therapist to determine how changes in one component may influence another component. This relationship will be depicted in case examples.

Environmental Interventions

The therapist can intervene at any level, but our primary focus when using MOHO is at the immediate environment level. Recommendations for environmental change can address home, school, community, work, hospital, day program, community, funding or policy, different age groups, a range of disabilities or health issues, and a variety of desires and challenges.

One example of a systematic MOHO-based approach to environmental analysis is the remotivation process (de las Heras et al., 2003). The remotivation process is a MOHO-based intervention process that was created in response to a lack of well-developed strategies aimed at people with very low volition. It supports the ongoing collaboration between the individual and the therapist, and the appropriate management of the physical, social, and occupational environment by describing a continuum of strategic interventions. These are arranged in a series of levels, stages, and steps designed to support progression through three modules: the exploration level, the competency level, and the achievement level.

Examples and cases follow, which illustrate the power of the environment in people's lives and how occupational therapists can influence the supportiveness of the environment. While these examples and cases are based on the authors' experiences, each individual can use them to generate examples that reflect their own cultural context and circumstances.

By evaluating the components and qualities of the environment (refer to Table 7-1) and working with clients, family members, and service providers to implement an environmental intervention plan, the occupational therapist can create a more supportive environment for the client.

- Following the occupational therapist's recommendations, a daughter caring for an aging parent who has fallen in the bathroom installs toilet handrails and increased lighting in the bathroom to prevent falls. Modification to improve *accessibility and safety of space* in the *immediate environment* is key to reducing fall risk and building self-efficacy.

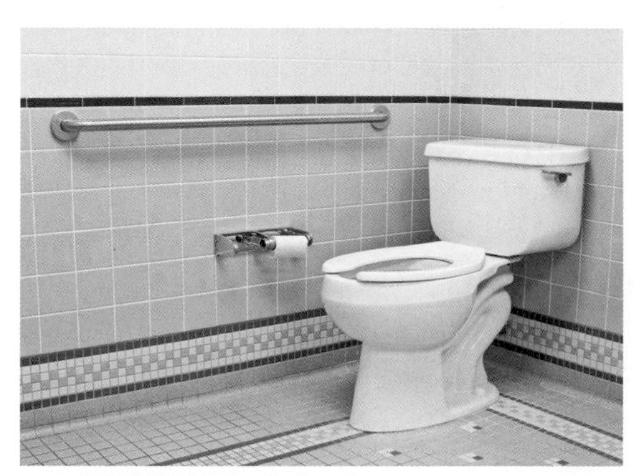

An accessible bathroom

- The occupational therapist assists a teacher in designing a quiet corner in the classroom with sensory objects such as a weighted blanket, soft cushions, and noise-reducing headphones. Providing a sensory-oriented space with adequate *availability of objects* can assist the students to recognize their need for certain types of sensory input and develop habits to take the initiative to meet that need independently.

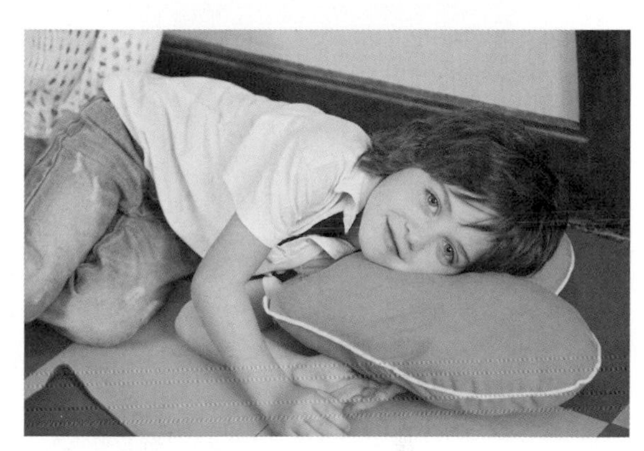

Sensory objects

- A nursing home provides a variety of craft materials in the day room that involve people working together to complete the activity, such as one person holding the pieces together while the other person applies glue. The occupational therapist can recommend *occupation and activity choices* that are well matched to the level of the clients, thus facilitating participation and enactment of interests.
- An inclusive playground is designed by the occupational therapist in consultation with a playground fabrication company. The therapist focuses on providing *choices of spaces* in the *local context* that maximize *accessibility* and teach children who use the park to respect each other's needs and play together.
- Occupational therapists incorporating the social model of disability (Oliver, 1990) can support *empowerment* through participation in collective action by connecting clients with disability advocates. Members and sympathizers of the disability community engage in demonstrations to raise awareness about disability and to protest against limits on *funding and policies* in the *global context* that disadvantage persons with disabilities, such as inadequate transportation services. In this way, they are having an impact on their community's *local environment*, rather than accepting the status quo.

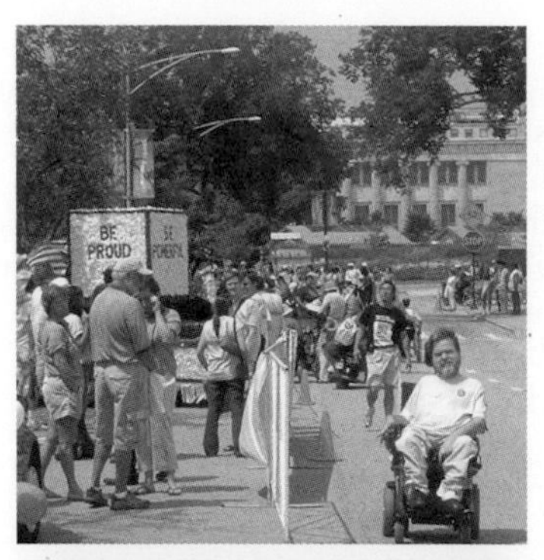

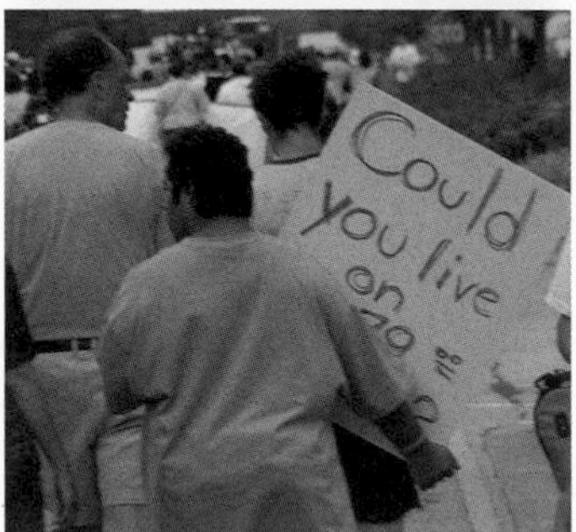

The annual Disability Pride Parade held in Chicago, Illinois

Case Examples

MOHO Problem-Solver Case: Supporting Participation at Home

Alex is an 8-year-old boy with severe intellectual disabilities and multiple physical disabilities. The referral requested occupational therapy involvement in Alex's care because it was thought that adaptive equipment was needed to support him in a functional position, to make his home accessible, and to ensure his safety. The occupational therapist used MOHO to guide her role of facilitating further changes in Alex's *social environment*. She knew that the robust management of *physical spaces and objects* would require a collaborative approach with all those involved in Alex's care, and so she provided information to help Alex's parents, taught them about Alex's condition, modeled how to interact with him, and trained them in moving and handling techniques. Once Alex's immediate physical and social needs were being met, she looked again to MOHO theory to guide her practice. She recognized that Alex's parents were doing a great deal to nurture their child and build his skills. They facilitated his *process* and *motor skills* in play and assisted his *performance* in activities of daily living, but he often seemed withdrawn and was sometimes agitated. She reasoned, "*Alex's wellbeing is dependent on the environment being adapted to meet his needs. How can he be helped to interact with the environment? How can he experience what it is like to make an impact on the environment? How can we support his active* participation?"

The therapist discussed Alex's *interests* with his mother to ensure a deeper understanding of the things of *value* to him, and together they found ways that would help Alex to be more in control of his physical space, objects, the social environment, and the activities he participated in. They asked themselves, "*How can we strengthen Alex's* personal causation? *How can Alex develop an understanding of his own abilities and what he is capable of? Ultimately, how can he gain a sense of his own* competence *when so much is being done for him?*"

For each of Alex's interests, they sought to help him experience cause and effect so that he could be more than a passive recipient. He delighted in music, and the occupational therapist was able to source a simple automatic control that Alex could use to switch his music on and off in his room. He had a warm and positive relationship with his parents, and the therapist reinforced the importance of them joining him in activities of apparent interest and employing intensive interaction techniques, such as mirroring Alex's vocalizations and movements so that he could engage in two-way *interaction*. She also made suggestions regarding a number of activities that would help to develop Alex's *coordination*: building towers of blocks for him to knock down; blowing bubbles for him to burst; utilizing a computer program with a touch screen that allowed him to manipulate images. Over time, his parents noticed an improvement in Alex's *communication*, as the items required for different activities could be used as objects of reference to help him choose between different options. He also appeared to have better knowledge of what was happening—*"We show him his washcloth, and he knows that it's bath time . . .He chooses the bath toys he wants to play with . . . He's so much more content and playful now that he is more in control."* The occupational therapist was able to document these changes, which showed improvements in *volition, habituation, and skills*, as well as the *environment*.

MOHO Problem-Solver Case: Making a Group Home More Resident Focused

A local agency running group homes for adults with moderate intellectual/developmental disabilities was reprimanded by the state public health department for not being sensitive to the residents' need for autonomy and empowerment. One of the homes had an inspection in 1 month, and the home administrator, Hector, contacted the occupational therapist for assistance because if they lost their approval from the state they would have to close. Hector also wanted to increase staff satisfaction and retention since the home had had a lot of staff turnover. Hector contacted an occupational therapist with a private consulting practice and stated, *"We really want to improve this home and not risk losing our approval and funding. We will hire you for 5-10 hours per week for the next month. I know most occupational therapists work with individuals, but I need you to work with the* environmental *problem that we have."*

Being well-versed in MOHO, the therapist was prepared for this consultation. She decided to begin by conducting an assessment of the environment using the Residential Environment Impact Scale (REIS), version 4.0 (Fisher et al., 2014). The REIS is a semistructured environmental assessment designed to examine the impact of various aspects of the physical, social, and occupational environment of an institutional setting on its inhabitants. The REIS uses four data collection methods to gather the information needed to comprehensively evaluate how well the facility provides support and opportunities in four areas: everyday space, everyday objects, enabling relationships, and structure of activities. Data are collected by a walk-through of the home, observation of three daily routines or activities, an interview of the residents, and an interview of a caregiver.

Findings from the REIS can be used to guide recommendations aimed at improving the residents' sense of identity and competence in meaningful and culturally appropriate activities. The REIS can be used with a range of residential settings, including group homes, nursing homes, and single-family dwellings serving individuals with a wide range of health and disability circumstances.

- Conducting this assessment allowed the therapist to get a full picture of how the group home's strengths and areas for improvement impacted the residents, both individually and collectively. The therapist used the results to identify the following priorities for a remediation plan: increase opportunities for residents to enact their personal causation, by increasing their exposure to desired objects, opportunities to personalize their living spaces, and opportunities to engage in activities of interest.

This process involved getting to know the interests and preferences of each resident, and providing time and resources for them to explore and engage in those interests incrementally over time.

- Create a nonstigmatizing integrated social context in which residents and staff interact with one another as respected peers.

Previously, the staff within the home interacted spontaneously with one another, only interacting with the residents when there were problems or assistance was needed. The rest of the time, the staff paid more attention to each other than to the residents. This had the effect of making the residents feel like they were second-class citizens within the home. The staff changed their behavior by interacting with the residents as their primary relationships, by acknowledging the residents' unique roles and interests and sharing their own interests and opinions with the residents.

Since the therapist only had 1 month, she began by providing staff with consultation regarding their daily *habits* and routines within the home. She asked each staff member to gather information about ways in which each resident might explore his or her interests and have the opportunity to make choices within their daily lives. An idea that emerged from the staff was to have the residents run their own weekly community meeting rather than having staff lead the joint meeting. This would allow the residents to have input on the activities and shopping trips planned for each week and policies of the home such as use of the telephone and hours for visitors.

Hector visited the home after 3 weeks and was pleased with the initial changes that had been implemented. The home manager told him, "*Having an outside person come in and see what we are doing through fresh eyes is very helpful. We are with the residents so much that we don't see what they are capable of.*" She noted that there was increased communication among the residents during group meetings and increased resident cooperation, with the residents talking to one another with more familiarity. She mentioned that there was a difference in the staff morale and interaction with the residents. Staff deferred to the residents, asking their preferences or opinions before making collaborative decisions.

Through evaluating the *physical, social, and occupational environment* and implementing changes, the therapist had solved the problem facing this organization. The home passed the inspection, allowing the residents to continue their community-based life in a supportive environment.

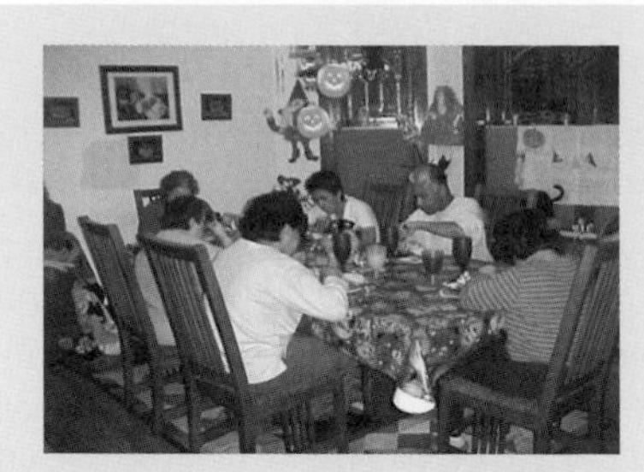

Residents sitting at the table having dinner

Conclusion

As these diverse examples and cases illustrate, modifying the environment can exert an all-important influence on occupation. Considering how the environment impacts occupation as well as how people interact with their environments is essential to providing environmentally focused recommendations and interventions that enable participation.

Acknowledgments

The authors acknowledge contributions from Helena Hemmingsson, Lucy Trevino, Joanne Lee, and Renée R. Taylor, and the mentorship of our treasured colleague, Gary Kielhofner.

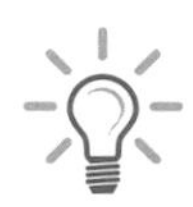

Chapter 7 Review Questions

1. Describe the different levels of environment: immediate, local, and global.
2. List examples of what is included in the physical environment, social environment, and occupational environment.
3. Provide an example of how the social environment can influence the occupational environment.
4. Explain how high environmental demands can be a positive influence on performance and participation.
5. Define and explain the concept of environmental impact.
6. a. Give three examples of how factors in the environment can be used to improve volition.
   b. Give three examples of how factors in the environment can be used to improve habituation.
   c. Give three examples of how factors in the environment can be used to improve skills.
7. Discuss how intervention at the different levels of the environment (immediate, local, and global) can support occupational participation.
8. Describe how someone's cultural background and beliefs can influence their physical, social, and occupational environmental needs.
9. Give examples of how the environment can be assessed using different methods for collection of information.
10. Choose one of the case studies and list the environmental contexts that were addressed by the therapist. What modifications did the therapist make to enable participation?

HOMEWORK ASSIGNMENTS

1. Analyze your own environment and determine if any changes can be made to make it more supportive for your occupational functioning. Include an analysis of your physical, social, and occupational environment.
2. Is your favorite restaurant or store accessible to wheelchair users? Are purchasing options available in alternative formats for people who have limited vision or hearing? What changes could be made to improve accessibility?
3. What policies support or restrict access to housing, health care, and employment opportunities for people with a mental illness?

thePoint® For additional resources and exercises, visit http://thePoint.lww.com

Key Terms

Culture: Beliefs and perceptions, values and norms, customs and behaviors that are shared by a group or society and are passed from one generation to the next through both formal and informal education.

Environment: Particular physical, social, and occupational features of the specific context in which one does something that impacts upon what one does, and how it is done.

Environmental impact: Actual influence (in the form of opportunity, resources, demand, or constraint) that the physical and social aspects of the environment have on a particular individual.

Objects: Naturally occurring or fabricated things with which people interact and whose properties influence what they do with them.

Spaces: Physical contexts that are bounded and arranged in ways that influence what people do within them.

REFERENCES

Altman, I., & Chemers, M. (1980). *Culture and environment*. Monterey, CA: Brooks/Cole.

American Occupational Therapy Association. (2014). Occupational therapy practice framework: Domain and process (3rd ed.). *American Journal of Occupational Therapy, 68*(Suppl. 1), S1–S48. doi:10.5014/ajot.2014.682006

Borell, L., Gustavsson, A., Sandman, P., & Kielhofner, G. (1994). Occupational programming in a day hospital for patients with dementia. *Occupational Therapy Journal of Research, 14,* 219–238.

Brake, M. (1980). *The sociology of youth culture and youth cultures*. London, United Kingdom: Routledge & Kegan Paul.

Bronfenbrenner, U. (1992). Ecological systems theory. In R. Vasta (Ed.), *Annals of child development: Six theories of child development: Revised formulations and current issues* (pp. 187–249). London, United Kingdom: Jessica Kingsley.

Bronfenbrenner, U. (1993). The ecology of cognitive development: Research models and fugitive findings. In R. H. Wozniak & K. W. Fischer (Eds.), *Development in context: Acting and thinking in specific environments* (pp. 3–44). Hillsdale, NJ: Lawrence Erlbaum Associates.

Csikszentmihalyi, M. (1990). *Flow: The psychology of optimal experience*. New York, NY: Harper & Row.

de las Heras, C. G., Llerena, V., & Kielhofner, G. (2003). *The Remotivation Process* [*Version 1.0*]. Chicago: Model of Human Occupation Clearinghouse, Department of Occupational Therapy, University of Illinois at Chicago.

Fisher, G., Forsyth, K., Harrison, M., Angarola, R., Kayhan, E., Noga, P., et al. (2014). *Residential Environment Impact Scale (REIS)* [*Version 4.0*]. Chicago: Model of Human Occupation Clearinghouse, Department of Occupational Therapy, University of Illinois at Chicago.

Gitlin, L. M., & Corcoran, M. (2005). *Occupational therapy and dementia care: The home environmental skills building program for individuals and families*. Bethesda, MD: America Occupational Therapy Association.

Hammel, J., Magasi, S., Heinemann, A., Gray, D. B., Stark, S., Kisala, P., et al. (2015). Environmental barriers and supports to everyday participation: A qualitative insider perspective from people with disabilities. *Archives of Physical Medicine and Rehabilitation, 96*(4), 578–588.

Heinemann, A. W., Magasi, S., Hammel, J., Carlozzi, N. E., Garcia, S. F., Hahn, E. A., et al. (2015). Environmental factors item development for persons with stroke, traumatic brain injury, and spinal cord injury. *Archives of Physical Medicine and Rehabilitation, 96*(4), 589–595.

Hemmingsson, H., Egilson, S., Hoffman, O., & Kielhofner G. (2005). *The School Setting Interview (SSI)* [*Version 3.0*]. Nacka, Sweden: Swedish Association of Occupational Therapists.

Jonsson, H., Josephsson, S., & Kielhofner, G. (2000). Evolving narratives in the course of retirement: A longitudinal study. *American Journal of Occupational Therapy, 54,* 263–270.

Kielhofner, G. (2008). *Model of human occupation: Theory and application* (4th ed.). Philadelphia, PA: Lippincott Williams & Wilkins.

Law, M. (1991). The environment: A focus for occupational therapy. *Canadian Journal of Occupational Therapy, 58,* 171–179.

Law, M. (2015). The environmental determinants of occupation. In M. A. McColl, M. C. Law, & D. Stewart (Eds.), *Theoretical basis of occupational therapy* (3rd ed., pp. 113–122). Thorofare, NJ: SLACK.

Lawton, M. P. (1980). *Environment and aging*. Monterey, CA: Brooks/Cole.

Lawton, M. P., & Nahemow, L. (1973). Ecology and the aging process. In C. Eisdorfer & M. P. Lawton (Eds.), *Psychology of adult development and aging*. Washington, DC: American Psychological Association.

Magasi, S., Hammel, J., Heinemann, A., Whiteneck, G., & Bogner, J. (2009). Participation: A comparative analysis of multiple rehabilitation stakeholders' perspectives. *Journal of Rehabilitation Medicine, 41*(11), 936–944.

Magasi, S., Wong, A., Gray, D. B., Hammel, J., Baum, C., Wang, C. C., et al. (2015). Theoretical foundations for the measurement of environmental factors and their impact on participation among people with disabilities. *Archives of Physical Medicine and Rehabilitation, 96*(4), 569–577.

Moore-Corner, R. A., Kielhofner, G., & Olson, L. (1998). *A user's manual for the Work Environment Impact Scale (WEIS)* [*Version 2.0*]. Chicago: Model of Human Occupation Clearinghouse, Department of Occupational Therapy, University of Illinois at Chicago.

Ogbu, J. U. (1981). Origins of human competence: A cultural-ecological perspective. *Child Development, 52*, 413–429.

Oliver, M. (1990). *The politics of disablement.* Basingstoke, United Kingdom: Macmillan.

Rapoport, A. (1980). Cross-cultural aspects of environmental design. In I. Altman, A. Rapoport, & J. F. Wohlwill (Eds.), *Human behavior and environment* (Vol. 4). New York, NY: Plenum.

World Health Organization. (2001). *International classification of functioning, disability and health: ICF.* Geneva, Switzerland: Author.

Zeisel, J., Silverstein, N. M., Hyde, J., Levkoff, S., Lawton, M. P., & Holmes, W. (2003). Environmental correlates to behavioral health outcomes in Alzheimer's special care units. *The Gerontologist, 43*(5), 697–711.

Dimensions of Doing

Carmen-Gloria de las Heras de Pablo, Chia-Wei Fan, and Gary Kielhofner (posthumous)

CHAPTER 8

EXPECTED LEARNING OUTCOMES

Upon completion of this chapter, readers will be able to:

1. Identify the three levels of doing that form the foundation of our understanding of occupation.
2. Provide examples of how people with diverse performance capacities engage in occupation.
3. Understand the complexity behind dimensions of participation in occupation.
4. Apply these expanded dimensions of participation to recognize the uniqueness of each client in practice.
5. Define the concept of occupational adaptation in practice with diverse populations.

Within the Model of Human Occupation, doing has been described at three levels (Haglund & Henriksson, 1995): occupational participation, occupational performance, and occupational skills (Fig. 8-1).

Occupational participation defines what we do in the broadest sense (Kielhofner, 2008). For this reason, it forms the focus of most of what will be explicated in this chapter. Participation describes our engagement in the broad categories of work (study), play, and the activities of daily living that undergird everyday life (Kielhofner, 2008). According to Kielhofner (2008), participation is collectively influenced by one's

- volition,
- habituation,
- performance capacity, and
- environment

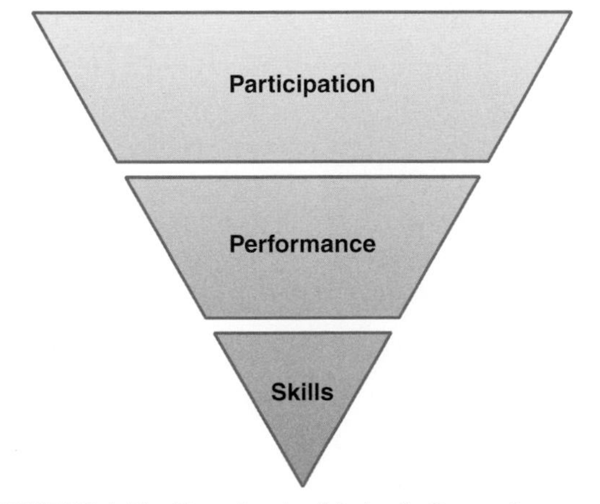

FIGURE 8-1 The Three Levels of Doing in Occupation.

As noted above, participation in an activity may involve doing a variety of things. **Occupational performance** comprises discrete acts, or units of doing, that are performed. Within the Model of Human Occupation (Kielhofner, 2008), occupational performance may be viewed as engaging in an occupational form (Nelson, 1988). Engaging in an occupational form involves completing (or literally going through the form of) a discrete act that may involve a series of steps that lead to a coherent whole or desired activity (Kielhofner, 2008). For example, as an occupational therapy student, your activities may involve not only reading this text, but also a wide range of other tasks (or occupational forms), such as studying for your medical conditions exam, preparing a research paper, and observing a practicing occupational therapist on fieldwork. Another example of an occupational form may involve one of your leisure activities, such as cycling. This may involve getting your bicycle serviced and ready to ride, planning where to ride, finding a friend with whom to enjoy the activity, and getting on the bicycle and pedaling at various speeds. In these ways, you are enacting the occupational form of bicycling. Your activities of daily living can include such things as bathing, checking your bank balance, and preparing dinner, all of which comprise various steps.

When these acts are repeated as part of a routine, they become habits. Habits are more likely to form when a person makes a volitional choice to engage in an act. Each act, and eventual habit of performance, takes shape within a social and physical environment that, hopefully, facilitates that act. Thus, in addition to volition and habitation, the environment is critically important in terms of its ability to enable (or restrict) one's performance. For example, powered mobility and a paved sidewalk may make it possible for a child to perform the act of touring a museum while attending a field trip with her classmates.

The observable, goal-directed actions that make up occupational performance are referred to as **occupational skills** (Fisher, 1999; Fisher & Kielhofner, 1995; Forsyth, Salamy, Simon, & Kielhofner, 1997). Within the Model of Human Occupation, three types of skills are recognized: **motor skills**, **process skills**, and **communication and interaction skills**. Motor skills define moving one's body or objects in one's environment. Specific motor skills include, but are not limited to, bending or stabilizing one's body and manipulating, lifting, or carrying objects. Process skills involve logically sequencing actions over time, selecting and using appropriate tools and materials, and adapting performance to overcome obstacles. **Communication and interaction skills** include being able to convey one's intentions and needs and to express oneself in a way that allows for involvement and coordinated social action with others (Forsyth et al., 1997; Forsyth & Kielhofner, 1999). Figure 8-2 presents a visual depiction of the skills included within the Model of Human Occupation (Kielhofner, 2008). Assessments that are based on MOHO, including the Assessment of Communication and Interaction Skills (Forsyth et al., 1997) and the Assessment of Motor and Process Skills (Fisher & Bray Jones, 2003), offer a detailed breakdown of additional skills that fall within each of these areas.

Participation in occupations has been conceptualized as involving the constant interaction of humans' feeling, thinking, and acting in and with the world. These three factors—feeling, thinking,

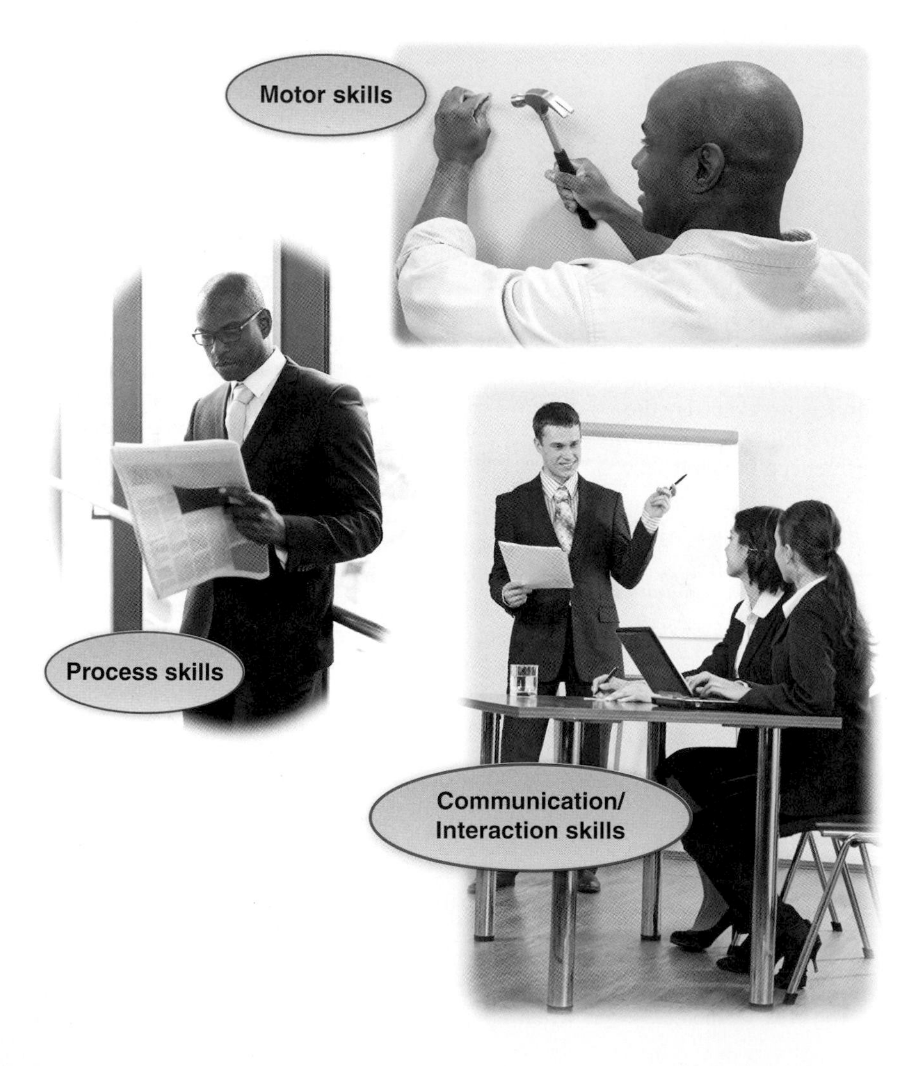

FIGURE 8-2 Three Types of Skills.

and acting—interrelate in different ways, and each one takes a more or less active role according to the unique person's reality of performance capacities, volition, habituation, and environmental impact (de las Heras de Pablo, 2011; Kielhofner, 2008, 1985). Coherent with this affirmation are occupational therapy principles that focus on the potentials and the essence of being in every person we work with (Kielhofner, 2008, 1985).

Ongoing studies on volition and the remotivation process (de las Heras de Pablo, Llerena, & Kielhofner, 2003), together with the evidence of practicing with persons of a wide range of performance capacities, have converged on the need to reframe concepts and expand the dimensions of doing presented previously in this chapter, in order to clarify and improve evaluation and intervention processes grounded in MOHO (de las Heras de Pablo, 2011, 2015; de las Heras de Pablo, Geist, Kielhofner, & Li, 2007; Melton et al., 2008; Parkinson, Cooper, de las Heras de Pablo, & Forsyth, 2014; Pépin, Guerrete, Lefebvre, & Jacques, 2008; Raber, Teitelmann, Watts, & Kielhofner, 2010).

CASE EXAMPLE: A WORKER RECOVERING FROM A MILD TRAUMATIC BRAIN INJURY

Alex is a 38-year-old mechanic in the process of replacing a leaking tire. The question "What is Alex doing?" might be answered in any of the following ways, depending upon one's perspective on doing (Kielhofner, 2008). For example:

- **Alex is making a series of calculated judgments and motor actions.**
- **Alex is changing a tire.**
- **Alex is engaging in a type of work.**

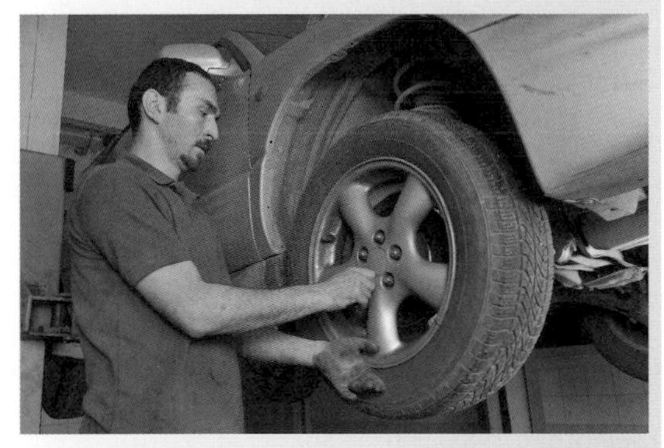

Alex changing a tire at work

In addition to these responses, we could also answer the question by placing Alex's actions into a larger context (Kielhofner, 2008). For instance, Alex is not only working, but he is also doing only one among many activities involved in his daily work routine as a mechanic: repairing and replacing tires. Within this activity, Alex uses motor skills to adjust the nuts on the tire with one hand, while he stabilizes the tire with the other. His process skills allow him to make a series of calculated judgments involving the weight and stability of the tire given its height above the ground, so that he may execute his fine and gross motor skills. These actions require intense concentration as he manages his balance on his feet and the slight tremor in his hands, both lingering effects of his head injury. At the same time, Alex demonstrates volition toward this activity because he enjoys what he is doing, feels responsible for doing it well, and is confident about what he is doing. Whenever he becomes fatigued or has a headache, his workplace environment allows him the accommodation of retreating to a break room to lie down in the dark. Once he feels better, he stays a little later to finish his work or comes in early the next day to get the job done. He interacts with his manager to negotiate when he needs a break, and communicates about when the job is finished and how it should be billed.

Within this example, we learn about Alex's daily work routine and about what motivates him to participate in work. He feels good about what he is doing and is responsible for his job. He demonstrates an ability to perform the act of changing a tire using his motor and process skills. His work environment provides adequate environmental supports that allow him to perform his work by taking quite rest breaks in a dark room, when needed. Taken together, all of the aspects of Alex's engagement in work demonstrate how volition, habituation, performance capacity, and the environment converge to positively affect Alex's work participation.

CASE EXAMPLE: AN OLDER ADULT WITH DEMENTIA

Now, let's shift from this image to another example.

Maria is a 77-year-old woman who had been a recognized artist in her country. Her life was dedicated to painting and to taking care of her children and husband. Due to Alzheimer's disease, she now stays at home and spends most of her time sitting on a sofa in her living room, close to a nursing aid who sits nearby. Her husband, a busy professional, does not take her into account. He

expects her not to bother him. Her occupational therapist has arranged a space at her home, for her, to explore and recapture part of her artist role through painting wooden boxes, frames, and small containers. Her space is organized in a room which was used as a library, with a flexible good-sized artist table, some of her paintings, a firm adjustable chair for her and another for her therapist or nursing aid. Her own brushes, painting, and other needed objects are organized over the table, close to her.

For today's session, the task that is chosen between Maria and her therapist consists of decorating useful wooden boxes using paint. This task has three recognizable steps: painting the box in one color, designing and painting designs over the already-painted box, and varnishing the box.

Every time Maria enters that space, she smiles and readily sits on the chair. Soon she begins painting the boxes or designing the motif (often stylized flowers) over the dried painted object, showing her competence that has accumulated through the years. When feeling tired, she leaves the space and goes back to her room, forgetting what she did. Each morning and afternoon her nursing aid invites Maria to this room so her quality time can remain regardless of the disease. Maria feels satisfied every time she spends her time there.

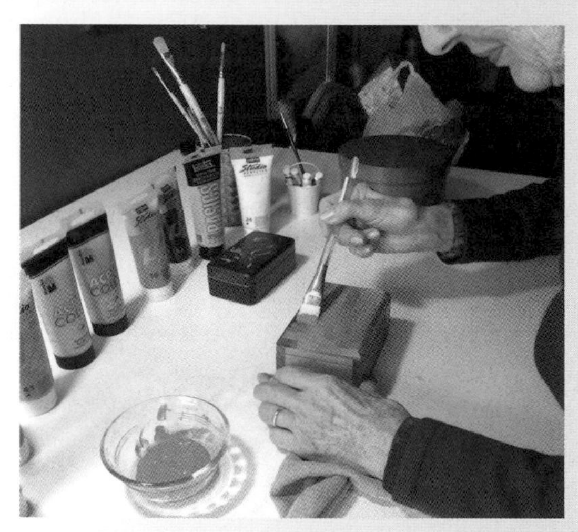

Maria painting a wooden box figure

What is Maria doing? Maria's doing may be explained as follows:

- Maria is performing the first and the second steps of something she used to do as part of the most important and pleasurable activity of her past role as an artist.
- Maria is using process skills (making judgments) when deciding what designs to paint and with which colors and ways she would do it, when adjusting the position of the box, or adapting her position and movements to effectively engage in painting. She is using motor skills when making motor actions by maintaining her arm position and smoothly combining movements to handle the brush when painting and designing the wooden box.

Maria is feeling pleasure, and is affectively connected with her life experience and history when engaging in painting, in her home.

A Cross-section of Occupation: Dimensions of Participation

The World Health Organization uses the term "participation" to refer to a person's involvement in life situations which makes him/her take part in society along with their experiences in their life contexts (World Health Organization [WHO], 2001). Currently, the Occupational Therapy Practice Framework uses the term "participation in occupations" as the way to achieve health, well-being, and participation in life (American Occupational Therapy Association [AOTA], 2014).

As reviewed at the beginning of this chapter and in Figure 8-1, the Model of Human Occupation has conceptualized three levels of doing: (a) occupational participation or participation in occupational roles; (b) occupational performance or the doing of occupational forms/tasks, and (c) occupational skills or actions with a purpose that are necessary for the completion of occupational forms/tasks (Kielhofner, 2002, 2008; Haglund & Henriksson, 1995).

A deeper reflection around the levels of doing and how the unique ways of feeling, thinking, and acting interrelate in each person was undertaken based on the occupational needs of persons with severe disabilities. These individuals had limitations in their cognitive capacities, limitations that interfered or inhibited with their possibilities of doing in the broadest sense, limitations of performance, and limitations of even engaging in an observable action. These people, nonetheless, had other potential for participating in occupations that had been observed through practice (de las Heras de Pablo, 2011, 2015; Kielhofner, 1985, 2008; Raber et al., 2010).

In this chapter, we have defined participation as persons' involvement in occupations. **Dimensions of participation** emphasize the diverse ways people become involved in occupations, considering their maximum potential for cognitive and physical capacity. This is acknowledged from the perspective of both objective measures of performance and the subjective experience of the client (de las Heras de Pablo et al., 2003, 2007; Goode, 1983).

Participation in occupation emerges from the constant interaction between persons' performance capacities, habituation, volition, and the environment. Therefore, it is both personal and contextual. It is personal in that the types of dimensions of participation in which a person will engage are influenced by the individual's unique motives, patterns of organization, and abilities and limitations. It is contextual in that the environment is part of a person's participation, providing conditions for either enabling or restricting it (Kielhofner, 2008). In this chapter, we define six dimensions of participation (Fig. 8-3). These dimensions reflect the systems perspective within the Model of Human Occupation, which calls for an integration of different aspects of volition, habituation, performance capacity, and environment when making sense of a person's occupational participation.

PARTICIPATION IN OCCUPATIONAL ROLES

Participating in occupational roles refers to engaging in occupations in the broadest sense. Performing the acts required for valued occupational roles (worker, player, amateur, student, family member, etc.) tells us that these could be desired and/or necessary to one's well-being. Participating in occupational roles involves taking part in long-term life projects that have a *personal and unique meaning* that pertains to work/productive activity, activities of daily living, or play/leisure occupations. Thus, no single categorization of occupations is proposed by MOHO. Readers may wish to examine the WHO classification and the AOTA practice framework classification (AOTA, 2014; WHO, 2001) as examples of how areas of participation can be identified. Participating in roles entails organizing and performing diverse activities for its fulfillment, conveying all dimensions of participation. Examples of participating in roles are volunteering for an organization, working in a full- or part-time job, recreating regularly with friends, doing self-care, maintaining one's living space, and attending school.

For example, a 10-year-old child may participate in the roles of family member, student, and amateur. As part of these roles the child would participate in activities like routine chores at home and family outings, school attendance and homework, sports and free play, and activities of personal hygiene and dressing. The child's school attendance and family activities are primarily shaped by societal expectations and social roles assigned to the child. What kind of sports the child plays may depend on capacities, interests, and available opportunities in the environment. Free play activities are a result of activity choices that reflect the child's personal causation, values, and interests as well as the opportunities provided in the physical and social environment. Thus, we can see that a complex interaction of personal and environmental factors ultimately shapes the full spectrum of occupational participation in a person's life.

VOLITIONAL PROCESSES, OBJECTIVE APPRAISAL, AND SUBJECTIVE EXPERIENCE: AN INTERACTION

Volitional processes can take diverse forms according to the persons' experience of his or her cognitive abilities, how he or she feels while engaging in occupations (subjective experience of performance capacity), and the opinions and feedbacks provided by an objective observer (objective appraisal of performance capacity). Volition may also vary in terms of the extent to which an activity is habituated, and with respect to the flexibility of the environment in terms of its affordances, restrictions, and mutability in response to the actor.

Based on these variables, an individual's volition toward participating in a particular occupation or occupational role follows a volitional process (Kielhofner, 2008), which may range from (1) merely experiencing the doing of an activity, to (2) experiencing and

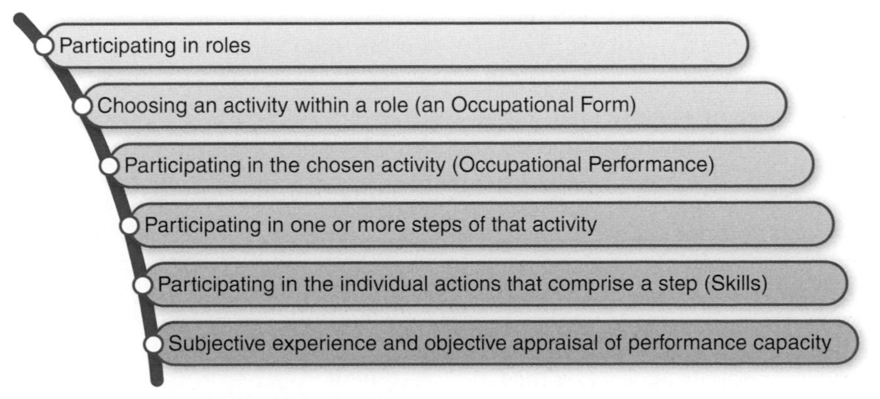

FIGURE 8-3 The Six Dimensions of Occupational Participation.

choosing, to (3) experiencing, interpreting, anticipating, and choosing. In the same way, an individual's volitional process progressively develops and unfolds through various periods in a person's life. It can retake simpler forms again, if abilities decrease or cease and/or environmental restrictions persist over time (de las Heras de Pablo, 2015). A larger number of people than we can imagine have difficulties even performing the skills required for the specific steps of a given activity (or occupational form).

MOHO Problem-Solver Case: A Mother with Lupus

Luisa is a 47-year-old widowed mother of two with systemic lupus erythematosus. In her role as a mother, Luisa used to perform all of the important activities with her children both at school and at home. This included taking them to school early in the morning and picking them up late in the afternoon, attending monthly meetings at school, rehearsing with them before participating in artistic or competitive events, helping them with some homework, facilitating their problem solving under stressful situations, doing housework with them, taking them to parties or extracurricular activities, and going shopping, among others. She also worked as a freelance writer and editor, which kept her awake until the middle of the night as she rushed to complete various deadlines.

After her diagnosis of lupus, she became progressively fatigued and developed severe, chronic pain. She was referred for physical therapy to manage the pain, and to occupational therapy to learn energy conservation strategies. However, her loss of energy and high levels of pain were not improved by these treatments and eventually inhibited her participation in all occupations. She was admitted into an intensive treatment center. She had to stay in bed for long periods of time, and quickly became demoralized. The only thing she was able to do was focus on the positive accomplishments of her children, sending them encouraging text messages and praising them on Facebook for their many accomplishments. Although she slowly began to recover her physical capacities through physical therapy, she had refused treatment with the occupational therapist, who began the relationship by inquiring about ways they might plan for Luisa's return to her worker role as a writer and editor.

Recognizing that she was not making any progress with Luisa, the occupational therapist decided to reconceptualize her disability experience from a MOHO perspective. The one thing that the therapist observed was that Luisa was content every time she was able to make a movement. Noticing the pleased expression on her face, she inquired as to what Luisa was thinking. Luisa responded that she was thinking that, perhaps on time, she would become a "full mother" again. Thus, the two of them began to focus their efforts upon recovering as much participation in the mother role as possible.

After a year, while still experiencing pain and fatigue, Luisa was able to invoke certain motor, process, and communication and interaction skills to perform some of the steps of some of the activities she used to do as a mother. For example, she enjoyed playing guitar with her youngest daughter, which used to be part of their many activities of rehearsing before an artistic event. The therapist provided her with an adaptation so that Luisa did not have to bear the entire weight of the guitar while playing and could remain seated upright rather than hunched over her knee. Luisa not only felt capable, valued, and joyful while playing guitar with her daughter, but the therapist reinforced both her and her daughter's abilities by offering a positive, objective appraisal.

The specific skills that made up Luisa's performance capacity were not the only attributes necessary for her to participate in valued tasks again. Her volition to sustain her role as a mother, which was initially noticed by her occupational therapist and reinforced by a number of environmental supports, sustained her occupational participation. These environmental supports were not only social, including her family and children's understanding, their emotional support, and the support of her therapist, but also physical, including the physical assistance she received from her family, and the adapted equipment for guitar playing, toileting, major hygiene, feeding, and other personal care tasks (Table 8-1).

As seen in this example, volition and environmental factors are also critical to whether and how impairments affect occupational performance. Positive volition, adapted equipment, and social support make possible for a person to complete an occupational form/task despite limitations of performance capacity.

Table 8-1 The Dynamics of Luisa's Participation in Occupation: Being a Mother

Dimension of Participation	Before First Episode of Systemic Lupus	While Living the First Episode of Systemic Lupus	A Year After First Episode of Systemic Lupus
Participation in an occupational role	Being a "full mother"	Could not participate in this role	Could not participate in role of mother
Choosing an activity within a role	Multiple activities as a mother	Could not participate in any activities	Could participate in five activities. A chosen activity was: Rehearsing with children prior to their participation in a musical event
Participating in that activity	Participates in all aspects of the activities of a mother	Could not participate in any aspects	One of the aspects of this activity: Helping daughter to learn playing the guitar
Participating in one or more steps of that activity	Participates on needed steps of each aspect of each activity	Could not participate in any steps, of any aspects, of any activities	Making a plan together for sequencing the common task, taking the guitar out of its container, tuning the guitar, playing the guitar
Performing one or more actions of a step	All process, motor and communication and interaction skills	Positioning, gazing, expressing through gesturing, speaking short phrases, collaborating, focusing, relating and respecting children when being helped and emotionally supported by them	Holding and lifting the guitar, positioning, coordinating, manipulating, attending, noticing, sequencing, asking, speaking, sharing, collaborating
Subjective experience and objective appraisal	Sense of commitment, pleasure, and efficacy that was also observed by others	Subjective sense of commitment while being with children. Helplessness	Subjective sense of commitment and satisfaction. Objective signs of appreciation from children

PARTICIPATION IN DEPTH

Examining participation in more depth leads us to consider the additional dimensions of occupational roles and of how a person's subjective experience (feelings about doing) and objective appraisal (others' evaluation of a person's doing) not only affect performance capacity, but also affect volition (Kielhofner, 2008). Table 8-2 summarizes this expanded configuration of participation.

This configuration considers participating in doing activities and participating in doing occupational forms/tasks as different, recognizing participation in activities of a role as a larger dimension of doing than performing occupational forms/tasks and as

Table 8-2 Defining Alex's Participation as a Worker

Participation	Participation in a specific occupational role • *Alex is participating in his worker role as an auto mechanic*
Performance	Performance of specific activities (i.e., occupational forms) within the occupational role • *Alex changes a tire* Performance of discrete steps, or units of action, that are required for changing a tire. • *Alex must diagnose the problem with the tire, determine if it should be fixed or replaced, position the jack, lift the tire off of the wheel, etc.*
Skills	Motor, process, and communication and interaction skills required for performance of the discrete steps • *Alex uses fine and gross motor skills to maintain his balance and manipulate the jack, wheel, and various aspects of the tire. Alex uses process skills to diagnose the problem with the tire and determine if it should be replaced. Alex uses communication and interaction skills to negotiate his break time and to notify his manager about job completion and billing.*
Subjective experience and objective appraisal	Subjective experience of the activity through Alex's feelings about his occupational circumstance (changing the tire) and objective appraisal by an independent observer (e.g., the approval of Alex's employer)

a smaller dimension than occupational participation. The specific acts that Alex had to perform in his worker role as a mechanic included diagnosing problems that customers identify, working with the electrical system, deep engine cleaning, repairing and replacing parts, changing oil and fluids, and replacing and repairing tires.

In the case example, Alex is performing just one aspect of his worker role, the act of changing a tire. The specific steps he needed to perform for changing a tire included: (step 1) diagnosing the reason for the flat tire, (step 2) determining if the tire could be repaired or if it needed to be replaced altogether, (step 3) positioning the jack that hoists the car into the air, (step 4) taking the hub cap off the defective tire, (step 5) removing the nuts that hold the tire to the wheel, (step 6) lifting the tire off the wheel, (step 7) examining the wheel for damage, (step 8) replacing the tire, (step 9) adhering the nuts back to the wheel, (step 10) adjusting the air pressure in the tire, (step 11) affixing the hub cap, (step 12) lowering the jack so that the car returns to the ground, and (step 13) communicating with his manager about job completion and billing.

As described earlier in the case example, each of these steps requires different combinations of motor, process, and communication and interaction skills. Integral to this process are Alex's unique experience and feelings while he is completing this activity, as well as his employer's objective appraisal of his performance.

Participation in Performing One or More Steps of a Task

Consider Maria and her participation in painting. She was able to perform two steps of a task: putting a base coat of paint onto a wooden box and designing the motif. These are steps she knew how to do and had incorporated through years of experience. She could follow this sequence of action because she was habituated to do it. When facing a similar physical context, she could recognize and complete simple designs and painting. Her social and physical environments supported the habituation of her painting, which demonstrated her maximum potential for performance capacity, reinforced by her positive and repeated volitional experience. All of these variables within MOHO made it possible for her to perform the steps of a meaningful task, thereby participating in her occupational role as an artist.

Maria did not have the cognitive capacity to learn new procedures, such as varnishing the box. However, she drew upon the existing process and motor skills that she needed for completing the first two steps. She also felt meaning and pleasure when sitting in her familiar environmental context and when participating in her specific occupational role as an artist every time she was exposed to it. Like Alex, she enjoyed and performed her job well, but in a different way. "Performance limitations may influence but not prevent, occupational participation, if a person can make volitional choices and has adequate environmental supports" (Kielhofner, 2008, p. 102).

The Changing Intensity of Participation

Intensity of participation refers to the performance of a group of actions necessary to participate in a given occupational role. When the actions required for a specific role are consistently performed, people feel a sense of accomplishment with respect to an occupational goal. As a mechanic, Alex might have three activities to complete in a given day: repairing and replacing tires, changing oil and fluids, and cleaning car engines. His ability to complete each of these activities in a given day allows him to participate in his worker role and provides him with a sense of achievement.

On the other hand, incremental, transformational, or catastrophic disability events cause people to adapt to new ways of participating in roles. Older adults, after living a life of full participation in different roles, get to a moment where they may not be able to meet the physical demands of their past roles. This prompts them to change their lifestyles for their own health and well-being. At the same time, they may arrange their routines so that they are able to perform some of the activities of some of their past roles. For example, a homemaker who used to do all of the home maintenance activities (e.g., laundry, cooking, cleaning of the house, and maintaining the outside garden) may be able to participate in cooking and light cleaning of the house, having some help from her grown children to complete the other activities.

Whereas in the past this same woman may have engaged in numerous leisure activities, now she may select only one entertaining activity that does not demand much physical or mental energy, such as going to the movies with a friend or her husband. In the past, she might have taken long walks or run every morning, played bridge with friends every Thursday, made crafts for charity fund-raising events every afternoon, and taken care of her grandchildren, all of them considered as part of her leisure role.

MOHO Problem-Solver: Shifting Generalized Expectations. Adults with Severe and Profound Developmental Disabilities

A professional team at a long-term psychiatric facility hired an occupational therapist. They told her: "these people don't do anything except engage in stereotypical behaviors all day . . . Working here will be easy for you. The only problem is that you have to expect that they will engage in resistance, like not wanting to go or stay in the program."

Other clients were described as not being able to comprehend what nursing aids and professionals told or asked them to do, and as not being able to engage in purposeful actions. Some were dressed, fed, and cleaned by staff, who commented that they were not able to note what was going on around them and that they were passive, and therefore "easy to manage." The section chief then advised: "Remember, they will do it again, so please use this technique consistently until they learn this repertoire." On mornings and afternoons, the more functional clients were led into rooms to copy actions of inserting objects in a wooden platform. Many of them looked down while staff assisted them with their actions. Ice cream or coffee was given if the clients stayed in their places during the entire routine.

After a month of relating with and observing residents' occupational needs, the occupational therapist met with the chief of the team in charge of the program to provide a needs assessment report and orient him about the perspective that MOHO offered with respect to people's participation. The occupational therapist then proposed a period of time to pilot a different program based on developing clients' intrinsic motivation. This approach replaced the operant conditioning approach that the team had been using (i.e., rewarding positive behavior with ice cream or coffee).

The section chief was dubious, but agreed to allow the therapist to proceed. For a period of 1 month, the therapist arranged a period of exploration during which the treatment team got to know the clients by observing the situations and tasks they chose spontaneously based on their personal interests and abilities. The team was amazed to discover that even the most passive and resistive clients demonstrated preferences. As the Remotivation Process and Volitional Questionnaire indicate, the therapists on the treatment team became experts in evaluating the subtle behavioral and emotional indicators in the clients that guided the process of offering relevant environmental opportunities which could evoke an optimal sense of pleasure and satisfaction through participation (de las Heras de Pablo et al., 2007; de las Heras de Pablo et al., 2003; Parkinson et al., 2014; Raber et al., 2010; Serratrice & Habib, 1997).

For example, the occupational therapist observed one profoundly impaired client while sharing her experience in different situations. The therapist discovered that the muscles of her body and face became tense when staff positioned her or moved her around in the wheelchair. Instead, she relaxed her face and body when the therapist took her smoothly to sit close to the sunlight reflected in the window, and when she selected light music of her old times and kept the radio turned on close to her. The occupational therapist shared with staff these findings and explained how motivation worked with people including with themselves. Nursing aids began a different routine with this client, and knew how to do it. They also derived a new satisfaction with what they were doing at work.

Similarly, the more active clients were able to perform discrete actions during the activities that were offered. For example, they were able to clap, verbalize, make sounds, and stomp their feet on the floor when listening to different types of music. They played with tempera paint by either spreading it or by covering a large piece of paper with their foot- and handprints while walking or positioning their body and hands over the paper. Other actions included rolling in the grass, pushing a ball with their bodies or extremities, and other actions within simple social activities.

The therapist informed the team about the impact of the clients' ability to choose activities on their satisfaction, and participation in all of the activities on the unit, including collaborating with staff in self-care tasks. The clients were smiling, looking at others, walking straight and faster. They found meaning through participating in pleasurable and dignifying actions.

This example reaffirms the importance of an emphasis on volition, as well as the importance of considering the social and physical environment in terms of providing significant opportunities for clients to perform activities and participate in occupations. Offering experiences of situations that evoke feelings of comfort and pleasure that clients may have felt in the past helps them reconnect with feelings and experiences in which they were able to participate more fully in occupations.

In this example, the level of clients' thinking and acting is not as high or present like it is for people in other case examples, demonstrating the various dimensions of participation in this chapter. However, feeling among the clients is very present (subjective experience). This last and more basic dimension of participation recognizes the potential that emotions and feelings have on the lived experience of meaning and therefore on the persons' active role on choosing occupational circumstances, independent of persons' capacity for thinking and acting.

Embedded Dimensions of Participation in Occupations

As discussed and illustrated in Figure 8-3, the six dimensions of participation in occupation are complementary and related with one another. Each dimension contributes to participation in relevant occupational roles (occupational participation). At the same time, participation in occupational roles requires the completion of activities necessary to meet occupational goals, activities, and the doing of occupational forms/tasks. In order to complete occupational forms/tasks, we need to follow and complete a sequence of steps that require purposeful actions (occupational skills) for achieving successful performance. Finally, while being part of the occupational context, persons feel the experience of meaning, pleasure, and confidence about what they do.

This comprehensive view of dimensions of participation recognizes persons' possibilities for participating in all dimensions, in some, or in the most basic one, respecting each person's unique performance capacities, volitional status, and environmental resources and impact (Table 8-1).

Occupational Adaptation: Occupational Identity, Occupational Competence, and Environmental Impact

As the previous discussion demonstrated, the act of doing, for all but the most severely impaired, includes numerous dimensions of participation in occupations. This participation results in occupational adaptation and the interrelated elements of which it is comprised, including occupational identity and occupational competence, both of which influence and are influenced by the environment (i.e., environmental impact).

The term "occupational adaptation" has been used in the literature to refer to the extent to which persons are able to develop, change in response to challenges, or otherwise achieve a state of well-being through what they do (Fidler & Fidler, 1978; King, 1978; Nelson, 1988; Reilly, 1962). In earlier versions of MOHO, adaptation was defined as meeting personal needs and desires while meeting reasonable environmental expectations through one's occupation (Kielhofner, 1985, 1995). Schkade and Schultz (1992, p. 831) first used the term "occupational adaptation" to refer to "a state of competency in occupational functioning toward which human beings aspire." Their definition suggested that adaptation involved dual aspects of competency and aspiration. Spencer, Davidson, and White (1996) added that occupational adaptation was a cumulative process emanating from one's life history. Mallinson, Mahaffey, and Kielhofner (1998) reported evidence from a study of life history interviews that a person's adaptation consists of two distinct elements, identity and competence. A subsequent study of persons' life histories generated further evidence of occupational identity and occupational competence as distinct components of occupational adaptation (Kielhofner, Mallinson, Forsyth, & Lai, 2001). According to Kielhofner (2008), **occupational adaptation** is composited by two interrelated elements: **occupational identity** and **occupational competence**. Kielhofner (2008) considered occupational adaptation as the development of a positive occupational identity, coupled with the experience of occupational competence over time within the context of one's environment.

Later, based on MOHO practice outcomes and practice systematization in different occupational therapy settings, de las Heras de Pablo (2015, 2011) explicitly considered **environmental impact** as a third crucial element for understanding occupational adaptation, arguing that opportunities, resources, demands, and restrictions of cultural, political, and economic conditions and social and physical environmental dimensions of different occupational settings play an active role in changing, for better or for worse, the course of occupational adaptation (de las Heras de Pablo et al., 2003; Kielhofner, 2008; Kielhofner, de las Heras de Pablo, & Suarez-Balcazar, 2011). According to the systems perspective embraced by MOHO (Kielhofner, 2008), aspects of the environment not only affect personal factors, such as volition, habituation, and performance capacity, but these personal factors also serve to change certain variables within the environment, to some extent. Consequently, contextualizing persons' identity and competence processes together with those characteristics of the environment became the key to conceptualizing occupational adaptation.

Building on this theoretical and empirical work, we present an expanded definition of occupational adaptation and its *three components: identity, competence,* and *environmental impact* (Fig. 8-4).

OCCUPATIONAL IDENTITY

Christiansen (1999) noted that identity refers to a composite definition of the self, including roles and relationships, values, self-concept, and personal desires and goals. He further argues that our participation in occupations helps to create our identities. Building on his argument, as well as the empirical work referred to earlier, occupational identity is defined here as a composite sense of who one is and wishes to become as an occupational being generated from one's history of occupational participation (Kielhofner, 2008). One's volition, habituation, and experience as a lived body are all integrated into occupational identity. Consequently, occupational identity includes an integrated composite of:

- One's sense of capacity and effectiveness for doing (personal causation).
- What things one finds interesting and pleasurable to do (interests).
- Who one is, as defined by one's roles and relationships (role identity).
- What one feels and thinks is important and therefore compromised to do (values).
- A sense of the desired routines of life (volitional anticipation of a preferred lifestyle).
- A sense of the supports and expectations of one's environment (volitional anticipation of environmental opportunities and demands).
- Personal occupational goals toward the future (volitional choice).
- Personal decisions regarding what to do in the immediate present (volitional choice).

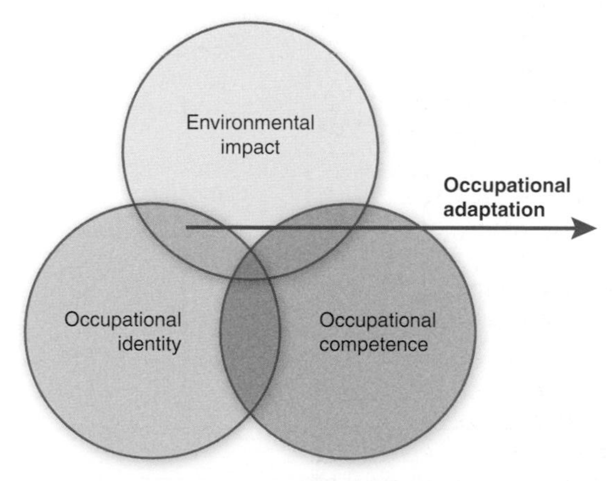

FIGURE 8-4 Occupational Adaptation.

Occupational identity reflects accumulated life experiences that are organized into an understanding of who one has been and a sense of desired and possible direction for one's future. Thus, occupational identity, on people whose objective performance capacity enables their thinking, serves both as a means of self-definition and as a blueprint for upcoming action being in the immediate, near, or further future. Preliminary evidence suggests that occupational identity is represented in a continuum that begins with self-appraisal and extends toward the more challenging elements of accepting responsibility for and knowing what one wants from life (Kielhofner et al., 2001). Current evidence confirms these findings by showing that building an occupational identity starts with developing awareness of our capacities and interests and extends to constructing a value-based vision of the future we desire. Even more, occupational identity is constructed through the continuous development and change of volitional process lived in the ongoing participation in occupations according to a person's age, abilities, and environmental impact (de las Heras de Pablo, 2015; de las Heras de Pablo et al., 2003, 2007; Parkinson et al., 2014; Pépin et al., 2008; Raber et al., 2010). The readers could refer to Chapters 14, 15, 18, and 19 for further information.

OCCUPATIONAL COMPETENCE

Occupational competence is the degree to which one sustains a successful pattern of occupational participation that reflects one's occupational identity (Kielhofner, 2008). Thus, while identity has to do with the subjective meaning of one's occupational life, competence has to do with putting that identity into action in an ongoing way.

Occupational competence, for persons whose objective performance capacity enables occupational participation, appears to begin with organizing one's life to meet basic responsibilities and personal standards and extends to meeting role obligations and then achieving a satisfying lifestyle (Kielhofner & Forsyth, 2001). Occupational competence in this group of people includes:

- Fulfilling the expectations of one's roles and one's own values and standards for performance (role performance)
- Maintaining a routine that allows one to discharge responsibilities (habits of routine)
- Participating in a range of occupations that provide a sense of ability, control, satisfaction, and fulfillment (participation in occupational roles)
- Pursuing one's occupational goals by taking actions to achieve desired life outcomes (habits of routine, habits of style)

Occupational competence, of people who could engage in the most basic dimensions of participation in occupation, could be demonstrated by:

- Completing the last step of chosen occupational forms done in groups, everyday at a community program.
- Following structured afternoons of preferred play/leisure activities according to a routine.
- Participating in doing two occupational forms/tasks of a meaningful family activity every Sunday and another pleasurable task every afternoon.
- Helping meaningful others with completing a step of a task, by holding or transporting relevant objects needed, every time he or she is invited and supported to do it.
- Enjoying particular occupational circumstances in which others participate in doing, every time he or she is included.

ENVIRONMENTAL IMPACT

Environmental impact refers to the manner by which personal and environmental characteristics integrate dynamically while a person is participating in occupations. Persons are in constant negotiation with themselves and with the opportunities and restrictions posed by the social, physical, cultural, economic, and political characteristics of the environment. While a majority of persons are able to fully participate in occupations, some are dependent on environmental supports mainly because of their limited performance capacity and reduced volition. No matter what the status of a person's performance capacity, habituation, and volition is, during the process of participation, both the person and his or her relevant social groups are challenged with changes they need or want to make in order to achieve the maximum compatibility between them (refer to Chapters 14 and 25 for further information).

OCCUPATIONAL ADAPTATION

Occupational adaptation is defined here as having a positive occupational identity and the correspondent occupational competence constructed over time through the dynamics of a constant interaction between personal factors and environmental impact (Fig. 8-5). While occupational identity and competence codevelop over time, one cannot operationalize a view of self and life that one has not developed. Evidence also suggests that while disability can affect both

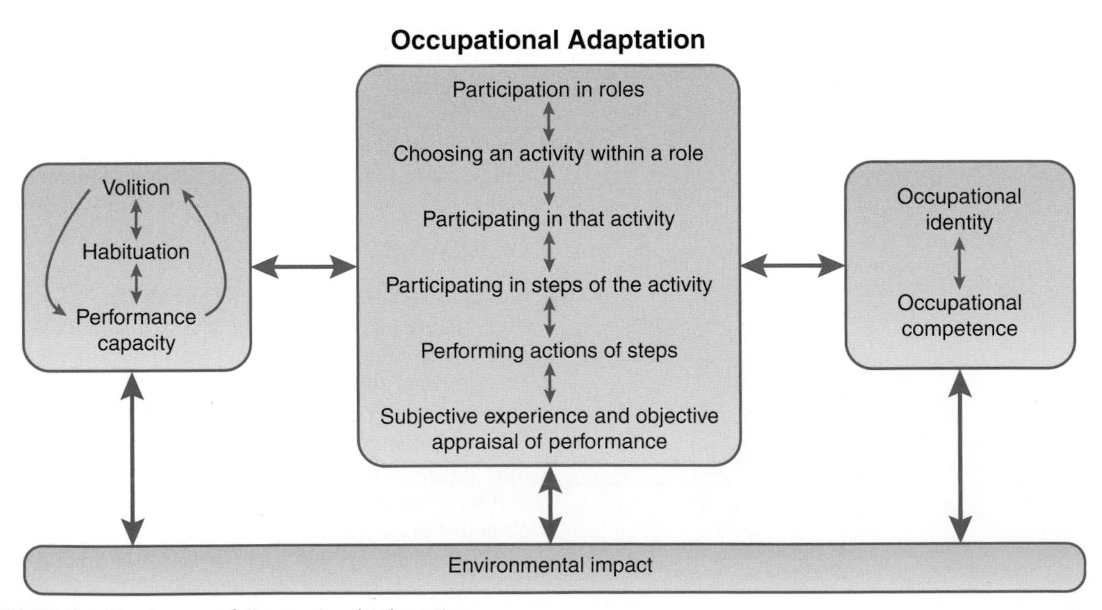

FIGURE 8-5 The Process of Occupational Adaptation.

identity and competence, its effects are more easily observed in the area of competence (Kielhofner et al., 2001; Mallinson et al., 1998). In addition, one person's correspondence between occupational competence and identity can vary significantly or subtly, from one occupational setting to another, and also from participating in one occupation, activity, or task into another. By considering this in practice, we can observe that the balance of occupational competence and identity generated from participating within different occupational settings is what makes a person feel satisfied or not with a particular occupational lifestyle. Moreover, the environmental impact in terms of affecting, and being affected by, a person's volition, habituation, and performance capacity is considerable. Thus, we can only understand occupational adaptation if we are able to reason about the unique significance that the interaction of these diverse experiences gives to each individual (de las Heras de Pablo, 2015, 2011, 1993). Figure 8-6 depicts a summary of the process of occupational adaptation as it incorporates the four essential elements of the Model of Human Occupation (volition, habituation, performance capacity, and environment).

Conclusion

As noted earlier, occupational adaptation is the consequence of one's history of participation in life occupations, enacting in occupational roles, choosing activities within those roles, participating in those activities, engaging in the steps of the activities, and performing the individual actions that comprise the steps. During this process, a person receives feedback from others within the social environment and feels the subjective experience of performance and of being in significant contexts within the physical

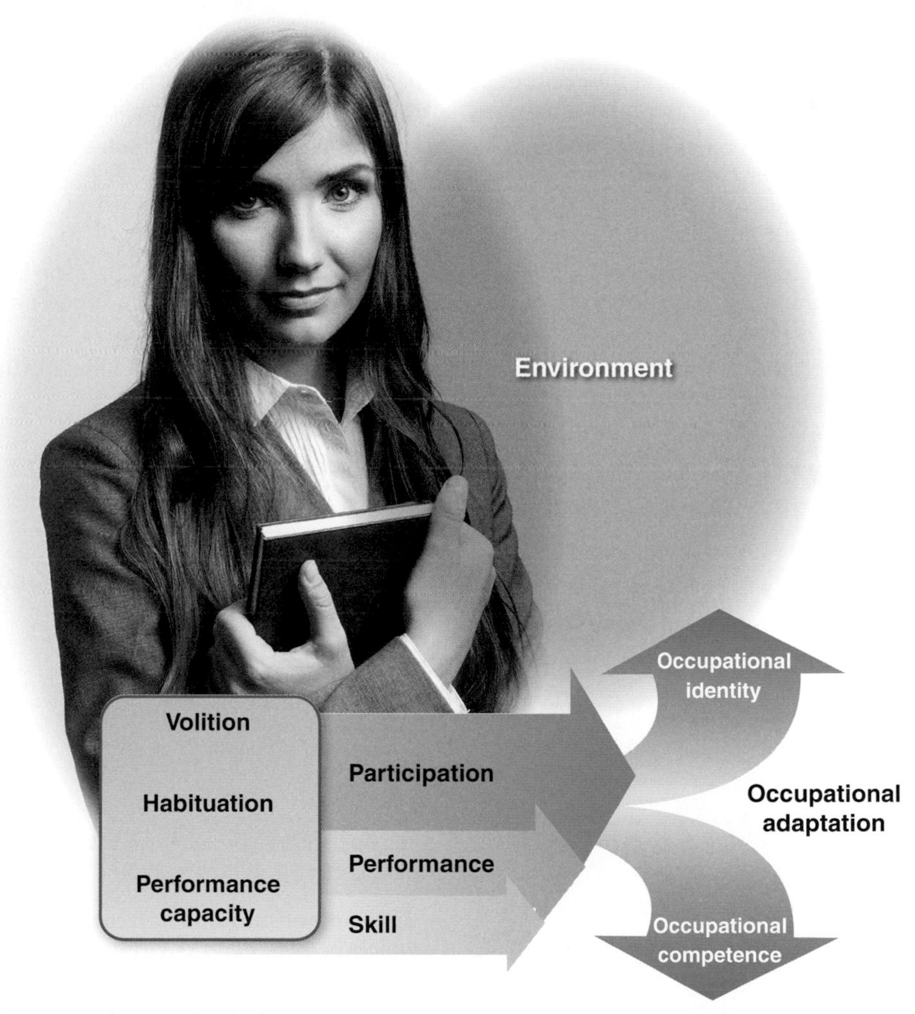

FIGURE 8-6 The Process of Occupational Adaptation.

environment. Our personal characteristics, in interaction with those of the environment, influence our participation in occupations. This occurs from the time we discover the physical and human world through our senses, learn our first actions, and begin to participate as one with the world by doing things. Through our participation, our own volition, habituation, and performance capacity are constantly shaped. Throughout this process of continuous interaction between ourselves and the environment, the environmental characteristics impact the development of our volition, habituation, and performance capacity. Over time, we construct our occupational identities and competence through ongoing participation in occupations. Occupational identity and competence are realized as we develop and respond to any life changes (including illness and impairment). Identity, competence, and environmental impact then unfold within the state in which we find ourselves at a changed point in our lives. Most persons will, at one time or another, experience either meaningful or positive moments of participation that reaffirm and enhance their identity and competence or a threat or problems in occupational adaptation requiring the rebuilding of occupational identity and competence, and support within the environment.

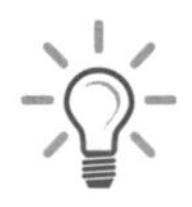

Chapter 8 Review Questions

Considering the perspective of MOHO, how would you respond to the following comments?

1. "My father became very lazy the past years. Since he retired he only does the garden at home. He does not do anything productive".
2. "Occupational therapists cannot work with patients who have severe problems in their cognitive abilities because they cannot participate in activities. So, we have to focus on working with those patients who are doing activities and can progress in their lives."
3. "This person participates in occupational roles, thus she does not feel what she is doing. It is automatic."

HOMEWORK ASSIGNMENTS

1. Reflect about a moment in your life where you participated in an occupation by feeling the ambience and remembering other significant lived experiences. Ask a friend about this too. What meaning did it have for you? What stories came into your mind?
2. Reflect about a friend or a family member who has had or has an illness or impairment. Describe the configuration of his or her participation in occupation?
3. Exercise:
    1. Identify a role you participate in.
    2. Identify the activities you need to do in order to accomplish this role.
    3. From these activities choose one.
    4. Identify the sequence of steps you need to do in order to complete the activity chosen.
    5. From these steps choose one.
    6. Identify the skills you need to perform in order to complete this step.

thePoint® For additional resources and exercises, visit http://thePoint.lww.com

Key Terms

Communication and interaction skills: Conveying intentions and needs, and coordinating social action in order to act together with people.

Dimensions of participation: Diverse possibilities in which people become involved in occupations, considering as a parameter their maximum potential of cognitive and physical capacity.

Environmental Impact: Refers to the manner by which personal and environmental characteristics integrate dynamically while a person is participating in occupations. The environment offers opportunities, resources, demands, and restrictions of cultural, political, and economic conditions, social and physical environmental dimensions of different occupational settings that play an active role in changing, for better or for worse, the course of occupational adaptation.

Motor skills: Moving self or task objects.

Occupational adaptation: Having a positive occupational identity and the correspondent occupational competence that have been constructed over time through the dynamics of a constant interaction between personal factors and environmental impact in the ongoing participation in occupation.

Occupational competence: Degree to which one is able to sustain a pattern of occupational participation that reflects one's occupational identity.

Occupational identity: Composite sense of who one is and wishes to become as an occupational being generated from one's history of occupational participation.

Occupational participation: Defines what we do in the broad areas of work (study), play, and activities of daily living.

Occupational performance: Defines discrete acts or units of doing.

Occupational Skills: Observable, goal-directed actions that a person uses while performing a step of a task.

Process skills: Logically sequencing actions over time, selecting and using appropriate tools and materials, and adapting performance when encountering problems.

REFERENCES

American Occupational Therapy Association. (2014). Occupational therapy practice framework: Domain and process (3rd ed.). *American Journal of Occupational Therapy, 68*(1), S1–S53.

Christiansen, C. H. (1999). Defining lives: Occupation as identity: An essay on competence, coherence, and the creation of meaning. *American Journal of Occupational Therapy, 53,* 547–558.

de las Heras de Pablo, C. G. (2011). Promotion of occupational participation: Integration of the model of human occupation in practice. *The Israeli Journal of Occupational Therapy, 20*(3), E67–E88.

de las Heras de Pablo, C. G. (2015). *Modelo de Ocupación Humana.* Madrid, Spain: Editorial Síntesis.

de las Heras de Pablo, C. G., Geist, R., Kielhofner, G., & Li, Y. (2007). *The Volitional Questionnaire (VQ)* (Version 4.1). Chicago: Model of Human Occupation Clearinghouse, Department of Occupational Therapy, College of Applied Health Sciences, University of Illinois.

de las Heras de Pablo, C. G., Llerena, V., & Kielhofner G. (2003). *Remotivation process: Progressive intervention for people with severe volitional problems: A user's manual.* Chicago: The Model of Human Occupation Clearinghouse, Department of Occupational Therapy, College of Applied Health Sciences, University of Illinois.

de las Heras de Pablo, C. G. (1993). *Validity and reliability of the volitional questionnaire* (Unpublished master's thesis, Tufts University, Medford, OR.

Fidler, G. S., & Fidler, J. W. (1978). Doing and becoming: Purposeful action and self-actualization. *American Journal of Occupational Therapy, 32,* 305–310.

Fisher A. G. (1999). *Assessment of motor and process skills* (3rd ed.). Fort Collins, CO: Three Star Press.

Fisher, A. G., & Bray Jones, K. (2010). *Assessment of motor and process skills: Vol. 1: Development, standardization, and administration manual* (7th ed.). Fort Collins, CO: Three Star Press.

Forsyth, K., & Kielhofner, G. (1999). Validity of the assessment of communication and interaction skills. *British Journal of Occupational Therapy, 62,* 69–74.

Forsyth, K., Salamy, M., Simon, S., & Kielhofner, G. (1997). *Assessment of communication and interaction skills.* Chicago: University of Illinois, Model of Human Occupation Clearinghouse.

Goode, D. (1983). Who is Bobby? Ideology and method in the discovery of a Down's syndrome person's competence. In G. Kielhofner (Ed.), *Health through occupation: Theory and practice in occupational therapy.* Philadelphia, PA: F. A. Davis.

Haglund, L., & Henriksson, C. (1995). Activity: From action to activity. *Scandinavian Journal of Caring Sciences, 9,* 227–234.

Kielhofner, G. (1985). *A model of human occupation: Theory and application.* Baltimore, MD: Williams & Wilkins.

Kielhofner, G. (1995). *A model of human occupation: Theory and application* (2nd ed.). Baltimore, MD: Williams & Wilkins.

Kielhofner, G. (2002). *A model of human occupation: Theory and application.* Philadelphia, PA: Lippincott Williams & Wilkins.

Kielhofner, G. (2008). *A model of human occupation: Theory and application* (4th ed.). Philadelphia, PA: Lippincott Williams & Wilkins.

Kielhofner, G., & Forsyth, K. (2001). Development of a client self-report for treatment planning and documenting therapy outcomes. *Scandinavian Journal of Occupational Therapy, 8,* 131–139.

Kielhofner, G., Mallinson, T., Forsyth, K., & Lai, J. S. (2001). Psychometric properties of the second version of the occupational performance history interview (OPHI-II). *American Journal of Occupational Therapy, 55,* 260–267.

Kielhofner, G., de las Heras de Pablo, C. G., & Suarez Balcazar, Y. (2011). Human occupation as a tool for understanding and promoting social justice. In F. Kronemberg, N. Pollard, & D. Sakellariu (Eds.), *Occupational therapies without borders: Towards an ecology of occupation based practices* (Vol. 2, pp. 269–277). London, United Kingdom: Elsevier.

King, L. J. (1978). Toward a science of adaptive responses. *American Journal of Occupational Therapy, 32,* 429–437.

Mallinson, T., Mahaffey, L., & Kielhofner, G. (1998). The occupational performance history interview: Evidence for three underlying constructs of occupational adaptation. *Canadian Journal of Occupational Therapy, 65,* 219–228.

Melton, J., Forsyth, K., Metherall, A., Robinson, J., Hill, J., & Quick, L. (2008). Program redesign based on the model of human occupation: Inpatient services for people experiencing acute mental illness in the UK. *Occupational Therapy in Health Care, 22,* 37–50.

Nelson, D. (1988). Occupation: Form and performance. *American Journal of Occupational Therapy, 42,* 633.

Parkinson, S., Cooper, J. R., de las Heras de Pablo, C. G., & Forsyth K. (2014). Measuring the effectiveness of interventions when occupational performance is severely impaired. *British Journal of Occupational Therapy, 77*(2), 78–81.

Pépin, G., Guérette, F., Lefebvre, B., & Jacques, P. (2008). Canadian therapists' experiences while implementing the model of human occupation remotivation process. *Occupational Therapy in Health Care, 22*(2/3), 115–124.

Raber, C., Teitelman, J., Watts, J., & Kielhofner, G. (2010). A phenomenological study of volition in everyday occupations of older people with dementia. *British Journal of Occupational Therapy, 73*(11), 498–506.

Reilly, M. (1962). Occupational therapy can be one of the great ideas of 20th century medicine. *American Journal of Occupational Therapy, 16,* 1–9.

Schkade, J. K., & Schultz, S. (1992). Occupational adaptation, Part 1: Toward a holistic approach for contemporary practice. *American Journal of Occupational Therapy, 46,* 829–837.
Serratrice, G., & Habib, M. (1997). Émotion et motivation. Encycl Méd Chir (Elsevier Paris). *Neurologie, 17-022-E-30,* 7.
Spencer, J. C., Davidson, H. A., & White, V. K. (1996). Continuity and change: Past experience as adaptive repertoire in occupational adaptation. *American Journal of Occupational Therapy, 50,* 526–534.
World Health Organization. (2001). *International Classification of Functioning, Disability and Health (ICF).* Geneva, Switzerland: Author.

Crafting Occupational Life

Jane Melton, Roberta P. Holzmueller, Riitta Keponen, Louise Nygard, Kelly Munger, and Gary Kielhofner (posthumous)

CHAPTER 9

EXPECTED LEARNING OUTCOMES

Upon completion of this chapter, readers will be able to:

1. Make meaning of their personal occupational life narrative within a point in time by defining the "plot" of the narrative and using metaphor to explain their story.
2. Describe the occupational narrative of others whose unique circumstances have been compromised through illness, disability, or other challenging circumstances.
3. Using the model of human occupation (MOHO) concepts, explain how an individual is challenged to craft or shape their occupational lives in order to participate in occupations that are important and satisfying to them.
4. Outline how occupational narratives evolve over time to craft an individual's occupational life.
5. Explain how an individual's self-awareness of their occupational life narrative can enable meaningful and sustainable occupational solutions for and with clients.

People craft their occupational lives through a dynamic system and ongoing process of generating and maintaining their occupational identity and competence. In Chapter 8 it was noted that occupational identity represents a composite sense of oneself and one's future generated from ongoing occupational participation. It further noted that occupational competence involves sustaining a pattern of participation that reflects one's identity.

The purpose of this chapter is to consider further how persons are challenged to organize, shape, or craft their occupational lives in order to participate in occupations which:

- An individual holds as important
- Support a person's unique sense of pleasure and satisfaction in doing things
- Reinforce knowledge of one's own capacities, limitations, and relative effectiveness
- Align with one's awareness of who one is in reference to the social world
- Have familiarity with the rhythms and routines of life
- Emanate lived experience as an embodied being
- Acknowledge apprehension of the world

Both occupational identity and competence encompass how the aspects of volition, habituation, and performance capacity collectively orient each person to his/her own unique life. These elements are always in the background, shaping how people craft their ongoing occupational lives in the stream of time and within their social and physical environment. Moreover, they are integrated into each person's unique **occupational narrative** or story of how a client's volition, habituation, performance capacity, and environment interact over time to influence what a client does with his or her life. This process forms a plot with a central metaphor that reflects a client's understanding of his or her own experience of disability.

MOHO Problem-Solver: Geriatrics

Cecil, a 70-year-old retired businessman, former amateur boxer, and widower waits patiently to be seen by an occupational therapist in an outpatient clinic. Although in his youth he was a high-achieving student and top athlete, he also carried a diagnosis of attention-deficit hyperactivity disorder. He has always struggled with issues of verbal impulsivity, organization, and focus. Recently, however, Cecil's difficulties with executive functioning have been escalating, causing him to lose things and forget to perform everyday tasks, such as paying bills and remembering to take his prescribed medications. Due to his history of having boxed when he was younger, he is also undergoing neurological and neuropsychological evaluation to rule out dementia. In addition to prescribing psychotropic medication to address his cognitive problems, Cecil's primary care physician has also recommended occupational therapy to assist him with organizational tasks at home.

During the occupational therapy consultation, the therapist asked Cecil a range of questions about his daily routine, responsibilities, and commitments. She then visited him in his home and conducted an analysis of his home and community environments. At the end of the multivisit consultation, the therapist came up with a series of adaptations and other recommendations that would allow Cecil to remain more organized at home and in the community, such as creating a filing system, purchasing see-through drawers and making labels for everything. The therapist also suggested a lanyard for Cecil's glasses and clips to secure his wallet and keys to his belt rings. A driving evaluation was also conducted, which Cecil passed effortlessly.

Unfortunately, the consultation did not result in Cecil making any significant changes in his daily habits or routines. Clips for his belt rings and a lanyard for his glasses were not consistent with his sense of style, and his fast-paced lifestyle did not always lend itself to placing objects into files or labeled drawers. When he provided this feedback to his referring physician, she was not surprised. Instead, she referred him to a different occupational therapist who was practicing from a model of human occupation (MOHO) perspective.

During their first meeting, the MOHO therapist asked Cecil a series of questions about his life story, beginning with his early interests in boxing and business. Cecil characterized his life in terms of a constant race in which he was "running to keep up." The son of a professional athlete, he grew up in an affluent neighborhood surrounded by peers who were highly achieving and competitive. As the only African American in his grammar school and high school classes, he described a constant need to prove himself in terms of his academic achievement and athletic prowess. Being gifted in both of these areas, it was never difficult for him to compensate for his difficulties with focus, organization, and impulsivity by relying on his peers and his teamwork mentality. He met his wife in college, whom he considered his soul mate. A highly organized and thoughtful person, she continually looked after him in terms of his daily routines. She took care of all of the household bills, appointments, and other necessary tasks of living, and his administrative assistant took care of his schedule and other organizational needs at work.

Now that Cecil's wife has died and he is no longer working, he finds that he is no longer surrounded by the infrastructures of peer support and structure once afforded to him by his social environment. He describes himself as no longer being able to "keep up" with the friends within his social networks and has a sensation that he is "backsliding." After hearing his therapist mirror this language and summarize his momentum-oriented metaphors of "not keeping up" and "backsliding," Cecil was able to identify his central limitations and make a commitment to structuring his daily habits and routines in a way that did not take much time and allowed him to preserve his sense of identity and personal style. Together with his therapist, he identified a need to establish new habits and a sense of a routine within his personal life. He purchased an iPhone watch and made use of the calendar, to-do lists, and reminder features. He learned to place important items, such as his smartphone, keys, wallet, and eyeglasses, in a specific tray that sat on a specific table within his home. He also purchased a stylish leather satchel to hold his personal items when away from home, which he strapped across his chest and took with him wherever he went.

When he returned to his physician for a follow-up appointment, he recounted a relationship with his occupational therapist, rather than a mere occupational therapy consultation. He told his physician that, in a single conversation with the new therapist, he learned a lot about himself and how much of a role his wife and professional peers had played in terms of helping him compensate for his lack of organization and structure. He reported that he has faced the fact that these people are no longer with him, and that he is now committed to maintaining certain habits and behaviors on his own that will help him stay more organized and not lose things so frequently.

Narrative Organization of Occupational Life

People conduct and draw meaning from life by locating themselves in unfolding narratives that integrate their past, present, and future selves (Aubin, Hachey, & Mercier, 1999; Geertz, 1986; Gergen & Gergen, 1988; Helfrich, Kielhofner, & Mattingly, 1994; Mattingly, 1991; Schafer, 1981; Spence, 1982; Taylor, 1989).

By considering each individual's volition, habituation, performance capacity, and unique set of environmental constructs, occupational therapy can facilitate making meaning of occupational life in changed or challenging circumstances. This leads to health- and well-being-promoting benefits as well as encouraging occupational participation (Fossey & Scanlan, 2014), an improved experience of occupational life (Mostert & Fossey, 2010), and a negotiated sense of managing personal occupational identity (Alasker & Josephsson, 2013; Lal et al., 2013; Price, Stephenson, Krantz, & Ward, 2011).

Two important features of narratives—plot and metaphor—synthesize and impart meaning on many elements and episodes of life. The following sections examine these two features of narrative.

PLOT

Gergen and Gergen (1988) refer to plot as the foundation of the narrative that determines how people think and talk when they use stories. The **plot** of a story represents the intersection between the progression of time and the direction (for better or for worse) that life takes. Consequently, the **narrative plot** is the way in which an individual characterizes the story of events that they are experiencing over time. It shapes events over time as they experience life in a variety of ways (Gergen & Gergen, 1988; Jonsson, Kielhofner, & Borell, 1997).

A narrative's plot reveals its overall meaning because it sums up where life has been and is going. For example, the tragic plot is found in a life when some event results in a steep downward turn in a previously good or improving life. It signifies a life ruined. The melodramatic plot involves a series of upward and downward turns. It reveals a life of struggle. In this way, plotting life events links them together in a way that makes sense of the life as a whole. Consequently, the various life episodes derive their meaning from the overall shape of the plot. One way of understanding narrative plots that have been used in occupational therapy research and practice is to characterize them as **regressive, progressive, or stability** narratives (Jonsson et al., 1997; Kielhofner et al., 2004). As shown in Figure 9-1 a progressive narrative is one in which the story is headed upward, a regressive narrative heads downward, and a stability narrative continues life in a constant direction.

People seek to evaluate life events in terms of their significance or impact on the unfolding life story. Most events represent a continuation of the basic direction of life. Others positively change or threaten where life is headed. In evaluating ongoing events of life, the underlying plot (the direction for better or for worse that life will take) is always at stake. For example, Cheah and Presnell (2011) demonstrated that older people's experience of acute hospitalization, while important for health, was, at a point in time, disruptive to their "normal" occupational life.

People evaluate each new unfolding circumstance of life in terms of how such things have gone before and in terms of where it might lead. For example, Jonsson et al. (1997) studied how older persons anticipated their retirement. What each person

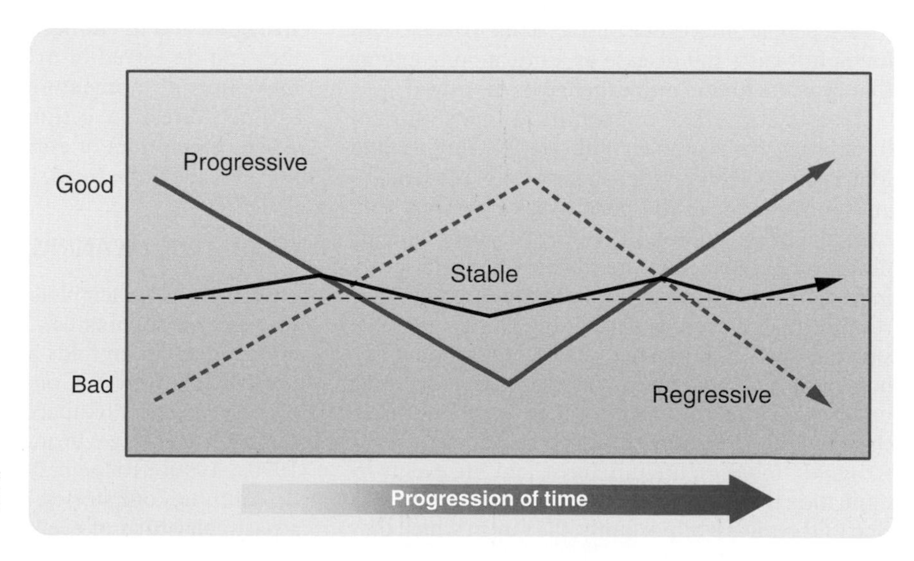

FIGURE 9-1 The Slopes of Progressive, Regressive, and Stable Narratives.

expected in retirement was always intimately tied to how past and present occupational life, especially work, had been experienced. If work was negative, then retirement could be seen as an escape. In this case, life after retirement could be expected to get better. If work was positive, then retirement could continue a good life by providing opportunities to do other valued things or it could be a loss that would make life worse.

How past and future are linked depends on and reveals the plot. If, for example, one is living a tragic narrative, past successes do not mean that things will necessarily go well in the future. On the other hand, if one is in a story where things are getting better, past failures will be lessons that provided the person with new strengths or obstacles that were overcome. The significance of the past for the present and the future depends on and reflects the narrative's plot. This is illustrated in Smith's (2008) account of powerful personal stories and the circumstances that influence the narrative plot. In a similar fashion, inevitable or likely events in the future take on their significance with reference to the past and present. How they are seen to relate to past or present also depends on and reflects the underlying plot.

METAPHOR

Stories are also given meaning by metaphors (Ganzer, 1993). **Metaphor** is the use of a familiar object or phenomenon to stand in the place of the less understood event or situation (Ortony, 1979). Metaphors succinctly characterize complex or emotionally difficult circumstances by evoking something familiar or readily understood to stand in the place of that which is difficult to grasp and/or face. Metaphors also provide a way of dealing with difficult circumstances. For example, when faced with serious, life-threatening illness, people often evoke the metaphor of battle. This metaphor casts the disease as a threatening enemy that must be fought and expelled or destroyed.

People also evoke metaphors to make sense of disabilities. For example, Mallinson, Kielhofner, and Mattingly (1996) identified metaphors of momentum and entrapment in the narratives of persons with mental illness. People hospitalized because of mental illness often referred to their lives in terms of speed, inertia, impetus, acceleration, and deceleration. They related images such as getting life going again, life slowing down, life passing one by, life grinding to a halt, or life going nowhere when they were summing up or evaluating the events of their lives. They used the metaphor of momentum to characterize their struggles, motives, life junctures, and life events by evaluating them in terms of the progression and direction of their lives. Importantly, the way in which they lived their lives also embodied such slowing down, coming to a halt, heading off in wrong directions, and so on. Other persons with mental illness described their lives as being severely restricted or confined by life circumstances. Their stories were imbued with the wish for escape or for finding a way out of the maze. They saw their situations as both intolerable and inexorable. Importantly, they also acted as individuals who were trapped. They could not make decisions. They sometimes exhibited symptoms of agoraphobia and were literally confined in their rooms or homes. They stayed in dissatisfying relationships, jobs, and life situations. Interestingly, similar broad themes emerged when Cheah and Presnell (2011) studied older people's experience of acute hospitalization. The participants described metaphors of suspension from normal life in relation to their own occupational roles, routines, choices, and environment and the incapacitating and unpleasant effect of this was evident.

How Metaphors Shape Narrative Meaning

Schön (1979) noted that metaphors are a primary vehicle through which persons comprehend things that have gone wrong in life. Consequently, when lives are troubled and when people are struggling to comprehend difficult, painful, and incomprehensible things that have happened, metaphors are effective ways of assigning meaning to them. Moreover, metaphors sum up "what needs fixing" (Schön, 1979, p. 255).

Metaphors have also been used to illustrate the learning experience of individuals in occupational groups. For example, occupational therapists have defined their developing familiarity with the use of MOHO theory in practice as a "journey," highlighting their participation struggle with "moving" from one practice to another (Melton, Forsyth, & Freeth, 2010). In pinpointing the essential nature of life's problems, struggles, and dilemmas, narratives also imply how they can be solved or overcome. For example, the metaphors of momentum imply solutions of going in a new direction, getting things going, or slowing down. Metaphors of entrapment suggest that one must escape or be freed.

NARRATIVE, MEANING, AND DOING

Narratives, with their plots and metaphors, shape how we perceive ongoing life. They are a way of making meaning as life unfolds and as new circumstances present themselves. Consequently, there is always openness in narrative that can take and make meaning of whatever emerges in an unpredictable life (Bruner, 1990a, 1990b; Ricoeur, 1984). Moreover, what we do continues our stories, sometimes aiming toward a particular turn of events or outcome, sometimes moving things along, and sometimes acquiescing to what seems inevitable (Jonsson, Josephsson, & Kielhofner, 2000; Jonsson et al., 1997). Occupation both emanates from and influences where one's story is going (Clark, 1993; Helfrich et al., 1994).

For this reason, narratives can either impede or focus action. For example, if someone already sees his or her life as a tragedy, there is little reason to work toward goals because the tragic plot pronounces that things are ruined. On the other hand, if someone sees his or her life as getting better, he or she will likely be motivated to work hard toward that outcome. For example, in a study of 129 participants with AIDS, Kielhofner et al. (2004) found that clients' narratives were significant predictors of whether people would remain in or drop out of a program of vocational services and of whether those who successfully participated in the program would achieve employment or other productive outcomes.

SUMMARY

The coherence and meaning people achieve in their lives is facilitated through narratives. The following features of narratives give them this integrating and meaning-making potential:

- Narratives tie together past, present, and future as well as integrate multiple themes of self and the world.
- Narratives integrate and impart meaning through the use of plot and metaphor.
- Narratives are open-ended and thus allow us to comprehend emergent events and circumstances of life, tying them to what has gone before and what might come next.
- Narratives are not only told but are also done.
- What one does continues the unfolding of one's narrative.

Given these considerations, an occupational narrative is defined as a story (both told and enacted) that integrates across time one's unfolding volition, habituation, performance capacity, and environments through plots and metaphors that sum up and assign meaning to these elements. Both occupational identity and our competence are reflected and enacted in occupational narratives.

Four Narratives

How occupational narratives figure in ongoing life can best be appreciated by detailed examination of such stories. The following sections present four occupational narratives. Each narrative tells about living with an impairment. Aaron's story is told by his mother, Roberta Paikoff, with liberal perspectives from Aaron. It illustrates the extent to which crafting an occupational narrative can involve the collective efforts of parents and child. Kelly's story is in the first person because she authored it. Leena's and Lisa's stories are rendered in the third person, because the text was shaped by someone other than the story's character.

Pediatrics Narrative

Aaron is currently planning his sixth birthday party, to which he plans to invite all the children in his mainstream kindergarten class, as well as a few friends from last year's preschool class. He has a clearly articulated theme (jungle animals) and place (home) where he'd like to have his party, as well as some ideas for things the guests will do (crafts and games where we make or pretend we are jungle animals).

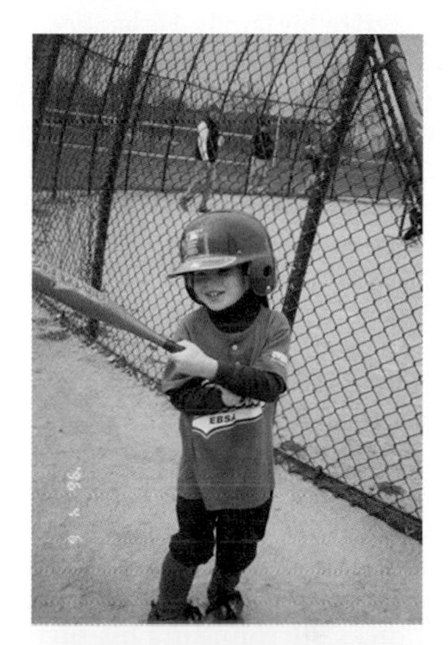

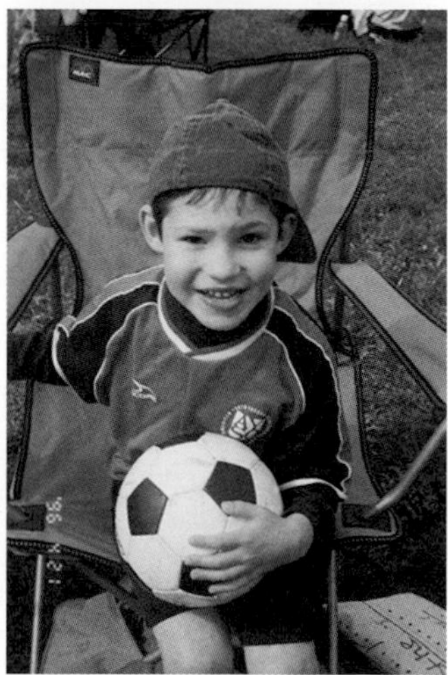

Aaron practices using his muscles by playing sports

One of the assignments Aaron had recently for kindergarten was to research and present to his class the kind of job he would like to have when he grows up. When I asked him what he would like to be when he grows up, his answer was crystal clear and instantaneous, "A Dad." On further probing, I asked him if he would like to do other work besides being a dad. He said, "Sure, I'll do my work." When I asked what kind of work it would be, he said, "Whatever they need me to do, I'll do." On still further probing, we discussed what his favorite part of school (stories) was, and when I suggested maybe he'd like to be a teacher, he answered, "or run the library." And so it happened that Aaron was the only one in his kindergarten class to research and report on two jobs: being a father and a librarian!

Aaron suffered diffuse brain injury during or before birth, because of causes that have never been specified to his family. He has been followed through early intervention since birth, and received a diagnosis of cerebral palsy when he was 1 year old. His cerebral palsy is relatively mild, in that he is able to walk without assistance, and to either perform or approximate many of the gross motor activities his nondisabled friends are doing. However, his gross and fine motor skills are well behind his age peers. His lack of motor control over certain muscle groups has not allowed him to predict bladder and bowel movements, so he has not yet been able to learn to use the toilet, the aspect of his cerebral palsy which bothers him the most right now. Cognitively, he is at or above his peers in reading and math skills, and his social development is right on target.

As Aaron's mother, I recall, with pain, the circumstances surrounding his birth. It was completely unexpected. An ultrasound at 12 or 13 weeks indicated everything was all right; I was so relieved. It never occurred to me that our story would be anything but the happy one most people take into a wanted, cherished pregnancy. When Aaron was born, at first I felt like a hero, because he had stopped moving *in utero*; I had called, come in, and was taken care of. Later that evening, when I called to the Infant Special Care Unit and was not able to talk with anyone, I still wasn't worried. But when my husband and I came down, and they told us he had had seizures and needed to be on a ventilator and have a series of tests (MRI, EEG), I became frantic. Suddenly, I got an image of my "special needs child" and thought of the many children we see out in the world, with serious limitations, and thought, "I am going to be one of those parents." I told one of my dear friends, "This is a life transforming experience," and it really has been.

At the juncture of Aaron's birth and his first few weeks of life, a couple of experiences really stand out for me. One was an occupational therapist who examined Aaron when he was 1 week old, and we were preparing to take him home for the first time. She told us, "You don't compare him to other children. You compare him to himself. If you continue to see progress, you are happy. If you see stalls or stagnation, you seek help." In addition, when we took Aaron for his first visit to our pediatrician, he said, "If you have to injure your brain, the best time in life to do it is in utero or at birth." He followed this up with, "If what happened to Aaron happened to us, the results would be catastrophic. But the infant brain is still developing, and very malleable, and you will be amazed at what he can do." And, indeed, we have been, and continue to be, amazed at what Aaron can do.

Both of these examples set me and my family (including Aaron) on a narrative course which is optimistic and full of possibility. Certainly, repeatedly over the last 6 or so years, we have been given less than sanguine news about Aaron. In some cases that news has proved to be incorrect, in other cases the jury is still out. But for us, these have been situations where we have considered the "bad news" and incorporated it into our overall, very positive views of Aaron and his growth.

Aaron will tell you that the hardest thing about having cerebral palsy so far has been "the potty." As early as last year, I suspected that Aaron's delay in toilet training might be in part muscle and sensation related. On the advice of my wise and thoughtful supervisor in the preschool where I work, I decided to tell Aaron that he had cerebral palsy just about a year ago, when he was about to turn 5. Her theory was that if we start "naming" the disability for him at this young age, it would become a normative part of his narrative, and I believe, for the most part we have been successful in this. When I first told him about his cerebral palsy, I asked if he had noticed that sometimes he had more trouble getting his muscles to do things than other kids in his class. He said "yes," and I followed up with, "there's a reason for that. You have something called cerebral palsy, which comes from having hurt your brain when you were a tiny baby." I then pointed out the many, many ways that cerebral palsy does not affect him (e.g., knowing his numbers and letters, making friends, being a good friend, enjoying stories) and highlighted the ways that we think it does (moving his body, especially his fingers, and using the potty).

The other thing that Aaron mentioned as being hard about cerebral palsy is actually a far more universal struggle. He said it is hard when Nathan (his older brother) "beats him up." I was alarmed when he first said this, but when I asked further, he said "Nathan beats me at everything—he dribbles around me, he beats me at basketball, soccer, and chess and he can bike." Since Nathan is an older brother, it is not hard to explain this as part of having an older brother. However, I do anticipate that as Aaron continues to mature, his ability to compete and participate in sports relative to his age-mates may continue to bother him. I have already been thinking about whether to have him continue in mainstream sports activities, or to begin thinking about participating in groups like the Special Olympics.

Aaron enjoys school very much. When I asked him what he liked best about it, he said, "the homework." Within school, he likes rug time, calendar and story time. An exciting part of kindergarten for Aaron has been learning to read, and he says he is a "pretty good reader." The topic he likes to learn about most is animals, because "some of them are wild and some of them are not—but I like them both the same." He is looking forward to first grade, where he hopes he will "read more books."

At home, Aaron enjoys playing all sorts of board games, including Sorry!, Chess, and checkers. He also loves pretend play. Just today, he created an aquarium in our playroom, a day after our visit to the real aquarium. His was far more elaborate, including marine life as well as a zoo! He was particularly delighted to show us his penguin, dolphin, and whale show. Aaron also loves to read books with his family, both books he can read and being read to.

I asked Aaron how he felt about talking about cerebral palsy. He said, "I like talking about cerebral palsy. When I talk about cerebral palsy I learn things." When I asked him about being different from others he said, it felt "good, especially having different hair." As a final question, I asked Aaron what he would say to another child who just found out he had cerebral palsy. His response was, "I have cerebral palsy too."

Aaron's Narrative in Perspective

This narrative illustrates how MOHO concepts can be considered and applied to an individual's characteristics, capabilities, and challenges to explain how the narrative of occupational life is being crafted. Aaron's story illustrates that an optimistic plot has been shaped by his mothers' information, honesty, hopefulness, and support. This has contributed to his positive progression through participation and inclusion in normal childhood occupations. As he is a child, his story is still partly located in his mother's memory and formulation. As his mother continues to nurture Aaron to achieve further occupational competence, she will guide him to take over his narrative and steer it into his chosen direction. Figure 9-2 shows Aaron's plot moving in a positive direction, steadily upward after his birth. Aaron is a child so his story is still partly located in his mother's memory and formulation. As she realizes and illustrates through his planned adult roles, it will eventually be his story to take over and in the direction he chooses.

Aaron's sense of his own capabilities for doing (personal causation) is being supported by how his mother provides him with information

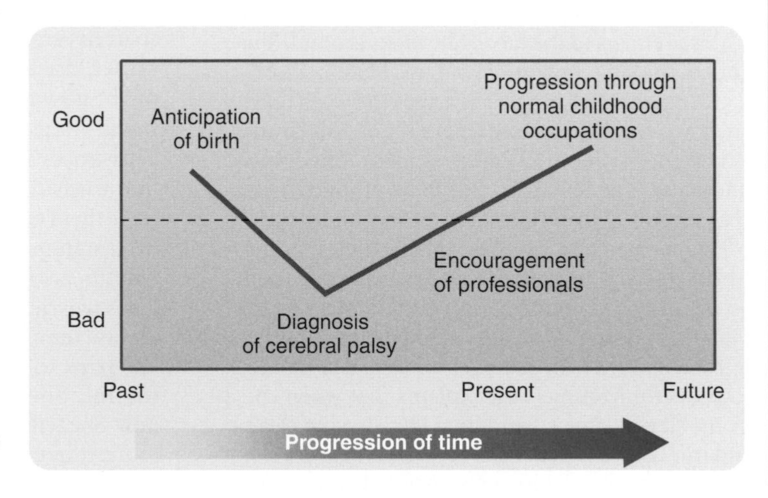

FIGURE 9-2 Aaron's Plot Moving in a Positive Direction.

about his situation framed in feedback about all the activities that Aaron is able to do despite the physical challenges. Subsequently, Aaron goes on to describe his belief in his ability to do many things as well as constructing understanding of his personal limits. Both Aaron and his mother described a wide range of his interests including specific board games, pretend play, and stories. Aaron also described his performance capacity in terms of the challenges to get his muscles to do things. Aaron identified that this had an impact on some of the things that he needed and wanted to do, for example, learning to use "the potty." However, the opportunity to gain understanding about how his body functions appears to have been empowering for Aaron. At a young age he can already account for his occupational performance and, with the insight and support of his mother, is crafting a positive occupational plot, and narrative for the future can include the identification of new strengths and overcoming obstacles.

Older Adult Narrative

A visitor has just come to talk with Lisa, who is 54, divorced, and lives by herself in her own house near her parents' home in a suburb of Stockholm. After greeting her guest, she sits down but rises immediately, asking, "Do you want a sandwich?"

"No thanks," the guest says.

Then she fetches some cookies and puts them on the table. She goes to the refrigerator, opens it, and looks inside, saying something to herself about buns. Then she seems to catch herself, embarrassed. Her guest wonders aloud what she said and Lisa responds, "I was looking for the buns, but I suppose I already ate them." Lisa takes some dark bread from the refrigerator and says, matter-of-factly, "Do you want a sandwich?"

The guest repeats, "No, thanks."

Lisa returns to the table. She looks around. She goes to the sink, saying, "What was I looking for?"

Later, after her lunch, she wipes the wash bowl and then says, "I wonder where I took this from? Where do I keep it? I have no idea!" She looks under the sink. She turns. She looks around more. "No, I think I keep it in the laundry," she says.

In her typically Swedish, practical view of the world, it is important for Lisa to remain active and be useful. She announces, "If there is laundry to do, I just start doing it." One of her favorite activities is ironing. When an observer notes that she looks so peaceful ironing, Lisa explains that when she irons, "It gets nice . . . and then I like having clean and ironed shirts in the closet . . . and then you feel useful doing it . . ." Lisa goes on to tell about how, on good days, she becomes adventuresome and goes into the city to shop for food on sale. Being practical and useful sums up much of how life should be in Lisa's commonsense view; however, she has a secret that makes this difficult.

In autumn 1990, Lisa's dementia first showed at work when she experienced depression, memory loss, and difficulty concentrating. Her symptoms were interpreted as depression and she began taking antidepressive medication without any benefit. Her difficulties increased and she was assigned to less demanding tasks. By the deep winter, she could not handle work at all and had to leave her job with disability benefits. By spring she was hospitalized.

At this time Lisa had severe memory deficits. She could not, for example, recall her own age. As Lisa describes it, she feels "somewhat of a chaos inside." Today, her cognition continues to deteriorate. Lisa is considered to suffer from a degeneration of the frontal cortex.

Lisa makes it clear that she must not show her disease to the world, but it is hard work to conceal her difficulties. She wonders, "Perhaps everybody can see I'm this dizzy and crazy," and then she repeats how hard she works to conceal what she is like. Even Lisa's mother, who is the person closest to her, is not entirely aware of her problems. Lisa considers aloud what might happen if her mother knew the facts of her dementia, "Maybe they would take my house away from me, or something like that, and believe I can't manage at all . . ." Then there is the worry about what will happen when her mother is no longer nearby as a source of support. "I worry about the day she dies. Then I will be all by myself with this sticky mess in my head. Then I won't manage and everything will fall apart."

The impending chaos when Lisa's life will come apart hovers relentlessly around her little house. It causes Lisa anxiety over all the many things that might go wrong and overwhelm her. Thus, "All small things become huge houses. I get a lot of Christmas cards, and I worry about having to first find cards to send in return, and then I have to write them out. And find addresses. And then they need stamps and I have to get out to buy stamps. And then I have to mail them and all . . ." So go Lisa's worries about how she is going to manage.

Lisa reminisces to her guest about the frequent bus trips to Stockholm that were a part of her routine. She is very hesitant to take these trips now. She tells how, a few weeks ago, she was going to meet her daughter in a large shopping center in the city. When the time came, she could not imagine how to get into the city or return home, so she did not go. Today, she starts to look for her telephone books so she can call the bus company with a question about the schedule. She finds the books in the cleaning cupboard but just stares at them, apparently wondering which one she should consult. Finally, she sighs, "No, today I feel bad. I don't want to do it." Then, as if to explain, Lisa tells her guest, slowly and solemnly, "I'm not that strong anymore. I'm weak and I can't make it. It feels like I just could break down. Before this I was strong, but I'm not anymore."

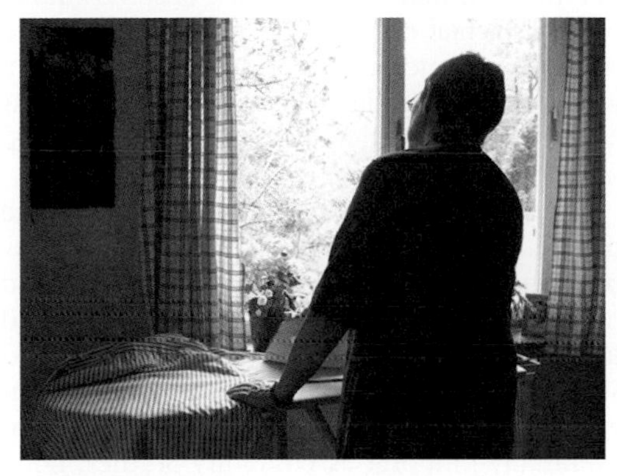

Lisa ironing at home

Lisa's Narrative in Perspective

The downward slope of Lisa's narrative takes her to the edge of a precipice (Fig. 9-3). In any moment she may be found out as incompetent, losing her house and her freedom as she had lost her job. One mistake, she believes, could bring her world crashing down on her. Lisa's story is largely lived and articulated only in sporadic bits. She does not employ a deep overriding metaphor but evokes the household images of a "sticky mess" in her head and the small tasks that become like managing big houses. At times Lisa expresses herself in a metaphor of feeling that things in her life are broken and "falling apart." Lisa's story illustrates a far less optimistic plot. Indeed the lived narrative suggests a plot of doom and loss. She describes being fearful of how her context might change and shatter the occupational life that she clings to. Her sense of chaos is tangible and the need for occupation-focused support to enable an experience of safety and acceptance is evident.

Nonetheless, her story illustrates that even persons with cognitive limitations manage to employ their occupational lives. Despite her prevailing gloomy narrative, Lisa is still able to articulate a sense of pleasure in some familiar occupational forms that she feels competent to perform (e.g., ironing). As Bruner (1990a) notes, narrative is basic to how we think about our lives.

Young Adult Narrative

Walking up the ramp and into the Hyatt hotel for the Society for Disability Studies (SDS) conference, I can feel a tingling of excitement. As a PhD student in this burgeoning field, I am surrounded on a daily basis by Disability Studies scholars (both impaired and "temporarily able-bodied"), many of whom are among my closest friends. Each new introduction to a disabled scholar at SDS signifies for me a reaffirmation of my involvement in and affection for the disability community. I feel a common bond with these individuals, one that extends far beyond our professional interests and deep into our identity as disabled people.

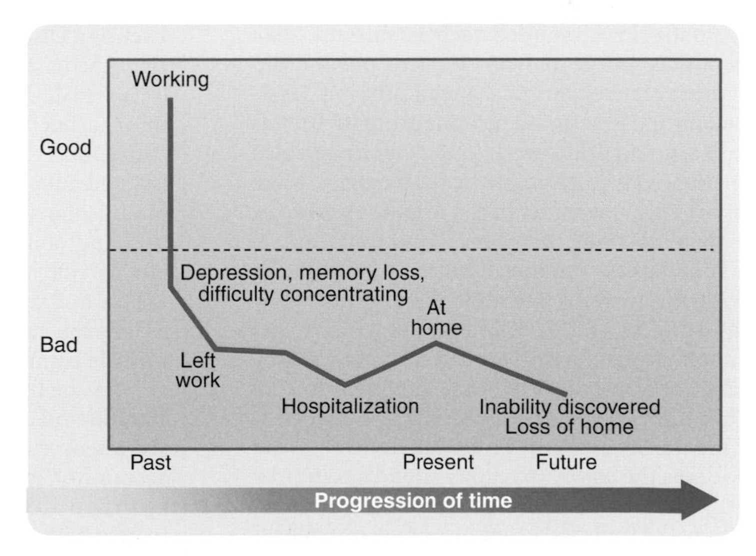

FIGURE 9-3 Lisa's Narrative Slope.

It wasn't always like this. For the majority of my brief 28 years in this world, I was largely cut off from, and therefore often wanted nothing to do with, others with disabilities. Of course, growing up with cerebral palsy I was exposed to other "handicapped" (still a common and largely acceptable label in the 1980s) children on an almost daily basis. At the local rehabilitation center I stretched alongside them on the blue foam physical therapy mats. I played board games with them as my occupational therapist unwaveringly tried to convince me to use my eternally clenched right hand rather than my relatively dexterous left one. As part of the recreational program I went swimming and even rode horses with other disabled children, all the while feeling removed and distant, and even embarrassed to be in their company. Instead, I longed to experience the "normalcy" of my nondisabled schoolmates. I longed to be integrated into their cliques, or just to have someone to eat lunch with; I longed to get into the girls' family Volvos and to play in their bedrooms after school instead of going to therapy. In high school, I longed to get into the boys' cars after school, to hang out with them downtown, to drink beer with them, to be invited to their parties, and to kiss and even to make love to them.

This pressure to be as "normal" as possible seemed to bombard me from all directions. I do not fault my parents, my teachers, or even my therapists for exerting this pressure. In fact, I commend them for it. My mother always says that all she ever wanted was for me to have "options." Certainly, my current options are numerous. Graduating with honors from a college prep school where I spent between 4 and 5 hours every evening on homework just to keep up with my able-bodied classmates, I was awarded a scholarship at a small liberal arts college for women. Here, not only did I remain very successful academically, but developed for the first time a genuine group of friends (with whom I still keep in close touch) and also experienced my first romantic relationship. More importantly, however, I began to truly explore the personal meaning of my disability.

For the first time in my life, I was living on my own; I was not attending therapy, not wearing orthotics, not depending upon my parents to cook for me, do my laundry, help me with my homework, or tell me when I should go to bed. While I cherished this freedom, it also made me all the more cognizant of my differences. What good was the ability to readily attend a fraternity party at the nearby men's college if no man would give me the time of day because of my difference? What good was working so hard to prove myself academically as long as I believed that I would still be counted among the 71% of people with disabilities (PWDs) who wanted to work but faced the barrier of discrimination?

I had no choice but to grapple with a harsh realization. Even if I did find a job and a partner, became famous, mothered 10 children, and made a million dollars, I'd never attain the normalcy I once so desperately desired. I simultaneously began to realize that I was not alone in my inability to "fit" into the mainstream. There were millions of us out there! Millions who, because of some kind of physical, mental, or behavioral "deficiency," suffered from unwarranted exclusion and discrimination, who were not afforded the same opportunities as "able-bodied" individuals, and many of whom lived in silence and shame because of it.

Thus began my second vigorous quest as a disabled person. This time I sought not to attain normalcy but rather to discover my history, my culture, and my community of fellow PWDs. At first I worked in relative isolation. Still the only visibly disabled student in my school, I looked to a still small but ever burgeoning field of knowledge, which I would eventually pinpoint as Disability Studies. Long after finishing my statistics assignment and my Spanish homework, I'd lie awake reading about the passage of the Americans with Disabilities Act and devouring personal narratives written by other disabled individuals. Although their backgrounds and their impairments varied widely, it was utterly amazing how much their experiences of disability seemed to resonate with my own.

Still, my own disability identity was not something I just fell into; acquiring it has been a very gradual process with many bumps along the way. Even as a Disability Studies scholar and disability rights activist, there are still times when I long to be "normal." I want not to be stared at when I walk into Starbucks (as if disabled people didn't need coffee too!). I want not to be spoken down to or ignored altogether when I try to order a meal or buy a gallon of milk. There are times when I worry about my ability to find a job, to find a partner, to be a parent. I occasionally still ask my mother the zillion-dollar question, "will I have a good life?" as if I expected her to look into a crystal ball and provide complete reassurance.

The one thing I have learned, however, is that there are no certainties in life. As trite as such a statement may seem, I cannot think of a more accurate or appropriate way to frame it. Growing up in a small town in Virginia, trying desperately to fit in with my able-bodied peers, I never would have thought that I would be in a doctoral program in Disability Studies in Chicago. Never would I have thought that I would intentionally seek out other adults with disabilities and that some of them would become such wonderful friends. Never would I have thought that I would come to view my disability not as an unwanted appendage but as an integral part of who I am.

I realize that my disability still leaves me much to grapple with, in terms of developing both my professional path and my personal identity. I hope that one day I can say that I am completely comfortable with myself, but I highly doubt that there are many people in this world, disabled or not, who can honestly make such a claim. Truly understanding disability, both professionally and personally, requires a learning curve, and so I have no choice but to do what I've done for my whole life: keep studying. Continuing to listen to others' experiences as well as to my own will, I believe, propel me a long way toward achieving such a goal. Indeed, it already has.

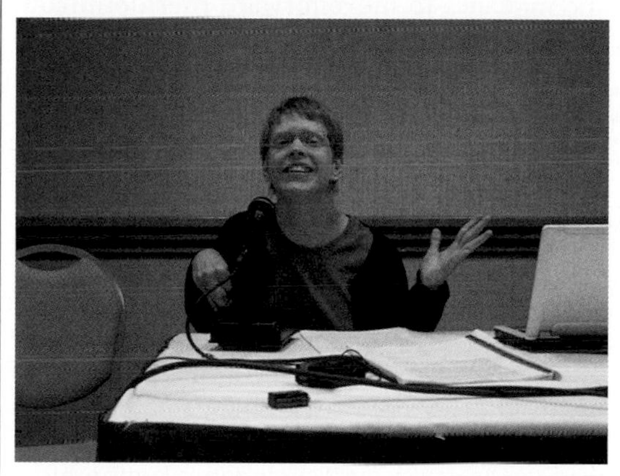

As a doctoral student, Kelly presents a paper at an international conference for Disability Studies scholars

Kelly's Narrative in Perspective

Kelly's narrative is one of searching and discovery. We see that the turning point for her was when she realized that it was not "normalcy" but identity she was seeking. Her narrative has an upward slope (Fig. 9-4) fuelled by the quest for that new identity. Kelly illustrates how an individual can relate the unfolding story of their occupational life experience through past, to present, and considering future possibilities. Narrative plot can and does change over time and is influenced by factors in the individual's physical and social environment as well as their characteristics of health and well-being.

Kelly describes a temporal journal of discovery; a journey that had obstacles (or "bumps along the way"); an experience of uncertain destinations and, at times, one of retracing steps. Her reflections are a valuable insight for occupational therapists. Kelly's story serves, in part, to remind us that health care professionals are generally a temporary guest to serve at a particularly vulnerable time in the life of an individual. It is from the individual's expertise in their own experience that sustainable solutions to enable their occupational performance in valued occupations can be drawn.

Adult Narrative

Leena graduated from high school with top grades and straightaway finished university studies. She always enjoyed the challenge of academic pursuits and thrived when challenged at work. Leena's greatest challenge has been to adapt to chronic pain. Ten years ago at age 35, she first had surgery on her back. Despite ongoing medical treatment the pain has never fully subsided and for the past 5 years she has suffered chronic, neurogenic pain.

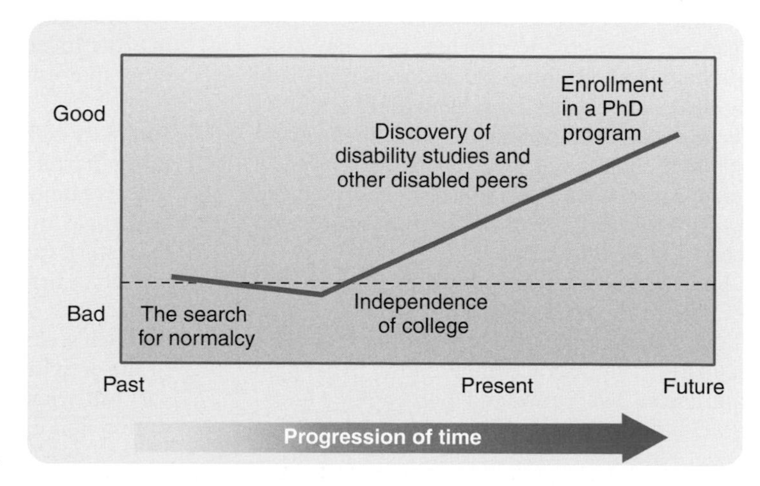

FIGURE 9-4 Kelly's Narrative Slope.

When attending the Pain Clinic the therapists asked Leena how she has come to deal with this pain in order to find a way forward. Leena used a metaphor of momentum, noting: "Even if there was a mountain in front of me I manage to find a route, a canyon—that's my way forward."

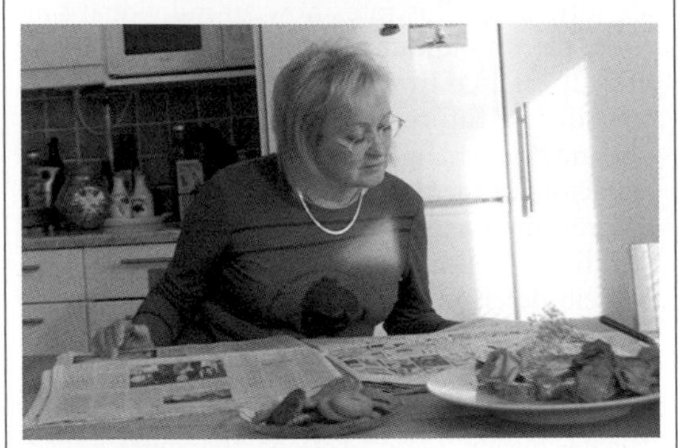

Leena reads the newspaper

Leena described how she had worked as a managing director in a big firm that does international trade. Her work demanded long hours and a lot of traveling. She had been a top performer in her field. After the onset of serious chronic pain, Leena knew she would not be able to go back to her old position. Instead, Leena chose to undertake studies in law with the aim of earning a doctoral degree. The following quote illustrates the extent to which she has had to be flexible in her narrative in order to maintain it: "When I began [university] this time, I decided I wanted a doctoral degree. Even if it took twenty years, I wanted a doctoral degree. After having studied law for a year, I realize I must be satisfied if I get a bachelor's degree. I think I can do a lot. When I have completed sufficient studies, I can work at home."

Leena's ability to continue the forward momentum of her life is also reflected in the way she has organized her life. She manages everyday tasks with help from her husband and a cleaning lady who takes care of her home few times a month. (Leena noted that one benefit is that her husband is a better cook than she is.) She attends physical therapy four times a week, which she has scheduled so as not to conflict with when she has to attend lectures at the university.

She reads voraciously both in Finnish and in English; the materials range from scientific articles to novels and detective stories. Even this occupation requires accommodation to her pain experience: "Every now and then I enjoy a newspaper. I like to read the newspaper sitting down but I am always in an awful agony afterwards. Nonetheless, every now and then I want to do it that way. Usually I read lying down and then I easily fall asleep."

Leena also described how she used to be a fast walker and that people found it hard to keep up with her pace. Nowadays she requires a cane to make walking bearable. She has found another way to go fast: "You go fast with a bike and although my legs get more sore [than from walking], I want to ride a bike, I can't help it. I have learned that I can't ride many days in a row, because if I do that my pain lasts longer and gets worse." By moderating how frequently, how long, or in what way she does what is meaningful, Leena can avoid a level of pain that makes activity impossible. She knows her body well. She assures that she can do important, enjoyable occupations by respecting the limits that her body sets for her.

Leena's Narrative in Perspective

Leena's story is a stability narrative in which she manages to move forward (her dominant metaphor) facing chronic pain like other life's challenges. Notably her narrative requires her to adapt her plans and her routines, and the flexibility to do so makes the narrative possible. Leena seeks to achieve occupational performance in activities that she has prioritized as important to her at a point in time, the present. Leena explains how she has achieved occupational adaptation to fulfill certain occupations and adjust to new circumstances. She has crafted a new narrative of recovering contemporary ordinary life *with* her lived experience of chronic pain. Particular activities that are pleasurable and volitional (e.g., reading the newspaper) come with a compromise of further experience of pain. Leena further illustrates occupational adaptation by forgoing activities generally defined in a homemaker role in order to be involved in other activities that are more interesting and fulfilling to her (Fig. 9-5).

Summary of Narratives

In the narratives described, every person's story reflects a unique and personal journey with its own challenges and accomplishments. Yet, woven into these stories are all the components of occupational identity. That is, each person seeks to make sense, subjectively, of his or her own performance capacity. Each seeks to find enjoyment and satisfaction in the activities that fill their lives. Each tries to sort out what is important to them. Each aims to find and enact roles. Each must deal with the

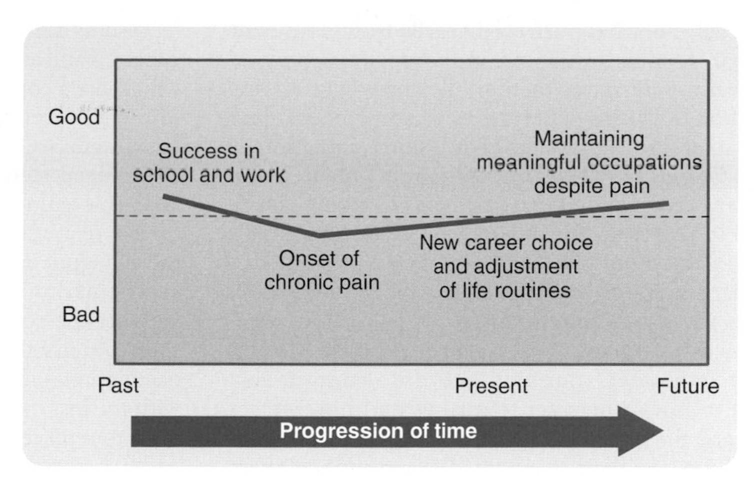

FIGURE 9-5 Leena's Narrative Slope.

routines of everyday life. Each experiences a body with physical or mental impairments.

These narratives make comprehensible the things each person does (or does not) do. For example, they reveal why Aaron uses and enjoys his swift imagination, how Leena manages to move forward through life, why Lisa gave up her habit of taking the bus into the city, and why Kelly is pursuing a PhD in disability studies. These decisions and actions all take meaning from and enact the fundamental plot of the narrative to which they belong.

Ultimately, how these persons go about life—their occupational competence—is tied to the underlying plots and metaphors of their stories. These persons all clearly conduct their lives in terms of their narratives.

Influences on the Occupational Narrative

Narratives are ultimately shaped by many things. Nonetheless, three factors appear to have an important impact. These are the unfolding events of life, social forces, and the presence or absence of an engaging occupation. The following sections examine each of these factors.

UNFOLDING EVENTS AND CIRCUMSTANCES OF LIFE

Each of the four narratives shared in this chapter so far indicates that ongoing events and circumstances of life insert themselves into narratives, having a significant influence on how they unfold. In a longitudinal study, Jonsson et al. (2000) examined how narratives shape and are shaped by what happens as lives unfold. The study began when a group of older persons was anticipating retirement and continued as they progressed into retirement. Over time, the actual direction that retirees' lives took was reflective of an interaction between their original narrative and unfolding events and circumstances. Subjects' narratives readied them to respond in particular ways to ongoing life events and circumstances. Nonetheless, differences in those external circumstances and events could also nudge the narrative in one direction or another. Thus, stories tended to be resilient, that is, to maintain their own plot. However, whereas life events and circumstances were usually integrated into the existing plot, they sometimes changed. In either case, the narrative had to come to terms with new events and circumstances.

SOCIOCULTURAL INFLUENCES ON NARRATIVE

A dynamic tension always exists between how we narrate our lives and what is around the next corner. While each person constructs his or her occupational narrative, there are also important and pervasive influences by the sociocultural context. First, each person derives a sense of narrative plot and various metaphors from surrounding cultures. The themes and images that populate our narratives are those derived from the kinds of discourse we encounter in our everyday worlds. Prevailing plots and metaphors that are part of the language and behavior of any culture serve as templates for how persons can make sense of and enact their lives. Moreover, in the course of socialization and throughout life, societies show to members what kinds of stories can be brought to bear on certain situations or problems.

Each story has borrowed heavily from dominant social themes. To the extent that societies provide prevailing narrative themes, they may have an impact on the kinds of narratives persons within them construct for themselves. For example, Kielhofner and Barrett (1997) document how a woman living in poverty is located in a narrative of seeking escape and refuge from the ongoing circumstances of her life in the inner city. Such a narrative arises out of social conditions and appears common among those who share such conditions.

Because our occupational lives unfold in interaction with others, our narratives are also invariably tied to how others act toward us and how we act toward them. Those who enter and find a place in our lives, and their characteristics and actions, affect our occupational narratives. This feature of narratives was illustrated in the study of retirees when family members were mobilized to do things that avoided the negative turn of events anticipated by their relatives (Jonsson et al., 2000). It is an important feature of social life that we note and seek to influence the occupational narratives of those whose lives intersect with our own. In the end, our stories are tied to theirs.

In sum, social influences on narrative are twofold. First, the content and shape of our narratives are provided by the social context. We invariably construct narratives that draw on socially available plots and metaphors. Second, since we live our occupational narratives in interaction with others, they inevitably affect our stories.

ENGAGING OCCUPATIONS

The third phase of the study of elderly retirees noted previously suggests that constructing a positive life story requires a person to find and participate in an engaging occupation (Jonsson, Josephsson, & Kielhofner, 2001). Engaging occupations evoke a depth of passion or feeling and become a central feature in a narrative. They are done with great commitment and perseverance and stand out from the other things a person does. They are infused with positive meaning connected to interest (i.e., pleasure, challenge, enjoyment), personal causation (i.e., one's sense of ability to do something), and value (i.e., one's belief that something is worth doing, important, and makes a contribution to family or society). Thus, the engaging occupation resonates with all aspects of volition. It is typically done with regularity over a long period of involvement and includes several occupational forms that cohere or constitute an interrelated whole. Involvement in an engaging occupation also represents a commitment or sense of duty to the occupation and a connection to a community of people who share a common interest in that occupation. In summary, an **engaging occupation** is a coherent and meaningful set of occupational forms that cohere and evoke deep feeling, a sense of duty, commitment, and perseverance leading to regular involvement over time in relation to a community of people who share the engaging occupation.

The narratives shared in this chapter appear to support the concept of engaging occupations and their potential centrality to achieving a positive occupational narrative. Each person was struggling with the loss of, the challenge of maintaining, or the need to replace an engaging occupation.

Conclusion

This chapter illustrated how people conduct and make meaning out of their occupational lives by locating themselves in an unfolding occupational narrative. Furthermore, engaging in occupations can evoke a depth of passion or feeling and become a central feature in a narrative. As each person lives life, he or she develops an occupational identity and occupational competence that represents ongoing patterns of thinking, feeling, and doing. Occupational identity is reflected in the relative success the person has in formulating a vision of life that carries him or her forward. Occupational competence is reflected in each person's relative success in putting that vision into effect. Occupational identity and competence are reflected in the telling and doing of the occupational narrative.

This is not to suggest that identity and competence are always integrated. Indeed, there are situations in which one is unable to enact the life story one envisions and desires. There is evidence that following the onset of disability, many persons may initially experience a gap between the identity reflected in their narratives and what they are able to enact (Kielhofner, Mallinson, Forsyth, & Lai, 2001; Mallinson, Mahaffey, & Kielhofner, 1998). These same studies also suggest that one cannot have competence without an intact identity. Crafting life appears to begin with what we imagine when we begin to fashion our occupational narratives. This reflects the fact that narrative is the great mediator between self and life. We always apprehend ourselves and the world around us in terms of our stories. Narrative is both the meaning people assign to occupational life and the medium within which they enact it.

CASE EXAMPLE TO TEST YOUR KNOWLEDGE: COMMUNITY-DWELLING ADULT

Gail described her reflections on her occupational adaptation to the occupational therapist: "I am 49 years old and live in a town house in England. I have many friends and colleagues but my pet dog, Nutmeg, and my two cats, Comfrey and Woodruff, together with a close friend, form the backbone of my social world. I have always maintained a belief that I can and should contribute to society through my work; it's part of the structure on which I judge my success. However, this belief and unexpected life circumstances took me in a direction that I would not have anticipated as a young woman.

After completing university training, I worked as an accountant. I chose accounting because of a love of mathematics that I had from childhood. I enjoyed and was successful at this work. However, my life took a downward tumble, I felt as though my foundations were being rocked and the cement holding everything together was cracking. For a period of time I experienced serious mental and physical illness. This was a low point in my life, but I managed to hold onto a belief that I could overcome this adversity. Eventually, I made a decision to dramatically change the course of my life; I was determined to rebuild my life in a new way. I did this through a change in career, entering an occupation where I encourage those experiencing similar mental illness to be advocates for their own needs. This occupation has greater meaning to me *because* of my own illness experience and my need to give back. My own disability experience has given me a unique understanding of the needs of people experiencing mental illness. I have come to see this as a gift that I can use to support others. Experiencing mental illness also helped me to recognize the importance of enjoying life and taking responsibility to do so. As part of this I went about constructing a full leisure life. My many leisure interests include, for instance, playing the clarinet and, more recently, learning to play the violin. In addition I satisfy my interest in mathematics by studying for a mathematics qualification at university. I relax through reading and gain a sense of adventure through traveling. All in all, the reconstruction of what I do everyday has been a helpful learning experience about myself and enabled me to adapt to my changed circumstances and insights."

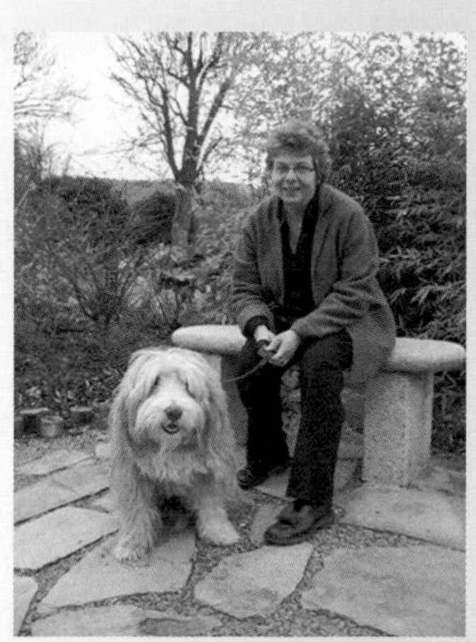

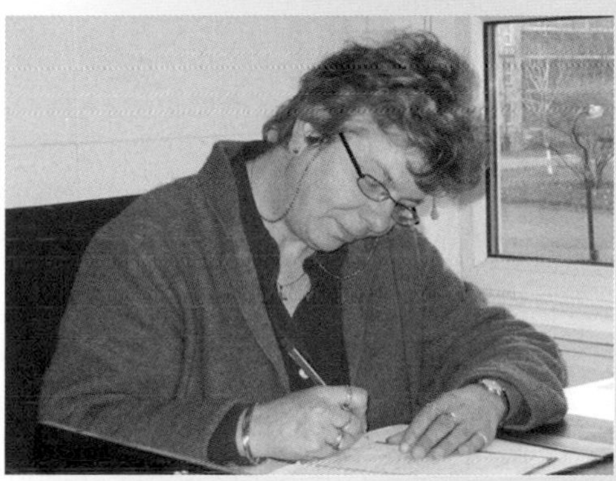

Gail on a daily walk with Nutmeg, and at work advocating for others with disabilities

Questions to Encourage Critical Thinking and Discussion

- Outline your assessment of the direction that Gail's story is taking at the points in time described. Illustrate your answer by drawing Gail's narrative slope with reference to the key features of her occupational narrative.
- What is the "plot" of the occupational life that Gail is describing? What could Gail's occupational outcome look like if a different plot were being described by Gail?
- Describe the metaphor that Gail uses in her occupational narrative description. How does

this help to illustrate the challenges and successes that she experiences?

- What key MOHO concepts can be extrapolated from Gail's description?

Review Questions

- Explain why it is important to elicit a client's occupational narrative in therapy? Evaluate the risks and benefits of this approach.
- Explain how a therapist might approach extracting a central metaphor from a client's self-described experience of chronic illness or disability. What value does knowing a client's metaphor have within the occupational therapy treatment process?
- Define a progressive narrative slope. How might knowing that a client's narrative is characterized in this way help facilitate the occupational therapy treatment process?
- Describe in detail an engaging occupation that you or someone you know is involved in. How did it evolve and what was the end product?

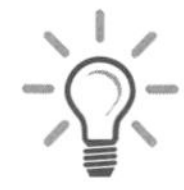

Chapter 9 Review Questions

1. Characterize how a person may be challenged to organize, shape, or craft their occupational life in order to participate in occupations that have meaning and importance to them.
2. Describe the two important features of narrative: plot and metaphor.
3. How might reflections on the "past," "present," and "future" affect a person's experience of the "plot" they are describing?
4. How would you describe the tension that always exists between how we narrate our lives and what is around the next corner?
5. What are the alternative plots that could have played out in the case examples provided in this chapter?

HOMEWORK ASSIGNMENTS

1. Reflect on your own experience of occupational adaptation over time. Consider and describe the plot of your narrative. Select and use a metaphor to describe your circumstances. Illustrate your answer by outlining a narrative slope for your life experiences.
2. Consider the nature of the relationship between what a person does, the context of their living circumstances, and their personal characteristics and capabilities. How has their occupational life been crafted over time? Apply this question to an individual that is known to you and has been challenged by their circumstances. Have occupational compromises been made? How has this affected their narrative "plot?"
3. Consider how understanding how people craft their occupational lives will shape your interactions with people in your role as therapist.

thePoint® For additional resources and exercises, visit http://thePoint.lww.com

Key Terms

Engaging occupation: A coherent and meaningful set of occupational forms that cohere and evoke deep feeling, a sense of duty, commitment, and perseverance leading to regular involvement over time in relation to a community of people who share the engaging occupation.

Metaphor: The use of a familiar object or phenomenon to stand in the place of the less-understood event or situation.

Narrative plot: The way in which an individual characterizes the story of events that they are experiencing over time.

Occupational narratives: Stories (both told and enacted) that integrate across time our unfolding volition, habituation, performance capacity, and environments through plots and metaphors that sum up and assign meaning to all these various elements.

Plot: Represents the intersection between the progression of time and the direction (for better or for worse) that life takes.

Progressive: A characterization of a narrative in which the story is headed in a positive direction.

Regressive: A characterization of a narrative in which the story is headed in a negative direction.

Stability: A characterization of a narrative in which the story is relatively constant, with minimal fluctuations from the positive to the negative.

REFERENCES

Alasker, S., & Josephsson, S. (2013). Negotiating occupational identity while living with chronic rheumatic disease. *Scandinavian Journal of Occupational Therapy, 10*, 167–176.

Aubin, G., Hachey, R., & Mercier, C. (1999). Meaning of daily activities and subjective quality of life in people with severe mental illness. *Scandinavian Journal of Occupational Therapy, 6*(2), 53–62.

Bruner, J. (1990a). *Acts of meaning*. Cambridge, MA: Harvard University Press.

Bruner, J. (1990b). Culture and human development: A new look. *Human Development, 33*, 344–355.

Cheah, S., & Presnell, S. (2011). Older people's experiences of acute hospitalisation: An investigation of how occupations are affected. *Australian Occupational Therapy Journal, 57*, 120–128.

Clark, F. (1993). Occupation embedded in a real life: Interweaving occupational science and occupational therapy: 1993 Eleanor Clarke Slagle lecture. *American Journal of Occupational Therapy, 47*, 1067–1078.

Fossey, E., & Scanlan, J. N. (2014). 2020 Vision: Promoting participation, mental health and wellbeing through occupational therapy: What are we doing and where are we heading? *Australian Journal of Occupational Therapy, 61*(94), 213–214.

Ganzer, C. (1993). *Metaphor in narrative inquiry: Using literature as an aid to practice*. Paper presented at the 15th Allied Health Research Forum, Chicago, IL.

Geertz, C. (1986). Making experiences, authoring selves. In V. Turner & E. Bruner (Eds.), *The anthropology of experience*. Urbana: University of Illinois Press.

Gergen, K. J., & Gergen, M. M. (1988). Narrative and the self as relationship. In L. Berkowitz (Ed.), *Advances in experimental social psychology*. San Diego, CA: Academic Press.

Helfrich, C., Kielhofner, G., & Mattingly, C. (1994). Volition as narrative: Understanding motivation in chronic illness. *American Journal of Occupational Therapy, 48*, 311–317.

Jonsson, H., Josephsson, S., & Kielhofner, G. (2000). Evolving narratives in the course of retirement: A longitudinal study. *American Journal of Occupational Therapy, 54*, 463–470.

Jonsson, H., Josephsson, S., & Kielhofner, G. (2001). Narratives and experience in an occupational transition: A longitudinal study of the retirement process. *American Journal of Occupational Therapy, 55*, 424–432.

Jonsson, H., Kielhofner, G., & Borell, L. (1997). Anticipating retirement: The formation of narratives concerning an occupational transition. *American Journal of Occupational Therapy, 51*, 49–56.

Kielhofner, G., & Barrett, L. (1997). Meaning and misunderstanding in occupational forms: A study of therapeutic goal setting. *American Journal of Occupational Therapy, 52*, 345–353.

Kielhofner, G., Braveman, B., Finlayson, M., Paul-Ward, A., Goldbaum, L., & Goldstein, K. (2004). Outcomes of a vocational program for persons with AIDS. *American Journal of Occupational Therapy, 58*, 64–72.

Kielhofner, G., Mallinson, T., Forsyth, K., & Lai, J. S. (2001). Psychometric properties of the second version of the occupational performance history interview. *American Journal of Occupational Therapy, 55*, 260–267.

Lal, S., Ungar, M., Leggo, C., Malla, A., Frankish, J., & Suto, M. J. (2013). Well-being and engagement in valued activities: Experiences of young people with psychosis. *OTJR: Occupation, Participation and Health, 33*(4), 190–197.

Mallinson, T., Kielhofner, G., & Mattingly, C. (1996). Metaphor and meaning in a clinical interview. *American Journal of Occupational Therapy, 50*, 338–346.

Mallinson, T., Mahaffey, L., & Kielhofner, G. (1998). The occupational performance history interview: Evidence for three underlying constructs of occupational adaptation. *Canadian Journal of Occupational Therapy, 65*, 219–228.

Mattingly, C. (1991). The narrative nature of clinical reasoning. *American Journal of Occupational Therapy, 45*, 998–1005.

Melton, J., Forsyth, K., & Freeth, D. (2010). A study of practitioners' use of the model of human occupation: Levels of theory use and influencing factors. *British Journal of Occupational Therapy, 73*(11), 549–558.

Mostert, E., & Fossey, E. (2010). Claiming the illness experience: Using narrative to enhance theoretical understanding. *Australian Journal of Occupational Therapy, 43*(3/4), 125–132.

Ortony, A. (1979). *Metaphor and thought*. Cambridge, MA: Cambridge University Press.

Price, P., Stephenson, S., Krantz, L., & Ward, K. (2011). Beyond my front door: The occupational and social participation of adults with spinal cord injury. *OTJR: Occupation, Participation and Health, 31*(2), 81–88.

Ricoeur, P. (1984). *Time and narrative* (Vol. 1). Chicago, IL: University of Chicago Press.

Schafer, R. (1981). *Narration in the psychoanalytic dialogue*. In W. J. T. Mitchell (Ed.), *On narrative* (pp. 25–49). Chicago, IL: University of Chicago Press.

Schön, D. (1979). Generative metaphor: A perspective on problem-setting in social policy. In A. Ortony (Ed.), *Metaphor and thought*. Cambridge, MA: Cambridge University Press.

Smith, G. (2008). Powerful stories and challenging messages. *Advancing Occupational Therapy in Mental Health Practice*, 147–157.

Spence, D. P. (1982). *Narrative truth and historical truth: Meaning and interpretation in psychoanalysis*. New York, NY: WW Norton.

Taylor, C. (1989). *Sources of the self: The making of the modern identity*. Cambridge, MA: Harvard University Press.

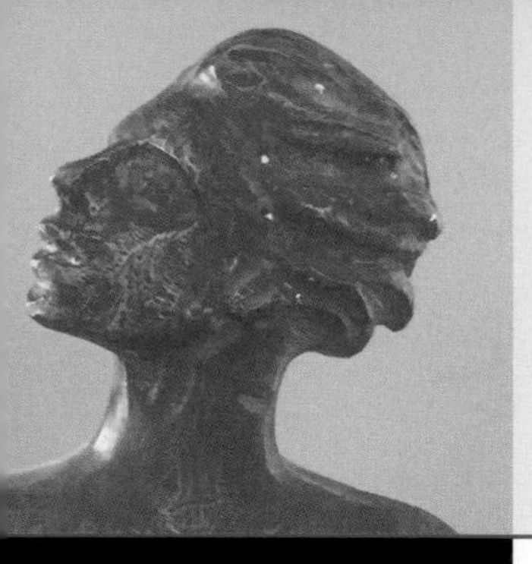

Doing and Becoming: Occupational Change and Development

Renée R. Taylor, Ay-Woan Pan, and Gary Kielhofner (posthumous)

CHAPTER 10

EXPECTED LEARNING OUTCOMES

Upon completion of this chapter, readers will be able to:

1. Describe the role of volition in the change process.
2. Describe the role of habituation in the change process.
3. Describe the role of performance capacity in the change process.
4. Describe the role of the environment in the change process.
5. Understand how a therapist works with the various elements of the model of human occupation (MOHO) so that they become reorganized and internalized into a new pattern of thinking, feeling, and performing.
6. Define each of the three elements of the change process according to MOHO.

Human development encompasses an ongoing process of multidimensional, multisystems change. This ongoing evolution becomes increasingly complex with the onset of a physical impairment or chronic illness. The following case example explains a process of change experienced by an older woman with cardiovascular disease.

MOHO Problem-Solver: An Older Adult with Cardiovascular Disease

Ms. Lu is an 86-year-old woman who had an active lifestyle throughout her life. She is highly independent and lives alone. Her son and one of her daughters live nearby. She has a strong will that led her to choose an exciting career, to get married, and to raise her children. Although her eyesight, hearing, and mobility have degenerated slowly over the years, before her stroke, she still attended choir group and a community-based program for older adults every week, which she accessed via public transportation and an electric scooter that was allowed on the trains.

Her mobility became very limited a year ago when she found it hard to breathe after a short walk. She was diagnosed as having "aortic stenosis" and received a TAVI (transcatheter aortic valve implantation) procedure. Following the procedure, she experienced a stroke (right cerebral thrombosis).

When she returned to her home, Ms. Lu was eager and intense about her anticipated recovery. Her physical therapist reinforced her feelings by encouraging her independence in gross motor functioning. Together, they performed exercises, and the therapist facilitated Ms. Lu's engagement in household chores, such as cooking, light cleaning, and using her powered mobility. Although she found these activities extremely fatiguing, Ms. Lu was able to perform them with minimal assistance from the physical therapist during the sessions.

In the absence of the physical therapist, the scenario was different. Without ongoing coaching, cheering, and other types of encouragement from the therapist, Ms. Lu struggled to complete the household chores by herself. Many days, she either forgot to perform an essential step of a chore or forgot to do the chore altogether. When she attempted to go to the grocery store, she forgot the train route and had to ask someone how to get there. Once she arrived at the store, she then forgot what to buy. In addition to these limitations, she had lost dexterity in her hand and could no longer sew, mend, and make clothing for her grandchildren as she usually did. Within a period of days of being home, she felt frustrated over these losses and quickly became demoralized during a subsequent session with her physical therapist.

A community-based occupational therapist soon became engaged in Ms. Lu's care. Familiar with MOHO, the occupational therapist began the treatment relationship by asking Ms. Lu to identify any activities or tasks that she felt were most important to do currently. Ms. Lu identified taking a bath by herself, instead of bathing in the sink, fixing her hair, washing her dentures, and being able to get groceries and cook for herself. The therapist modified her home environment by getting her a bath stool and adapting the shower head with a hose. Ms. Lu also learned how to wash her dentures and fit them into her mouth. Although she was not able to fix her hair on her own at this time, the therapist accompanied her to the hairdresser, where she received a haircut that made it easier for Ms. Lu to wash and care for her own hair. Over time, Ms. Lu began to gain perspective on her evolving occupational competence and identity. Increasingly, she took more responsibility for herself in her self-care activities. As she built proficiency within her home environment, she began to ride her scooter outside in the community, following a map that her occupational therapist had drawn for her. During the whole rehabilitation process, Ms. Lu made her own choices to engage in certain activities, just as she had chosen to receive the TAVI procedure.

Through participating in those meaningful activities in her life, Ms. Lu got back in touch with herself again. She rebuilt her daily routines in her own way and on her own terms. Her skills became more fluent and gradually, she felt more competent. She gradually regained her identity and sense of competence by participating in meaningful occupations (Fig. 10-1).

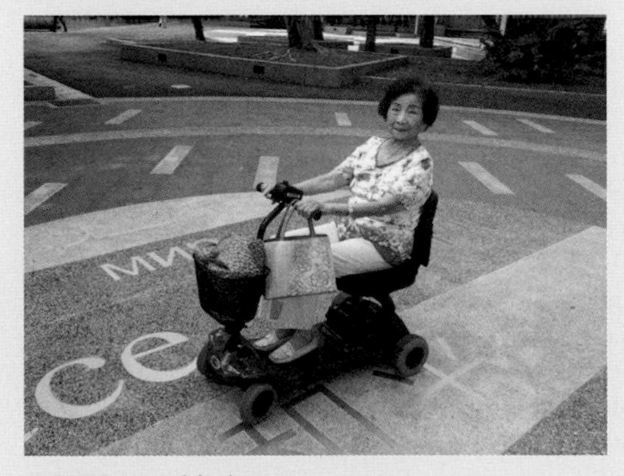

FIGURE 10-1 Ms. Lu.

What people do propels them through a trajectory of lifelong change. Fidler and Fidler (1983) referred to this process as "doing and becoming," underscoring how the course of life is shaped by occupation. When people work, play, and perform activities of daily living, they shape their capacities, patterns of acting, self-perceptions, and comprehension of our world. To a large extent, people author their own development through what they do.

Change Processes Underlying Development

Occupational development involves complex processes of change in volition, habituation, and performance capacity. Chapter 3 identified the elements involved in any permanent change (Fig. 10-2). First, an alteration of some internal or external component contributes something new to the total dynamic, out of which new thoughts, feelings, and actions emerge. Second, when these conditions are repeated sufficiently, volition, habituation, and/or performance capacity coalesce toward a new internal organization. Third, ongoing interaction of the new internal organization with consistent environmental conditions maintains a new stable pattern of thinking, feeling, and acting.

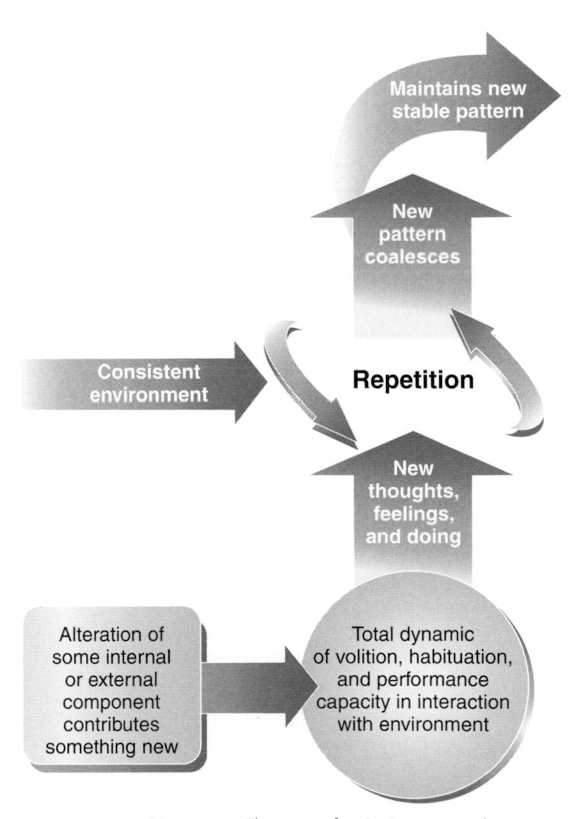

FIGURE 10-2 Necessary Elements for Permanent Change.

Ordinarily, volition, habituation, and performance capacity change in concert and are supported by the physical, social, and occupational environment. This is not to say that they change in an even or linear way; each element of the model of human occupation (MOHO) may be weighted differently at different times within the change process. From the therapist's perspective, change is about seeing a window of opportunity among the four dimensions of MOHO (volition, habituation, performance capacity, and environment). As the therapist facilitates the client to move through one pathway of least resistance, the other pathways for change are affected and engaged.

VOLITION AS AN INITIAL PATHWAY FOR CHANGE

Recall that, in MOHO, *volition* comprises three interacting elements: *interests ("I enjoy")*, *personal causation ("I can")*, and *values ("This matters")*. For many clients and their therapists, volition is the starting point for change. If a therapist can tap into what a client feels he or she is able to do and finds interest and value in doing, then that activity is volitional for the client. Clients are attracted to doing things that are volitional in nature. As a result, enabling a client to discover, identify, and practice activities that are volitional is often the starting point with many clients.

Volition is intricately related to the other MOHO contributors to occupational engagement (habituation, performance capacity, and the environment). As a person encounters an occupation that generates interest, pleasure, and feelings of ability and accomplishment (*volition*), the desire to continue to engage in that activity grows so that it becomes patterned over time (*habituation*). As the activity becomes a habit, it also becomes socialized into formal and informal roles. As healthy habit patterns form and roles are developed or revitalized, one's subjective experience while performing the activity (*performance capacity*) becomes increasingly positive. As performance capacity increases, the client's motivation to seek out contexts (*environment*) that facilitate and support this new process of engagement grows accordingly.

CASE EXAMPLE: AN ADULT WITH COMPLICATED BEREAVEMENT

It had been 2 years since her spouse's death in a motorcycle accident, and Anna, a schoolteacher, was still experiencing recurrent, major depressive episodes. Although she was able to teach her classes during the day, she often struggled to get dressed in the morning, progressed through her lessons in a robotic fashion, and then returned home to dose off in front of the television. Her most recent episode was so severe that she had not been eating and sleeping regularly, had become socially disengaged, and had found herself extremely sad and apathetic nearly all of the time. The episode had struck during the summer, when classes were out and her days became unstructured.

She had been taking antidepressant medication and seeking psychotherapy from a licensed clinical psychologist, but she had reached a point of diminishing returns. She was tired of talking about her spouse and the horrific circumstances surrounding his death. Yet she could find nothing else to talk about during her psychotherapy sessions. It was at that time when her psychotherapist recommended that Anna enroll in an intensive partial-hospitalization day treatment program.

The occupational therapist at the day program ran a daily group grounded in MOHO. Its only requirement was to bring in pictures from magazines, newspapers, or digital images from social media or other online news outlets that represented an image of something intriguing, valuable, or pleasurable. For the first few days, Anna arrived empty-handed. After her spouse died, she did not find that anything held her interest, and really did not care to aspire toward anything. Nothing in life mattered to her. Because Anna was not able to think of anything that she currently aspired toward, the OT suggested that she bring in a picture of an aspiration or interest she once had in childhood. Anna texted her sister that evening and asked her to remind her of what she seemed to care about as a child. Her sister reminded her that, for years, her walls were covered with pictures of dogs and other animals and that Anna's favorite activity as a child was going to the zoo. As an adolescent, she also worked at an anticruelty shelter for dogs and cats.

Anna was slightly embarrassed when she showed up to the group the following day with pictures of dogs, exotic cats, and a range of birds. However, she now had a starting point for conversation and participation within the group context. As members of the group asked her more about her *interests* in animals, Anna disclosed her sense of competency with animals and described how interacting with them always seemed to come naturally to her. As she reclaimed her sense of *personal causation*, she began to gain more insight into her own interests, values, and perceived capacities. She shared a long-standing *value* that she always felt protective toward those she considered the "innocents," which included

all animals, but particularly dogs. As a result of suggestions made by group members and a family connection that a group member had with the owner of a dog grooming school, Anna's participation in the group, which began with a volitionally based exercise, led her to planning what would eventually become a life-changing and meaningful occupation as a dog groomer.

HABITUATION AS AN INITIAL PATHWAY FOR CHANGE

For others, habituation may be the starting point for change. Habituation comprises habits and roles. Once solidified, these habits and roles become regular aspects of a person's life routines. When first learning MOHO, one might ask why a therapist would wish to begin the change process for a particular client with habituation (rather than volition). A therapist may see that a client is a person who enjoys order, ritual, and repetition but is uncertain about or unable to demonstrate or express specific interests, capacities, or values at a given point in time. In this case, the therapist may come to discover what the client enjoys by first learning about, observing, and supporting certain patterns of behaviors in which the client engages. As these behaviors are repeated over time, positive habit patterns are likely to form. At the same time, the client's volition and capacity for performance are revealed within that activity.

CASE EXAMPLE: AN ADULT WITH ASPERGER'S SYNDROME AND LEARNING DISABILITIES

Ben, a 30-year-old man with Asperger's syndrome and learning disabilities, has training and experience working as a security guard. He lost his most recent job at a shopping mall because of having lost control of his emotions in front of a group of customers. Currently, he is attending a work rehabilitation program, and many of the approaches used in the program are grounded in MOHO. Ben has been unable to identify his interests and has expressed concerns about returning to work as a security guard, mentioning that having to confront shoplifters and being called to resolve other conflictual situations causes him to experience nightmares and numerous other symptoms of stress.

The occupational therapist leading the program noticed that Ben would often arrive at the program at least 30 to 60 minutes before the other clients began to arrive. He enjoyed standing near the door to the facility, greeting, and chatting with each person arriving to work. At mealtimes, he would often circulate the cafeteria, stopping at each table to make small talk. Noticing the regularity at which Ben engaged in these behaviors, the occupational therapist designed an adapted work simulation activity for Ben, which involved serving as a host at a restaurant. Eventually, as Ben moved into an apprenticeship at a local family restaurant chain, he developed an interest in the restaurant business and built his sense of ability as a host. Over time, this grew into a formal employment opportunity as a host at a Disney resort near his home.

PERFORMANCE CAPACITY AS AN INITIAL PATHWAY FOR CHANGE

According to MOHO, performance capacity comprises objective and subjective elements. The objective elements are the aspects of performance capacity that are observable and measurable from outside of the person. An example is a goniometer reading that measures the range of motion of a given joint. A goniometer reading provides an objective numeric estimate upon which a therapist can base treatment plans and make preliminary predictions about therapy outcomes. The subjective aspects of performance capacity involve a person's felt, internal, and lived experience of performance. These include, but are not limited to, a person's unique thoughts, perceptions, feelings, and sensations while performing a task or activity.

According to MOHO, the objective and subjective elements of performance capacity need not mirror each other at all times. For example, an objective measure administered by a therapist may underestimate a young child's ability to feed herself within a clinical setting, but the same client appears to defy all odds by demonstrating this ability within her natural environment. Conversely, this dichotomy between the objective and subjective elements also explains situations where a client may determine that an activity is impossible despite the fact that all objective measures indicate that she is more than able to perform the activity.

Because MOHO emphasizes adaptation rather than remediation, a MOHO therapist does not hold a preconceived notion or agenda of what performance must look like in an objective sense. In MOHO, importance is placed on the act of execution rather than on a normalized standard of correctness in execution. MOHO accepts performance as it is volitionally experienced and habituated by the client, ultimately, within her natural physical, social, and occupational environments. Thus, a therapist might choose performance capacity as the starting point for change if a client is observed to have or reports a subjective experience of ability and gratification in performance.

MOHO Problem-Solver: A Young Man with a Traumatic Brain Injury

Casey grew up on a dairy farm with 600 head of cattle, three-dozen chickens, and alternating crops, including soybeans and corn. At the age of 18, he experienced a head injury when struck by a front-end loader on a Bobcat machine that his younger brother was operating. After several weeks in inpatient rehabilitation, his safety and future in farming initially appeared questionable to his occupational therapist. He had lost vision in one eye, had difficulty with executive functioning and visual motor planning, and exhibited difficulties with balance on all objective tests. He was discharged from the hospital with the recommendation to continue with home visits from an occupational therapist and a physical therapist.

The physical therapist focused on improving Casey's core strength and balance with a number of exercises and a balance board. Being a cooperative and engaged client with a strong desire to improve, Casey followed all of the therapist's instructions and performed his recommended homework exercises religiously between visits. His progress was slow, but he did show development in his core strength, with less improvement in his coordination and balance over time.

Having read the chart notes from the inpatient rehabilitation unit, Bill, the occupational therapist, did not know what to expect before his first visit with Casey.

Bill began the visit by asking Casey some general questions about his daily activities and occupational roles before and after the accident. Being a man of few words, Casey consistently reported, "All I have ever known is farming. . . It is the only thing I know how to do." Casey had little insight into his other interests, and cited his strong sense of family as a singular value in life. Having been trained in MOHO, Bill understood that Casey's occupational identity was as a farmer. Bill decided that therapy in this case was best conducted outside of the home environment and instead within the fields and barns that comprised Casey's family farm.

Bill began therapy by asking Casey for a tour of the farm. During that tour, Bill asked Casey a number of questions about each aspect of the farm, from the crop-farming machinery to the milking operation, to the doctoring of the heifers and the care of the steer. As Casey described each element, he spoke proudly of his many abilities on the farm. Although he and his family were respectful and cooperative with the recommendations from his neurologists and therapists at the hospital, who recommended that he not engage in farming until further notice, Casey reported that he has felt "useless" to his family ever since his accident and knows he could be helping more. At that moment, Bill observed Casey's younger brother pouring feed into the chicken feeder. Bill suggested that Casey give it a try and offered a small coffee container as a makeshift feed scoop. Casey approached the feeder, hung on to the side of the barn with one hand, and scooped the chicken feed out into the feeder with the other. Although some feed fell onto the ground and Casey struggled to maintain his balance, he performed the job successfully and reported an experience of freedom and mastery while completing the task. Casey's subjective experience of performance capacity, in that moment, led to countless additional opportunities for rehabilitative activities and built adaptations around the farm, which Casey and Bill created together during subsequent visits. Soon, the physical therapist also became engaged in this form of work rehabilitation. Casey developed a daily routine, recovered specific roles within the family unit, and rediscovered a sense of self-efficacy and interest in his work.

ENVIRONMENT AS AN INITIAL PATHWAY FOR CHANGE

According to MOHO, various aspects of a client's physical, social, and occupational environment act as facilitators or barriers to engagement in occupation. Changes in environmental impact are also an important part of any change trajectory. An aspect of the environment may initiate change by imposing an expectation or offering a unique opportunity. For example, an occupational environment of a factory offers machinery, work outputs, and a pace of work that cannot be duplicated within a clinical environment. The social environment comprised by a client's family may offer a constraint if family members are overly protective, thereby interfering with the client's capacity for independence in a particular area of occupational performance. Alternatively, a client's family may act as a facilitator for occupational performance and participation if they collaborate with the client in ways that promote engagement. Change usually involves interacting with different aspects of the environment, modifying surroundings, seeking out new settings, or avoiding past contexts. The influence of these altered person–environment interactions is essential to the change process and, eventually, to the maintenance of new patterns of thinking, feeling, and doing that are the result of change.

MOHO Problem-Solver: A Middle-School Child with Cerebral Palsy and a Nonverbal Learning Disability

Ali is a 9-year-old boy with moderate athetoid cerebral palsy and a nonverbal learning disability. Having grown up receiving treatment from a range of occupational, physical, and speech therapists, Ali dreaded his appointments with his school-based occupational therapist. The occupational therapist was assigned to work with Ali, consistently a straight A student, on developing better social skills so that he could form friendships at school.

In the past, Ali's family had facilitated some of Ali's friendships, by encouraging Ali to invite his classmates to visit him at the family's extravagant estate, which featured an indoor swimming pool, a game room, and a garage full of muscle cars (a special collection belonging to Ali's father). This strategy was partially effective for a while, but Ali could not consistently maintain a friendship. What resulted were single visits from individual classmates, with reciprocal invitations for visits at the classmate's home being absent. In addition to the ephemeral nature of these visits, Ali did not exert good judgment about whom to invite, resulting, during one visit, in his classmates taking advantage of the family's generous nature and leaving trash and damage to the walls of the home.

Ali's occupational therapist, Jenna, understood that the strategy that the family had been using was ineffective. At the same time, Ali did not demonstrate a lot of interest or self-confidence when it came to social relationships. Moreover, he exhibited poor judgment when selecting potential friends and often did not recognize the social cues of boys who would later bully or humiliate him, resulting in feelings of hurt and betrayal. Initially, Jenna attempted to teach and coach Ali to develop specific social skills, including how to read facial expressions, how to interpret body language and tone of voice, how to share and act reciprocally, and how to resolve conflicts. Although Ali understood and could repeat the concepts on an intellectual level, he lacked the interest (*volition*) and practice (*habituation*) necessary to enact what he learned within his daily relationships at school, maintaining that his peers would reject and humiliate him no matter what he did.

For these reasons, Jenna decided to craft a unique social environment for Ali at school. First, she collaborated with Ali's teacher to provide an advocacy-based, educational session to the entire class about children with disabilities, specifically, cerebral palsy. In addition, a zero-tolerance rule was put into place within Ali's classroom that resulted in an automatic detention for any student caught behaving in a disrespectful or discriminating manner toward another student. Jenna then collaborated with Ali's teacher to offer an "extra credit" opportunity to a selected group of Ali's classmates who were known to show a capacity for sharing, understanding, and openness toward others. Ali was placed into this group, and they were charged with planning and enacting a school play using a script that had a disability advocacy, antibullying theme. Thus, Jenna had constructed not only an optimal social environment in which Ali could socialize, but also an occupational environment within which themes of disability advocacy and self-preservation were reinforced within the classroom and school.

SUMMARY

During change, volition, habituation, and performance capacity can resonate with and sometimes amplify each other. For example, increases in capacity tend to be accompanied by stronger personal causation. The latter leads to choices to do things that further develop that capacity. The process can also go in the other direction. For instance, older persons whose diminished capacities increase the risk of falling may develop, as part of personal causation, a fear of falling that leads to choices to curtail their movement and other activities. However, by engaging in an exercise program, older adults may reduce their risk of falling (Fuzhong et al., 2016).

In any process of change, multiple factors will intersect, contributing both synergistic and divergent forces. For example, adolescents discover new capacities and begin to see themselves as more autonomous. Such volitional changes lead adolescents to interpret what they do differently (refusals and defiance, previously viewed as transgressions, now become assertions of autonomy) and to select new action that tests limits and explores risk. Parents and others in the environment may not consistently agree with the adolescent's desires for autonomy and risk-taking. Moreover, the adolescent's own habituation may assert old patterns such as childhood habits of reliance on parents. Accordingly, the process of change can sometimes be characterized by disorganization, alterations in the pace of change, and backsliding. Change is seldom neat and orderly.

MOHO: A Continuum of Change

Change ordinarily occurs across a continuum from exploration to competence to achievement (Reilly, 1974). This continuum, which has been adopted as a descriptor for change within the MOHO, is usually involved in transformational and catastrophic change. That is, people typically progress through these levels of function when they move into new roles, encounter new environments, and make lifestyle changes, or when they reorganize their lives in response to a major disruptive circumstance or event.

This continuum of development may involve all areas of one's occupational life, as when persons who have acquired a major disability must reorganize how they view themselves and their abilities, how they achieve satisfaction and meaning in life, and how they go about their work, leisure, and activities of daily living. The continuum may also apply to only one aspect of a person's occupational life. The person who is retiring, the mother who decides to return to work after her children have left home, and the person who takes up a new serious hobby are examples of persons who may develop new occupational participation through the stages discussed below.

According to MOHO, **exploration** is the first stage of change in which persons try out new things and, consequently, learn about their own capacities, preferences, and values. Persons explore when they are learning to do new occupational forms, making role changes, or searching for new sources of meaning. Exploration provides the opportunity for learning, discovering new modes of doing, and discovering new ways of expressing ability and apprehending life. It yields a sense of how well one performs, how enjoyable the task is, and what meaning it can have for one's life. Exploration requires a relatively safe and undemanding environment. Since a person who is exploring is still unsure about capacity or desire, the resources and opportunities in the environment are critical.

CASE EXAMPLE: EXPLORATION

Sam, a 12-year-old boy, has been invited by his father to escort him on a business trip. Part of the time will be spent on a sailboat. Having never sailed before, Sam is apprehensive. Before accompanying his father, he decides to surf the Internet to learn more about the sport of sailing (Fig. 10-3). Once he arrives at the harbor, he remains in his chair and watches while others make their way onto the boats and push away from the dock. After nearly 20 minutes, Sam decides to board the boat, but with his father close at hand.

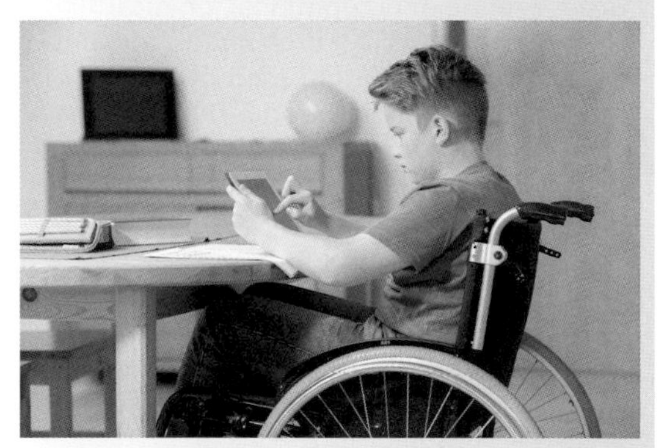

FIGURE 10-3 Exploration: Sam Learns About Sailing on the Internet.

Competency is the stage of change when persons begin to solidify new ways of doing that were discovered through exploration. During this stage of change, persons strive to be adequate to the demands of a situation by improving themselves or adjusting to environmental demands and expectations. Individuals at a competence level of change focus on consistent, adequate performance. The process of striving for competence leads to the development of new skills, the refinement of old skills, and the organization of these skills into habits that support occupational performance. Competency affords an individual a growing sense of personal control. As persons strive to organize their performances into routines of competent behavior that are relevant to their environment, they immerse themselves in a process of becoming, growing, and arriving at a greater sense of efficacy.

CASE EXAMPLE: COMPETENCY

Delois, a 34-year-old attorney, has always been self-conscious about dancing. After her diagnosis with multiple sclerosis, her self-consciousness has grown. At the same time, one of her friends from law school has invited her to stand up to her wedding. Knowing that she will be required to dance as a member of the bridal party, Delois decides to take dance lessons. During the lessons, her instructor encourages her to focus on the precise movements and steps and to practice the steps at home between lessons. Although she has not mastered the dance movements by any means, Delois is adequately prepared to dance with Curtis, a friend she meets at the reception (Fig. 10-4).

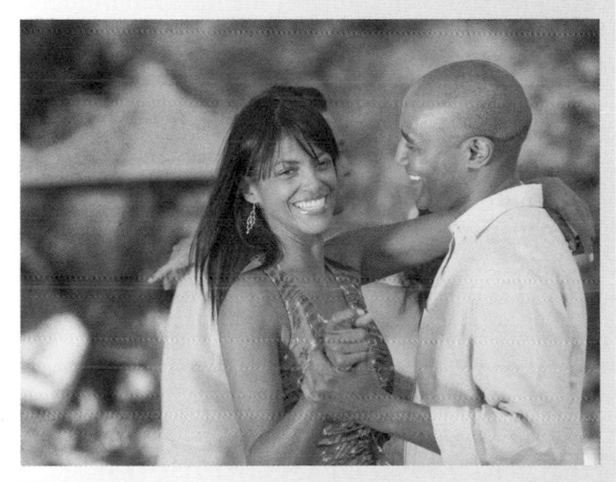

FIGURE 10-4 Competency: Delois Takes Lessons to Overcome Her Concerns About Dancing.

Achievement is the stage of change when persons have sufficient skills and habits that allow them to participate fully in some new work, leisure activity, or activity of daily living. During the achievement stage of change, the person integrates a new area of occupational participation into his or her total life. Occupational identity is reshaped to incorporate the new area of occupational participation. Other roles and routines must be altered to accommodate the new overall pattern to sustain occupational competence.

In the case in which all areas of a person's occupational participation are changing, some areas may attain achievement before others. For example, following a traumatic spinal cord injury, a person may first concentrate on redeveloping ways to manage activities of daily living that include moving to an independent living setting after a period of rehabilitation or living in an institutional setting. Developing patterns of leisure in the new context and returning to work may come later.

CASE EXAMPLE: ACHIEVEMENT

Nearly 2 years after her injury, Angela now finds joy and mastery in caring for her adopted infant (Fig. 10-5).

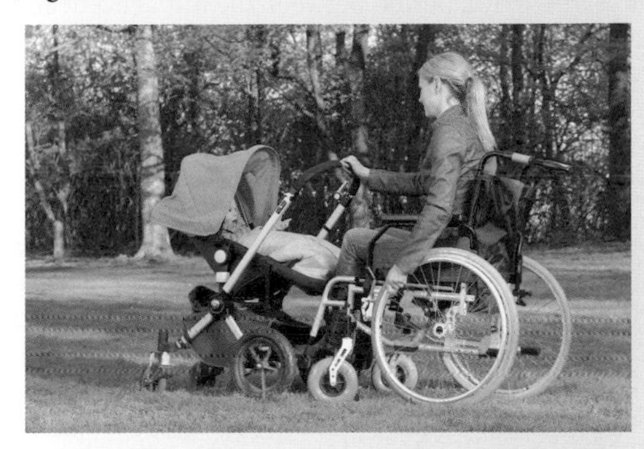

FIGURE 10-5 Achievement: Angela and Her New Baby Girl.

PROGRESSION THROUGH THE STAGES OF CHANGE

It should also be recognized that persons might move back and forth between stages. For example, having explored various career options and made a choice to enter an educational program, students sometimes find that the choice was not right and return to exploration. As another example, Hammel (1999) observed that persons with spinal cord injury often moved back and forth between these stages.

The three stages of change broadly describe the trajectory that occupational change is likely to take. The actual pattern of events, actions, thoughts, and feelings that transpires when someone goes through change will be unique for each person and for each episode of change.

READINESS FOR CHANGE

The three stages of change describe a typical pathway once a person has embarked on the process of change. This presumes that a person is ready to begin making change. For a variety of reasons, this may not be the case. Even persons whose occupational participation is not adaptive are sometimes reluctant to make a change or do not believe that a change is possible in their lives. Another factor limiting readiness to change may be proximity to a catastrophic event. Hammel (1999) found that following spinal cord injury, people went through a process of adjustment that preceded concrete steps toward change. At first, people were dominated by the sense of loss and a disruption of previous life. Following this, she observed that persons entered a period of reaction marked by strong feelings of anger, frustration, fear, and/or depression. Next, they began to acknowledge going on with life and to formulate intentions to make change. Following this, they began the exploratory stage of change. Such research suggests that catastrophic change may be marked by a period between the initial event and circumstance that precipitates or necessitates change and the beginning of making the change.

CENTRALITY OF THE ENVIRONMENT IN CHANGE

As already noted, the environment has a pervasive influence in any process of change. The environment can be the source of alterations that precipitate change. Many of the changes that occur in the course of development occur according to socially defined timetables and expectations for change.

The environment can also be a barrier to change. Social definitions of a person's identity or expected behaviors can conflict with personal desires and attempts to change. Realizing change is difficult when the environment fails to support or reward the alterations a person is trying to make. The stages of change presented earlier also suggest that appropriate environments exist for persons to advance through the stages. For example, to engage in the process of exploration or competency, the environment must allow for persons to try out and/or strengthen new action.

Contributions of Change to the Course of Development

As noted previously, the course of development is characterized by an ongoing process of change. The course of any life involves ongoing **incremental** and **transformational change**. Most lives will be affected by one or more periods of catastrophic change.

A cross-sectional view of development will show that, at any point in the life cycle, aspects of one's occupational life will be at different stages. For example, the older child who has mastered self-care and has integrated it into daily routines (achievement) will be at the beginning of exploring the vocational interests in play and school. Achievement in work will follow years later. Underlying development, then, is a complex collection of change processes that follow one another, overlap, and interweave.

Transformation of Work, Play, and Activities of Daily Living

Discussions of development often emphasize that particular courses or processes of development are normal. For example, most discussions of childhood development describe various attainments that, on average, have occurred by a particular age. However, great variation in the course of development occurs across persons. Too much emphasis on norms can distract us from the more important change processes that underlie development. Development is first and foremost a change process through which the individual is transformed throughout life.

The most obvious outward manifestation of occupational development is that persons engage in different occupations over the course of their lives. For example, younger children play, older children and adolescents attend school, and adults work. The transformation of occupation across the life span reflects an underlying order realized in the individual but sustained by the sociocultural environment. Socially established and culturally defined patterns of work, play, and self-care over the life span influence the sequence of occupational participation reflected in development.

The following sections provide an overview of the course of occupational development using the typical divisions of childhood, adolescence, adulthood, and later adulthood. The discussions are not meant to be exhaustive or detailed accounts of occupational development. Rather, they offer a perspective from which to consider how volition, habituation, performance capacity, and environment contribute to and undergo change throughout the life course.

Ongoing Tasks of Occupational Adaptation: Identity and Competence

During each stage of development, as internal changes occur and as the environments in which we do things change, we face two fundamental tasks. These are as follows:

- Constructing an occupational identity by which we know ourselves and our lives
- Establishing occupational competence in our patterns of doing

In each culture, the pattern of development is narratively structured. That is, the culture carries a dominant narrative describing the life course (Luborsky, 1993). Nonetheless, these dominant narratives are, to varying degrees, ill-suited to define the individual life course (Luborsky, 1993). For example, dropping out of school, changing career choices, getting divorced, becoming widowed, or being fired or laid off from a job all present variations in the life course story that people grapple with in forming their identity. More dramatically, being homosexual, having or acquiring a disability, or wanting to live life outside the culturally defined narrative present major challenges for achieving an occupational identity. Consequently, dominant cultural narratives can be sources of constraint that hinder adaptation.

How each person constructs an occupational identity and realizes it in everyday patterns of doing will vary from person to person. Some will more or less readily accept the dominant narratives shared by the group to which they belong. Others will choose a more individualistic course. Still others will be thrust by life circumstances into charting a different path for themselves. Nonetheless, the challenge of adaptation remains the same: to identify and enact a self and a way of living that is experienced as good, yields a sense of accomplishment, provides grounding in familiar routines, and allows one to realize one's unique potentials, limitations, and desires.

Childhood

Through the course of childhood, extensive transformation of volition, habituation, and performance capacity takes place. These changes allow the child to emerge as an occupational being with personal ways of doing, thinking, and feeling. Childhood occupation is both unique in its own character and serves as a foundation for later competence (Case-Smith & Shortridge, 1996; Hurt, 1980).

VOLITION

As children experience themselves doing things, their personal causation, interests, and values emerge. The volitional choices of early childhood are mainly activity choices. Later, children begin to make occupational choices to take on personal projects (e.g., learning to play a musical instrument) or discretionary roles (e.g., joining scouts, a club in school, or a sports team). Occupational choices may be, at first, assisted or coached by parents who supply for children the rationale for projects, habits, and roles.

Play is a major vehicle through which the child first develops a sense of personal causation (Bundy, 1997). As noted in Chapter 4, personal causation begins with children's awareness that they can cause things to happen. The desire to have effects in the environment becomes a strong motive and manifests itself in the child's play (Bundy, 1997; Ferland, 1997). Children's awareness of their capacities is gained through engaging with the environment in play, in social interaction, and eventually in other occupational spheres (Lindquist, Mack, & Parham, 1982). At first, children's sense of their abilities is very general (e.g., effort and capacity are not distinguished and not always accurate) (Nicholls, 1984). Through the child's experiences of failure and success, the child's knowledge of capacity and feelings of efficacy become more complex and accurate.

Cultural messages about values influence the child early in life. Adult approval and disapproval of actions guide the child's understanding of the social value of doing certain things. Growing awareness of what parents, siblings, and others value increasingly influences activity and occupational choices. For example, as children learn the value of being productive in occupations (e.g., chores and schoolwork), they increasingly assume responsibility for such behaviors and, in turn, experience the approval of others that solidifies the commitment to behave accordingly.

Childhood interests reflect expanding capacities. Children are attracted to activities that allow exercise of capacity and yield new experiences. Much of childhood pleasure comes from the mastery of new actions (Mailloux & Burke, 1997). As new capacities emerge, interest turns toward their utilization and expansion. For example, increased hand dexterity invites, and results from, the child engaging in play requiring fine motor control, such as constructing simple projects. Linguistic competence leads to interest in verbal humor and rhymes. Children find particular interest in those activities that provide optimal arousal by challenging capacity (Burke, 1977, 1993; Ferland, 1997).

HABITUATION

The young child's major occupational roles are player and family member (Florey, 1998; Hinojosa & Kramer, 1993). Parents and others see play as the normal business of the child. The player role has its own expectations, as when parents specify where and with what objects children may play. In addition, play is a means of trying out roles in sociodramatic play and games.

The family member role emerges as parents expect and value productive contributions of the child to the routines of family life by engaging in such occupational forms as picking up toys, doing small chores, and carrying out self-care. As childhood progresses, the range of roles increases to include the student role and the role of friend and membership in various childhood groups.

Biological rhythms provide the child's first consistent patterns. Environmental rhythms allow the child to internalize routines such as sleeping, waking, bathing, eating, playing, and self-care. In time, the child becomes more and more able to organize behaviors to accomplish chores and routines of self-care. Moreover, children find repetition a source of security, predictability, and comfort. Many habits that will be resources throughout life are acquired in childhood. Although the major influence on habits is the family routine, the child is affected by each new occupational setting, such as day care and school.

PERFORMANCE CAPACITY

Performance capacity undergoes dramatic transformation as the child gains experience, especially from play (Pierce, 1997; Robinson, 1977). Throughout childhood, increasing competence for interacting with the environment leads to the desire and capacity to seek out novel experiences. As children's capacities increase, their world expands (e.g., entering formal education). This process results in exposure to new environments that further impact on the development of capacity.

OCCUPATIONAL IDENTITY AND COMPETENCE

Occupational identity emerges in childhood. As children acquire the ability to integrate past, present, and future and to imagine themselves in an unfolding story, they begin to narrate parts of their lives and to sort out meanings through stories (Burke & Schaaf, 1997). By late childhood, children have a fairly developed sense of who they are. The occupational competence developed during childhood similarly tends to follow social norms and expectations. Nonetheless, each child begins to discover and pursue unique interests and aptitudes that individualize identity and competence.

Adolescence

Adolescence is typically a period of stress and turmoil due to both intrapersonal and sociocultural factors (Hendry, 1983). In addition to being a time of accelerated and dramatic biological change, adolescence can also be an uncertain social transition from childhood to adulthood. The beginning of adolescence is associated with both biological (puberty) and institutional (junior high school) changes. The end of adolescence was traditionally associated with entry into the worker role, but the timing of work entry can differ radically depending on whether one works directly after high school, attends college, or obtains postgraduate education. Consequently, adolescence has no firm boundaries.

VOLITION

Adolescence is characterized by an increasing drive for autonomy (Mitchell, 1975; Santrock, 1981). Adolescents must successfully learn to make activity and occupational choices that bring personal satisfaction and meaning yet meet expanding environmental expectations. The most pressing occupational choice of adolescence is selecting a type of work (Allport, 1961).

Adolescents are challenged to maintain a sense of efficacy while facing new social expectations for responsibility and having to acquire an expanding repertoire of occupational forms. Adolescents also begin to assess their capacity in terms of expected performance in future roles. During adolescence, belief in one's ability to control life outcomes ordinarily increases (Hendry, 1983). Increased freedom of choice challenges adolescents to clarify and establish their values. Rejection of some previous or parental values leads to a more personalized worldview and confirms for adolescents that their values are their own. Establishing values is challenging since the sources of values in society are many and sometimes contradictory. Not surprisingly, many adolescents experiment and struggle in the process of value formation, often moving between ideal values and the realities of life (Florey, 1998).

Interests also undergo substantial transformation during adolescence. What interests emerge depend very much on the social context. One of the primary influences on interest change is movement out of the family setting, where interests are often family centered, into a peer group where new interests are espoused. Interests also change because the adolescent can do new things such as dating and driving a car. Adolescents' interests also become more of an expression of identity (Csikszentmihalyi & Rochberg-Halton, 1981). What one enjoys becomes a kind of statement about what kind of person one is.

HABITUATION

Adolescence is a period of transformation in the roles and habits that regulate everyday behavior. Adolescents try out many of the roles they will hold as adults. Such role experimentation fills several needs for adolescents. It helps them to consolidate their identity, to satisfy the desire for status and independence, and to recognize their abilities for particular roles.

Although some roles continue from childhood into adolescence, the nature of those roles and the expectations associated with them begin to change. For example, in the family context, adolescents become more responsible for taking care of themselves (e.g., buying their own clothes, cooking meals for themselves) and contributing to household (e.g., through part-time work). Although there are increasing opportunities to try on a variety of roles, adolescents may be frustrated that certain adult roles are not yet available to them (Hendry, 1983).

For the adolescent, the peer group is a source of information about the world outside the family and is a testing ground for new ideas and behaviors. The role of friend is increasingly important and may undergo several changes during adolescence. Part-time jobs and volunteer work expose many adolescents to the work world and afford the opportunity to develop skill in getting and keeping jobs, budgeting time and money, and taking pride in accomplishments. Volunteer work can also serve as a means for exploring future vocations.

New habits are required for the changing circumstances of adolescence and for the world of work. Adolescent habits take over much routine behavior that was previously externally regulated in the family and by the other social contexts. A major impact on the habits of the adolescent is the movement from grammar school to junior high and high school. No longer in a single classroom with a series of daily activities for the entire class, students have individual schedules and must be responsible for being in the right place at the right time. More of adolescents' time is at their personal discretion. They must use time to establish a routine for the student and other roles.

PERFORMANCE CAPACITY

Physical growth and change is central to the transformation of performance capacity in adolescence. Adolescents reach or approximate their adult size and begin bodily processes that characterize adulthood. Intellectual, cognitive, and emotional capacities expand in adolescence, allowing greater depths of awareness and comprehension of the world (Mitchell, 1975; Santrock, 1981). The adolescent also expands capacities for communication and interaction.

OCCUPATIONAL IDENTITY AND COMPETENCE

Adolescents begin to seriously see themselves as the authors of their own lives and to connect present actions with future outcomes and possibilities (Case-Smith & Shortridge, 1996). Adolescents' need to craft their own occupational identity and competence culminates in several important occupational choices, such as selecting a career and finding a partner.

The early adolescent's identity is more concerned with issues of enjoyment. Later, the adolescent gives increasing consideration to sense of capacity and feelings of efficacy and chooses occupations according to internalized values. By late adolescence, occupational identity is much more sophisticated and centers on the occupational choices necessary to enter adult life. Nonetheless, this process is highly variable and proceeds at different paces for different persons (Ginzberg, 1971). In fact, because identity and competence are continually evolving and changing with growth and experience, the process of occupational choice is continuous and dynamic.

Adulthood

The boundaries of adulthood are closely tied to one's working life. Adulthood typically begins with the assumption of a more or less permanent full-time job or other productive occupation and ends with retirement (Hasselkus, 1998). Adulthood is the longest period of life. Contrary to popular views of adulthood as a period of stability or a state of maturity that is achieved and sustained, adults undergo considerable change. Some of these changes are externally recognizable, as the person passes through a series of steps, crises, or transitions: marriage or divorce, starting a family, changing jobs, and bidding farewell to grown children. Other changes are internal, as the individual sorts out the various meanings, goals, and purposes that guide choice and self-evaluation in adult life.

VOLITION

Diverse factors such as economic constraints and obligations of parenthood affect adult decisions, but for most people, adulthood is the time when one truly begins to live one's own life. Adulthood ordinarily is accomplished by an increasing desire to achieve and to work autonomously. For most people, this is accompanied by an increased sense of efficacy.

Early adulthood is generally a period of acquiring and refining abilities for one's line of work. Young workers see themselves as learning and increasing their efficacy. By middle adulthood, individuals have generally realized their peak performance. Although the sense of efficacy is often dominated by work, other adult experiences such as rearing a family and maintaining a household are also areas that evoke strong feelings about one's effectiveness. Parents often find themselves facing great responsibilities with minimal preparation, such as the challenge of a newborn or confronting an adolescent's rebelliousness. Similarly, such adult responsibilities as maintaining a household and managing personal finances can be sources of stress, accomplishment, and failure.

During adulthood, values usually become increasingly important as a motivating force and a source of self-evaluation. Although personal values related to occupation tend to remain relatively stable throughout adulthood, a generalized shift does often occur. The goals of early adulthood are focused on instrumental and material values, such as getting ahead at work and earning a satisfactory living. Middle-aged workers may begin to focus more on humanitarian concerns and on themes of legacy (e.g., what one will leave to the future or how one will be remembered by children). Although this particular pattern of value change will not characterize all adults, some shift in values is likely in the course of adult life.

Leisure and work interests are relatively stable. Many adults entered their work because it embodied the opportunity to channel and develop personal interests. However, it is not a universal phenomenon that adults find their work interesting. Many adults pursue their interests avidly and seriously during their leisure time. Other adults use interests as a means of relaxing and regenerating themselves for work.

HABITUATION

Adulthood is characterized by a variety of socially prescribed and individually chosen roles that structure the adult's daily life and provide identity. Apart from family roles, most of these roles are enacted in community settings (Hasselkus, 1998). Typical adult role transitions include the initiation or end of partnerships, parenthood, changes in work roles, and joining civic and social organizations.

The one pervasive feature of adult life is work. Working requires learning new behaviors, forming new interpersonal relationships, reapportioning one's use of time, and, frequently, developing a new identity. The work role also influences other adult roles, especially friendship and leisure roles. Workers often share confidences and decision making with coworkers and may develop strong friendship ties with colleagues.

Most adults have to divide their time among work, family, community, and leisure roles. Participation in organizational and social roles, volunteering, and participating in religious organizations are other roles that many adults pursue. Because each of these roles can involve substantial investments of energy and time, a large number of people find inevitable conflicts in their use of time. Despite the potential for conflicts in time use, having a combination of roles appears to enhance well-being (Baruch, Barnett, & Rivers, 1980).

Habits of adulthood are necessarily concerned with the efficient allocation of time to various roles and the occupational forms they require. The division of the weekly routine into time for work, play, rest, self-care, and family is to some extent contingent on the norms of society (e.g., the typical 9-to-5, Monday-through-Friday work week). Adult habits are influenced by their context in other ways as well. For example, factory and hospital work requires a rather rigid adherence to schedules, whereas farmers and university professors must develop their own routines around seasonal variations in work. Marriage, purchasing a home, and the arrival of children also place demands on persons to develop habits for home maintenance and caretaking. Previously accustomed to a routine organized around personal needs and desires, adults typically find themselves having to orient their routines to a broader set of concerns.

PERFORMANCE CAPACITY

Adulthood represents both the peaking and the declining of abilities. Young adults are still acquiring new abilities, whereas middle and later adulthood is characterized by some waning in capacity (Bonder, 1994). Physical changes affect the occupational performance of adults. Over time, adults experience a decrease in energy and strength along with some decrement in sensory perception. For example, it is in adulthood that many people first require glasses or bifocals. Others find that they must cut back on some rigorous activities.

IDENTITY AND COMPETENCE

Adults assess and reassess their unfolding life stories (Handel, 1987; Kimmel, 1980). Narrative reassessment typically reflects a transformation from an early concern with competence and achievement to a later concern with value and personal satisfaction. This transformation, sometimes referred to as a midlife crisis, may lead persons to recraft their stories, change work careers, or enact similarly drastic alterations in their occupational lifestyles. Whatever life course they choose or life events they must grapple with, adults continue the narrative process of knowing themselves, exploring the worth and meaning of their lives, and seeking to control the circumstances and direction of their lives. For some adults, this struggle results in a high level of well-being. Others fail to find a satisfactory and meaningful life course and, instead, live lives characterized by compromise, conflict, or catastrophe.

Later Adulthood

Later adulthood is defined by both biological changes and social convention. Retirement and eligibility for social benefits demarcates entry into this period of later adulthood (Bonder, 1994). It is difficult to define later adulthood by chronologic age alone. Rather, it is useful to think of later adulthood as demarked by changes in lifestyle as determined by waning capacity, personal choice, and social convention.

VOLITION

Older adults' volition is important to help direct the many choices that drive or are in response to necessary changes in lifestyle. Old age is generally accompanied by losses of capacity, and lack of opportunities to use abilities can lead elderly persons to experience diminution of personal causation. Since the loss of capacity may have important implications for independence and lifestyle, some older adults may be especially inventive in sustaining a sense of efficacy, whereas others may hold unrealistic views of their abilities.

Values typically undergo some transformation and have a pervasive influence on occupational choices in old age. One view holds that older adults shift from instrumental values such as being ambitious, intellectual, capable, and responsible toward terminal values such as a sense of accomplishment, freedom, equality, and comfort. Although this pattern may be true of many older adults, it is most accurate to say that the nature and direction of any value change depend on past and current life circumstances. Nonetheless, for most older adults, the importance of work and achievement wanes, while other values concerning family, community, and leisure become more significant (Antonovsky & Sagy, 1990). As abilities decline, elderly persons must redefine their standards and revise the way in which values are satisfied. Nonetheless, value commitments are important to maintaining morale in later life.

For many older adults, the relative freedom from obligations in old age provides the opportunity to pursue a variety of interests more seriously or fully than before. However, constrained capacity and resources in later life can prevent some persons from pursuing interests. For example, some older adults are involved in solitary and passive occupations although they prefer to be involved in social and more active occupations (McGuire, 1980). Older adults can be constrained in their activity choices by a lack of transportation, facilities, money, and companions; by fears of injury, learning new things, or disapproval; and by no longer feeling a sense of satisfaction (McAvoy, 1979; McGuire, 1983).

HABITUATION

Role changes in later life can sometimes be involuntary and unpleasant. For example, elderly persons may lose the spouse and friend roles through death. Many lost roles are not easily replaced. Older adults who cannot replace lost or diminished roles may experience boredom, loneliness, and depression. Many older adults rely on family, community, or other institutions to provide roles. For example, Elliot and Barris (1987) found that older adults' role identification was greater in nursing homes that provided more opportunities for activity.

Some persons continue to work beyond ordinary retirement age for income; to feel satisfied, useful, and respected; and/or to have a major role in organizing their lives (Sterns, Laier, & Dorsett, 1994). When it does occur, retirement can be a far-reaching event, because so much of life is geared toward preparation for, entry into, and advancement in work and because work structures a great deal of time and activity. Consequently, the transition from work to retirement is full of both possibilities and pitfalls. Retirement is an entirely individual process (Jonsson, Kielhofner, & Borell, 1997). For one individual, it may mean escape from arduous labor and an opportunity to devote time to occupations of a higher priority, such as family involvement, a second career, or hobbies. For another, it may mean loss of social contact and severance from a primary source of self-worth and meaning. Whatever the implications, retirement is a major life event that reshapes an individual's occupational life.

Family roles and relationships are important and often change dramatically in the lives of older adults (Cutler-Lewis, 1989). Older adults often spend significant time with adult children and grandchildren. Relationships with adult children can be an important source of gratification sustained by a reciprocal exchange in the form of affection, gifts, and services. For example, older adults often act as babysitters, confidantes and advisors, house sitters, and providers of income. As older adults become frail, disabled, or chronically ill, adult children may assume responsibility for the care of their aging parents. This role reversal is often complicated and challenging for all involved.

Friendship is another important role of older adults. Although having extensive friendships is not necessary, the person who has a number of friendships is less vulnerable to loss of friends through death. Loss of one's partner in old age may severely disrupt life. One may lose a friend, homemaker, financial supporter, and caretaker, depending on the nature of the relationship. Other role changes may accompany the loss of a partner. The surviving partner may have to take over many things previously done by the spouse.

Elderly persons often possess habits developed over a long period in a stable environment. Changes in underlying capacity and changes in environment can challenge these habits. At the same time, changing circumstances, such as widowhood or retirement, often impose demands for acquiring new habits. Moreover, as capacities decline, habits become increasingly important to sustain functional performance and quality of life.

PERFORMANCE CAPACITY

Aging involves a natural decline in performance capacity and is associated with a high frequency of health conditions that affect capacity (Kauffman, 1994; Riley, 1994). However, substantial losses of ability are not inevitable and may be forestalled if the elderly person remains active. Consequently, age-related changes are unique to each person. Moreover, the impact of such decrements may be mitigated by adapting one's habits and environment.

OCCUPATIONAL IDENTITY AND COMPETENCE

With aging, the composition and telling of one's life story seems to gain importance. As older adults approach the end of life, both the need to make the most of the time one has and the need to make sense of the life one has lived become important (Ebersole & Hess, 1981; Hasselkus, 1998). The sense of whether one's life story has fulfilled the cultural ideal can be a source of comfort and fulfillment or of distress (Luborsky, 1993).

For most older adults, the central fixture in the life narrative is the transition to retirement, which can mean vastly different things to retirees (Jonsson et al., 1997; Jonsson, Josephsson, & Kielhofner, 2000, 2001). As discussed in the previous chapter, a major factor affecting the extent to which occupational identity and competence are positive for the elderly person appears to be whether the person has an engaging occupation (Jonsson et al., 2001).

Conclusion

This chapter identified some of the major transformations and patterns that characterize the course of occupational development. In attempting to portray what may be typical or ordinary in the developmental course, individual differences were necessarily ignored. However, these differences are critical to development. Indeed, the most remarkable characteristics of any individual journey through life are the singular incidents, the crises, the personal transformations, the setbacks, and other features that deviate from any neat or normative portrayal of development. Moreover, these unique events, struggles, and transformations give each life its special direction, pace, and meaning and hold the key to understanding that particular life.

CASE EXAMPLE: FOR LEARNING AND REFLECTION

Robert, a retired professional soccer player, worked in pharmaceutical sales for approximately 30 years following his soccer career. He lives alone and has one adult child, who works as a surgical nurse at a local hospital, and has three grandchildren. Now 74 years old, he is also retired from sales but enjoys coaching his granddaughter's soccer team. Since his mid-50s, Robert has been experiencing severe rheumatoid arthritis, gout, and kidney disease. Recently, he had a kidney transplant. Natasha, an occupational therapist, has been assigned to work with Robert following surgery. After surgery, Robert appears to be going through the motions of therapy, appears demoralized, and does not appear to be eager to return home. He is concerned that he will not be able to help his granddaughter with her soccer-related aspirations and that his family will no longer see any use for him.

REVIEW QUESTIONS

1. **What do you see as Robert's biggest obstacle to recovering and being able to re-engage with his granddaughter's soccer team?**
2. **As a MOHO therapist, which component of MOHO would you use to begin the treatment relationship with Robert? Explain your rationale.**
3. **At what stage of the change process is Robert? Justify your answer.**

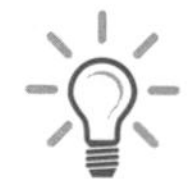

Chapter 10 Review Questions

1. Provide an example of how volition enabled you, a client, or someone you know to undertake an important occupational change.
2. Under what circumstances might it be useful to initiate the change process by focusing on a client's habituation?
3. Explain why the subjective elements of performance capacity might be important in the change process.

4. Provide an example of your own or another person's physical, social, and occupational environment. Describe how each of these elements of the environment might serve as facilitators or barriers to an important occupational change.
5. Think about an important occupational change that you need to make in your own life. At what stage of the change process do you find yourself? Explain your answer.

HOMEWORK ASSIGNMENTS

1. Describe a time in your life when you faced a significant occupational change. In being able to manage that change process, which aspects of MOHO were important? At what stage of the change process are you in? Please discuss your reflections in detail.

thePoint® For additional resources and exercises, visit http://thePoint.lww.com

Key Terms

Achievement: The stage of change when persons have sufficient skills and habits that allow them to participate fully in some new work, leisure activity, or activity of daily living.

Catastrophic change: Stage of change that occurs when internal or external circumstances dramatically alter one's occupational life situation, requiring a fundamental reorganization.

Competency: Stage of change when persons begin to solidify new ways of doing that were discovered through exploration.

Exploration: First stage of change in which persons try out new things and, consequently, learn about their own capacities, preferences, and values.

Incremental change: A gradual alteration such as change in amount, intensity, or degree.

Transformational change: Change that occurs when one fundamentally or qualitatively alters an established pattern of thinking, feeling, and doing.

REFERENCES

Allport, G. (1961). *Pattern and growth in personality*. New York, NY: Holt, Rinehart & Winston.

Antonovsky, A., & Sagy, S. (1990). Confronting developmental tasks in the retirement transition. *Gerontologist, 30*, 362–368.

Baruch, G., Barnett, R., & Rivers, C. (1980, December 7). A new start for women at midlife. *New York Times Sunday Magazine*, pp. 196–200.

Bonder, B. R. (1994). Growing old in the United States. In B. R. Bonder & M. B. Wagner (Eds.), *Functional performance in older adults* (pp. 4–14). Philadelphia, PA: F. A. Davis.

Bundy, A. C. (1997). Play and playfulness: What to look for. In L. D. Parham & L. S. Fazio (Eds.), *Play in occupational therapy for children* (pp. 52–66). St. Louis, MO: Mosby.

Burke, J. P. (1977). A clinical perspective on motivation: Pawn versus origin. *American Journal of Occupational Therapy, 31*, 254–258.

Burke, J. P. (1993). Play: The life role of the infant and young child. In J. Case-Smith (Ed.), *Pediatric occupational therapy and early intervention* (pp. 198–224). Stoneham, MA: Andover Medical Publishers.

Burke, J. P., & Schaaf, R. C. (1997). Family narratives and play assessment. In L. D. Parham & L. S. Fazio (Eds.), *Play in occupational therapy for children* (pp. 67–84). St. Louis, MO: Mosby.

Case-Smith, J., & Shortridge, S. D. (1996). The developmental process: Prenatal to adolescence. In J. Case-Smith, A. S. Allen, & P. N. Pratt (Eds.), *Occupational therapy for children* (pp. 46–66). St. Louis, MO: Mosby.

Csikszentmihalyi, M., & Rochberg-Halton, E. (1981). *The meaning of things*. Cambridge, MA: Cambridge University Press.

Cutler-Lewis, S. (1989). *Elder care*. New York, NY: McGraw-Hill.

Ebersole, P., & Hess, P. (1981). *Toward healthy aging: Human needs and nursing response*. St. Louis, MO: C. V. Mosby.

Elliot, M. S., & Barris, R. (1987). Occupational role performance and life satisfaction in elderly persons. *Occupational Therapy Journal of Research, 7*, 215–224.

Ferland, F. (1997). *Play, children with physical disabilities and occupational therapy: The ludic model*. Ottawa, ON: University of Ottawa Press.

Fidler, G., & Fidler, J. (1983). Doing and becoming: The occupational therapy experience. In G. Kielhofner (Ed.), *Health through occupation: Theory and practice in occupational therapy*. Philadelphia, PA: F. A. Davis.

Florey, L. (1998). Psychosocial dysfunction in childhood and adolescence. In M. E. Neistadt & E. B. Crepeau (Eds.), *Occupational therapy* (pp. 622–635). Philadelphia, PA: Lippincott Williams & Wilkins.

Fuzhong, L., Eckstrom, E., Harmer, P., Fitzgerald, K., Voit, J., & Cameron, K. A. (2016). Exercise and fall prevention: Narrowing the research-to-practice gap and enhancing integration of clinical and community practice. *Journal of the American Geriatrics Society, 64*(2), 425–431.

Ginzberg, E. (1971). Toward a theory of occupational choice. In H. J. Peters & J. C. Hansen (Eds.), *Vocational guidance and career development* (2nd ed.). New York, NY: Macmillan.

Hammel, J. (1999). The Life Rope: A transactional approach to exploring worker and life role development. *Work: A Journal of Prevention, Assessment, and Rehabilitation, 12*, 47–60.

Handel, A. (1987). Personal theories about the life-span development of one's self in autobiographical self-presentations of adults. *Human Development, 30*, 83–98.

Hasselkus, B. R. (1998). Introduction to adult and older adult populations. In M. E. Neistadt & E. B. Crepeau (Eds.), *Occupational therapy* (pp. 651–659). Philadelphia, PA: Lippincott Williams & Wilkins.

Hendry, L. B. (1983). *Growing up and going out: Adolescents and leisure*. Aberdeen, Scotland: Aberdeen University Press.

Hinojosa, J., & Kramer, P. (1993). Developmental perspective: Fundamentals of developmental theory. In P. Kramer & J. Hinojosa (Eds.), *Pediatric occupational therapy* (pp. 3–8). Philadelphia, PA: Lippincott Williams & Wilkins.

Hurt, J. M. (1980). A play skills inventory: A competency monitoring tool for the 10-year-old. *American Journal of Occupational Therapy, 34,* 651–656.

Jonsson, H., Josephsson, S., & Kielhofner, G. (2000). Evolving narratives in the course of retirement: A longitudinal study. *American Journal of Occupational Therapy, 54,* 463–470.

Jonsson, H., Josephsson, S., & Kielhofner, G. (2001). Narratives and experience in an occupational transition: A longitudinal study of the retirement process. *American Journal of Occupational Therapy, 55,* 424–432.

Jonsson, H., Kielhofner, G., & Borell, L. (1997). Anticipating retirement: The formation of narratives concerning an occupational transition. *American Journal of Occupational Therapy, 51,* 49–56.

Kauffman, T. (1994). Mobility. In B. R. Bonder & M. B. Wagner (Eds.), *Functional performance in older adults* (pp. 42–61). Philadelphia, PA: F. A. Davis.

Kimmel, D. C. (1980). *Adulthood and aging* (2nd ed.). New York, NY: John Wiley & Sons.

Lindquist, J. E., Mack, W., & Parham, L. D. (1982). A synthesis of occupational behavior and sensory integration concepts in theory and practice, Part 1: Theoretical foundations. *American Journal of Occupational Therapy, 36,* 365–374.

Luborsky, M. (1993). The romance with personal meaning: Gerontology, cultural aspects of life themes. *The Gerontologist, 33,* 445–452.

Mailloux, Z., & Burke, J. P. (1997). Play and the sensory integrative approach. In L. D. Parham & L. S. Fazio (Eds.), *Play in occupational therapy for children* (pp. 112–125). St. Louis, MO: Mosby.

McAvoy, L. L. (1979). The leisure preferences, problems, and needs of the elderly. *Journal of Leisure Research, 11,* 40–47.

McGuire, F. (1980). The incongruence between actual and desired leisure involvement in advanced adulthood. *Active Adaptive Aging, 1,* 77–89.

McGuire, F. (1983). Constraints on leisure involvement in the later years. *Active Adaptive Aging, 3,* 17–24.

Mitchell, J. J. (1975). *The adolescent predicament.* Toronto, ON: Holt, Rinehart & Winston.

Nicholls, J. G. (1984). Achievement motivation: Conceptions of ability, subjective experience, task choice, and performance. *Psychological Review, 3,* 328–346.

Pierce, D. (1997). The power of object play for infants and toddlers at risk for developmental delays. In L. D. Parham & L. S. Fazio (Eds.), *Play in occupational therapy for children* (pp. 86–111). St. Louis, MO: Mosby.

Reilly, M. (1974). *Play as exploratory learning.* Beverly Hills, CA: SAGE.

Riley, K. P. (1994). Cognitive development. In B. R. Bonder & M. B. Wagner (Eds.), *Functional performance in older adults* (pp. 4–14). Philadelphia, PA: F. A. Davis.

Robinson, A. L. (1977). Play, the arena for acquisition of rules for competent behavior. *American Journal of Occupational Therapy, 31,* 248–253.

Santrock, J. W. (1981). *Adolescence: An introduction.* Dubuque, IA: Brown.

Sterns, H. L., Laier, M. P., & Dorsett, J. G. (1994). Work and retirement. In B. R. Bonder & M. B. Wagner (Eds.), *Functional performance in older adults* (pp. 148–164). Philadelphia, PA: F. A. Davis.

PART II

APPLYING MOHO: THE THERAPY PROCESS AND THERAPEUTIC REASONING

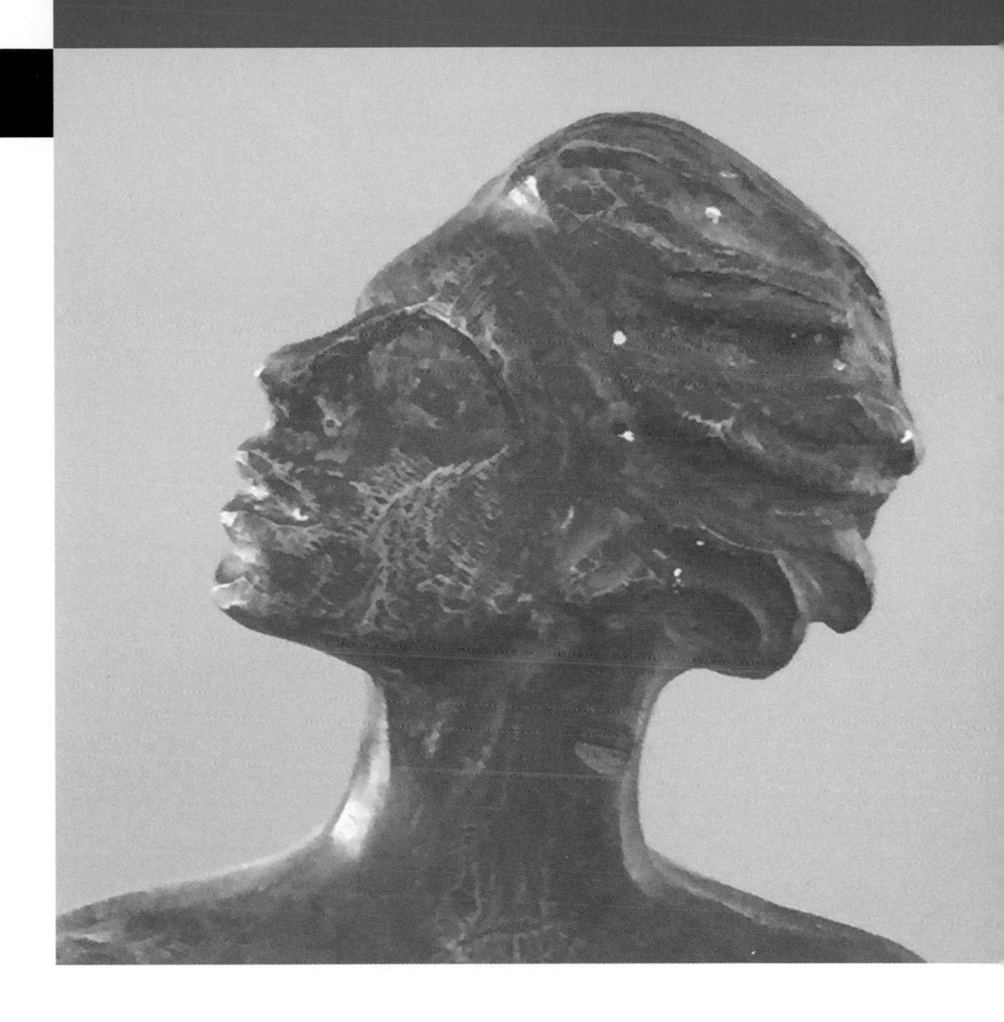

Therapeutic Reasoning: Planning, Implementing, and Evaluating the Outcomes of Therapy

Kirsty Forsyth

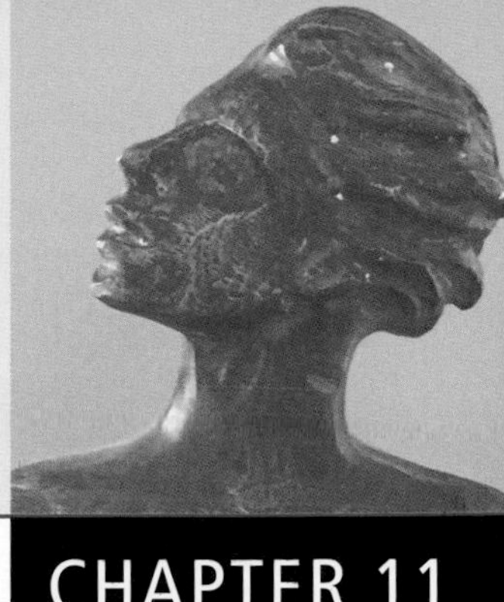

CHAPTER 11

EXPECTED LEARNING OUTCOMES

Upon completion of this chapter, readers will be able to:

1. Understand how model of human occupation (MOHO) is client centered.
2. Understand how to generate theory-driven questions.
3. Be aware of how to approach clients to complete standardized assessments.
4. Be able to define an occupational formulation.
5. Describe the components of measurable goals.
6. Understand the dynamics of intervention.
7. Identify ways to evaluate the outcomes of intervention.

Chapters 2 to 10 presented model of human occupation (MOHO) theory. This chapter begins describing how MOHO is put into practice. It discusses **therapeutic reasoning**, which is how therapists use the theory to understand a client and to develop, implement, and monitor a plan of therapy with a client. Therapeutic reasoning using MOHO should be client centered and theoretically driven. These two issues will be discussed next. (Note: The term "clinical reasoning" is used by authors to refer to the process by which therapists generate an understanding of clients and make decisions in therapy (Mattingly, 1991; Mattingly & Fleming, 1993). The term "therapeutic reasoning" is used here, instead, to avoid medical model connotations of the term "clinical" and to highlight the client-focused collaborative nature of the proposed reasoning process.)

Client-Centeredness in Therapeutic Reasoning with MOHO

MOHO is inherently a client-centered model in two important ways:

- It views each client as a unique individual whose characteristics determine the rationale for and nature of the therapy goals and intervention.
- It views what the client does, thinks, and feels as the central mechanism of change.

Therapeutic reasoning with MOHO focuses on understanding clients in terms of their own values, interests, sense of capacity and efficacy, roles, habits, and performance-related experiences within the relevant environments. Therefore, the concepts of the theory call attention to the importance of knowing the details of a client's experiences. Moreover, since the logic of intervention emanates from a conceptual understanding informed by client characteristics in combination with the theory, the client's unique characteristics always define the goals and strategies of intervention.

The client's occupational engagement (i.e., what the client does, thinks, and feels) is the central dynamic of therapy. MOHO-based intervention supports the client's doing, thinking, and feeling in order to achieve change desired by the client and indicated by the client's situation. The therapist must understand, respect, and support client choices, actions, and experiences. The therapist must communicate with the client, seeking client input and validation, and engaging the client to collaborate in planning, implementing, and evaluating therapy.

Client-centeredness should extend to those clients who are unable to verbalize and be active in collaboration. The therapist must work to understand the client's view of the world, what matters to the client, what the client enjoys, and how the client feels about his or her abilities. The therapist can also collaborate with family members or others who care about and can serve as advocates for the client.

Theory-Driven Therapeutic Reasoning

Using MOHO as a practice model requires understanding of its underlying theory. Learning to think with theory evolves over time as the therapist uses it in practice. Importantly, engaging in therapeutic reasoning also enriches the therapist's understanding of the theory. Reasoning involves moving between theory and the circumstances of clients. Thus, one's knowledge of theory grows as one sees it represented in different clients' circumstances. For example, each client reveals a unique instance of personal causation. By seeing how numerous clients conceive of, understand, and feel about their capacity and efficacy, a therapist's understanding of personal causation is enriched.

Therapists' growth in knowledge of MOHO theory will also include a deepened appreciation of its implications in practice. For example, experience will reveal what therapeutic processes and strategies are generally most helpful for particular kinds of client problems. Notably, having a consistent set of theoretical concepts allows the therapist to think more systematically about clients and the therapy process, thereby enhancing what the therapist learns from experience.

Therapeutic Reasoning Process

The therapeutic process has seven steps (Forsyth, 2000a; Fig. 11-1), namely generating theory-driven questions, administering standardized assessments, occupational formulation, identifying occupational changes, developing measurable goals, implementing interventions, and assessing outcomes of intervention. Importantly, these steps are not sequential. Therapists generally move back and forth between steps over the course of therapy. Each step will now be described below.

GENERATING THEORY-DRIVEN QUESTIONS TO INFORM NONSTANDARDIZED ASSESSMENT

Therapists must get to know their clients. Getting to know clients is facilitated when one asks questions about the client. MOHO theory allows the occupational therapist to generate these questions. That is, the major concepts of the theory (volition, habituation, performance capacity, occupational participation, occupational performance, skills, environment, occupational identity, and occupational competence) orient the therapist to be concerned about certain things when getting to know a client. As shown in Figure 11-2, these concepts raise broad questions about clients. These questions can be specifically developed for different populations, for example, questions about children (Table 11-1) including:

- What is the child's sense of who she/he has been, is, and wishes to become in relation to family life, school, friendships, hobbies, and interests?
- To what extent has this child sustained a pattern of satisfying occupational participation over time?

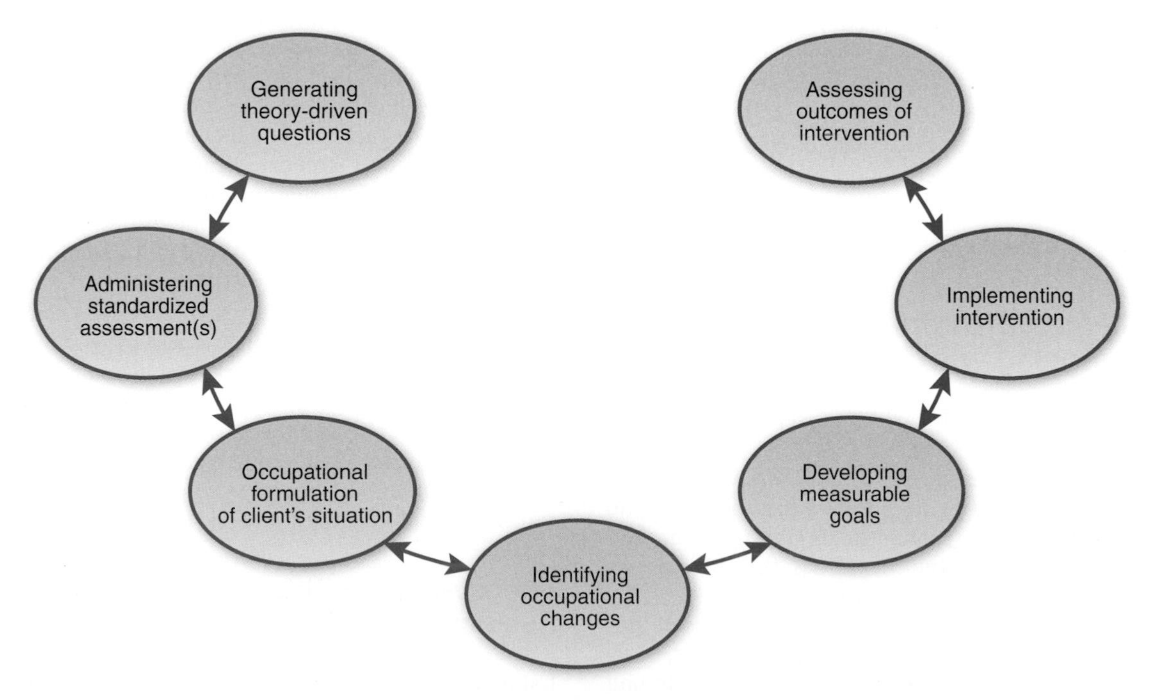

FIGURE 11-1 Therapeutic Reasoning Process. (From Forsyth 2000a, with permission.)

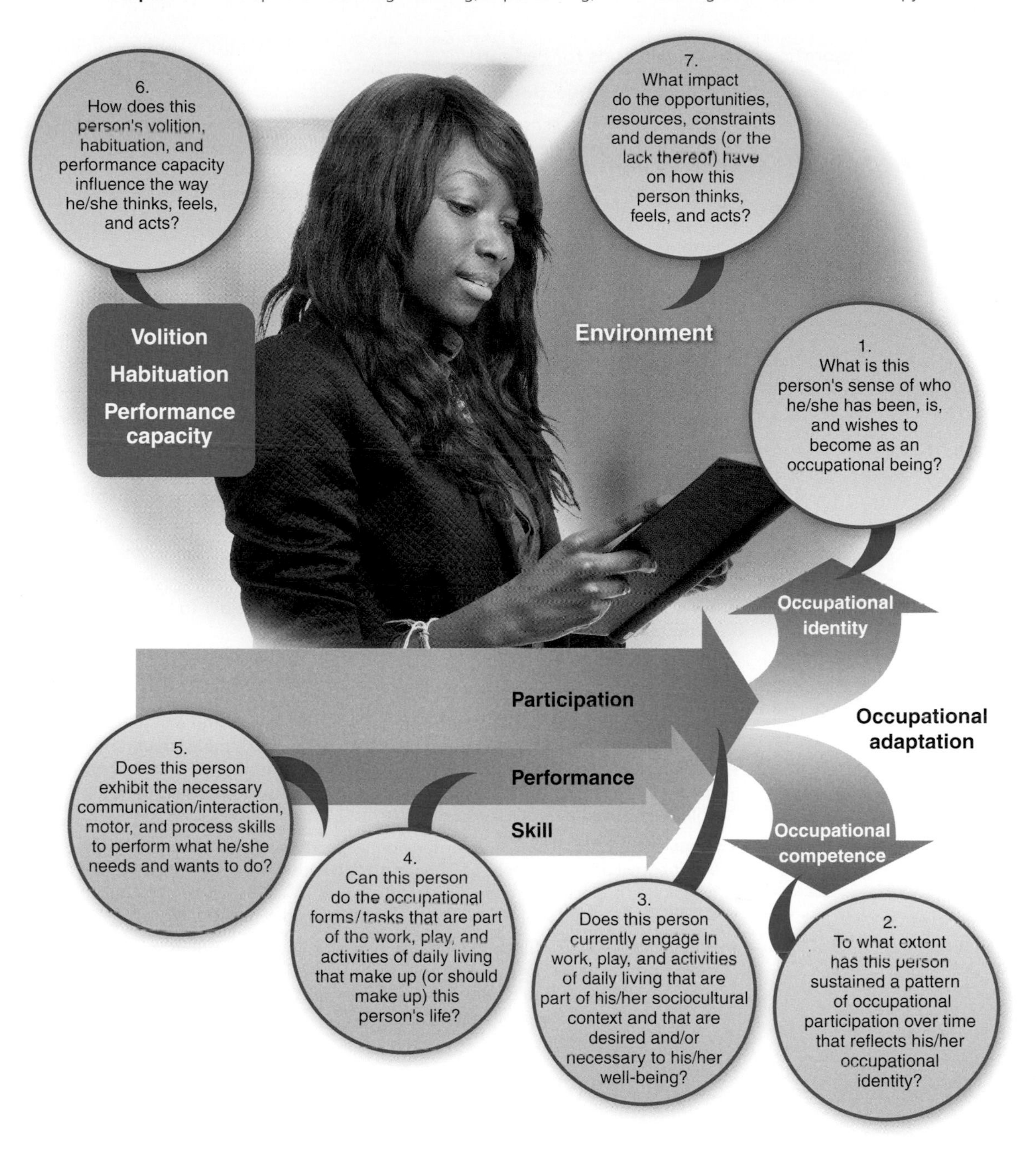

FIGURE 11-2 Theory-Driven Questions.

- Does the child currently engage in work, play, and ADLs that are part of his/her sociocultural context and that are desired and/or necessary for his/her well-being?

Specifically developing questions for older adults (Table 11-2), including the following:

- How does this older adult view themselves? Do they perceive themselves to be a grandparent, mother, volunteer, church member, activist? Do they view themselves as not contributing to society or friends and family? Do they view themselves as failing to remain active and engage with life?
- What is the family's sense of who this older adult is? How does this affect the older adult's view of themselves?

Table 11-1 Theoretical-Driven Questions for Pediatric Practice

MOHO Concept	Corresponding Questions
Occupational identity	• What is the child's sense of who she/he has been, is, and wishes to become in relation to family life, school, friendships, hobbies, and interests? • What is the family's sense of who this child has been is, and what do they wish her/him to become? How does this affect the child's occupational identity?
Occupational competence	• To what extent has this child sustained a pattern of satisfying occupational participation over time? • Does this child feel he/she can do the things he/she needs to do in school, with friends, and in the community? • To what extent have important people in this child's life sustained patterns of occupational participation over time that reflect their occupational identity in relation to this child (i.e., care giving, playmate)?
Participation	• Does the child currently engage in work, play, and ADLs that are part of his/her sociocultural context and that are desired and/or necessary for his/her well-being?
Performance	• Can this child do the things that are part of the work, play, and ADL activities that make up, or should make up, their life? • Can the child do the things that the family expects the child to do as part of their work, play, and ADL activities?
Skill	• Does the child exhibit the necessary communication/interaction, motor, and process skills to perform what she/he needs and wants to do?
Environment	• What work, play, and ADL activities does the family consider to be desired and/or necessary for the well-being of this child? • Does the family support the child in developing the necessary volition, habituation, and communication/interaction, motor, and process skills needed for participation and development? • What impact do the opportunities, resources, constraints, and demands (or lack of demands) of the environment have on how this child thinks, feels, and acts? • How do the opportunities, resources, constraints, or demands provided by spaces, objects, occupational forms/tasks, and social groups affect the child's skill, performance, and participation?
Volition	• What is this child's view of their personal capacity and effectiveness? • What convictions and sense of obligations does this child have? What does she/he think is important? • What are this child's interests? What does this child enjoy doing?
Habituation	• What routines does this child participate in and how do routines influence what she/he does? • What are the roles with which this child identifies with and how do they influence what she/he routinely does?

Table 11-2 Theoretical-Driven Questions for Older Adult Practice

MOHO Concept	Corresponding Questions
Occupational identity	• How does this older adult view themselves? Do they perceive themselves to be a grandparent, mother, volunteer, church member, activist? Do they view themselves as not contributing to society or friends and family? Do they view themselves as failing to remain active and engage with life? • What is the family's sense of who this person is? How does this affect the person's view of themselves?
Occupational competence	• Has the older adult been able to meet their responsibilities over time? • Does the older adult perceive themselves to be able to do the occupations they need and/or want to be able to do? • Does the older adult feel competent within their occupational life?
Participation	• Does the older adult currently routinely engage in productive activities, leisure and self care activities that he/she needs and/or wants to be able to do

Performance	• Can this older adult do the self-care, productivity, and leisure that make up their life? • Can the older adult perform their daily activities to a standard they are happy with?
Skill	• Does the older adult exhibit the necessary communication/interaction, motor, and process skills to perform what she/he needs and wants to do?
Environment	• What daily activities does the family consider to be desired and/or necessary for the well-being of this older adult? • Does the family support the person in their efforts to engage in daily activities? • What impact do the opportunities, resources, constraints, and demands (or lack of demands) of the environment have on how this person views themselves and their abilities? • How do the opportunities, resources, constraints, or demands provided by spaces, objects, occupational forms/tasks, and social groups affect the older adult's participation in daily life?
Volition	• Does this older adult have appropriate confidence in their abilities? • What is the set of driving principles this person lives by? What is important to them and how does this affect their choices to engage in daily activities? • Does the older adult do activities they find enjoyable and satisfying?
Habituation	• What is the daily routine of this older adult and how do routines influence what she/he does? • How does the older adult feel about the routine? • What are the responsibilities the person holds and how does this affect their daily routines?

The Therapeutic Reasoning Table in this book (Appendix A) also lists a wide range of questions that might be asked about any given client. Thus, therapists are encouraged to use this table as a resource when first learning how to translate MOHO theory into client questions. It is important to note, however, that these questions are not exhaustive and will need to be tailored to each client.

When you ask questions, more specific questions are likely to emerge. For example, the occupational therapist may ask, can this person identify personal interests? The therapist may find that their client cannot identify any interests. In this instance, it is important to understand why they cannot identify interests. Thus, the following questions might be relevant to ask depending on the client: Has the client lacked opportunity to develop interests? Or has the client lost interests because of the interference of an impairment? On the other hand, if a client identifies several interests, the therapist may wish to go on to ask whether the client participates in these interests and what common themes, if any, exist in the interests. How one proceeds with a line of questioning is always informed by the answers to previous questions.

This approach to generating questions is nonstandardized. A therapist using this approach takes advantage of naturally occurring opportunities to gather information. These approaches capitalize on opportunities for obtaining useful information in informal and spontaneous ways. Every opportunity the therapist has to observe and/or talk with a client will potentially yield useful information. If therapists use such opportunities wisely, they can gather a wealth of information efficiently and effectively. Reasons for choosing this approach and how to ensure dependability are described in Chapter 12.

CASE EXAMPLES: ILLUSTRATING NONSTANDARDIZED APPROACHES TO ASSESSMENT

An Adult with Multiple Sclerosis

Sara is a college-educated, 44-year-old woman recently diagnosed with multiple sclerosis. Her therapist introduced MOHO as follows:

As an occupational therapist, I work from a perspective that is concerned with how multiple sclerosis has affected your ability to participate in the things that are important to you—for example, your work, taking care of yourself, and your leisure activities. I'll want to get to know what is important to you and how you feel your illness has affected your ability to do what you need to do and like to do. I will also want to know something about your major life responsibilities and your everyday routines.

We'll work together to figure out ways we can to minimize any problems in your everyday life and how you can best go on with life in a meaningful way. We can make changes in your environment or in how you go about doing things that allow you to be more effective in getting done what you need and want to do. Can you let me know how you spend a typical day? What do you do from the time you get up in the morning until you go to bed at night?

An Adult with Alzheimer's Disease

Melissa is a 65-year-old woman who had limited cognitive capacities due to Alzheimer's disease. Her therapist used a much briefer explanation:

My job is to help you manage things and be able to do what's most important and enjoyable to you. What do you enjoy doing?

ADMINISTERING STANDARDIZED ASSESSMENT(S)

A therapist can move past a nonstandardized approach as described above and choose a standardized assessment(s). These are assessments that follow a set protocol that has been developed and tested through research. Standardized assessments guard against bias and provide information that is readily interpretable. Standardized assessments have reliability and validity. As will be discussed in later chapters, a wide range of MOHO-based standardized assessments have been developed and are available to therapists. How to choose a standardized assessment is described in Chapter 12. MOHO standardized assessments have been developed in partnership with therapists. Subsequently, there is a range of flexibility built into how the assessment is administered to ensure the assessment can be used within the reality of tight timeframes within practice, and the therapist can use their own therapeutic style within the assessment process. For example, The OCAIRS (Forsyth et al., 2005) has a structure for asking questions; however, the occupational therapist is encouraged to use their own style as to what questions to ask first, the sequence of questions, how to phrase the question, and whether to conduct the interview formally or informally while dong an activity. The MOHOST (Parkinson, Forsyth, & Kielhofner, 2006) was specifically developed to have as much flexibility as possible within its administration and has multiple data gathering methods to facilitate this. Once the standardized assessments have been administered there will be a wealth of information available to make sense of the person's occupational situation.

CASE EXAMPLE: THE OCCUPATIONAL SELF-ASSESSMENT

When administering the Occupational Self-Assessment (OSA) (Baron, Kielhofner, Iyenger, Goldhammer, & Wolenski, 2006), the therapist may say the following to the client:

"It would be very helpful if you would complete a short form called the Occupational Self Assessment. It will take you about 10 to 15 minutes. The form asks you to look at a number of statements about how you do things in your everyday life. You will indicate on the form how well you do the things listed and how important they are to you. I'm asking you to fill out this form because I want to know what's important to you. I also want to know where you think things are going okay and where you might feel you have some problems. When you have finished this part of the form, we will look at it together and then you and I will use it to decide what things you would most like to change about your life."

OCCUPATIONAL FORMULATION OF THE CLIENT'S SITUATION

The occupational therapist needs to make sense of all this assessment information and create an understanding of what the assessment information is telling them. The term "occupational formulation" was coined by Forsyth (2000b) and describes how an occupational therapist takes all the assessment information for a client and pulls it together in order to create a set of arguments about their unique perspective of their client's occupational situation. The occupational formulation will guide the next step of identifying occupational changes that are possible and developing measurable goals. It is, therefore, an important part of the occupational therapy process, and it is important to get the occupational formulation right (i.e., to accurately understand the client's situation). For this reason, therapists should involve clients to the extent possible. By working together, the therapist and client can often generate insights into a client's situation that neither had at the outset. Clients know their own experiences. However, clients do not always have a clear picture of all the factors that are contributing to that experience. The aim of the occupational formulation, then, is to generate new insights that will form the basis for formulating a course of action to achieve desired occupational change. An occupational formulation can be generated by using the reflective questions in Table 11-3 (Forsyth, 2000b).

CASE EXAMPLE: OCCUPATIONAL FORMULATION

How can I say complex information quickly? In a time-pressured situation, OTs often need to be able to share their occupational formulation in a very concise way. An occupational formulation will support a summary statement being developed, which allows the OT to say complex information very quickly. See the following for an example of John, who has been hospitalized due to depression.

John is a 55 year old man who in the past has been a husband, father, brother, son, worker, friend, rugby player. He values these roles and is keen to return to them in the future. Currently in the ward he has limited awareness of his abilities/limitations leading to few choices to engage in activities and this in turn has resulted in an empty unstructured routine. John wants to work with OT to set goals towards regaining his roles.

IDENTIFYING OCCUPATIONAL CHANGES

When setting goals, it is more straightforward to reflect on the occupational formulation and identify what occupational changes may be possible during occupational therapy. This gives the occupational therapist the basis for the measurable goal and ensures the therapist is thinking in an occupation-focused way.

Below are *examples* of occupational changes:

- Personal causation: Enhancing the person's understanding of their abilities and limitations
- Value: Increase the person's ability to identify and prioritize what is important
- Interest: The client has an increased participation in things of interest
- Habits: An increase in a client's organization of daily routines that improves effectiveness in managing role-related responsibilities
- Roles: Improved awareness of responsibilities associated with success in roles
- Skills: Learning to use more adaptive skills to compensate for weaker skills

Table 11-3 Occupational Formulation Questions

Occupational Formulation
Which assessments were used?
What is the person's identity? The person's view? The therapist's view?
What is the child's competence? i.e., skills, participation in activities The person's view? The therapist's view?
What are the participatory issues the person is having difficulty with? (think across community, work/school, and home) The person's view? The therapist's view?
What are the positive participatory issues for the child? (think across community, work/school, and home) The person's view The therapist's view?
Why is the child unable or having challenges with participation? *(Think about influencing factors, i.e., confidence, routines, responsibilities, motor skills, social skills, organizational skills, physical environment or social environmental issue, or a combination of these.)*
Reflect on the above information and identify three key issues
Key area 1: What is the participatory issue? Why is this situation occurring?
Key area 2: What is the participatory issue? Why is this situation occurring?
Key area 3: What is the participatory issue? Why is this situation happening?
Summary: Identify the person's name, age, and past roles that summarize the above key issues in one or two sentences

From Forsyth (2000b), with permission

- Social environment: Increase in information to family about client's needs and desires
- Physical environment: Change the physical spaces to facilitate moving around when doing things

The next step is to develop measurable goals with/ for the client.

DEVELOPING MEASURABLE GOALS

Measurable goals indicate the kinds of occupational change that the intervention will aim to achieve. Change is required when the client's characteristics and environment are contributing to occupational challenges. For instance, if a client feels ineffective, intervention would seek to enable the client to feel more effective. If a client has too few roles, intervention would seek to enable the client to choose and do new roles. Or, if the environment was impacting on the client's performance in a negative way, therapy would seek to modify that environment. To develop a measurable goal it should contain the flowing elements:

- Occupational change: What the client will do to demonstrate that the occupational goal has been achieved
- Setting: The specific setting where the client will do it (e.g., within the ward or within the client's home environment)
- Degree: The circumstances under which the client will do it (e.g., independently, with physical support, with verbal cueing, using equipment)
- Timeframe: The timeframe within which the client will be able to do it

A goal with all these elements clearly indicates what intervention aims to accomplish and provides a way of determining if clients are achieving their goals.

CASE EXAMPLE: WRITING A THERAPY GOAL

Following a stroke, a client, Beatrice, who was 70 years old, stated that she was anxious about doing daily activities. Having assessed Beatrice's motor and process skills, the occupational therapist further noted from some informal observations that Beatrice's inaccurate sense of her abilities was leading her to avoid choosing to do things that were well within her ability. Consequently, the therapist identified the following goal:

> **Within 7 days [timeframe], Beatrice will independently [degree] choose to engage in personal and domestic activities in line with her abilities & limitations [occupational change] in the ward [setting].**

IMPLEMENTING INTERVENTION

Occupational therapy is fundamentally about facilitating clients to engage in occupations in order to achieve the outcome of intervention, which is being able to effectively engage in meaningful occupations. Our health is restored by doing everyday things that support us to have a sense of our occupational identity and competence. By playing a guitar, typing on a computer keyboard, or driving a car, people internalize the forms of behavior maintaining themselves as guitarists, typists, and drivers. We are not born carpenters, teachers, therapists, guitarists, fishers, writers, dancers, gardeners, poets, typists, and singers. But we may become them by behaving as such.

Applying therapeutic reasoning within intervention is complex because how our clients engage in occupation is spontaneously organized in real time and in the context of action. It could be the anxiety from a lack of belief in one's skill interfering with performance, the force of old habits resisting new volitional choices, or the pull of values to keep going despite pain and fatigue. We, therefore, have to simultaneously be reasoning about the dynamic interactions between elements within the person and those in the environment. The therapeutic reasoning is focused on altering for and with the person their volition, habituation, performance, or the environment, in order to create a set of circumstances that improve the person's ability to engage in occupation. An example is outlined below.

CASE EXAMPLE: INTERVENTION FOCUSING ON PERSONAL CAUSATION?

Peter is 39 and was diagnosed with rheumatoid arthritis 10 years ago. Currently, his personal causation challenge is evidenced by his anxiety and his reluctance to choose to do things well within his performance capacity. Improving Peter's personal causation requires that he experience success in doing more challenging things that he is currently avoiding. Peter will need to choose more challenging activities and reexamine his thoughts and feelings about his capacity for and effectiveness in doing things. To support Peter, the occupational therapist will create the environmental circumstances and encourage him to try to do them, pay attention to the dynamics of his attempts, and support success and provide him feedback on his success. This plan might be communicated to Peter as follows: "Peter you and I discussed you sometimes feel anxious about doing things that you probably can do OK. The best way to overcome this is to do these things

with support. I will be with you and make sure they go okay. If you are feeling anxious, just let me know and we will adjust what we are doing so you feel OK. After you try out something we can sit and chat about how you feel it went."

The occupational therapist would structure his experience within the intervention to include a volitional cycle of

- **Choosing: Facilitating Peter to choose an activity that doesn't match the person's perception of their ability using encouragement and persuasion**
- **Experience: Supporting Peter within the experience of doing the activity by making incremental adjustments to his environment when he is showing signs of anxiety**
- **Feedback: Providing feedback through providing opportunities to evaluate/reflect on the outcome of their doing with the OT. Stating how he/she feels the person performed and, if needed, challenging the person's perceptions of their performance**
- **Anticipation: This would lead to discussion to support Peter anticipating doing the activity again in a more positive light**

This cycle of occupational performance was repeated until Peter was confidently making spontaneous choices to do the activity.

There may be one occupational change targeted (as with Beatrice above) within intervention or there may be a range of changes targeted within interventions. It may, therefore, be more appropriate to use a program of intervention that describes more complex therapeutic reasoning related to intervention. The below are examples of programs that are available from kforsyth@qmu.ac.uk which outline more complex therapeutic reasoning related to intervention. They cover the areas of child and family, working aged adults, and older adults.

CHILD AND FAMILY INTERVENTIONS

The CIRCLE Collaboration is an academic practice partnership between occupational therapy colleagues and education colleagues. There are manualized interventions (*i*) for teachers and (*ii*) complementary mutualized interventions for occupational therapists. The main aim of the CIRCLE Collaboration is to promote collaborative working between occupational therapists and schools to support children's participation in the classroom.

The teacher manuals include: (a) Up, Up and Away! Planning to meet the need (0–5 years), (b) Teachers' ideas in practice—Inclusive learning and collaborative working: 5- to 11-year-old children, (c) Teachers' ideas in practice: Inclusive learning and collaborative working: 12- to 18-year-old children. These are used alongside CIRCLE assessments and the ACHIEVE assessment.

a. *Up, Up and Away! Planning to meet the need: 0- to 5-year-old children*

   The "Up Up and Away!" manual outlines ideas to optimize opportunity for children (aged 0–5 years) at risk of poor learning. The resources aim to improve participation of children through early intervention. The "planning to meet the need" manual aims to provide practical, stage-appropriate principles and strategies to meet needs once they are identified, help staff and carers to engage with parents, share ideas for building the foundations to participation in school, and highlight and promote diversity at all times. The MOHO is used as a guiding structure.

b. *Teachers' ideas in practice—Inclusive learning and collaborative working: 5- to 11-year-old children*

   This manual is aimed at teachers and brings together good practice focusing on advice and strategies for improving the participation and achievement of pupils who have special educational needs in the 5 to 11 age range. They provide a theory-driven intervention structure based on the MOHO focusing on the physical and social environment, structures and routines, motivation and skills. The manuals include practical supports and strategies across common "area of challenge" in the classroom. The manual also provides guidance on collaborative working with occupational therapists and other services.

c. *Teachers' ideas in practice: Inclusive learning and collaborative working: 12- to 18-year-old children*

   This manual is aimed at teachers and brings together good practice focusing on advice and strategies for improving the participation and achievement of pupils who have special educational needs in the 11 to 18 age range. They provide a theory-driven intervention structure based on the MOHO focusing on the physical and social environment, structures and routines, motivation and skills. The manuals include practical supports and strategies across common "areas of challenge" in the classroom. The manual also provides guidance on collaborative working with occupational therapists and other services.

The occupational therapist manual is described below.

CIRCLE Therapy Manual: Occupational Therapy

The Occupational Therapy Manual describes the key techniques that therapists use during intervention based on the MOHO. The manual explains (with practical examples) what the therapist does to help children participate in the classroom and school. The theoretical background literature underpinning each technique is also included. The manual is designed to be used by therapists, especially newer therapists and those working with students or mentoring colleagues. The manual includes short intervention descriptions using everyday language to describe how occupational therapy techniques are applied in schools, which can be used directly with teachers when working together. The manual also includes a collaborative communication chart which highlights the issues Occupational therapist think about when determining the type of intervention required, including decisions between whether intervention takes place in class or out of class, one to one or in a group, its intensity, and when discharge will happen.

WORKING-AGED ADULTS

Wayfinder: Rehabilitation for People with Complex Needs; A User's Guide for Occupational Therapists

The Wayfinder initiative is focused on developing methods of empowering people to stay healthy and living in the community engaging in meaningful everyday activities. It is focused on ensuring the person is effectively supported by their environment to be able to lead a meaningful life within the community. This manual is for occupational therapists who are working in complex rehabilitation which spans from institutional care to community care. It defines a graded approach to support and interventions for people with complex needs based on the MOHO. It describes intervention principles at each stage of rehabilitation and provides insight into the appropriate environments which are needed to support people in the community more effectively.

Activate: Vocational Rehabilitation Intervention Manual

Vocational rehabilitation is an area occupational therapists have worked within for some time. There hasn't, however, been an intervention manual which provides MOHO-based principals to guide this intervention and return people back to work. This manual provides evidence-based set of intervention strategies for occupational therapists who are advocating for and supporting people to participate in productive work. It provides interventions that can be used to support people to achieve their vocational goals (entering, reentering, returning to, or remaining in work). A full range of interventions are described relative to volition, habituation, skills, and environment.

OLDER ADULTS

MOHO ExpLOR Intervention Manual

People who have complex needs have historically not had occupation-focused intervention programs which are specifically targeted to their needs. The MOHO ExpLOR intervention manual has been designed to structure an environmental intervention for people when their occupational participation is severely impaired. For people whose overall developmental level means that changes are expected to be exploratory in nature, the MOHO ExpLOR manual has been designed to support intervention at this stage. The MOHO ExpLOR intervention manual will also help the therapist to support the people in the client's environment to better support the individual participate in everyday activity.

Making It Clear Manual

There has been a move within occupational therapy to deliver a more preventative approach. This would try to support people to participate in the communities before they become unwell and need more health service supports. This manual provides a preventative occupational therapy approach to supporting older adults at risk in the community. From the literature on resilience in older people it became clear that there is a need to better understand resilience from the viewpoint of older people living in our communities. The occupational therapist supervises the deployment of the intervention with volunteers. The manual provides volunteers with guidance about how to support older people to participate in everyday life and their communities in order to improve older people's resilience.

ASSESS OUTCOMES OF INTERVENTION

Determining intervention outcomes is an important final step. Typically, intervention outcomes are documented by:

- Examining the extent to which measurable goals have been achieved (called goal attainment)
- Readministering standardized assessments to measure change

Both these approaches are valuable in documenting outcomes. Assessing outcomes by examining goal attainment is helpful in reflecting on the extent to which the therapeutic reasoning process resulted in good decisions for interventions. Since goals are formulated in collaboration with clients, examining the extent to which goals have been attained allows a determination of how much the client's desires were achieved.

Structured assessments can provide useful measures of change. Typically, structured assessments are given at the beginning and the end of intervention and differences in the client's score or measure are used as indication of how much change was achieved. MOHO-based assessments are designed to capture one or more of the concepts from the theory (e.g., volition, skill, or participation). Using these assessments is particularly useful when the concept was a target of therapy. Thus, for example, if an aim of therapy was to improve volition, skill, or participation, then assessments which measure these constructs can be used to demonstrate whether there was improvement. Using structured assessments also allows one to compare change across different clients or when different strategies are used. In this way, they can contribute to evidence-based therapy.

CASE EXAMPLE: GENERATING THEORY-DRIVEN QUESTIONS TO INFORM NONSTANDARDIZED ASSESSMENT

Dan is a client in a long-term treatment facility for adolescents with psychiatric disabilities. Dan had experienced difficulties in his student role related to depression. He also had a history of substance abuse. Dan appeared nervous and uneasy most of the time. The concept of volition naturally led the therapist to wonder about several things about Dan:

- **What are Dan's thoughts and feelings about his abilities and limitations, and do they account for his anxious demeanor?**
- **Does Dan have interests and act on them, and does he enjoy the things he does?**
- **What are Dan's values, and is he able to realize them in what he does?**
- **What kinds of decisions does Dan make about doing things, and how do his personal causation, values, and interests influence these decisions?**

ADMINISTERING STANDARDIZED ASSESSMENT: The therapist observed Dan in several situations using the AMPS assessment (Fisher, 2003). The therapist also interviewed Dan about the things he did in his life using the OCAIRS (Forsyth et al., 2005), his experiences at home, in school, and with friends. Finally, Dan filled out a couple of paper-and-pencil assessments that allowed him to tell the therapist about his interests and values including interest checklist (Matsutsuyu, 1969) and the OSA (Baron et al., 2006).

OCCUPATIONAL FORMULATION: Guided by the MOHO concept of volition, the therapist was able to use the information to construct the following understanding of Dan. Dan is a 16-year-old boy who is a son, sibling, friend, and school student. He was referred to occupational therapy because his depression was impacting on his ability to effectively engage with his roles. Dan's experience was dominated by anxiety over his performance. His anxiety was fueled at home by an extremely critical parent who constantly anticipated and pointed out Dan's failures. Moreover, because Dan had gained a reputation in school as a difficult student, he faced a similar judgmental attitude from several teachers. Dan felt much pressure by these attitudes because he disliked very much the feeling that others perceived him as "bad." Finally, Dan's peers tended to view him as different and did not readily include him in the things they did. Subsequently, his personal causation was dominated by a sense of incapacity and inefficacy. He felt very little control over most aspects of his life. He showed little interest in most of the things other adolescents enjoyed, and even when doing something that he felt some attraction to. Because of his anxiety over performance, Dan was unable to feel a sense of enjoyment or satisfaction in doing most things. His few interests were solitary, since he was fearful of performing around peers. He very much valued and wanted to be able to do the same things as other adolescents and to be included by them. Because he viewed himself as lacking capacity for these things, he devalued himself, often making disparaging comments about his own performance.

IDENTIFYING OCCUPATIONAL CHANGES: According to MOHO theory, volition—in combination with environmental conditions—influences occupational choices. The therapist observed the following characteristics of Dan's choices that emanated from his volition and environment. He consistently avoided doing anything new or facing any kinds of performance demands. When allowed to make his own choices he always chose to do things that were familiar, safe, and solitary. He was extremely uncomfortable around peers and put forth a great deal of effort to avoid situations

in which peers could judge his performance. For example, he would sometimes privately admit his lack of confidence about performance to the therapist, but in a group therapy session with peers present, he insisted that all the things available to do were "stupid," thereby avoiding having to perform in front of his peers.

With this additional information, the therapist could recognize how Dan's volition, along with corresponding environmental conditions, was sustaining him in a negative situation. That is, his choices to do things were designed to avoid failure and judgment of others, but these choices also assured he would neither learn new skills nor develop a stronger sense of capacity and efficacy.

Occupational changes that would support Dan were identified as

- Increasing Dan's belief in skill and sense of efficacy so that he could make choices to do things he valued and that would lead to improving his performance
  - Increasing his range of interests and ability to enjoy doing things, both alone and with peers
  - Enabling him to gain competence, and thereby a feeling of efficacy, in doing what he most valued.

Develop Measurable Goals: The therapist shared his understanding of Dan's situation with him to determine whether he agreed. This served not only to make sure that the therapist had accurately comprehended Dan, but also to inform Dan, in terms he could understand, of the theoretical ideas the therapist was using. Dan reluctantly agreed with what the therapist proposed and added some of his own concerns and interpretations. This discussion gave the therapist further insights into Dan and helped Dan learn more about himself. As they came to a mutual understanding of Dan's situation, they discussed some ideas for goals in therapy. This discussion informed Dan of how the therapist was thinking about his situation.

Using the theory to make sense of Dan's situation and sharing the therapist's occupational formulation with him helped them arrive at mutually agreeable goals for his intervention. Dan's long-term volition-related goals included:

- Within 12 weeks, Dan will be able to independently engage in one new interest (woodwork) within the occupational therapy department and find it enjoyable
- Within 12 weeks, Dan will be able to spontaneously make statements of competence in doing woodwork within the occupational therapy department

Intervention: Next, the therapist and Dan had to decide how to go about achieving these goals. MOHO theory indicates that these volitional changes require the following process. First, environmental conditions outside Dan needed to change to allow a new dynamic out of which new volitional thoughts, feelings, and actions could emerge for Dan. Second, the therapist needed to repeat this situation sufficiently so that Dan's volition could begin to reorganize around a sense of capacity, a desire and enjoyment of doing things, and a positive valuation of himself.

Consequently, the therapist began with the therapeutic strategy of advising and encouraging Dan to choose projects in which he could readily succeed and that he saw as valuable. Dan decided to engage in woodwork. This involved the use of tools—something important to Dan. Handling the tools symbolized competence to him. Moreover, they allowed Dan to create products that would tangibly affirm his competence. During therapy the therapist gave him constant feedback on his successes and invited Dan to review each session, identifying what he had enjoyed, accomplished, and learned. They dealt with problems and challenges that arose by working together to see how he could achieve good outcomes by problem solving and asking for help. This meant redefining help-seeking from being a sign of failure to being yet another method Dan could choose and use to accomplish what he wanted. Dan's intervention began with individual sessions in which he could be free of the worry about what his peers would think about his performance. He progressed to doing things in parallel groups when he had developed sufficient capacity and belief in his own abilities to demonstrate his newfound competence in front of peers.

The therapist's understanding of Dan's volition also guided the therapist in the details of his intervention. The therapist knew that when he was reluctant to engage in activities it was because they were too threatening. The therapist observed Dan carefully for signs of anxiety in performance and consistently reoriented him to simply enjoy the activity.

Assess Outcomes of Intervention: Within 12 weeks, Dan achieved his goals. The therapists completed a repeat OCAIRS and identified an improvement in Dan's occupational engagement. As they began to plan for Dan's discharge from therapy, the therapist also knew that maintaining the volitional changes he had gained in therapy would require consistent, supportive environmental conditions to allow him to continue his new pattern

of thinking, feeling, and acting. Consequently, the therapist made recommendations for Dan's parents and teachers, which were shared with them by the psychologist who managed Dan's case and conducted family therapy with Dan and his parents.

CRITICAL REFLECTION

- **Describe how you might share your view of Dan with him, how would you approach him, what phrases would you use, and how would you handle his questions.**
- **How might you approach supporting someone like Dan to do an activity they were feeling anxious about? What would you say, how would you support him to make this choice?**
- **When a client is experiencing anxiety when they are doing a valued activity, how would you handle this, what would you say, what would you do to support them to continue and feel calmer?**
- **What kinds of things would you want to feedback to Dan after each session, what would you say, how would you challenge Dan's negative views of himself?**
- **How might you document Dan's intervention in a final report?**

Chapter 11 Review Questions

1. What is therapeutic reasoning? And why is it not called clinical reasoning?
2. How is therapeutic reasoning client centered?
3. Can you identify a theory-driven question for each main element of MOHO theory?
4. How would you phrase an introduction to the OSA assessment?
5. What is an occupational formulation?
6. Can you identify four occupational changes?
7. What are the elements of a measurable goal?
8. Describe two ways to evaluate the outcomes of intervention.

HOMEWORK ASSIGNMENTS

1. Think of a person who has received occupational therapy services whereby MOHO was used:
   - What questions were asked of them to help build an understanding of their occupational situation?
   - Were there any standardized assessment used?
   - What was the identified occupation-focused changes?
   - Were the goals structured to be measurable?
   - Can you identify how the elements of the person—their volition, habituation, performance or the environment—were altered, in order to create a set of circumstances that improve the person's ability to engage in occupation?

DIDACTIC CLINICAL INFORMATION

2. Therapeutic reasoning comprises of
   - Generating theory-driven questions to Inform nonstandardized assessment
   - Administering standardized assessment(s)
   - Occupational formulation of client's situation
   - Identifying occupational changes
   - Develop measurable goals
   - Implementing intervention
   - Assess outcomes of intervention
3. Occupational formulation: The term "**occupational formulation**" was coined by Forsyth (2000b) and describes how an occupational therapist takes all the assessment information

for a client and pulls it together in order to create a set of arguments about their unique perspective of their client's occupational situation.

4. Measurable goals consist of
   - Occupational change: What the client will do to demonstrate that the occupational goal has been achieved.
   - Setting: The specific setting where the client will do it (e.g., within the ward or within the client's home environment).
   - Degree: The circumstances under which the client will do it (e.g., independently, with physical support, with verbal cueing, using equipment).
   - Timeframe: The timeframe within which the client will be able to do it.
5. Implementing intervention requires a detailed focus on simultaneously reasoning about the dynamic interactions between elements within the person and those in the environment.
6. Assessing outcomes of intervention can be achieved by
   - Examining the extent to which measurable goals have been achieved (called goal attainment)
   - Readministering standardized assessments to measure change

thePoint® For additional resources and exercises, visit http://thePoint.lww.com

Key Terms

Therapeutic reasoning: Is how therapists use the theory to understand a client and to develop, implement, and monitor a plan of therapy with a client

Occupational formulation: As a term was coined by Forsyth (2000b) and describes how an occupational therapist takes all the assessment information for a client and pulls it together in order to create a set of arguments about their unique perspective of their client's occupational situation.

REFERENCES

Baron, K., Kielhofner, G., Iyenger, A., Goldhammer, V., & Wolenski, J. (2006). *The Occupational Self-Assessment (OSA)* [Version 2.2]. Chicago: Model of Human Occupation Clearinghouse, Department of Occupational Therapy, College of Applied Health Sciences, University of Illinois.

Fisher, A. G. (2003). *Assessment of Motor and Process Skills (AMPS)* (5th ed.). Ft. Collins, CO: Three Star.

Forsyth, K. (2000a). *Therapeutic reasoning process.* Dunblane, Scotland: Scottish Centre of Outcomes Research & Education.

Forsyth, K. (2000b). *Occupational formulation.* Dunblane, Scotland: Scottish Centre of Outcomes Research & Education.

Forsyth, K., Deshpande, S., Kielhofner, G., Henriksson, C., Haglund, L., Olson, L., et al. (2005). *The occupational circumstances assessment interview and rating scale* [Version 4.0]. Chicago: Model of Human Occupation Clearinghouse, Department of Occupational Therapy, College of Applied Health Sciences, University of Illinois.

Matsutsuyu, J. (1969). Interest checklist. *American Journal of Occupational Therapy, 23,* 323–328.

Mattingly, C. (1991). The narrative nature of clinical reasoning. *American Journal of Occupational Therapy, 45,* 998–1005.

Mattingly, C., & Fleming, M. (1993). *Clinical reasoning: Forms of inquiry in a therapeutic practice.* Philadelphia, PA: F. A. Davis.

Parkinson, S., Forsyth, K., & Kielhofner, G. (2006). *The model of human occupation screening tool* [Version 2.0]. Chicago: MOHO Clearinghouse, University of Illinois.

Assessment: Choosing and Using Standardized and Nonstandardized Means of Gathering Information

Kirsty Forsyth

CHAPTER 12

EXPECTED LEARNING OUTCOMES

Upon completion of this chapter, readers will be able to:

1. Understand when and how to use nonstandardized assessment.
2. Understand what to consider to ensure nonstandardized assessment is dependable.
3. Understand when and how to use standardized assessment.

As noted in Chapter 11, therapists gather information to create an understanding of the client's situation. Effective assessment is critical to understanding clients and their occupational needs. Moreover, assessment is essential to making effective decisions about the goals and strategies of occupational therapy. As Trombly (1993) notes, "we cannot ethically treat what we do not measure" (p. 256). This chapter will examine choosing both nonstandardized and standardized assessment approaches.

Most of the validated, standardized, and semistructured model of human occupation (MOHO) assessments are available via the UIC Model of Occupation Clearinghouse at http://www.cade.uic.edu/moho/. Other assessments are accessible via the reference with which they are cited in this chapter. This is a critical set of issues within occupational therapy practice because not seeking adequate information within an assessment can result in poor outcomes for our clients. The following case illustrates a poor outcome for Henrietta and identifies what information could have been gathered in the assessment that would have led to a different and more positive outcome.

MOHO Problem-Solver: An Older Adult with a Bone Fracture

Henrietta is 75 years old and has osteoarthritis. She was referred for occupational therapy. The referral stated that Henrietta had recently been hospitalized after sustaining a fractured femur. At their first meeting, Henrietta indicated that she was familiar with occupational therapy. Several months ago, she first received occupational therapy as an inpatient following a mild stroke. She remembered that the therapist had asked her about "getting in and out of the bath," her physical difficulties, and then recommended that Henrietta receive a bath board and bath seat. Henrietta recalled, "initially I was extremely excited about being able to bathe again." Henrietta then came to the occupational therapy department, where the therapist demonstrated how to use the bath board and seat. She then asked Henrietta to try using the equipment to get in and out of the bath. Henrietta remembered, "I managed this well," and she never saw the occupational therapist again. In fact, the therapist had documented in Henrietta's file that she was able to "transfer in and out of the bath using the bath board and seat." After Henrietta was discharged, another community-based occupational therapist had visited her home once to install the bath board and seat. When asked where the bathing equipment was now, Henrietta answered, "under the bed . . . I never use it."

Why was this happening? Instead of using the bathing equipment, Henrietta had been washing herself at the bathroom sink. The following is why Henrietta had abandoned the bathroom equipment and begun washing at the sink. First, Henrietta's bathroom at home was much smaller than the one in the hospital. Consequently, she had difficulty maneuvering into position while using her walking frame. Second, she could not gather and organize all the needed bathing objects within reach, which frustrated her.

Third, Henrietta had attempted to bathe in the morning, as had always been her habit. However, because this was before her pain medication had begun to have an effect, she was in pain. Fourth, Henrietta found it very anxiety-provoking to do the routine she had simulated in the hospital with the bath full of hot water and steam. Despite these factors and because bathing was so important to her, Henrietta chose to continue with the bath. As she proceeded, she realized that she had forgotten some of the therapist's instructions for how to use the bath board and seat. Consequently, she was only able to maneuver part way onto the bath equipment. After several attempts, her skin became sore and she decided she could not manage and gave up. Henrietta was so flustered by this negative experience and so unsure of her capacity to use the bathing equipment that she resolved never to try bathing with the equipment again. So, she asked a neighbor to remove the bathing equipment. Then she put it permanently under the bed. Following this, Henrietta chose to bathe in the best way she could: washing at the bathroom sink. However, her endurance was severely taxed by this bathing process. It was during this morning wash at the bathroom sink that Henrietta, exhausted, slipped and fractured the neck of her femur.

Poor outcome: While obviously not intended, the two occupational therapists' failure to gather information could have contributed to Henrietta's fall and fracture.

What MOHO approach would have helped? The therapists needed more information about Henrietta than they gathered. They might have recognized the need to gather more information had they generated the following MOHO-based questions:

- When the new equipment (objects) is put into the physical space of Henrietta's bathroom along with other objects (her walking frame, soap, shampoo, towels, robe, etc.), how will the overall bathroom space and objects collectively impact her performance?
- What was Henrietta's daily habit of bathing? How would this habit influence her success in bathing?
- How will Henrietta experience her first attempt to bathe at home?
- Will she feel an adequate sense of efficacy to continue using the equipment?

Gathering adequate information to answer these questions would have pointed to the utility of:

- Solving problems of dealing with limited maneuvering space
- Helping Henrietta find a way to transport/arrange her bathing objects in reach of the bathing seat
- Altering daily habits so that she could bathe in the afternoon or evening when she had less pain
- Providing further training and practice in the use of the adaptive equipment under real-life conditions
- Giving her verbal encouragement and reassurance to reduce her anxiety

Even if Henrietta had not been able to bathe with these interventions, the therapist could have worked with her to establish a different, safe way of getting washed. Certainly, the additional time and cost of doing adequate information gathering would have been substantially less than the expense of Henrietta's hospitalization for the hip fracture. As this case illustrates, taking time to do adequate information gathering can be very cost-effective. Failing to gather adequate information can have high human and economic costs.

Deciding When and How to Use Nonstandardized Assessment

It is critical that an occupational therapist gathers information as efficiently as possible. However, it is important to make sound decisions about what information to gather and how to gather it. Therapists must always balance limitations on practical constraints (i.e., time) with the need to learn as much as possible about the client. Decisions about information gathering focus on three interwoven issues (i.e., getting the most important information; assuring that the information is complete and accurate; choosing the best means of gathering the information). The best way to assure that one is gathering the most important information is to generate clear questions that will be answered by assessment. Chapter 11 discussed this process of generating questions using MOHO theory. Generating these questions is a necessary step to gathering information. From the perspective of MOHO theory, comprehensive assessment means that a therapist will minimally raise and seek answers to questions pertaining to the client's engagement in occupation and their volition, habituation, performance capacity, and environment. The questions that the therapist raises will indicate the kind of information that needs to be gathered to generate an adequate understanding of the client's situation. Assuring that the information is complete and accurate requires therapists to secure information from a range of sources. Choosing the best means of gathering information should be guided by the questions the therapist wants to answer and by considerations of what means of information gathering the client can effectively engage in. As noted in Chapter 11, therapists can draw on both nonstandardized and standardized means of assessment. Both are considered below.

Therapists can use nonstandardized approaches to gathering information. **Nonstandardized approaches** are informal methods of assessment, for example, having a conversation with a client while beginning a therapy session, observing a student's performance when visiting the classroom, listening to a client's comments about the workplace where he/she was injured, noting the affect of a client during a group session, and listening to a client's narratives about what happened since the last therapy session. From the perspective of MOHO theory, comprehensive assessment means that a therapist will minimally raise and seek answers to questions pertaining to the client's engagement in occupation and their volition, habituation, performance capacity, and environment. The questions that the therapist raises will indicate the kind of information that needs to be gathered to generate an adequate understanding of the client's situation.

Nonstandardized approaches to gathering information are useful as supplements to standardized approaches, for taking advantage of unexpected opportunities to obtain useful information. Sometimes, nonstandardized approaches are the only option available to the therapist. As noted previously, nonstandardized approaches to gathering information take advantage of natural circumstances that arise for learning about a client. The following are some common circumstances in which therapists will decide to make use of nonstandardized methods:

- There is no appropriate standardized assessment available for the question(s) one wants to answer or for the ability of the client one has
- The client is uncomfortable with or unable to complete a standardized assessment
- The therapist wishes to augment information collected by standardized assessments
- An unexpected opportunity to obtain useful information arises

Unstructured methods of information gathering are particularly dependent on identifying questions that one wants answered. When guided by such questions, therapists can be more vigilant to look for opportunities to find information. For instance, if a therapist has generated questions about a client's volition, then any informal conversation the therapist has with that client can be directed to answering those specific questions. On the other hand, if a therapist has not consciously generated questions about the client, there are likely to be lost opportunities to learn critical things about the client. Generating theory-based questions is an important step to doing nonstandardized information gathering in a systematic and disciplined way.

ASSURING DEPENDABILITY WHILE USING NONSTANDARDIZED ASSESSMENT

When using nonstandardized methods to gather information, therapists must ensure that the information gathered is accurate and dependable (Denzin & Lincoln, 1994; Hagner & Helm, 1994; Hammersly, 1992; Krefting, 1989; Miles & Huberman, 1994; Wolcott, 1990). There are three important strategies for assuring dependability of information gathered by nonstandard methods of assessment.

- Evaluating context
- Triangulation
- Validity checks

Evaluating Context

Circumstances have an important influence on the information gathered. For example, a client struggling with some problem suddenly confides in a therapist about all his fears for the future. From such an encounter, the therapist may have much more honest and useful information than the information previously gathered in a formal interview. On the other hand, circumstances may make the information unreliable. For example, if a client is reporting on her performance in a group where it is clear he/she is trying to impress another group member, the therapist may have reasons to suspect that the report is exaggerated. Circumstances often tell the therapist how much confidence to place in the information.

Triangulation

Triangulation is a method of helping to assure that information is accurate by comparing it with information from another source (Denzin & Lincoln, 1994). Thus, for example, one may compare what clients say they can do with observation of their performance or with what a spouse or caretaker says the person can do.

Validity Checks

When using nonstandardized methods, therapists should be vigilant to assure that their interpretation of the meaning of the information is valid. First, a therapist should ask whether an interpretation corresponds logically and structurally with the general picture obtained from earlier information. If it does, then one has a stronger basis to consider the interpretation. The therapist may also ask whether the interpretation corresponds with case examples and other discussions offered by the theory that guided the information gathering. Another important method of checking the validity of one's interpretations is to continue to collect information that will either support or refute the interpretation of the previous information's meaning. Finally and importantly, one can and should check interpretations of information by asking the client if the interpretations are valid. For example, observation of a client's behavior in a task situation suggests that the client was anxious, and the therapist interprets this information as meaning the client's sense of efficacy in a particular task is poor. The therapist can check the validity of this interpretation by sharing it with the client to ask whether he or she agrees.

Deciding Which Standardized Assessment to Choose

Other chapters in this book present **standardized assessments** that have been developed for use with MOHO. These assessments are designed to provide therapists with the best possible means of gathering relevant, sound, and thorough information. Table 12-1 lists these assessments and the MOHO concept on which they provide information. Each of these assessments reflects years of development, and the assessments have been studied and refined to varying extents to enhance their dependability and practical value. These assessments range from a few minutes to over an hour to complete. The amount of time and effort each assessment takes is generally proportional to the amount of information it gathers. Thus, in selecting which of these assessments to use for a given client, therapists will need to carefully think about the kind and depth of information needed and the time available for assessment. The below are a series of questions and answers that will help guide the choice of standardized assessment, related to age, client ability, time to complete, client centeredness, incorporating non-MOHO assessments, considering diagnosis, considering culture, and a strategy for choosing which assessment to choose. These issues will now be explored.

AGES COVERED BY MOHO ASSESSMENTS

Table 12-1 also indicates the age groups with which the assessments are used. More specific information on the age-appropriateness of each assessment will ordinarily be covered in the manuals or texts that present the assessments. In the end, appropriate use of the assessments in terms of age will depend on a therapist's judgment. For example, the appropriateness of some assessments that require more abstract thought and self-reflection will depend less on chronological age and more on intellectual development and personal maturity of the client. Therapists should always be vigilant to consider a client's developmental readiness and ability to participate in any assessment process.

CLIENT CAPACITY FOR MOHO ASSESSMENTS

Another important consideration is the client's capability for participating in the assessment. MOHO-based assessments range from those that require clients to actively participate in self-assessment to those that require minimal or no action on the part of the client. In a number of instances, the administration of assessments can be altered to accommodate client limitations. For example, a client whose motor abilities impair speech could respond to an interview using augmented communication, or a client with motor limitations that prevent writing can respond to self-reports verbally. Most manuals for MOHO-based assessments provide guidelines for whether and how the administration can be accommodated and still maintain the psychometric properties of the assessment. Whenever client limitations are of the kind that such an accommodation of the assessment cannot be made, there are still often alternatives. For instance, therapists have often found it useful to ask family members to respond to assessments on behalf of the client.

CLINICAL EFFICIENCIES WITHIN THE MOHO ASSESSMENTS

Table 12-2 indicates the minimal type of effort and time required of the therapists and the requirements for client participation of the MOHO-based structured and semistructured assessments. In thinking about which assessments to choose, this table can be a helpful guide. Whatever assessment(s) therapists choose, there are a number of additional strategies that can make assessment more efficient. Some of the assessments are designed so that they can be administered simultaneously and self-administered assessments can be incorporated into groups. Standardized assessment should be separate from intervention to ensure you

Table 12-1 MOHO-Based Assessments, Concepts on Which They Provide Data, Methods They Use, and Populations for Which They Are Designed and Where They Are Discussed in This Text

Concepts Addressed by the Assessment	Occupational Adaptation		Volition			Habituation		Skills			Performance	Participation	Environment		Method of Data Gathering			Population			
Assessment	**Identity**	**Competence**	**Personal Causation**	**Values**	**Interests**	**Roles**	**Habits**	**Motor**	**Process**	**Communication/ Interaction**			**Physical**	**Social**	**Observation**	**Self-report**	**Interview**	**Children**	**Adolescents**	**Adults**	**Elderly**
ACHIEVE assessment	X	X	X	X	X	X	X	X	X	X	X	X	X	X		X		X			
Assessment of communication and interaction skills										X					X			X	X	X	X
Assessment of motor and process skills								X	X						X			X	X	X	X
Child occupational self-assessment		X	X	X	X	X	X	X	X	X	X	X				X			X	X	X
CIRCLE	X	X	X	X	X	X	X	X	X	X	X	X	X	X	X			X			
ESPI													X	X	X			X	X	X	X
Interest checklist					X											X			X	X	x
Making it clear			X	X	X	X	X	X	X	X	X	X	X	X		X			X	X	X
Model of human occupation screening tool			X	X	X	X	X	X	X	X	X	X	X	X	X		X		X	X	X
MOHOxpLOR			x	X	X	X	X	X	X	X	X	X	X	X	X				X	X	X
NIH activity record			X	X	X	X	X				X	X				X			X	X	X
Occupational circumstances assessment interview and rating scale			X	X	X	X	X				X	X	X	X			X		X	X	X
Occupational performance history interview-II	X	X	X	X	X	X	X				X	X	X	X			X		X	X	X

(continued)

Table 12-1 MOHO-Based Assessments, Concepts on Which They Provide Data, Methods They Use, and Populations for Which They Are Designed and Where They Are Discussed in This Text (continued)

Concepts Addressed by the Assessment	Occupational Adaptation		Volition			Habituation		Skills			Performance	Participation	Environment		Method of Data Gathering			Population			
Assessment	**Identity**	**Competence**	**Personal Causation**	**Values**	**Interests**	**Roles**	**Habits**	**Motor**	**Process**	**Communication/ Interaction**			**Physical**	**Social**	**Observation**	**Self-report**	**Interview**	**Children**	**Adolescents**	**Adults**	**Elderly**
Occupational questionnaire			X	X	X	X	X					X				X			X	X	X
Occupational self-assessment		X	X	X	X	X	X	X	X	X	X	X	X	X		X			X	X	X
Occupational therapy psycho-social assessment of learning			X	X	X	X	X				X	X	X	X	X		X	X			
Pediatric interest profile		X	X		X	X						X						X	X		
Pediatric volitional questionnaire			X	X	X								X	X	X			X			
Role checklist				X		X										X			X	X	X
Residential environment im-pact scale													X	X	X	X	X	X	X	X	X
School setting interview											X	X	X	X			X	X	X		
Short child occupational profile			X	X	X	X	X	X	X	X	X	X	X	X	X		X	X	X		
Volitional questionnaire			X	X	X										X				X	X	X
Worker role interview			X	X	X	X	X						X	X			X			X	
Work environment impact scale													X	X			X			X	

Table 12-2 Therapist and Client Requirements for MOHO Assessment Administration

Assessment	Therapists' Requirements for Administration	Client Requirements to Participate	Estimated Total Therapist's Time[a]
ACHIEVE assessment	Parent and teacher complete form	Parent/teacher – concentrate, read, and write	15 minutes
Assessment of communication and interaction skills	Observe client in a goal-oriented activity that involved social interaction, complete[b] scale	Engage in some social interaction	20–60 minutes
Assessment of motor and process skills	Observe client in a goal-oriented activity that involved social interaction, complete motor and process scales	Perform an occupational form (simple to complex)	30–60 minutes
Circle	Teacher completes the form	Minimally interact with the environment	15 minutes
Child occupational self-assessment	Introduce assessment and give directions, provide support to complete self-report, review ratings with client	Concentrate, read, and write	15–20 minutes
ESPI	Collect information via interview, observation, and from key informants and then complete scale	Minimally interact with the environment	15–30 minutes
Interest checklist	Explain instructions and discuss client responses	Read and write	
Make it clear	Explain instructions and discuss client responses	Concentrate, read, and write	10 minutes
Model of human occupational screening tool	Collect information via chart review, interview, observation, and from surrogates and then complete scale	Minimally interact with the environment	15–30 minutes
MOHOxpLOR	Collect information via chart review, interview, observation, and from surrogates and then complete scale	Minimally interact with the environment	15–30 minutes
NIH activity record	Explain instructions and discuss client responses	Concentrate, read, and write	15–20 minutes
Occupational circumstances assessment interview and rating scale	Conduct a semistructured interview and complete scale	Answer questions	20–40 minutes
Occupational performance history interview-II	Conduct a semistructured interview, complete three scales, and complete a life history narrative slope	Answer questions	45 minutes to 1 hour
Occupational Questionnaire	Explain instructions and discuss client responses	Concentrate, read, and write	15–20 minutes
Occupational self-assessment	Explain instructions and discuss client responses	Concentrate, read, and write	15–20 minutes
Pediatric interest profiles	Explain instructions and discuss client responses	Look at pictures or read, use a crayon, or write (depending on which profile is used)	15–20 minutes

(*continued*)

Table 12-2 Therapist and Client Requirements for MOHO Assessment Administration (continued)

Assessment	Therapists' Requirements for Administration	Client Requirements to Participate	Estimated Total Therapist's Time[a]
Pediatric volitional questionnaire	Observe client and complete scale	Minimally interact with the environment	20–40 minutes
Residential environmental impact scale	Collect information via interview, observation, and from key informants and then complete scale	Interact with the environment	15–30 minutes
Role checklist	Explain instructions and discuss client responses	Concentrate, read, and write	10–15 minutes
Short child occupational profile	Collect information via chart review, interview, observation, and from surrogates and then complete scale	Minimally interact with the environment	15–30 minutes
School setting interview	Interview student	Answer questions	20–40 minutes
Volitional questionnaire	Observe client and complete scale	Minimally interact with the environment	20–40 minutes
Worker role interview	Conduct semistructured interview and complete scale[c]	Answer interview questions	30–45 minutes
Work environment impact scale	Conduct semistructured interview and complete scale	Answer interview questions	30–45 minutes

[a]Does not include time for clients to complete self-administered assessments.
[b]Completing MOHO instrument scales ordinarily involves using a 4-point rating scale and entering clarifying/qualifying comments.
[c]There are interview formats available that allow the WRI to be combined with the OCAIRS or the WEIS saving administration.

secure an accurate baseline assessment. However, assessments can accomplish therapeutic aims. For example, during an interview, the therapist builds rapport with a client, and as part of the assessment, the therapist provides feedback to a client or shares information about the client's situation. Engaging in an assessment helps a client clarify values. Participating in an assessment process gives a client a more realistic view of personal capacity. Completing an assessment and discussing results can be used to collaborate on treatment goals and strategies.

CLIENT-CENTEREDNESS OF THE MOHO ASSESSMENTS

Client-centered practice requires that therapists chose the form of assessment that maximizes client involvement to the greatest extent possible. Where direct involvement of the client in the assessment process is not possible, therapists should make every effort to construct an understanding of the client's perspective. Clients who are least able to self-advocate deserve the most careful assessment of their volition. There are ways that a therapist can readily gain insight into the volition of lower functioning clients. The Volitional Questionnaire (VQ) and the Pediatric Volitional Questionnaire (PVQ), the Model of Human Occupation Screening Tool (MOHOST), the Short Child Occupational Profile, and MOHOxpLOR work well with such clients. Additionally, therapists can make good use of nonstandardized means of assessment for such clients.

COMBINING MOHO AND NON-MOHO ASSESSMENTS

Therapists often use MOHO in combination with other practice models or with theories borrowed from other disciplines or professions. When this is the case, assessments that correspond to those models and theories may be used alongside the MOHO assessments. Occupational therapists also use assessments other than those based on MOHO because they are part of an interdisciplinary approach or because administration requires their use. For a variety of reasons, then, therapists basing practice on MOHO will use assessments other than those presented in this book. When this is the case, it is important to consider why one is using the assessment, what kinds of information it provides, and how it can best be used in relationship to the model and the MOHO-based assessments that are being used. For example, they are using MOHO in association with other conceptual practice models that have their own assessments. They may also choose other assessments that specifically target occupational performance in ways that MOHO-based assessments do not. Such assessments include activities of daily living assessments, standardized development assessments, and formal work evaluations. These kinds of assessments are used when the therapist needs information on the client's capacity to do specific occupational performance such as dressing, bathing, or driving. Although such assessments were not developed specifically for use with MOHO, they are certainly compatible with it.

MOHO ASSESSMENTS ARE NOT DIAGNOSIS DRIVEN

None of the MOHO-based assessments are designed for use with clients from a specific diagnostic group. MOHO focuses on understanding the impact of a disease or impairment on the person's occupational participation, not on the disease or impairment itself. Therefore, most of the assessments will work with clients who have a wide range of diagnoses. This is not to say that the therapist should ignore the diagnosis or impairment in selecting assessments. Two important considerations in selecting assessments that do emanate from the client's diagnosis or impairments are:

- Whether the diagnosis or nature of the impairment has implications that are better addressed by certain assessments
- Whether the client's impairment limits the client's ability to do what is necessary to participate in the assessment

Some MOHO-based assessments are particularly relevant to a given population. For example, the NIH Activity Record (ACTRE; Chapter 16) gathers information on pain and fatigue. Therefore, for clients who are likely to experience pain and fatigue that impacts their occupational participation, the ACTRE would be the better choice.

When a diagnosis is known to routinely produce certain kinds of occupational consequences, it may warrant use of particular assessments. For example, chronic, severe depression typically results in severe volitional problems. For this reason, the VQ is frequently an assessment of choice for clients with severe depression. Another example is that traumatic injuries or catastrophic illnesses that significantly alter a person's life (e.g., persons with spinal cord injury or persons with AIDS) often produce changes in interests and participation in interests, changes in roles, and changes in occupational identity and occupational competence. For this reason, such clients would be good candidates for use of the Modified Interest Checklist, the Role Checklist, and the Occupational Performance History Interview, Second Version (OPHI-II), since all three assessments provide information on changes that occur as a result of diseases or impairments that change a person's life.

Knowing what implications for assessment emanate from a client's diagnosis or impairment requires that the therapist have two kinds of information. First, the therapist must have some knowledge of how the diagnosis or impairment is likely to impact the client occupationally. Second, the therapist must know the content and organization of the MOHO-based assessments. When these two factors are known, the therapist can make effective matches.

CULTURAL DIFFERENCES

Most MOHO-based assessments have been developed in collaboration with persons representing multiple cultures and languages. Research indicates that many of the MOHO-based assessments do not reflect cultural biases. For example, studies of the Assessment of Motor and Process Skills (AMPS; Fisher, 1999) have indicated that it is free of cultural bias (Fisher, Liu, Velozo, & Pan, 1992; Goto, Fisher, & Mayberry, 1996). Studies of the Worker Role Interview (WRI; Haglund, Karlsson, Kielhofner, & Lai, 1997), the Work Environment Impact Scale (WEIS; Kielhofner et al., 1999), the OPHI-II (Kielhofner, Mallinson, Forsyth, & Lai, 2001), the ACIS (Kjellberg, Haglund, Forsyth. & Kielhofner, 2003), and the OSA (Kielhofner & Forsyth, 2001) indicate that these assessments are valid cross-culturally and when administered in different languages.

Assuring that assessments are relevant and valid with persons from diverse cultural backgrounds requires ongoing development and research. Such work is being undertaken across the MOHO-based assessments. Nonetheless, therapists should always be vigilant to consider whether an assessment is valid for clients based on their cultural background.

A further point needs to be made about MOHO-based assessments in relation to culture. Because the theory of this model incorporates culture into its concepts (e.g., volition and social environment), many of the assessments are specifically designed to capture a client's unique cultural perspective. For example, the OPHI-II elicits and considers culturally influenced values, interests, roles, and occupational narratives. For this reason, such assessments are particularly useful when therapists desire to gather information about the client's culturally influenced thoughts, feelings, and actions.

MOHO ASSESSMENTS AS MEASURES OF CHANGE

A number of MOHO-based assessments can be used to document change in clients and to evaluate the impact or outcomes of therapy. Table 12-3 lists the assessments that provide data relevant to evaluating client change and demonstrating impact. It also indicates the type of change that the assessment would capture. Which assessment one chooses for capturing change or demonstrating program outcomes depends on what changes services are designed to achieve. Outcome measures should be targeted to those aspects of clients that the services aim to achieve.

Choosing MOHO Assessments

Choosing which assessments to use routinely is one of the most important decisions therapists make about their practice. The following steps are helpful in making an informed decision:

- Becoming familiar with all potentially relevant MOHO assessments and identifying those that appear most suitable for use
- Piloting these assessments in practice to evaluate their utility
- Developing an assessment strategy that allows flexibility to meet individual client needs

Table 12-3 MOHO Assessments Suitable for Indicating Client Change and Program Outcomes

Assessment	Type of Change Captured by Assessment
ACHIEVE assessment	Change in occupational participation
Assessment of communication and interaction skills	Change in skill
Assessment of motor and process skills	Change in skill
Circle	Change in occupational participation
Child occupational self-assessment	Change in values and competence
ESPI	Change in occupational participation
Make it clear	Change in occupational participation
Model of human occupational screening tool	Change in how volition, habituation, skill, and environment support participation
MOHOxpLOR	Change in occupational participation
NIH activity record	Change in participation and in fatigue, pain, perceived competence, interest, and value in what one routinely does
Occupational questionnaire	Change in participation and in competence, interest, and value in what one routinely does
Occupational case analysis interview and rating scale	Change in how volition, habituation, skill, environment, and goal setting support participation
Occupational performance history interview, version II	Change in narrative slope before and after intervention
Occupational self-assessment	Change in values and competence as well as in environmental impact
Pediatric interest profiles	Change in children's and adolescent's interests, perceived competence, and participation
Pediatric volitional questionnaire	Change in children's volition (motivation to do things)
Residential environment impact scale	Change in residential environment
Role checklist	Change in roles and value assigned to roles
Short child occupational profile	Change in how children's volition, habituation, skill, and environment support participation
School setting interview	Change in student–environment fit to support participation
Volitional questionnaire	Change in volition (motivation to do things)
Worker role interview	Change in psychosocial readiness for work

LEARNING ABOUT THE ASSESSMENTS

This first step involves simply becoming familiar with the range of assessments developed for use with MOHO. Table 12-1 provides an overview of the assessments and Table 12-2 indicates the time, effort, and client participation required for each assessment. These tables will help to identify those assessments that are potentially most suitable to one's population and context. Another resource for identifying potentially relevant assessments is Figure 12-1. The figure categorizes MOHO-based assessments according to whether they are general (providing data on many MOHO concepts and designed for use across practice settings) or specific (focused on one or a few concepts and/or designed for specific practice settings).

In situations where there is only time for a single evaluation or for doing an initial evaluation, it is recommended that therapists select an assessment from the first row that will provide more comprehensive information (i.e., cover all or the majority of the MOHO concepts). If one's clients tend to have specific challenges, you may choose an assessment that focuses on that specific area (see middle of Figure 12-1). Such assessments are often completed after an initial more comprehensive assessment, but may be used alone if appropriate to the focus of the intervention. If working in a specialized setting, such as a school or a work rehabilitation program, consider the assessments listed at the bottom of Figure 12-1. These assessments may be either used in combination with comprehensive assessments or used alone.

Once one has selected potentially relevant assessments, the next step is to become familiar with them. Examining copies of the assessments and reading articles that discuss the assessment's development and/or use in practice are also recommended. Additional information may be obtained at the University of Illinois at Chicago MOHO Clearinghouse website http://www.cade.uic.edu/moho/. An evidence-based search engine at the website provides access to comprehensive bibliographies for each assessment.

PILOTING ASSESSMENTS IN PRACTICE

With the exception of the AMPS (Chapter 15), therapists can learn to administer MOHO-based assessments from manuals that have been developed for each assessment or from available guidelines. (Information on purchasing manuals and accessing guidelines can be found at www.moho.uic.edu) After accessing the relevant information for administration, one should try out an assessment. This allows one to determine how an assessment works in one's context. Piloting a few potentially relevant assessments provides an

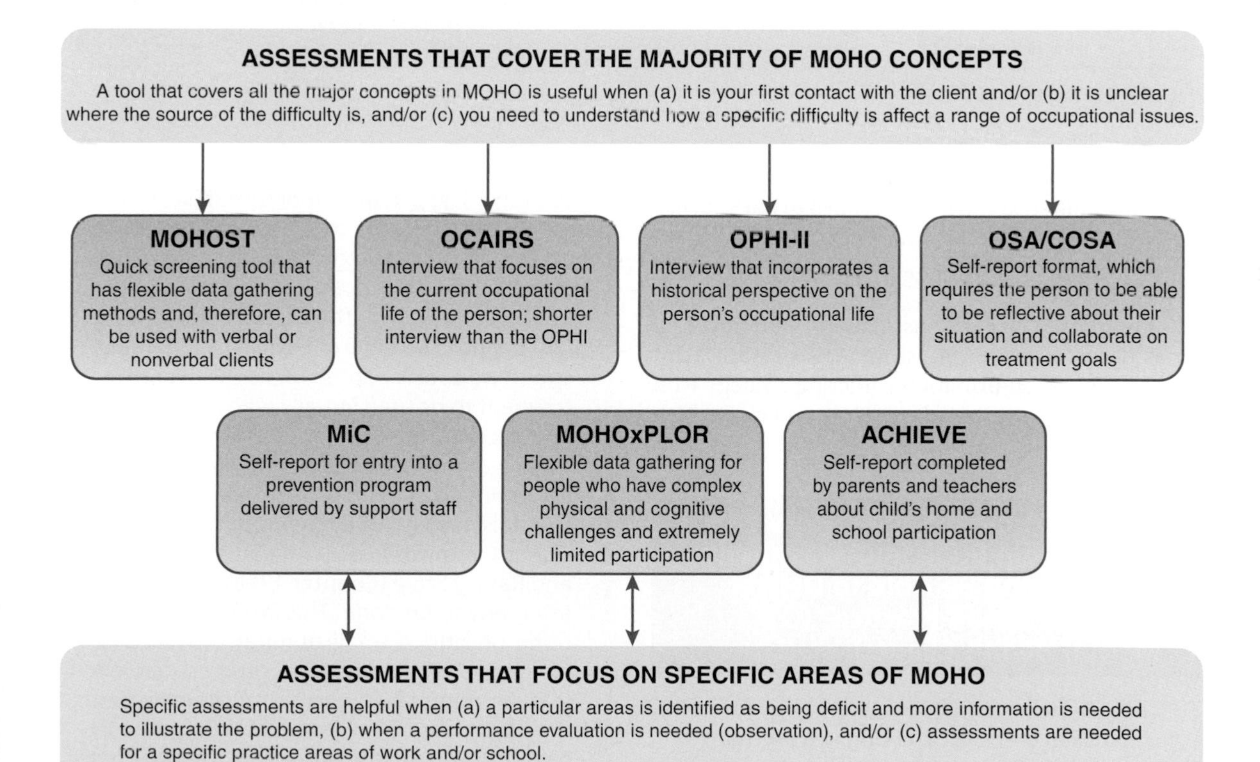

Continued on next page

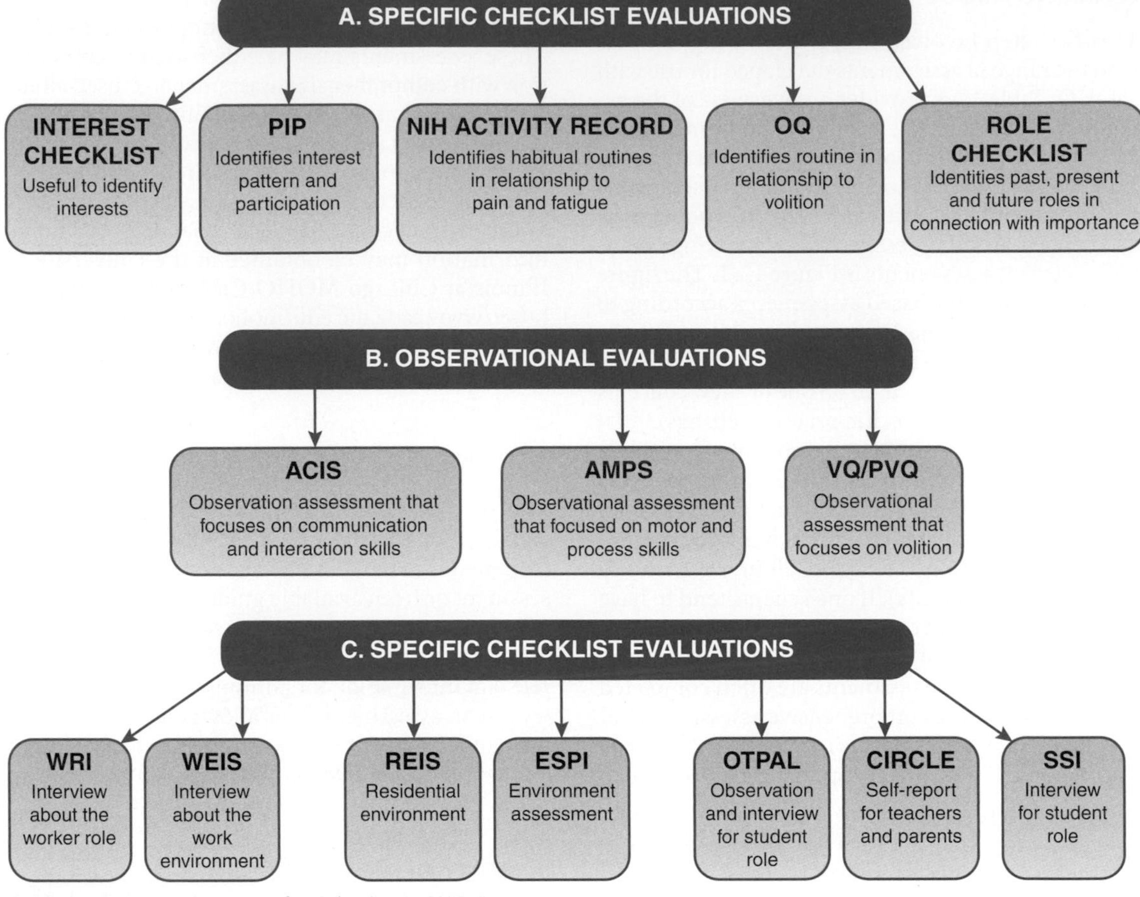

FIGURE 12-1 A Decision Tree for Selecting MOHO Assessments.

opportunity to test out which assessments best meet one's working style and are best suited to one's clients.

DEVELOPING AN ASSESSMENT STRATEGY

A single MOHO-based assessment may meet all one's needs. However, most therapists find it helpful to create an information gathering strategy with optional assessments and a means to decide which to use for specific clients.

MOHO Problem-Solver: How Can MOHO Help Build an Assessment Strategy and Be Able to Deliver Evidence-Based Practice? (OT, Mental Health Clients)

The chapter author was supporting an occupational therapist working in a psychiatric rehabilitation setting to develop an assessment strategy. The occupational therapist stated, "Most of the clients coming into our service are initially not able to complete an interview or a self report."

The therapist was therefore guided toward identifying the Model of Human Occupational screening tool (Chapter 18) as the overall assessment to be used initially with most clients. The occupational therapist then indicated, "there are a few clients who initially have the ability to engage in an interview," so the therapist was guided to choose the Occupational Circumstances Assessment-Interview and Rating Scale (Chapter 17) as the primary interview to be done. This interview may be done on only a small number of clients as an initial assessment, although the interview may be done later with some clients when they progress to the point of being able to participate in an interview. The occupational therapist indicated, "we have a significant number of clients who progress and identify the goal of returning to work or achieving employment," and the Worker Role Interview or the Work Environment Impact Scale were identified as appropriate. Since the latter is designed to interview clients concerning a specific job setting or type of job setting, only those clients with previous employment will ordinarily be candidates for this assessment.

The occupational therapist stated that "our clients often have significant challenges in their skills to participate in occupation." The assessment strategy also indicates that when the MOHOST identifies problems in skills, the AMPS or the Assessment of Communication and Interaction Skills may be done. Finally, the occupational therapist stated, "we do have some clients who show more extreme problems in motivation to engage in occupation," the Volitional Questionnaire was therefore identified to use with these clients. Since these are observational assessments, they can be done on clients who are at a lower level of functioning than is required for the interviews.

The occupational therapists stated, "I am really happy with the choices of assessments; it allows our assessment strategy to have many different configurations of assessments to be done according to client needs and characteristics." One client may be assessed only through repeated applications of the MOHOST to monitor progress and identify intervention needs. Another client, who showed clear challenges in communication/interaction, may be assessed with the ACIS following the MOHOST. Repeated use of the ACIS may help monitor the client's response to intervention and need for further intervention or support. Still another client who shows some impairment that affects occupational participation but wants to live in the community may be assessed (following the MOHOST) with the OCAIRS and the AMPS to gather critical information for intervention and discharge planning. Developing an assessment strategy will take some time and experimentation, but it is the surest means of doing optimal assessment for clients.

CRITICAL REFLECTION

What are the benefits of having a MOHO assessment strategy?

Reflection points include

- Why would the above assessment strategy be efficient?
- Why would the above assessment strategy be client centered?
- Why would the above assessment strategy be comprehensive?

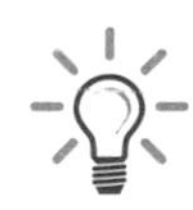

Chapter 12 Review Questions

1. Why would you use a nonstandardized assessment approach?
2. How can you assure dependability when using a nonstandardized assessment approach?
3. Describe how you can be client centred using MOHO standardized assessments.
4. How can you increase efficiency when using MOHO standardized assessments?
5. What role does diagnosis have to play when choosing MOHO standardized assessments?
6. Describe the cultural considerations when choosing MOHO standardized assessments.
7. Name three MOHO standardized assessments and what outcomes they capture.

HOMEWORK ASSIGNMENTS

1. Reflect on a post or a fieldwork placement and develop a MOHO assessment strategy to meet the needs of the clients.
2. Pair with another person and complete an OCAIRS interview, then a MOHOST on each other and complete an OSA. Then, i) compare the time it takes to complete, ii) reflect on the experience of the assessment from a service user's perspective, iii) discuss why you might want to use one assessment over the others.

DIDACTIC CLINICAL INFORMATION

Choose a nonstandardized approach to assessment when

1. There is no appropriate standardized assessment available for the question(s) one wants to answer or for the ability of client one has.
2. The client is uncomfortable with or unable to complete a standardized assessment.
3. The therapist wishes to augment information collected by standardized assessments.
4. An unexpected opportunity to obtain useful information arises.

Choose a standardized approach to assessment by considering

1. client age,
2. client ability,
3. time to complete,
4. client centeredness,
5. considering diagnosis,
6. considering culture.

thePoint® For additional resources and exercises, visit http://thePoint.lww.com

Key Terms

Nonstandardized approach: Uses naturally occurring opportunities to gather information in a fluid way. This approach capitalizes on opportunities for obtaining useful information in informal and spontaneous ways.

Standardized assessment: Follows a set protocol that has been developed and tested through research.

RESOURCES

Most of the validated, standardized, and semistructured MOHO assessments are available via the UIC Model of Occupation Clearinghouse at http://www.cade.uic.edu/moho/. Other assessments are accessible via the reference with which they are cited in this chapter.

REFERENCES

Denzin, N. K., & Lincoln, Y. S. (Eds.). (1994). *Handbook of qualitative research.* Thousand Oaks, CA: SAGE.

Fisher, A. G. (1999). *Assessment of motor and process skills* (3rd ed.). Ft. Collins, CO: Three Star Press.

Fisher, A. G., Liu, Y., Velozo, C. A., & Pan, A. W. (1992). Cross-cultural assessment of process skills. *American Journal of Occupational Therapy, 46*, 876–885.

Goto, S., Fisher, A. G., & Mayberry, W. L. (1996). The assessment of motor and process skills applied cross-culturally to the Japanese. *American Journal of Occupational Therapy, 50*, 798–806.

Haglund, L., Karlsson, G., Kielhofner, G., & Lai, J. S. (1997). Validity of the Swedish version of the worker role interview. *Scandinavian Journal of Occupational Therapy, 4*, 23–29.

Hagner, D. C., & Helm, D. T. (1994). Qualitative methods in rehabilitation research. *Rehabilitation Counseling Bulletin, 37*, 290–303.

Hammersly, M. (1992). Some reflections on ethnography and validity. *Internal Journal of Qualitative Studies in Education, 5*, 195–203.

Kielhofner, G., & Forsyth, K. (2001). Development of a client self-report for treatment planning and documenting therapy outcomes. *Scandinavian Journal of Occupational Therapy, 8*(3), 131–139.

Kielhofner, G., Lai, J. S., Olson, L., Haglund, L., Ekbadh, E., & Hedlund, M. (1999). Psychometric properties of the work environment impact scale: A cross-cultural study. *Work, 12*, 71–78.

Kielhofner, G., Mallinson, T., Forsyth, K., & Lai, J. S. (2001). Psychometric properties of the second version of the occupational performance history interview (OPHI-II). *American Journal of Occupational Therapy, 55*, 260–267.

Kjellberg, A., Haglund, L., Forsyth, K., & Kielhofner, G. (2003). The measurement properties of the Swedish version of the assessment of communication and interaction skills. *Scandinavian Journal of Caring Sciences, 17*(3), 271–277.

Krefting, L. (1989). Disability ethnography: A methodological approach for occupational therapy research. *Canadian Journal of Occupational Therapy, 56*, 61–66.

Miles, M. B., & Huberman, A. M. (Eds.). (1994). *Qualitative data analysis.* Thousand Oaks, CA: SAGE Publications.

Trombly, C. (1993). The issue is—anticipating the future: Assessment of occupational functioning. *American Journal of Occupational Therapy, 47*, 253–257.

Wolcott, H. F. (1990). On seeking and rejecting validity in qualitative research. In E. W. Eisner & A. Peshkin (Eds.), *Qualitative inquiry in education: The continuing debate* (pp. 121–152). New York, NY: Teachers College Press.

Occupational Engagement: How Clients Achieve Change

Genevieve Pépin

CHAPTER 13

EXPECTED LEARNING OUTCOMES

Upon completion of this chapter, readers will be able to:

1. Understand and explain the key factors influencing change.
2. Describe the barriers and enablers of change.
3. Identify the barriers and enablers of change in a range of scenarios.
4. Identify factors supporting changes in a range of scenarios.
5. Understand the role of volition process in supporting change.

The purpose of this chapter is to examine how clients achieve change in therapy. Volition, habituation, and performance capacity are fashioned, maintained, and altered by what people do and how they think and feel about their doing. Environmental conditions in which people engage in occupation are also key determinants of whether and how change takes place. Therefore, change depends on the multiple and complex interactions between volition, habituation, performance capacity, and environmental conditions.

The foundations of this chapter rest on the core belief that change in occupational therapy can only happen when driven by the client's occupational participation, engagement, and choices. This implies that therapists understand what supports occupational participation and engagement, what motivates occupational choices, and how they occur in therapy.

Occupational Participation

Occupational participation promotes and facilitates change by considering the social and cultural aspects of occupation. The World Health Organization (WHO) defines participation as "involvement in a life situation" (World Health Organization, 2002, p. 100). Participation is also conceptualized and defined as participation in society, which includes the "ability to engage in community, civil and recreational activities" (Bedirhan et al., 2010). Consistent with these descriptions of participation, and as discussed in Chapter 8, occupational participation involves "work, play and activities of daily living that are part of one's socio-cultural context and that are desired and/or necessary to one's wellbeing" (Kielhofner et al., 2008, p. 101). This is important to understand when considering change. This means that an activity or an occupation might not be personally meaningful but might hold important social or cultural value for someone (Hitch, Pepin, & Stagnitti, 2014a, 2014b).

For example, consider Joshua, who has difficulties at school. He finds concentrating on tasks and reading challenging and doesn't like doing his homework. While personally, homework might not be meaningful, Joshua knows it is important and he knows doing his homework helps him at school. Similarly, Alexandra doesn't find cleaning her room and putting her toys away enjoyable or meaningful. However, she does it because her parents expect she will keep her room clean.

Occupational Engagement

Change is also driven by the client's occupational engagement. Occupational engagement refers to "clients' doing, thinking, and feeling under certain environmental conditions in the midst of or as a planned consequence therapy" (Kielhofner, 2008, p. 184). Therefore, engagement is a function of the personal and sociocultural meaning of an occupation. As specified by Kielhofner, 2008:

> An engaging occupation is a coherent and meaningful set of occupational forms that cohere and evoke deep feeling, a sense of duty, commitment and perseverance leading to regular involvement over time in relation to a community of people who share the engaging occupation. (2008, p. 124)

Occupational engagement is associated with the emergence of emotions and feelings which for the most part are positive and contribute to the development and determination of a sense of self and identity. Engagement has also been associated with a sense of pleasure and happiness (Hitch et al., 2014b). To engage in occupation requires continuous interactions between volition, habituation, and performance capacity. For example, Kielhofner and Forsyth (2008) identified key dimensions of occupational engagement, of which one was experiencing a level of satisfaction/enjoyment (or dissatisfaction/displeasure) with occupational performance. Other key dimensions of occupational engagement may be:

- Drawing on performance capacity to exercise skill in occupational performance
- Evoking old habits that shape how the occupational performance is done
- Enacting or working toward a role
- Assigning meaning and significance to what is done (i.e., what this means for the client's life)
- Feeling able (or unable) in doing the occupational form

Occupational Choices

Occupational choices, as they have been explained previously in this book, are deliberate decisions made by someone to initiate or terminate activities or occupations whether it is based on personal or sociocultural meaning or a combination of both. This decision is the result of the volitional process, where the thoughts and feelings that occurred through experience, interpretation, and anticipation are assessed by a person to decide whether to begin, continue, or end an activity or occupation.

For example, Gladys, while recovering from a total hip replacement, was concerned and anxious as she showered and dressed herself in the morning (experience). After her shower and once dressed, Gladys reflected on her performance and talked to her husband about what she did and how she felt while completing her self-care activities (interpretation). The next morning, Gladys remembered how exhausted she was after completing her self-care activities. She also remembered feeling anxious about whether or not she would be able to do these activities as she prepared to shower and get herself dressed (anticipation). Gladys thought about the relief of realizing she was able to shower and dress independently. She remembered the conversation with her husband and his suggestions to make things easier for her. Upon reflection, Gladys decided to continue to complete her self-care activities independently using some of the strategies suggested by her husband (occupational choice).

Therapists, when working with clients toward their occupational goals, will need to consider the client's personal circumstances and determine if an occupation is personally meaningful and associated with positive feelings, if it has strong social and cultural meaning, or if it has both personal and sociocultural meaning. This knowledge can help a therapist better understand the motivation of a client for doing. As occupational therapists, we support clients' occupational engagement while acknowledging that some occupational forms might not generate the same meaning and be socially and culturally significant.

The intricate and essential relationship between volition, habituation, performance capacity, and environment will also help both the therapist and the client in planning and implementing therapy. Considering contexts and environments in which occupations are taking place will facilitate change.

In the following section, we will consider the different steps of the volitional process in relation to occupational participation and occupational engagement. We will explore strategies to identify barriers to change and actions to facilitate change, as well as important factors to consider. In this chapter, we will illustrate the intricate relationships between volition, habituation, performance capacity, and the environment by providing different examples.

EXPERIENCE

What is important to remember when conceptualizing "experience" is the impression that it leaves on the person. An experience includes the actual event or occurrence combined with the emotional response the event or occurrence creates for someone.

The environment in which the experience takes place allows for experimentations, trials, and errors to occur. The environment can be natural or constructed. An event, or an occupational form, can take place in a client's natural environment like their home, workplace, school, a family or a friend's house, or shops. In a therapeutic context, the environment is usually unfamiliar or constructed.

CASE EXAMPLE: AN ADOLESCENT WITH SOCIAL ANXIETY

Alannah is 17 years old. She has been playing the clarinet for 4 years. When she plays the clarinet in the school orchestra, the emotional experience is positive. She feels satisfaction and enjoyment. Music is an individual experience as much as a social experience for her. Her environment provides

her with the support and opportunities she needs and she knows the school music teacher or her peers will help her if she asks them to. She feels safe and comfortable enough in her group to ask for help when she needs to.

In comparison, let's look at what happens for Alannah, who still enjoys playing the clarinet, but feels anxious when playing her instrument or when playing in formal performances in front of people. Alannah feels uncomfortable and too shy to ask for help. She believes everyone else is better than her. These feelings negatively impact her overall experience of playing the clarinet. The impression and emotional response to playing her instrument is negative.

As occupational therapists, we would ask ourselves why this experience would be difficult or easy for Alannah. What is affecting Alannah's emotional response? Is it volition— Alannah's personal causation, interests, and values? Is this related to her performance capacity? What elements of her environment are limiting or supporting her occupational experience? Therapists will use therapeutic reasoning to answer these questions and guide their actions. Therapeutic reasoning, in this context, means that a therapist will closely monitor the client's process of occupational engagement to determine the barriers and facilitators of occupational engagement.

INTERPRETATION AND REFLECTION

Interpretation takes place once the experience has occurred and is completed. It involves reflecting on occupational performance and the corresponding emotional response. The process of reflection has been described as detailed thinking about an experience (Bruce, 2013). Reflection incites change by critiquing actions, their relevance and effectiveness, and their purpose (Larkin & Pépin, 2013) and by stimulating the emergence of new actions or perspectives (Bruce, 2013). Some authors have warned that reflecting on experiences may be testing because it can highlight areas of conflicts and difficulties and be associated with strong emotions (Bruce, 2013). The role of the therapist will be to ensure proper support is provided and that the reflection is comprehensive, including strengths and progress as well as challenges. In reflecting on and interpreting an experience, a client will ask themselves what went well, what was more difficult, what could be done differently, and how they felt.

MOHO Problem-Solver: An Older Adult with Rheumatoid Arthritis

Liz has a long-standing history of rheumatoid arthritis and often experiences severe pain. During her next flare-up, Liz sought assistance from a model of human occupation (MOHO)-based occupational therapist, whose focus was on understanding how Liz interpreted and reflected upon her occupational engagement. The new therapist learned that one of the most fundamental occupations for Liz, preparing meals, was difficult, painful, challenging, and tiring. Nevertheless, Liz continued to prepare meals for herself and her husband as she had done for over 50 years now. From talking with Liz, the therapist understood that meal preparation was an important part of her role as a wife and mother. She prepared her husband's meals for as long as she remembered. For Liz, this was an occupation that was fully engaging for her, and one that she never wanted to abandon.

As her arthritis flared up and her symptoms increased, Liz found herself of two minds about many of her occupations. On the one hand, she valued them and saw them as an integral part of her identity and roles. On the other hand, she increasingly wondered how she could keep going, and what she could do differently while maintaining her role as a wife and a mother.

Motivated to support Liz's occupational engagement, the therapist asked the following questions: What influences Liz's interpretation of her experience of preparing meals? What are the different factors involved? Does the environment provide opportunities or constraints? What can we say about Liz's personal causation, values, and beliefs? What is the importance of this occupation with regard to Liz's occupational identity and roles? How does Liz's performance capacity shape her interpretation of her experience? What could be done differently to support her occupational engagement? What support or strategies can I provide Liz with to facilitate her occupational performance?

ANTICIPATION

Anticipation is closely related to possibilities and expectations we are presented with (Kielhofner, 2008). It has also been described as an emotion that can involve pleasure, excitement or anxiety, and discomfort associated with speculation and planning about the future (Sadock & Sadock, 2007). Anticipation has also been linked to the creative process of inferring intentions or outcomes to model one's behavior (Angus, deRosnay, Lunenburg, Terwogt, & Begeer, 2015). In therapy, a client's anticipation will be based on their lived experience of an event and how it was interpreted. The event could have taken place within a therapeutic context with the support of the therapist or in the client's own environment where there might or might not have been support available.

CASE EXAMPLE: A SCHOOL-AGED CHILD WITH CEREBRAL PALSY

Tim is 10 years old. He has cerebral palsy (with spastic diplegia). Tim usually uses elbow crutches for mobility. Recently, Tim fell down the stairs at school when three older students ran past him and bumped into him. Tim needed shoulder surgery. He is currently using a manual wheelchair with assistance. Tim has been back to school only once since the surgery to meet with his teachers and discuss accessibility to the different rooms and parts of the school. When he was there, he found it quite confronting having to depend on someone to get around. He also felt uncomfortable in the wheelchair, having the sensation that he was stuck between people who wouldn't move or who were staring at him. Tim is supposed to go back to school next week. He is dreading going back and has been saying he doesn't feel well enough to go. He has asked his parents that he not go back until he doesn't need the wheelchair.

Tim's occupational therapist asked herself a few questions, with the goal of facilitating Tim's occupational engagement in mind. How can Tim's environment be modified to enable him to participate in school-related activities? What strategies could be implemented to educate teaching staff and students about accessibility and environmental design? How can we build Tim's confidence and sense of control so that he may return to school with more confidence and desire to participate?

OCCUPATIONAL CHOICES

A client's choices and decisions are central to effective therapy. Our preferences and choices of one activity over another shape what we do in the immediate future. Such choices and decisions are often the first step toward change. Such choices as selecting what to do, how to do it, and what to aim for are also central to therapy, as they represent the client's volitional involvement in the therapy process. Persons choose or decide when they anticipate and select from alternatives for action. A wide range of choices and decisions may take place in the therapy context. By making such choices and decisions, clients can shape the nature of their own therapy and what that therapy aims to accomplish. The very process of making choices can help clients feel more in control of their lives. Often, when the client has limited performance capacity, making choices and decisions is one of the most empowering things the client can do. Finally, choices and decisions are critical, since they influence what will change, what will remain the same, and how the change will unfold.

CASE EXAMPLE: AN OLDER MAN WITH CARDIOVASCULAR DISEASE AND ANXIETY

Costa is an 89-year-old widower. He lives in the suburbs with his daughter, Anastasia, her husband, and their 5-year-old son. Costa had open heart surgery 3 months ago. He is now back home and eager to resume his activities. Costa loves to meet his friends at the local Greek Club. They play cards, talk about a variety of things, and have a bite to eat. There were a few complications following Costa's surgery, which necessitated more hospital admissions. A community nurse comes to Costa's house daily to take care of an infected scar on his chest that is not healing properly. The complications, pain, and stress associated with the entire experience has left him cautious and disillusioned. Additionally, he feels tired very quickly, unsteady in his balance at times, and breathes heavily. He is afraid to leave home and relies heavily on his daughter.

As part of his cardiac rehabilitation, Costa was referred to see an occupational therapist. Together, they identified activities that were important for Costa. He talked about his friends at the Greek Club at length. He also said he was concerned about what would happen if he felt unwell while he was there and had to tell his friends he couldn't do certain things. Costa is a very proud man. Costa's occupational therapist provided him with a walker, which they practiced using in his environment. The occupational therapist also went to the Greek Club and assessed the accessibility of that environment. Looking at the activity schedule of the club, Costa and his occupational therapist identified quieter days of the week, where there was still enough staff to help Costa if he needed. Costa's daughter also identified days where it was possible for her to drive her dad to and from the club.

With these provisions in place, Costa chose to return to the Club for the first time since his surgery-related complications occurred. He enjoyed his time with his friends and was very happy to spend time with them. At the same time, he was tired when he came back home, had little appetite, and went to bed very early. He expressed concern about the impact of these activities on his heart and health. For these reasons, Costa decided to keep to the schedule he and his occupational therapist put together and go to the Greek Club twice a week for the time being. He also kept using his walker to get around. The therapist supported him in making these decisions.

In her interactions with Costa, the occupational therapist made sure she explored Costa's interests, beliefs, and values. Acknowledging Costa's fears based on his experience of the open heart surgery, as well as his concerns about going back to the Greek Club, the therapist conveyed her empathy toward Costa and provided him with the equipment and strategies that would support his occupational engagement.

Promoting Change

Alannah, Liz, Tim, and Costa's stories demonstrate three essential elements of occupational engagement and change according to MOHO. First, they illustrate the influence that volition, habituation, performance capacity, and the environment have on the volitional process, overall. Second, they highlight the intricate relationships between volition, habituation, performance capacity, and environment and the roles they play in promoting occupational participation and engagement. Third, it shows the interaction between the volitional process, occupational engagement, and change.

The therapeutic environment gives therapists opportunities to plan, create, organize, and provide experiences with their clients. Through doing, clients, with the support of the therapist, can experiment, explore, and try different activities or occupational forms in a variety of environmental contexts. The experience becomes that of learning where both client and therapist discover strengths and areas to further develop, with the ultimate goal of facilitating occupational engagement.

One way in which therapists can be especially attentive to the dynamics of occupational engagement is to compare the major (versus minor) efforts that clients make when they are engaging in a range of occupations. Attending to the client's occupational choices can be an important variable when facilitating the process of change. Providing diverse experiences gives the client opportunities to (1) explore and (2) practice, which are two important elements that contribute to change.

As discussed previously in this book, the first stage of change involves exploration. Exploration includes investigating new objects, spaces, and/or social groups and occupational forms. It includes doing things with altered performance capacity, trying out new ways of doing things, and examining possibilities for occupational participation in one's context. Clients practice in therapy when they repeat a certain performance or consistently participate in an occupation with the effect of increasing skill, ease, and effectiveness of performance. Practice aims to enhance effectiveness in doing an occupational form and/or participating in an area of occupation, such as self-care, work, school, or leisure.

While the client interprets the experience with the support of the therapist, reexamination can take place. Clients will leave behind perceptions, feelings, beliefs, and patterns of acting that are no longer valid or have led to difficulties. Reexamination, then, involves critically appraising and considering alternatives to previous beliefs, attitudes, feelings, habits, or roles. Reexamination allows for new experiences modeled on what has been left behind and modified. Reshaping the experience will be done with the client's involvement and through negotiation.

When possible, the client should be involved in a process of negotiation throughout therapy. The onset of disability often results in new situations and experiences that create a gap between the person with the disability and others' perspectives, desires, and expectations. Moreover, it is anticipated that the client will differ with the opinion of the therapist concerning the nature of his or her impairments and their consequences. This will play out in two ways. First, it will reveal itself in the client's volition, specifically in terms of the client's sense of personal causation (sense of self-efficacy). Second, it may be observed in the client's self-report of his or her subjective experience when performing certain occupations (i.e., subjective experience of performance capacity). A necessary process of negotiation involves give and take between the client and the therapist (or others in the client's environment) that places empathic understanding of the client's choices as the priority, and at the same time creates a transparent, mutually agreed-upon middle ground between different expectations, plans, or desires.

Ultimately, the desired outcome of the volitional process is the occupational engagement that is achieved through the client's ultimate occupational choice or decision to pursue an activity or occupation. For long-term change to occur in therapy, it is important that occupational engagement be sustained. One of the challenging aspects of therapy is sustaining effort over time despite such things as difficult environmental barriers, pain, failures, and slower-than-expected progress. By its nature, therapy is taxing for clients. Therefore, to sustain change, a client must persist in occupational performance or participation despite uncertainty or difficulty.

For example, despite the pain Liz felt from rheumatoid arthritis, she made the decision to maintain some of her occupations, such as preparing meals for her husband, because it was a meaningful occupation that encompassed her roles, values, and beliefs. It is also important that a client commits to undertake a course of action for accomplishing a goal or personal project, fulfilling a role, or establishing a new habit. Occupational choice always involves commitment, because it requires one to sustain action over time. Committing to a course of action is also an act of hope, since the client's intention is to achieve some goal, occupy a place in the social world, or modify their lifestyle in anticipation of improving life. After Costa's experience of going to the Greek Club, and working collaboratively with his occupational therapist, he decided to continue with what the therapist planned to sustain his occupational engagement.

The previous section explored barriers and enablers of change. It identified and explained important elements (exploration, practice, reexamination, negotiation, sustainability, and commitment) to consider in promoting occupational engagement and change in therapy. The next section presents a synthesizing case example that illustrates how occupational participation, engagement, and change were hindered and eventually supported through therapy.

CASE EXAMPLE TO TEST YOUR LEARNING: AN ADULT WITH SCHIZOPHRENIA

Eileen is a 28-year-old mother. She separated from her husband recently. Her daughter, Alice, is 9 months old. Eileen was diagnosed with schizophrenia in her early 20s. She experienced paranoid ideation and delusions of persecution. She used to hear voices telling her she was in danger, and that others were plotting to punish her for things she did in the past. Because of these ideas and rigid beliefs, Eileen was reluctant to engage in treatment and suspicious of the prescribed medications and their side effects. She has a long history of repeated hospitalizations in the psychiatric unit, and managing her symptoms has been difficult. Eileen always struggled socially. She had very few friends going through school. As her symptoms increased, she isolated herself from others. She was fearful and felt people were conspiring against her. Despite her illness, she maintained her interest in the outdoors and in a range of physical activities. Her family has been supportive but also challenged by Eileen's symptoms.

When Eileen met her ex-husband, Johnny, her parents were a bit concerned. However, it looked like he made her feel good about herself. Eileen said she felt normal and safe with him. They went hiking together and took long walks in parks around the city. A few months later, Eileen and Johnny were engaged, and they married within a year. Once they were married, Johnny became increasingly controlling. He didn't allow her to go hiking and walking or do any other outdoor activities. He was often verbally abusive toward her. Eileen became more anxious while being afraid Johnny would leave her if she didn't do what he said. Eileen became pregnant quickly. She thought a baby would help their relationship. However, the abuse continued throughout the pregnancy.

After the birth of their daughter, Eileen felt a strong bond and loved her daughter. Those feelings made her acutely aware of her own challenges and difficulties. Her psychotic symptoms increased, as did her anxiety. She wondered how she would cope and if she would be able to take care of a child in the environment they were in. Eileen became increasingly suspicious of Johnny. The context in which Eileen was living increased her thought disturbances. Voices were telling her to save herself and that other people were after her and her daughter. Desperate, Eileen set fire to the garage next to their house to distract her husband, and ran away, leaving her daughter with her parents.

Eileen lived on the street for 2 weeks and she was eventually taken to the hospital by the police. She was admitted to the psychiatric unit of a large state hospital. Eileen refused treatment, medications, and stayed in her room. She didn't want to see or talk to anyone except her family and her daughter. Eileen was labeled as a difficult patient by the medical team. Progress notes highlighted that Eileen did not engage or participate in treatment activities. She refused to take her medication as prescribed and had very limited contact with the people around her.

The occupational therapist assigned to work with her observed from a distance that Eileen

seemed to get great pleasure from the visits from her daughter and family. She held her daughter closely and affectionately, played with her, and cared for her. She talked to her parents, asking how they are and asked about her daughter when she was not present. These were the only times where Eileen seemed less anxious and actively engaged in any activity or occupation. Each time her daughter and family left, Eileen returned to her room and isolated herself.

During a team meeting, Sarah, the occupational therapist, asked the team to include her parents in helping Eileen to get out of her room and play with her daughter in another part of the ward. She hypothesized that modifying the environment where Eileen engaged with her daughter and family members would be an important first step in promoting change. At the same time, it would allow Sarah to complete a volitional questionnaire and attempt to determine where Eileen sat along the volitional continuum. Sarah explained that, once more is known about the nature and level of Eileen's volition, she will be better equipped to facilitate occupational engagement at a level that is appropriate for her. The social worker also noted how different Eileen was around her family, and especially her daughter Alice. Together, Sarah and the social worker reminded the medical team of Eileen's past relationship with her husband and difficulty trusting others. Sarah added information about Eileen's previous interests in outdoor activities. The team started discussing Eileen's previous experiences of engaging in relationships with others and how these relationships turned out to be negative or challenging—at times because of the symptoms of schizophrenia and at other times because of the attitude and behavior of other people. Sarah explained how, in her opinion, Eileen had learned not to engage as a result of previous negative experiences interpreted as dangerous, unsafe, or difficult.

The next time Eileen's parents came to visit, Alice was a bit restless and, as she was attempting to walk, she crawled to the door of Eileen's room to get out. The social worker suggested that they guide Alice into a small room overlooking a garden close to Eileen's room, using her favorite toys to keep her interest. Eileen reluctantly agreed, keeping a very close eye on her daughter. With her parents, Eileen sat on the floor playing with her daughter and talking to her parents. Shortly thereafter, Sarah, the occupational therapist, walked past the room. Alice attempted to crawl after her. Eileen quickly became agitated and brought her daughter back closer to her. This gave Sarah an opportunity to introduce herself and talk with Eileen and her family. At the same time, she was able to observe Eileen engaging with her daughter in play. After her visitors left, Sarah asked Eileen if she'd like to use the same room again next time Alice and her family came to see her. Sarah noted how Alice seemed to be alert and curious and comfortable around Eileen in that room. Eileen agreed and said she was comfortable there, too, but didn't want to go to the bigger lounge room where everybody was. That room is not safe, said Eileen.

Critical Thinking Questions

- Based on Eileen's story, what do you think are the barriers to her occupational engagement?
- Discuss each component of the volitional process in relation to Eileen's personal circumstances.
- Eileen seems to be reluctant to change her behaviors. She mistrusts people and refuses treatment. Using the volitional process, explain why Eileen reacts this way.
- Which of Eileen's strengths might promote change and occupational engagement?
- Reflecting on the components of the volitional process, what could Sara do to facilitate change and support Eileen's occupational engagement?

Conclusion

This chapter examined the process of change in therapy, focusing on two key points. First, change involves complex reorganization in which multiple, simultaneous alterations in volition, habituation, performance capacity, and environmental conditions resonate with each other. Second, the process of change is always driven by the client's occupational engagement. The true dynamic of change involves what the client does, thinks, and feels. This chapter presented how the volitional process can explain barriers and enablers of change and guide therapeutic strategies to facilitate change. It offered important elements (exploration, practice, reexamination, negotiation, sustainability, and commitment) that represent contributors to change. Any therapist who seeks to facilitate a client's change process will do well to pay attention to the unfolding dynamics of change and to the client occupational engagement that fuels that change process (Fig. 13-1).

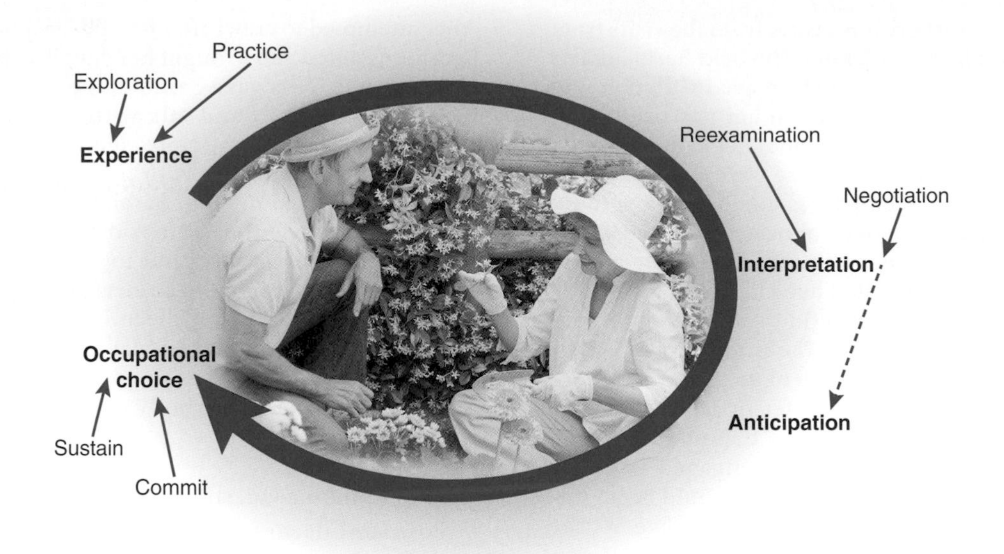

FIGURE 13-1 How Occupational Engagement Facilitates the Process of Change.

thePoint® For additional resources and exercises, visit http://thePoint.lww.com

REFERENCES

Angus, D. J., deRosnay, M., Lunenburg, P., Terwogt, M. M., & Begeer, S. (2015). Limitations in social anticipation are independent of imagination and abilities in children with autism but not in typically developing children. *Autism, 19*(5), 604–612.

Bedirhan Üstün, T., Chatterji, S., Kostanjsek, N., Rehm, J., Kennedy, C., Epping-Jordan, J., et al. (2010). Developing the World Health Organization disability assessment schedule 2.0. *Bull World Health Organization, 88*, 815–823.

Bruce, L. (2013). *Reflective practice for social workers: A handbook for developing professional confidence.* London, United Kingdom: Open University Press.

Hitch, D., Pepin, G., & Stagnitti, K. (2014a). In the footsteps of Wilcock, Part 1: The evolution of doing, belonging, and becoming. *Occupational Therapy in Health Care, 28*(3), 231–246.

Hitch, D., Pepin, G., & Stagnitti, K. (2014b). In the footsteps of Wilcock, Part 2: The interdependent nature of doing, being, becoming, and belonging. *Occupational Therapy in Health Care, 28*(3), 247–263.

Kielhofner, G. (2008). *A model of human occupation: Theory and method in action.* Philadelphia, PA: Lippincott Williams & Wilkins.

Kielhofner, G., Borell, L., Holzmueller, R., Jonsson, H., Josephsson, S., Keponen, R., et al. (2008). Chapter 9: Crafting occupational life. In G. Kielhofner (Ed.), *Model of human occupation: Theory and application* (4th ed.). Philadelphia, PA: Lippincott Williams & Wilkins.

Larkin, H., & Pépin, G. (2013). Becoming a reflective practitioner. In K. Stagnitti, A. Schoo, & D. Welch (Eds.), *Clinical and fieldwork placement in the health professions* (pp. 31–42). Melbourne, Australia: Oxford University Press.

Sadock, B., & Sadock, V. A. (2007). *Kaplan and Sadock's synopsis of psychiatry: Behavioral sciences and clinical psychiatry* (10th ed.). Philadelphia, PA: Lippincott Williams & Wilkins.

World Health Organization. (2002). The World Health Report 2002: Reducing risks, promoting healthy life. Retrieved from http://www.who.int/whr/2002/en/

Intervention Process: Enabling Occupational Change

Carmen-Gloria de las Heras de Pablo, Sue Parkinson, Genevieve Pépin, and Gary Kielhofner (posthumous)

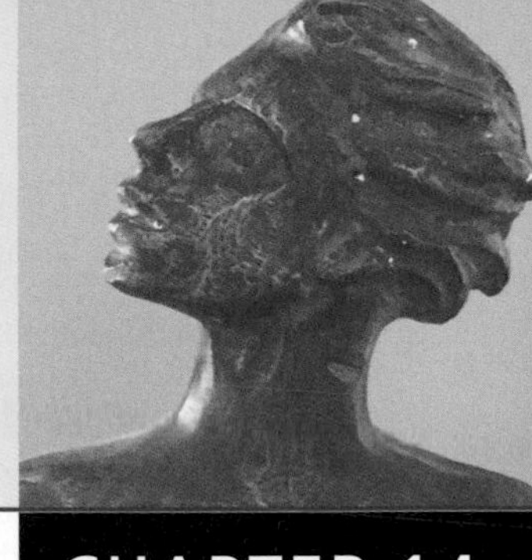

CHAPTER 14

EXPECTED LEARNING OUTCOMES

Upon completion of this chapter, readers will be able to:

1. Understand the premises that underpin the intervention process.
2. Identify updated MOHO intervention methods for facilitating change with diverse populations.
3. Realize the possibility of applying these methods in practice.
4. Appreciate how different methods can be selected and integrated to support participation in occupation.

MOHO provides occupational therapists with the theory and the practical tools to promote participation in occupations, whether with people whose occupational concerns affect an incremental process of change, with people who are at risk of having occupational adaptation problems, or with people who experience long-standing problems with occupational adaptation (de las Heras de Pablo, 2011, 2015; Kielhofner, de las Heras de Pablo, & Suarez-Balcazar, 2011).

Enabling occupational change with MOHO begins when therapists first make contact with a person and continues during the intervention and evaluation process. As a conceptual practice model based on human occupation and centered on the person, MOHO expects that each action with a person contributes to an alliance that promotes participation in occupation. To enable occupational change with efficacy and efficiency, occupational therapists must respect MOHO theory, its main principles, and the particular occupational needs of each person or collective. They must integrate these throughout the intervention process, which implies maintaining MOHO's dynamic vision of the change process. Flexibility is therefore required when making decisions about the best alternatives for therapeutic action and when analyzing the multiple personal and environmental variables impacting occupational situations and their interaction during the intervention process.

Approaching the Intervention Process

As already stated, to be effective and efficient when approaching the intervention process, using MOHO requires the dynamic use of therapeutic reasoning that integrates theory and practice at all times. Four premises should be borne in mind:

- *Premise 1: A Systems Perspective.* MOHO draws on concepts from dynamic systems theory to provide us with an understanding of the dynamics of human occupation and of the occupational process of change. Hence, MOHO principles emphasize the simultaneous and interactive adjustments that take place in a person, in the environment, and in the relationship between a person and the environment. MOHO theory also states that change is continuous over time, meaning that change is a natural part of life as it progresses. So, when guided by MOHO, personal and environmental factors should be considered in equal measure throughout the therapeutic process. Personal and environmental changes will be facilitated in parallel, and the focus of therapy may switch between the two. For instance, a MOHO-based therapist may work with a person, with the person's family, and with other relevant active participants in the client's social group—both in their own processes of change and also as facilitators of the change process for the individual (Table 14-1).
- *Premise 2: Empathy as a Foundational Ideology.* MOHO stresses the importance of "supporting persons to do what they need to do in order to achieve their goals and changes in their occupational lives" (Kielhofner, 2002, p. 351). Thus, when applying MOHO, a therapist must develop an ability to establish and maintain a meaningful working relationship with each client. Two main attitudes are highlighted by MOHO: empathy

Table 14-1 Model of Human Occupation Intervention Principles

Working with Clients	Working with Environment
• *Change is dynamic*, involving *simultaneous and interactive alterations* in people, the environment, and the relationship between the person and the environment	• *Change is dynamic*, involving *simultaneous and interactive alterations* in people, the environment, and the relationship between the person and the environment
• *Change occurs in a person's life in progress,* and therefore meaning is attributed to unfolding events, leading to on a sense of *occupational identity* and *competence*	• *Facilitating change in social groups* requires an approach that takes into account their culture and life circumstances
• *Progressive facilitation of motivation for doing* (volition), particularly of personal confidence (personal causation), constitutes the basis of achieving empowerment and self-advocacy skills	• *Facilitating change in social groups and organizations* needs to consider their members' *volitional characteristics*
• *Peoples' active participation* in developing self-knowledge and assessing environmental realities is crucial to achieving change in their occupational circumstances	• Changes in occupational circumstances need to consider the *strengths* of social groups' members and to build new relationships through participation in common projects
• *Peoples' active participation* in opening up occupational opportunities and obtaining resources from social groups and organizations allows change in their occupational circumstances	• Changes in social groups are based on *exploring* alternatives and solutions together with therapists and clients
• *The therapeutic relationship* and the person's *participation in meaningful occupations* are pivotal to the intervention process	• *Use of self* (empathy, confidence) and meaningful relationships are pivotal to intervention with social groups
• *Collaborative work between the person or groups of people and the therapist* (doing, thinking, and feeling with) is a central aspect of the change process	• Changes in any physical environment need to respect a person's *culture* and *social and economic reality*
• The process of change focuses on *reaffirming occupational strengths* and facilitating the development of *new ones*	• *The main focus of making changes in physical environment is on how* the existing resources, spaces, and objects can be arranged to have the *best impact* on participation in occupations
• The process of change is based on *exploring* alternatives and solutions, and on *experiencing* them in *relevant contexts*	• *Prioritization* of diverse resources and objects that meet several objectives facilitates a more effective use of people's skills and their development
• Serious consideration of environmental dimensions and their characteristics, *and the unique impact they have* on the persons' personal occupational factors is fundamental to directing therapy goals	

Adapted from de las Heras de Pablo, 2015 (p. 164–165).

and professional confidence. Therapists are empathetic when they make genuine efforts to understand a person's unique feelings, thoughts, and ways of doing and when they communicate this understanding to the person, either verbally or nonverbally. Therapists develop professional confidence when they are able to clearly explain critical aspects of a person's occupational life with honesty and respect, and using understandable language to explain theory. Confidence between therapist and the person promotes mutual collaboration, maximizes participation in occupations, and increases commitment to the process of change.

- *Premise 3: The Client Leads in His or Her Own Stages of Change.* A crucial competency for occupational therapists using MOHO is being able to understand the flow of stages of change, from exploration, to competency, to achievement, within the unique reality of an individual. The unique reality refers to each person's particular personal and environmental characteristics, his or her "microreality" or own world (de las Heras de Pablo, Llerena, & Kielhofner, 2003). In practice, this implies focusing on the *singular potential* of each person with regard to his or her feelings, thoughts, and behaviors, which ultimately make his or her participation unique. That is, a person who can only participate in the most basic dimension of participation could still be conceptualized as being within an achievement stage if this is his or her maximum potential for participation. This last point of view is the one that allows us to accomplish a successful, client-centered, therapeutic intervention (de las Heras de Pablo, 2011, Raber, Teitelman, Watts, & Kielhofner, 2010).

- *Premise 4: Understanding the Role of Performance Capacity.* Finally, if practice is to be based on MOHO, occupational therapists must understand how underlying capacities (i.e., the objective appraisal of performance capacity) are conceptualized by MOHO. The model considers a person's underlying capacities to be important personal factors that impact participation in occupation, but MOHO-based evaluation and intervention methods do not address them in an isolated or singular way. Instead, MOHO considers a client's performance capacity from a systems perspective (described in Premise #1). Depending upon the desires of the client and the overarching treatment agenda, an occupational therapist must determine if there is a need to use other conceptual practice models that specifically approach objective performance capacities in combination with MOHO.

Methods for Facilitating Change

The methods for facilitating change presented in this chapter comprise a group of interrelated actions and intervention procedures that are integrated in a unique and flexible way for each person (or a particular group). These include: (1) therapeutic strategies; (2) specific interventions; and (3) MOHO-based protocols of intervention specifically designed for groups with common occupational needs (Figs. 14-1 & 14-2).

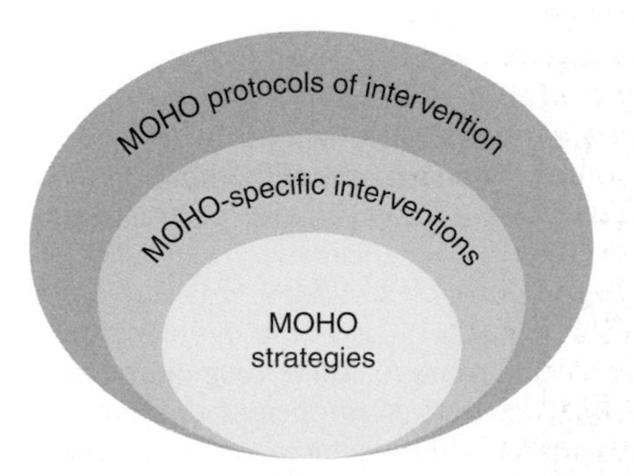

FIGURE 14-1 MOHO Intervention Methods.

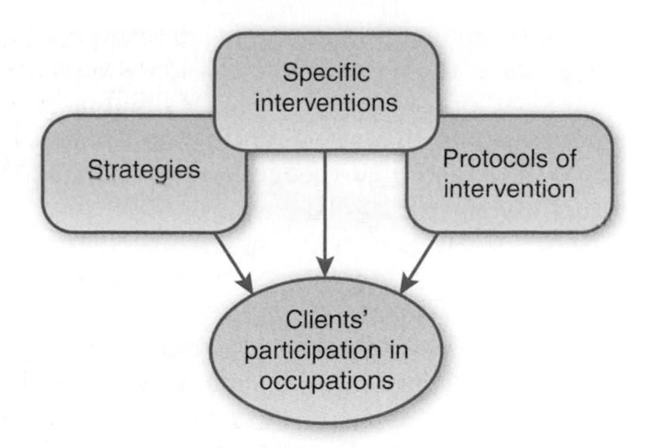

FIGURE 14-2 Intervention Methods Support Client's Participation in Occupations.

THERAPEUTIC STRATEGIES

A **therapeutic strategy** is a therapist's action that influences positively a person's doing, feeling, and thinking to facilitate participation in occupation and desired change. The nine strategies that are identified in MOHO are: validating, identifying, giving feedback, advising, negotiating, structuring, coaching, encouraging, and providing physical support (Kielhofner, 2008). Although the concepts of these strategies have been bounded to clarify their use during the intervention process, they may be used simultaneously and in conjunction with the specific interventions described later in this chapter. Strategies should be used genuinely and naturally as situations arise, but it is important for therapists to be reflective about using them. Wherever possible, this will involve anticipating the kinds of strategies that might benefit a person, and moving fluidly between the strategies as the intervention unfolds.

Validating

Each moment of the occupational change process is potentially charged with thoughts and feelings that accompany what a person does. Validating these experiences is essential to effective therapy. *To* ***validate*** *is to convey respect for the client's experience or perspective regardless of therapists' personal biases or reactions about such experiences or perspectives.* Therapists must carefully attend to and acknowledge the client's experience whether it is the lived body experience or the experiences associated with volition like enjoyment, sense of capacity, boredom, frustration, investment, or excitement.

Validation can take place in different occupational circumstances and contexts, involving things as simple as acknowledging the presence and unique identity of a person, accompanying a person without talking, listening actively to peoples' stories during a conversation or interview, reassuring the way persons go about doing a task, taking into consideration some of their ideas for solving a problem, or simply asking the person about themselves and demonstrating a genuine interest in their thoughts and feelings.

Identifying

To ***identify*** *refers to providing the person with knowledge of personal and environmental opportunities and resources and options for enhancing participation in work, play/leisure, and activities of daily living that clients wish and need to do.* This information may include the identification of strategies to use when approaching occupational situations where the person may fulfill their goals. This information may also include identifying strategies when approaching resources, including social services (e.g., other professionals or community agencies) and physical resources (e.g., equipment or funding). When identifying these things, therapists will also give the person the opportunity to identify alternatives or contribute their own ideas, before supporting them to make a choice.

Giving Feedback

To ***give feedback*** *refers to sharing information with the person about their occupational situation in order to enhance their participation in occupations.* For example, feedback occurs when therapists: share their overall conceptualization of a person's situation, or their understanding of the person's ongoing action, and indicate the progress that a person has made. Providing feedback helps people to understand the value (positive or negative) of certain behaviors by explaining their impact on themselves and other persons, and can help to reframe their interpretation of their thoughts and feelings about themselves. Consequently, feedback can provide information that enhances volition, habituation, skill, and performance.

Advising

To ***advise*** *refers to recommending intervention goals and strategies by sharing information and suggestions about the outcomes that appear feasible and desirable or indicating possible options for achieving outcomes in therapy.* These recommendations ordinarily contain information or insights beyond the person's own thoughts and feelings. Therefore, sharing the advice with a client can serve to broaden or change the client's perspective. It should be noted, however, that advice is not the same as persuasion, in that the individual may change their own mind freely. This is important for client-centered practice because it allows people to make informed decisions based on a rationale explained by the therapist.

Occupational therapists usually advise people when they hesitate, have difficulty making choices about activities or tasks to perform in the short term, or have problems committing to a particular long-term goal such as a personal project, taking on new roles, or changing their lifestyle. In order to effectively advice, the therapist needs to consider the state of persons' volition and the factors of habituation, performance capacity, and environment that could be impacting such state of volition. By doing so, the therapist can give honest advice with empathy for the client's perspective and desires.

Negotiating

Negotiating refers to the give and take process with the person or their relevant social groups about what they will or should do in the future. It occurs when a person (or group) and a therapist have differing information or viewpoints about certain aspects of the person's occupational circumstances. It may be necessary to resolve disagreement between the therapist and the person or groups, or to simply compare and reconcile their different perspectives. The process may help to facilitate the person's achievement of their occupational goals and be useful when advocating for a person's occupational opportunities, when working with caregivers and family members on how to best support their family member's participation in occupations, or when setting relevant goals and actions with the person.

To effectively **negotiate**, the therapist must be aware of and elicit the views of all concerned. Without such efforts the others' viewpoints can be obliterated and, as consequence, create frustration, feelings of personal devaluation, loss of confidence in the therapist's professionalism, or failure to open occupational opportunities for people. Thus, negotiation *always requires a respectful elicitation and understanding* of a person's thoughts and feelings about the situation, and the therapist's willingness to compromise to see things differently, or to depart from usual procedures. A successful negotiation can be very important for empowering people, as it facilitates taking ownership of their own viewpoints, openness to learn about selves and others, taking responsibility for own decisions, and openness for working with others toward same goals.

Structuring

To ***structure*** *refers to establishing clear expectations of performance by offering people alternatives, setting limits, or establishing ground rules.* Structuring can often serve to create reasonable demands for people to make choices, perform activities, maintain habits, and fulfill roles. Structuring looks for giving a person a sense of control and safety by making opportunities and constraints in the environment clear. It can be useful for helping people to internalize role responsibilities (role scripts) and to learn to be effective members of groups. Moreover, external expectations can be a support to volition (de las Heras de Pablo, 2015; de las Heras de Pablo et al., 2003; Jonsson, Josephsson, & Kielhofner, 2000; Raber et al., 2010). That is, people can find it easier to be motivated to do things when others have reasonable expectations of them, when good judgment has been shown in inviting them, or when the right people provide company and support.

Coaching

*To **coach** refers to assisting or supporting people by instructing, demonstrating, or cuing how to use or display their abilities and skills in various therapy or occupational settings.* For example, a therapist may choose to demonstrate assertive behavior to a client with social difficulties in a role play situation, and then makes suggestions to the client about how to assert himself when taking his turn in the role-play situation.

Encouraging

*To **encourage** refers to providing emotional support and reassurance to people when exploring new situations, choosing to take risks, and sustaining effort in the face of difficulty.* Encouraging is ordinarily necessitated because of difficulties with self-confidence (personal causation) and/or because of existing gaps between performance capacity and the things a person is attempting to do. Encouragement allows the person to feel greater confidence, to relax and enjoy themselves, and to recall why something is worth the effort. To effectively encourage, therapists need to be flexible in how they demonstrate it, basing their judgment on the person's culture, age, and personality, as well as the seriousness or playfulness existing within the occupational context, and the social characteristics of the occupational forms or tasks.

Providing Physical Support

***Physical support** refers to when an occupational therapist uses their body to provide support* for a client to complete an occupational form/task, or a step of an occupational form/task when the person cannot or will not use their own motor skills, or when the person needs volitional affirmation in order to try to do something relevant. Ways of providing physical support may include assisting people by putting the hand on persons' back, or taking their hand to enhance their initiative to do things, or help their stability and walking while participating in occupations. It may also include physically accompanying a person, or taking a person somewhere. Thus, physical support can be useful for different purposes according to a person's occupational needs.

SPECIFIC INTERVENTIONS

***Specific interventions** refer to defined sets of procedures and strategies that foster occupational adaptation.* These interventions have successfully enhanced MOHO practice over many years and have been practiced with people of diverse ages, with diverse occupational needs, and within different contexts, countries, and cultures. Practice settings have included public hospitals, jails, correctional facilities, and community centers, as well as diverse community settings including homes, neighborhoods, streets, schools, universities, workplaces, and recreational or cultural settings (de las Heras de Pablo, 2006, 2011, 2015; Girardi, 2010; Kielhofner, 2002, 2008, 2009; Kielhofner et al., 2011; Poletti, 2010).

Specific interventions include:

- Evaluation doubling as intervention
- Participation in meaningful occupations
- Facilitation of exploration
- Occupational consulting
- MOHO-based skills teaching
- Peer support educational groups
- Occupational self-help groups
- Social groups education
- Environmental management
- Occupational role development and habit change

Evaluation Doubling as Intervention

With MOHO the evaluation process may be considered as an intervention too. From the first contact the occupational therapist has with a person, they start to build their mutual knowledge of each other and develop their initial rapport that further evolves into a therapeutic relationship. The therapeutic relationship is nurtured by a client-centered evaluation process that facilitates the active participation of the person in therapeutic reasoning by linking his or her thoughts and feelings about life to his or her own occupational reality, fostering self-knowledge, and engendering occupation-focused goal setting. Inevitably, MOHO-based interviews and self-assessments, because of their aims, design, and application procedures, become instruments for establishing rapport and a collaborative relationship. They empower people to explore and clarify their own occupational strengths and weaknesses; they facilitate the dynamics of the volitional process; and they inspire the planning, organizing, and pursuit of occupational participation and performance.

The evaluation is an ongoing process that, during intervention, takes the form of informal observation and conversations with individuals. Therapists open themselves to their clients' lived experiences and observe their clients' process of change in order to ensure a dynamic intervention process. In each follow-up evaluation, therapists and clients reassess the progress being made in achieving goals and objectives, review interventions and strategies used to facilitate change, and make decisions about the course of therapy. Alternatively, there are situations in which the only contact the therapist has with the person will be to assess their needs and make recommendation together, when it is all the more important that evaluation doubles as intervention. Finally, there are some people who might have personal queries related to their incremental changes, unsatisfactory occupational lifestyles, or doubts about taking on personal goals, and who only need a single consultation to clarify their occupational needs (de las Heras, 2011, 2015).

CASE EXAMPLE: AN ADOLESCENT WITH OCCUPATIONAL CONCERNS

Jaime finished high school when he was 18 years old. He belonged to a family whose culture emphasized preserving traditions and valuing professional studies like medicine, law, and engineering, which all his older siblings had done. Due to his excellent grades at school, his parents insisted that he study medicine. However, before taking the obligatory exams to enter university programs, his mother decided to consult an occupational therapist. The mother described her son as becoming increasingly anxious and withdrawn, and acknowledged that he did not feel like studying for the upcoming exams. She placed much importance on what his father was going to feel after all he had done for his son so that he would pursue a profession of prestige.

After the first informal conversation with Jaime and his mother, the therapist asked her to come back in an hour and a half when they could share their conclusions. This allowed her to spend time with Jaime. She provided *validation*, by letting him know that this was his space in which to relax and talk freely. She also introduced herself as an occupational therapist and a fellow human being, and invited him to sit comfortably. The therapist decided that the best instrument to use was the Occupational Performance History Interview (OPHI-II). This interview would let him go through his occupational life, reflecting on his participation in different occupations and activities and his appreciation of volition within them. While interviewing, Jaime showed most excitement when describing certain activities that matched his skills with his sense of pleasure and significance. Therapist *feedback, structure, and validation* helped him to *identify* the occupational contexts that allowed him to be spontaneous and open about his thoughts and feelings, and facilitated his participation in interests. Having shared his narrative and clarified his sense of competence and identity using criteria statements on the OPHI-II Scale, he felt *validated* in relation to his preferred occupational choices.

Using a master list of options for major areas of study at universities, the therapist *structured* a prioritization exercise of majors that universities offered. Jaime was able to decide which career he wanted to apply for. It was not Medicine, it was Physical Therapy. "I am calm now. I have the confidence I needed to explain to my parents what it is that I want to study." So, when his mother came back Jaime told her about his decision, expecting to have to *negotiate* a way forward. Surprisingly, his mother hugged him and congratulated him for making a decision, and for telling her that he was now ready to study for the exams. "Well, let me convince your father now. But you can explain things to him, just as you did with me."

Participation in Meaningful Occupations

Doing refers to exploring one's own capacity and practicing skills in order to test out, respond to, and solve any daily occupational circumstances. Through one's own experience and with feedback from others in various occupational contexts, one gets to know one's own strengths and limitations and those in the environment. Natural learning occurs, which sustains our occupational lives.

Occupation-based models (Scaffa, Reitz, & Pizzi, 2010) remind occupational therapists to focus on *participation in daily life occupations* that are relevant to a person. MOHO emphasizes that this participation in daily life occupations be relevant to a *person's life in progress*. It does not matter if the person is in the process of improving, building, or rebuilding their meaningful life routines, as long as participation in occupations facilitates the ongoing person's occupational narrative. In doing this, participation in personal or shared occupational projects, as well as in exploratory experiences that are consistent with a person's occupational goals or daily activity choices, strengthens **occupational identity** (i.e., a person's entire construction of who he or she is and wishes to become as an occupational being) and **occupational competence** (i.e., the actual actions taken to sustain a pattern of participation in occupations that is reflective of one's occupational identity).

By considering thoughts and feelings as well as performance when people participate in occupations, it reassures that, occupational therapists are going to provide them with opportunities of *active participation in their own process of change*. This is easy enough to say but can be difficult to internalize in daily practice. Therapists need *to do, feel, and think with* the person, instead of *doing for or to* the person. This ensures a mutual collaboration throughout the process of change and enables therapists to validate and reassure a person's volitional experience while they participate in occupations (de las Heras, 2010, 2015).

Participation in occupations may take place in

a. diverse occupational settings, assembling occupations into significant routines, and adapting both occupations and routines in a progressive way, according to unique personal needs;
b. transitional environments such as hospitals, day hospitals, rehabilitation centers, community centers, other facilities, where contexts for participation allow people to build or rebuild a continuum of change toward a full participation in relevant occupational settings; or
c. sheltered communities or protective residential environments should people need to live with the assistance of others, whether in a home, a residential facility or their close neighborhood.

Facilitation of Exploration

Facilitation of exploration *refers to a group of procedures and strategies that are used to foster people's desires to investigate aspects of the environment, their own abilities or skills, or their interests and values that support decision making and their activity and occupational choices.* Exploration is needed at any stage and moment of the dynamic occupational change process, which was explained at the beginning of this chapter.

Each new challenge implies a new exploration of alternatives, contexts, skills, and possible steps to achieve it. There are many situations that necessitate exploration. In fact, it can be said that life is an ongoing process of exploration, as each moment brings novelty with it. However, examples of specific situations that demand exploration include:

- participating in the evaluation process, in which one is supported to reveal self-knowledge;
- reflecting on one's own occupational situation;
- searching for one's own goals;
- undertaking roles alongside other people;
- entering into new occupational settings;
- expanding one's range of occupational skills;
- learning new things; or
- having the opportunity to do something on one's own for the first time.

Exploration is always positive because it is focused on the process itself and not on the results. Thus, facilitating exploration requires that therapists generate an exploratory context. This will offer opportunities for discovery, foster curiosity and decision making, and promote the absolution of failure, a sense of pleasure, and an absence of time limits (de las Heras et al., 2003; Reilly, 1974). Having an *exploratory attitude* is crucial for generating an exploratory context. This should include:

- having the *conviction* that mistakes are just as valuable as successful performance,
- *letting go* of one's own thoughts and feelings of fear regarding an individual's frustration; and
- having *confidence* in people's trial attempts.

"Let's try," "Let's see what we can find out," "Go ahead, it is your turn," "We are only going to investigate the possibilities, we are not going to commit to anything," "Let's have fun," "We are not going to test you on this, you know?" "What do you want?, this or that?" "How would you do this?" "Good try," and other expressions are commonly used within an exploratory context.

Exploration may be facilitated at *varying tempos*—slowly or quickly. This will depend on the unique personal and environmental occupational factors that shape a person's occupational circumstances. While some people would respond rapidly to *encouragement, validation, advice, or structure*, others, whose sense of capacity is not internalized yet, might need a precise way of delivering this intervention including using advocacy-detailed instructions and *gradual feedback*.

To effectively facilitate a sense of capacity in people who have severe difficulties in their motivation for doing (volition), occupational therapists should follow the Exploratory Module of the Remotivation Process (de las Heras et al., 2003).

Occupational Consulting

Occupational consulting refers to a social space constructed by the occupational therapist and the person to share and discuss individual occupational circumstances and upcoming issues related to a person's change process. The main goal of occupational consulting sessions is to work as a team in the development of occupational identity and **competence** by approaching critical aspects that may include: the planning and management of meaningful routines; the establishment of occupational goals and the planning of strategies to work toward their accomplishment; exploring and choosing strategies for enhancing motivation; planning and negotiating role performance and habit change; decision making and problem solving; identifying and planning the process of learning skills or tasks; and working on understanding and reviewing the person's own volitional process. MOHO concepts are addressed and MOHO strategies may be integrated to facilitate persons' active participation according to their needs.

When offering occupational consulting it is crucial to incorporate three ongoing and interrelated moments during the session. The first, allowing *a space for personal narrative*; the second follows on from the narrative content, with the *identification of agreed-upon goals* and the *analysis of goal accomplishment*; and a third moment for collaboratively *choosing and planning future actions and strategies*. These three instances are combined according to the volitional state of the person, using different therapeutic strategies selected for each moment and topic approached. The use of self-assessments and other MOHO assessments are considered important means of evaluating progress with the person, and of providing them with *structure* to foster their reflective thinking about their occupational circumstances (de las Heras, 2010, 2015).

Occupational consulting with MOHO is flexible in terms of its frequency and duration. Both are established with the person and vary according to the stage of change the person is going through. For example, at the beginning of the **competency stage**, more frequent and shorter sessions may be needed. In general, as the competency stage progresses and becomes more direct and frank, an optimal frequency would be once a week. Later still, follow-up sessions may be set less frequently.

During the **occupational consulting sessions**, the therapist regularly *designs a plan* with the person, outlining the next steps to be taken and the most effective ways to learn, based on their shared perception of the issues. Skills to be learned are *identified, negotiated, and prioritized* according to the person's abilities and volitional status, the physical contexts, and social expectations of performance. These unique skills must be achievable and realistic, and need to be relevant to the person and to the environment where they choose or need to participate in. Once skills have been determined, the therapist and the person *analyze personal and environmental assets* to establish measurable goals that can be accomplished.

Providing *structure* becomes a key strategy for the learning process during the *implementation phase of the plan. Structure must foster maximum volitional autonomy and performance independence*, avoiding doing too much for the person. To ensure this happens, the therapist must provide, as many as possible, opportunities for exploration of the chosen strategies, allowing trial and error while giving just enough *feedback* to facilitate initiative, decision making, and problem solving. Whenever possible, *providing structure* also requires that, the therapist gives the person the opportunity **to choose** the coaching approach that fits better with their style of learning. If the person is not able to choose, then the therapist may discover the most appropriate teaching strategies by liaising with family members and others close to the person. The therapist must *grade the process of learning* according to the person's abilities and desire to explore new ways to do things before commencing the coaching process.

Family MOHO-based consulting follows the same procedures. Family members or other close social groups are encouraged to actively participate, providing subjective and objective information, collaborating with their own strategies, learning MOHO and new strategies for facilitating their family member's participation in occupation, as well as *participating in their own process of occupational change*. In this respect, it is crucial to respect the time that family members may take to explore new occupational goals and ways of doing things, as their family member progresses. Fostering the satisfactory occupational participation of the caregiver (being a member of the family or staff) is of first priority. Therapists must validate, reaffirm, and facilitate a caregiver's sense of efficacy and satisfaction (de las Heras, 2015).

Peer Support Educational Groups

***Peer support educational groups** are sessions where participants with common occupational needs learn about diverse occupational topics that are relevant to enhance their daily participation in occupations.* Ideally, these are chosen by the participants themselves and planned with them in response to their needs. The peer support educational group offers an opportunity for sharing, discussing, giving, and taking information and advice from one another with regard to aspects related to occupational performance and participation. Common objectives might include increased self-knowledge, working toward personal goals, confronting challenges (and related problem solving and decision making), developing strategies to maintain a healthy lifestyle, and embedding general health management skills (e.g., symptom and stress management, or energy conservation) into occupational routines.

The key ingredients of peer support groups are the active participation of participants in sharing information with their peers, and considering *the lived experience of participants as the main resource for learning*. This, translated into practice, means that occupational therapists act as facilitators of the participants' active participation through *validating, encouraging, and structuring* communication among members, and sharing pertinent subjective and objective information. They may also introduce relevant MOHO evaluation tools and summarize the participants' contributions using appropriate MOHO terms when the meetings conclude. Meanwhile, members of these groups may assume the role of secretary, moderator, or other roles agreed upon depending on their interests and skills.

In accordance with the ethos of peer support, the groups would not traditionally be organized around modules that continue for a certain number of sessions. However, the involvement of the therapist may be time limited, or the duration of the group may be determined by the institution or financial considerations.

As we can see, *peer support educational groups* are different from traditional educational groups or psychoeducational groups, in that the latter focus on providing information to participants in a format decided by professionals as an instructional experience. In these cases, doing, thinking, and feeling with interested people is not the main priority.

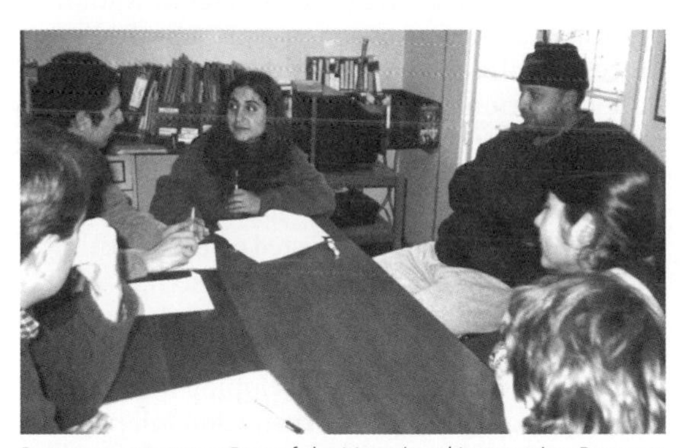

Peer support group: Part of the Vocational Integration Program at Reencuentros

Occupational Self-Help Groups

Occupational self-help *groups refer to meetings of people who have similar occupational needs that are organized by participants to share diverse occupational lived experiences and topics.* These may be related to common interests, challenging situations lived, accomplishments, problems experienced during daily participation, useful strategies to solve these problems, and planning collective projects related to specific shared goals. These groups emphasize problem solving, decision making, and learning from their peers' experiences. They offer ongoing support, contributing to stress management by knowing that one is not alone, and by pooling ideas for confronting the challenges that commonly occur when participating in occupations.

As mentioned previously, these groups may include the planning, organization, and implementation of projects, for example, to combat social stigma around certain illnesses or diverse gender and sexual issues; to help other people to set out on and continue their journey of recovery; to work on occupational justice; to design adapted objects for those with disabilities; to overcome poverty; or to advocate for their right for medication and treatment.

Within the context of projects aimed to help other people to overcome adversity, individual participants may offer help as volunteers or workers to support the process of change. They may have their own experiences of overcoming difficult conditions and may still be on their own recovery journey. As such, they become important partners in facilitating exploration and sharing specific strategies with those who have not yet reached the same point of recovery. Peer guides may participate as leaders of self-help groups, coleaders of peer support educational groups, facilitators of motivation and of learning skills, or givers of individual support or assistance with certain actions, tasks, or activities that are difficult for others (e.g., going shopping, initiating participation in groups, using public transportation, practicing conversational skills; Deegan, 1988; de las Heras, 2015).

At Reencuentros, a community integration center (de las Heras, 2006, Kielhofner, 2002), people who were starting work or commencing study in the community came together once a month to share their experiences. They empowered each other to continue facing challenges and maintain their assertive performance at their respective occupational settings. Moreover, others that were hesitant about taking on the same challenges were able to attend and gain *encouragement and validation* from their peers to explore possible options for them.

Therapists must remember that occupational self-help groups are implemented by and for the participants. They may offer a space for the group to have their meetings and take an observer role if, on occasion, they need to be present. At most, they may facilitate the flow of the group process by *validating, encouraging, and coaching the leader* or other members who have responsibilities within the group.

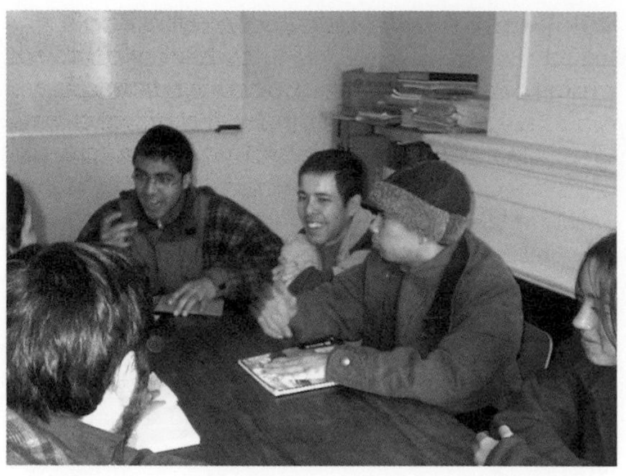

At Reencuentros, adolescents studying at different educational settings participated in their monthly self-help group

MOHO-based Skills Teaching

People may need to learn new skills, relearn skills that had been forgotten, or learn how to manage challenging situations better than before. These needs will depend on the occupational settings where they want or need to participate in, the activities or occupational roles they want or need to perform, and the goals agreed upon in therapy. With joint participation of therapist with family members, their peers, close friends, or health staff, this can be accomplished. *MOHO-based skills teaching refers to a progressive process of teaching purposeful actions and strategies that are critical for a person's daily participation* (de las Heras, 2015).

MOHO-based skills teaching may take place in three different formats, depending on a person's occupational circumstances: (1) through occupational consulting and independent practice by the person, (2) through *occupational consulting* and *coaching* of the person directly while they participate in occupation, or (3) through *coaching* the person directly while they participate in occupation. In all formats, the person practices critical skills while participating in occupations in the context of their daily life, *a context that gives meaning to learning.*

Coaching is based on a dynamic combination of *step-by-step instruction* using verbal and/or written indications, demonstrations, environmental cues, and doing tasks or steps together with the person. Coaching strategies must be chosen based on the person's possibilities to engage in the different dimensions of participation, the person's learning style, and the motivation and abilities demanded by the occupational forms/tasks.

CASE EXAMPLE: A YOUNG ADULT WITH TRAUMATIC BRAIN INJURY

Joseph was a 22-year-old man whose occupational life was characterized by successful occupational participation in a series of productive, ADL, social, and leisure roles. He was the best student in the 4th year of an engineering degree, the cohousekeeper and big brother of three siblings at home, and a volunteer who regularly helped adolescents at risk. He also practiced several sports, loved music and dancing, had many friends, and used to organize social gatherings and parties.

It was while practicing one of his favorite sports that he had a dramatic accident, causing severe brain damage. He was in a coma for 6 months. After that, he received physical and occupational therapy every day for 2 years. His mother was told that the rehabilitation had accomplished all that was possible in terms of neurologic recovery. Joseph had lost all his roles, mainly because of his cognitive deficits, but his mother never stopped looking for new alternatives. Because of her persistence, Joseph was referred by his neurologist to a community integration center, where his potential for participating in daily occupations was evaluated. It was found that he was able to attend to a valued and interesting task for 4 minutes, and presented severe volitional problems. His main desire was to continue to maintain a process of *"being productive."*

At the center, Joseph began participating with his therapist in an intensive process of remotivation, beginning at the fourth step of the Remotivation process' exploratory module ("Pleasure and efficacy in action") (de las Heras et al., 2003). He was given opportunities to participate in leisure activities that were compatible with the attraction of his past interests, and was *validated* for his occupational values. Joseph insisted on participating in administrative activities and studying. This was a challenging situation because these activities happened to be the most difficult for him to perform, and he was still developing a sense of capacity and had very low frustration tolerance. Despite this, the therapist trusted Joseph's strong values about persistence toward overcoming barriers and feeling productive. Based on this reasoning, the occupational therapist allowed him to participate in some administrative tasks that were needed for the administration of the center, and were graded to match his cognitive abilities. These administrative tasks included: (1)

keeping the attendance list updated by entering the names of participants on a spreadsheet using a computer; (2) collating two-page documents, and filing materials in administrative folders. He needed direct teaching to relearn these tasks. For him, because of his short attention span, *coaching* required direct verbal instructions given step by step, while demonstrating how to do each task. In addition, Joseph needed somebody close to him while he practiced the two steps required for each task, both to *assist him physically* when needed and to *encourage and validate him.* Progressively, he learned to follow the sequence and did not need a person with him. His therapist only had to leave written instructions by his side as a reminder in case he lost attention, or went for breaks to regain his energy. Later, when Joseph improved his process skills and felt more confident, he was coached by one of his peers to learn more complex tasks.

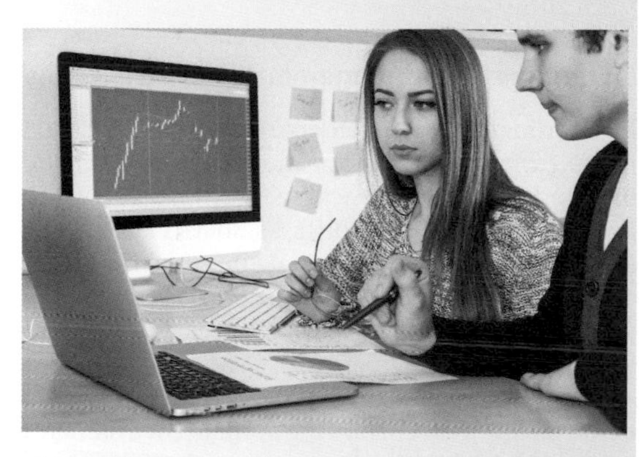

Joseph: Relearning skills with his occupational therapist

Social Education

Social education with MOHO takes the form of *participatory education* (Freire, 2000; Larsson, n.d.). This approach highlights the importance of empathy, and of developing a significant and respectful relationship based on teamwork, *fostering a sense of control and autonomy with those who could be* facilitators of change. Its goal is to promote participatory learning with family members, friends, neighbors, institutions' representatives, working teams, social and political organizations, and other crucial social groups that naturally enable a person to participate in occupations within a social context. This process includes the sharing of concepts and processes of participation in occupation and occupational adaptation. Depending on the nature of the social group, it may also involve sharing MOHO assessment tools, the results of assessment and reassessment, as well as *negotiating* the most feasible and meaningful strategies and procedures that would allow each social group to practice facilitating participation in occupation.

Social education can be delivered by formal or informal means, depending on the situation, on the characteristics and needs of the intended groups and on their goals. *Formal social education* may be accomplished in the context of meetings, speeches, presentations, or media interviews. *Informal social education* is contextualized in daily life such as inviting social groups to participate together in occupations of interest and cultural value; active community participation and involvement in improving health services; telling stories among friends, family members, workmates, or classmates; or occupational therapy initiatives of *informing and giving feedback* when walking through institutions or diverse community spaces (de las Heras, 2015; Kielhofner et al., 2011).

CASE EXAMPLE: A CAREGIVER WITH CUMULATIVE STRESS

Joseph's family had experienced nearly 3 years of uncertainty and pain. Firstly, not knowing if he was going to live, then not knowing if he would come out from the coma, and finally not knowing what his future would be. "Is my brother going to study again or help me with my school assignments?" "When will we know if Joseph will be as he was before?" "How can we help him?" "We don't know if we should get upset and angry at him when he does things we don't like." These were constant inquires that Joseph's siblings presented to Alice, their mother.

Joseph's therapist invited Alice to meet with her on a regular basis. From the very first moment, Alice had declared that she knew her son "will get back to be who he was before." She could not accept the tremendous change her son had gone through. Her situation led to the therapist deciding to extend the process of participatory education with Alice. Their first meetings gave Alice an opportunity to talk about her feelings, her expectations of her son's future, the ways she supported Joseph to do things, and the ways she managed his altered behavior that, in fact,

corresponded to an expression of frustration and pain for all he had lost. In these sessions, the occupational therapist shared openly all the outcomes of a comprehensive occupational evaluation, and explained MOHO's vision of the intervention process. Doing this helped Alice to make sense of things, and to open herself to a new possibility for her son. She demonstrated a keen interest to understand things better. The therapist gave her the last edition of the MOHO textbook to read, translated into Alice's first language: Spanish. They then spent a session learning the Remotivation Process, centering on Joseph's occupational circumstances. The therapist also gave her a copy of the Volitional Questionnaire (VQ), after teaching her how to complete it at home. In return, Alice brought the therapist all the information she had *identified* as being of interest that was related to neurological recovery. These participatory, social educational sessions were held once a week, in which therapist *validated* her efforts, *advised* her about how to supplement what she was doing already, *suggested* new strategies that she could undertake, and *encouraged* her while she was facing challenging circumstances.

As Alice became more confident as a mother, the therapist decided that it was the moment to approach a topic that was very sensitive. This topic related to the way Alice managed Joseph's behaviors when he was frustrated. Joseph used to spit all over the house, and bother his siblings by disconnecting their computers, or turning the radio to the highest volume when they were studying for school, or constantly making acute guttural sounds. Alice could not set limits (*give structure or boundaries*) as she felt guilty, knowing he had brain damage and that he had been her "right hand" at home since his father left when the younger children were in primary school. This was the most difficult task for her. The therapist *validated* her feelings and *advised* her, explaining to her that Joseph benefited from having clear and healthy limits and that home was the only place he behaved like he did.

The therapist began to support a progressive process of change with Alice, *exploring* strategies and *negotiating* the situations where she felt less challenged so that she could begin to practice them. After a period of practicing the agreed-upon strategies, the therapist followed this up by phone and e-mail communication. Alice now knew what to expect from Joseph and showed that she understood, as she was making long-standing changes in the way she interacted with him (habits of interaction). It took several occasions for Joseph to accept Alice's limits, but Alice persisted in *practicing* the strategies. Over time, experiencing these changes, and learning that Joseph could change his behavior and even contribute to valued tasks, Alice developed clearer expectations about her son's future and accepted her son's changed identity and competence.

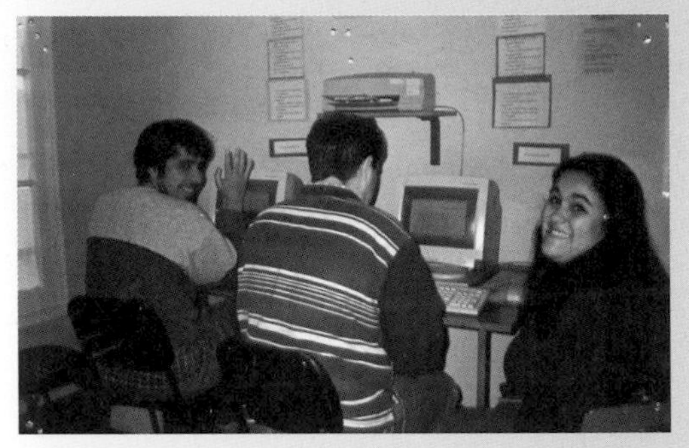

Joseph: Proud of being able to participate with his peers

Environmental Management

Environmental management refers to structuring or restructuring relevant occupational settings by changing or adapting the physical space and objects within it, the characteristics of the tasks, social expectations, and opportunities to participate in occupation. In so doing, the occupational therapist must be clear about the environmental dimensions and their characteristics and the degree of compatibility needed between these and a person's abilities, motivation, and patterns of performance. This enables the optimal environmental impact to be achieved, allowing participation in occupation to be enhanced in each moment of the change process. The MOHO tools based on the concept of environmental impact include the Residential Environment Impact Scale (REIS), the Work Environment Impact Scale (WEIS), and the School Setting Interview (SSI), as well as the VQ. These provide explicit and relevant information to develop a plan with the person and their meaningful social groups, in order to accomplish the best solution for them.

To develop and maintain a facilitating environment, it is necessary to *promote a balance between the opportunities and demands* of the occupational context, not only for the person but also for the therapists, the wider team, caregivers, family members, and the rest of the community.

The *physical environment* has a direct influence on performance, motivation, and developing a sense of identity. *Privacy*, for example, needs to be considered in all situations, even in reduced spaces. Therapists must be creative in how they adjust the physical space and give opportunities to clients to design their own personal spaces. The *availability of objects* must be considered: not only their presence but where and how they are distributed and organized in the space, avoiding unnecessary cluttering. In addition, it is crucial to preserve a person's dignity and identity by considering the *symbolic meaning of objects*. Wherever occupational therapists work, they must take into account the importance of the selection of objects according to culture, general interests, and characteristics of a person's abilities. *The message given by the types of objects and their distribution in the space are crucial aspects that could either facilitate or inhibit a person's initiative for doing* (de las Heras, 2011, 2015).

The adjustments that are needed in the physical environment when working with individuals who have physical disabilities are widely discussed in the occupational therapy literature, and therapists can draw on other models of practice to understand the full complexity of environmental adaptation. MOHO gives additional attention to the *experience and familiarity* that people have in the physical space and in using objects, which directly influences their range of complexity.

In considering *activities, occupational forms and tasks,* and their motivational properties, the therapist must reflect on the powerful relationship between a person's motivation for doing the task, the complexity of the task, and the quality of the person's performance. The best performance often occurs when motivation is in a medium range, when the person is interested in the activity or values it and feels sufficiently able to do it. High motivational levels may benefit the performance of simple tasks, but risks restricting the quality of performance in complex tasks if the person is not relaxed. At the same time, the task's degree of *complexity* has an important influence on a person's motivation for doing it. An optimal level of motivation occurs when the degree of complexity is compatible with personal abilities, and at the same time provides novelty or an appropriate level of challenge (de las Heras, 2010; Dunn, 1991). The *temporal dimension of a task*, or the duration of a task, must also be optimal for a person's abilities and motivational status.

Activity analysis using MOHO allows therapists to address relevant questions that support their decision making when facilitating satisfactory performance (Kielhofner, 2009). By observing the person's performance and volition, therapists are able to prevent a task from becoming so complex that it provokes a loss of interest in participating. It is important that their insights are shared with the people, so that they can develop their own mechanisms for regulating their time and adapting their participation in certain tasks (de las Heras, 2015).

Social groups are one of the most powerful environmental dimensions for facilitating or restricting the process of occupational change. *Social groups' permeability, expectations of participation and performance, norms and climate are crucial in facilitating or restricting participation in occupations.* Occupational therapists must bear in mind that they are part of the social environment, too, so the therapeutic relationship and the ways that they give feedback, validate, or assist can shape the social context. Very often, people may feel ambivalent about being more independent or being supported by others. This is a delicate situation where the balance between the opportunities and demands needs to be managed carefully with them and their significant others. Precise verbal and nonverbal communication is needed to foster clear and assertive messages. The therapist may also utilize the attitudes and specific procedures described in the Remotivation Process Manual and the strategies reviewed earlier in this chapter, to facilitate *empathy and permeability*, thereby promoting self-confidence, communication, and interaction.

CASE EXAMPLE: REFLECTION

Let's reflect on how the space, the objects, the social expectations, and support were managed to facilitate Joseph's best participation in significant tasks. In order to keep his attention on tasks, he needed an environment with the fewest distractions possible. This was very difficult to arrange in a center where several other people shared each space. For this reason *a desk was placed against a wall* which was opposite to the entrance of the office. *Only the objects and materials that he would use were placed on this desk, along with* the written instructions he needed. For example, when collating two-page documents, copies of each page were arranged on either side of the desk, and a stapler was placed on the right. The instructions, with the steps and actions he would need to follow, were placed in a visible position on the wall above the desk.

The person who worked alongside him, ready to assist or support when needed, communicated with him using clear *and short phrases*. This was the only person who talked to him when he was working. Therapists and other participants coordinated and respected this plan, and he was *validated and encouraged* by his peers and therapists when he took his breaks. As he progressed, he started to share workspaces with others. He also chose the peer who would become his main support, because he respected and shared his seriousness and his attitude toward helping others.

Occupational Role Development and Habit Change

During the competency stage of occupational change, roles and habit patterns begin to take form. People must confront challenges and *negotiate* between their internal expectations and desires and the expectations of social groups and conditions of the physical environment. When performing roles they also need to integrate their skills and motivation for doing (volition). It is in this ongoing process that occupational competence starts to take shape through a progressive learning and internalization of occupational participation patterns over time.

As MOHO theory explains, *roles and habits are difficult to change*. Because of this, when established patterns are not satisfactory or useful, either for people themselves or for their significant social groups, occupational therapists need to approach the process of change as soon as possible. The process of entering into new roles or reentering past roles is necessarily interwoven with the development and discontinuation of habits. In practice, the *acquisition of new roles* must follow the natural sequence of exploration, learning, and sustained practice, until internalization is achieved. The following entails a summary of procedures that would be implemented flexibly in line with the outcomes of any previous MOHO assessment (de las Heras, 2015).

The first phase of role development is for people to explore their internal expectations (what they want from a role and want to achieve in a role) and their external expectations (the real demands that these roles and specific occupational settings pose). In other words, the goal of this step focuses on initiating the process of role identification and gaining a preliminary knowledge of role scripts. The *exploration* of internal and external expectations of roles is supported by the following:

- *Use of selected self-assessments* and the corresponding *validation, feedback, and advice.*
- *Exploration of the significant occupational settings* with the person to identify their opportunities and demands.
- *The person's* ***progressive participation activities, tasks, or steps*** needed for significant roles, framed within a personal or collective project.
- *Construction of personal routines* that include participation in tasks of corresponding activities.

The combination of these procedures facilitates the progressive coming-together of chosen roles, performance, a sense of continuity of doing, self-knowledge of personal abilities and skills, and early development of the needed flexibility toward contingencies or changes in circumstances (disposition to change). These are all *basic aspects that are required for role internalization.*

The second phase of role development has the goal of internalizing the role, in other words, incorporating role scripts. The process of role internalization is benefited by the following sequence of procedures:

- *Planning and structuring* with the person their participation in relevant activities, and organizing them according to the person's progress, on a daily, weekly, or monthly basis (habits of routine).
- *Encouraging the person's* ***progressive participation*** *in role-related activities* and all tasks needed for their completion according to plan.
- *The person practicing* these routines until they feel confident and accomplish personal goals *negotiated* with the therapist.
- *Planning and structuring* performance standards according to personal and environmental expectations.

Internalizing a role implies a higher challenge because people have to take on more responsibilities, confront multiple barriers and setbacks, and persist in participating despite them. Thus, in this process, the therapist must use diverse *therapeutic strategies* and other *specific interventions* according to the occupational needs that have been assessed (de las Heras, 2015).

As mentioned earlier, when people participate in roles, in role-related activities, or in tasks, they begin *to organize their routines* (habits of routine) and *display or develop* their own ways of doing things (habits of performance), as well as showing specific characteristics that identify them, while doing (habits of style). *Changing habits* is considered to be one of the most difficult challenges for people who are changing them and also for people who facilitate change (de las Heras, 2010). This process requires a *constant negotiation* either daily or over time. This is because habits are intimately intertwined with motivational aspects (volition) and with physical and social environmental dimensions, which makes the process intensely complex.

There are many examples of habit change. Among them, changing schedules for getting up in the morning and going to bed at night; changing the way we react to unpleasant situations; learning new ways of doing certain tasks to achieve better efficiency or energy conservation; changing attitudes and actions toward others; or, even more complex, changing a whole lifestyle.

Habit change begins with *personal invalidation*, when people note that the way in which they used to organize themselves or perform tasks does not benefit them or help with achieving their personal goals or activity choices. This represents a challenge to their personal confidence (personal causation), personal values, or both. For habits to change, people need to have a *meaningful reason for doing it*, and at the same time, their significant social groups (including therapists) need to share consistent and logical expectations. If not, habits lose personal value. As commented on previously, the therapist must offer opportunities *to explore* and *identify* diverse alternatives and strategies, *encouraging* the person to choose one, and experience it in their relevant contexts. This is required to continue with sustained *practice* in similar situations, and, in so doing, to foster the internalization of a new pattern of performance (Kielhofner, 2008; Kielhofner, Barris, & Watts, 1982).

The habit change process requires occupational therapists to work very closely with a person's significant social groups, using *occupational group consulting* and social education with them to get clarity regarding their change expectations and develop common criteria for change facilitation. Therapists must *validate, advise,* and *negotiate* with these groups to achieve consistency in their expectations and in their understanding of the volitional process involved (refer to Alice's example in this chapter; Fig. 14-3).

There are three indispensable aspects that an occupational therapist must consider when facilitating habit changes:

- Therapists must foster change *according to the culture and characteristics* of relevant occupational settings, these being the places where the person participates or will participate in life occupations, including the specific spaces that support the process of change.
- When *prioritizing with the person and their relevant social groups* regarding which habits really need to be changed and which ones are possible to change, therapists need to *effectively negotiate,* leaving aside personal parameters or generalized standards. This can be achieved by considering the person's *unique occupational history and learning why and how habits were formed* and maintained.
- Therapists need to understand the process of habit change. To accomplish this difficult task, becoming familiar with the Remotivation Process guidelines, described later in this chapter, is highly recommended.

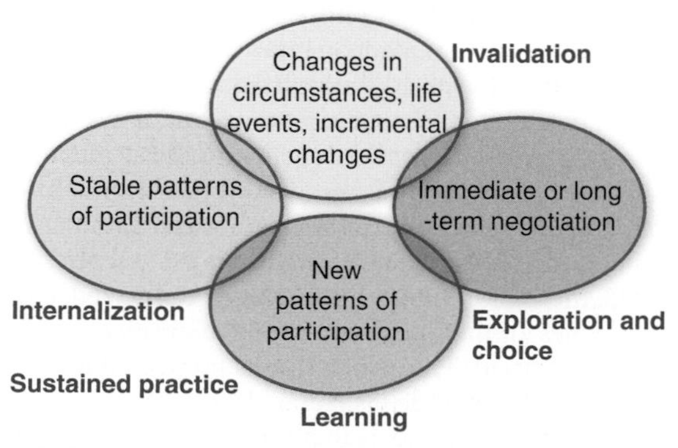

FIGURE 14-3 Occupational Role Development and Habit Change.

MOHO-based Protocols of Intervention

A ***MOHO-based protocol of intervention*** *refers to a set of specific procedures, which interweaves specific interventions and therapeutic strategies through the intervention process.* Protocols of intervention have been systematized through practice to approach occupational needs that are common to a group of people. Their intention is to be *a guide for occupational therapists or other facilitators on their implementation.* As each person and targeted group of people and their contexts have specific needs, the way in which these needs are approached should be flexible and guided by the results of an exhaustive evaluation process with MOHO.

REMOTIVATION PROCESS

The Remotivation Process is a continuum of strategic interventions designed to enhance motivation to engage in occupations. It is used with individuals who have varying skills, abilities, impairments, and illnesses but who share a marked reduction in their motivation to act on the world. The Remotivation Process is a key strategy that enables people to develop their occupational performance and participation. It is based on the natural continuum of volitional development through life, whereby people go through the stages of **exploration**, **competency**, and **achievement**, referred to as stages of volitional change (Kielhofner, 2008; see Table 14-2).

Exploration represents the first stage of volitional change. In this stage, people are not fully committed to their desires and are unsure about their capacities. Because the individual lacks certainty in this stage, the social and physical resources and opportunities available within an emotionally safe and undemanding environment are critical in order for progress to be made (Kielhofner, 2008). Intervention within this stage consists of providing opportunities for the person to try out new things, thereby learning more about their own capacities, preferences, and values (Kielhofner, 2008).

Competency is the middle stage of volitional change. In this stage, people focus on practice, consistency, and adequacy in performance. New approaches to performance or new activities that were discovered previously (e.g., during the Exploration Stage) are practiced and habituated. As demands and expectations within social and physical environments increase, the person strives to meet those demands

Table 14-2 Remotivation Process: Generalities

The Remotivation Process		
Modules	***Stages***	***Goals***
Exploration Module	1. Validation 2. Disposition for environmental exploration 3. Choice making 4. Pleasure and efficacy in action	Facilitate sense of capacity, a sense of personal significance, and a sense of security with the environment
Competency module	5. Internalization of self-efficacy 6. Living and telling own story	Developing a sense of efficacy, reaffirming sense of capacity and sense of control over own decisions and occupational performance
Achievement module	7. Self-monitoring and identification of critical skills 8. Self-advocacy	Integrating new areas of occupational participation into total life

by adjusting or improving upon their occupational performance. Therapists work to enable their clients to organize their occupational performance into established routines of behavior that allow them to feel increasingly competent and in control of their own lives (Kielhofner, 2008).

Achievement represents the final stage of volitional change. In this stage, people have reached a higher degree of competence in their skills and they have formed habits that allow them to participate in some new work, leisure activity, or activity of daily living (Kielhofner, 2008). During this stage, the therapist aids the person in integrating a new area of occupational participation into their lifestyle as a whole, reshaping the person's occupational identity in some small or large way (Kielhofner, 2008). To sustain the person's overall experience of occupational competence, a person must actively modify other roles and routines to accommodate the new area of occupational participation (Kielhofner, 2008).

When applying the Remotivation Process (de las Heras et al., 2003), emphasis is given to the importance of recognizing each individual's unique progression through the continuum and using interventions that are matched to the person's volition, both in terms of the person's unique volitional characteristics and in terms of the person's volitional status. When a life-changing illness or injury occurs, it is often the case that all areas of a person's occupational participation change. In these cases, a person may progress to the achievement stage in one area but remain in the exploration stage in another (Kielhofner, 2008). For example, after a hemorrhagic stroke, a person may focus on redeveloping approaches to completing activities of daily living, with the ultimate goal of moving from a skilled nursing facility into independent living. Areas of leisure and return to work may remain at the exploration or competency stage and may develop at a later time point (Kielhofner, 2008).

The Remotivation Process can be used by therapists, other health workers, family, or significant others seeking to help individuals develop volition. This process uses the VQ as the main MOHO tool to guide intervention through the whole process, but other MOHO assessment tools may be integrated through the process if possible and when needed.

History of the Remotivation Process

The Remotivation Process development began in 1989 with the goal of helping people who did not show a desire to explore and act, by reconstructing their motivation for doing. The first author of the Remotivation Process and a group of colleagues first practiced this approach with 50 institutionalized adults who had schizophrenia. They lived in a large psychiatric hospital and shared similar motivational problems. The colleagues explored specific strategies and procedures and observed people's responses closely. Data were collected using field notes and a preliminary version of the VQ. Procedures and strategies that had the most impact on improving volition were identified and selected through a qualitative analysis of the data. After observing positive outcomes when applying the procedures and the specific strategies that had been selected, the Remotivation Process was also piloted with people who experienced other psychiatric conditions, and with people who had dementia. In 1993, the exploratory module was systematized, and guidelines for the competency and achievement stages were identified. This protocol was published for the first time in 1999 (de las Heras, 1999).

After applying and evaluating the impact that the Remotivation Process had in occupational adaptation process of 200 adults living in the community, the exploratory process was refined and completed. Interventions and strategies for advanced stages of change were identified through practice, and the evaluation was completed with the third version of the VQ (de las Heras, Geist, & Kielhofner, 1993) and other MOHO assessments, like the OPHI-II, the Role Checklist, and the Occupational Self-Assessment (OSA). The first edition of its manual was published in 2003, and this attracted the interest of occupational therapists from all over the world (de las Heras, 2006; de las Heras et al., 2003).

The Remotivation Process: Application to Adults with Treatment-Resistant Depression

The occupational therapists who started using the Remotivation Process in Quebec, Canada, noted positive changes in their clients' engagement in occupation. Clinicians, psychiatrists, nursing staff, and occupational therapists worked together and developed a longitudinal study that aimed to measure the effects of participating in the Remotivation Process on people with depression, for whom psychiatric treatment had limited or no benefits. More specifically, the study used MOHO-specific assessments and psychiatric assessments to measure changes in volition, occupational performance, and symptoms according to the remotivation process stages of exploration, competency, and achievement. A total of 13 adults, with a mean age of 50.8 ($SD = 7.1$), participated in the study. All had been diagnosed with depression and were receiving treatment at the Institut Universitaire en Santé Mentale de Québec. All participants engaged in the Remotivation Process for approximately 20 weeks. During this period, measures were repeated at the beginning, midway through, and the end of the intervention. For most clients, overall improvement was noted, and the total scores of the OPHI-II and the VQ increased. Engagement in occupations also increased as well as the ability of participants to make choices about daily life. Their volitional stage also evolved over time (progressing from exploration to competency to achievement). This study provided specific evidence about a client-centered, occupation-focused intervention process based on occupational therapy core concepts (Pépin, Guérette, Lefebvre, & Jacques, 2008).

The Remotivation Process: Application to Dementia

A group of occupational therapists from Shawnee State University in the United States have since carried out phenomenological studies to understand volition in older adults with dementia. They sought to understand the dementia experience using the Remotivation Process and the VQ. The findings of these studies revealed important and detailed information to consider when applying the process in dementia (Raber et al., 2010; Raber, Quinlan, Neff, & Stephenson, n.d.).

Ongoing International Research

The Remotivation Process continues to be widely used and integrated as part of program development in countries with different cultures and languages (de las Heras, 2015; Kielhofner, 2008; Poletti, 2010; Quick, Melton, Critchley, Loveridge, & Forsyth, 2012).

MOHO Problem-Solver: Applying the Remotivation Process with Anorexia Nervosa

Joanne is a 26-year-old woman with an 8-year history of anorexia nervosa. She lives with her parents in a suburb of a large city, and has two older brothers who live on their own. She studies architecture at a university, but has had to have breaks in her studies and study part-time while struggling with anorexia. Joanne's parents have had difficulty understanding and dealing with their daughter's eating disorder, reporting that she was controlling the entire family.

When Joanne was younger, family-based therapy was tried with little success. The intensity of this intervention, especially surrounding mealtime, was too much for everyone and often resulted in a lot of fighting and little progress. She has had several hospitalizations since then and has received services in both private and public health care systems. She has worked with several practitioners, some of whom were specialists in eating disorders. Joanne is currently attending a day program for people with eating disorders, where a multidisciplinary team provides services and she receives enhanced cognitive behavioral therapy (CBT-E). CBT-E is supported by strong evidence and is described as one of the leading empirically supported treatments for eating disorders. One of the characteristics of CBT-E is that it provides treatment for eating disorder psychopathology rather than for a specific eating disorder diagnosis, and is applicable across a range of eating disorders. Despite this, Joanne's psychologist noted her slow progression, and she was labeled by some members of the team as being "treatment resistant" and "noncompliant."

The occupational therapist on staff was invited to explore Joanne's treatment resistance and noncompliance further. The OT was interested in understanding Joanne's motivation and decided to apply the Remotivation Process with her. She explained to the rest of the team that, by encouraging Joanne to explore her environment, giving her the opportunity to make decisions, and encouraging her to test her volition by trying activities that were not focused on food and calories or eating disorders, she was hoping to help Joanne become more motivated and engaged with her environment. She also decided to explore other aspects of Joanne's occupational life, including her interest in architecture.

The first step in applying the Remotivation Process was to understand more about the different dimensions of Joanne's volition (i.e., determine where Joanne was on the volitional continuum). After considering some of the other MOHO assessments, including the OPHI-II, the OT decided to administer the VQ because it is a brief observational assessment (as compared with an interview) and due to its singular focus on volition. Joanne was observed while attending a gardening activity in which five other young women with eating disorders were participating.

The scoring of the VQ revealed that Joanne was in the early stages of competency. With encouragement from the group facilitator, Joanne indicated some goals and stayed engaged for short periods of time. With the support of other group members, she showed some pride in the tasks being completed. Joanne also seemed to be comfortable with most of the other members of the group. Together, they attempted to solve some of the problems they encountered. These observations led the therapist to reason that Joanne's needs of constant *encouragement* to get involved, and not showing pleasure while participating, meant that the activity itself was not significant to her. Instead, what was valued by her was being close to people that appreciated her and cared for her.

Based on these findings, the therapist decided to talk with Joanne informally about what she had observed and to *validate* her opinions. She also shared what she had in mind in terms of doing. Because Joanne was still going through the exploratory phase of her volitional process development, it was agreed that the therapist would provide *opportunities for participation in activities* that would build Joanne's sense of capacity, and personal significance, and that would allow her to experience pleasure and efficacy in her actions. During the first few sessions, the therapist *facilitated Joanne's exploration* of her most valued occupation, studying architecture. She gave her the option to talk about her study choices, what interested her in that field, and how studying a topic that she loved made her feel—*validating and giving feedback to her*. They also looked at some of her favorite architecture books together, and decided to go for walks around the grounds of the outpatient clinic where Joanne could identify some architectural features in the surrounding buildings. These shared tasks, based on Joanne's interests, values, and successful past experiences, contributed to establishing her uniqueness and to building trust between them through consistency and continuity.

During **occupational consulting sessions,** Joanne and her therapist reviewed advances in her volition while participating in different daily activities. They reviewed the VQ that had been completed and noted Joanne's need for support when facing mistakes and problems. Joanne would ask the OT for understanding and advice at these times, but *the VQ showed that her volitional process was definitively at the competency stage.* Based on these findings, the therapist decided to use the OPHI-II with her. The interview and the subsequent analysis served as a vehicle for Joanne to begin working on linking her past and present volitional experiences with her interpretations and anticipation for future participation.

Within 2 months, Joanne became more active in her routines at home and at the outpatient clinic, agreeing with the psychologist to participate in group psychotherapy, albeit only as an observer. After few more sessions with the therapist, Joanne expressed her desire to return to university and continue her studies. Within the next two **occupational consulting sessions,** they *identified and negotiated* the activities that she would need to include into her routine *to return to her major role on a progressive* *basis.* They agreed to Joanne having some time dedicated to review university subject matter and books, every 2 days, and to enroll for a course of her choice. These *two activities related to her role as student,* and helped her to *explore* her volition while participating in the university setting again. To be able to face this new challenge, Joanne *decided* to get in touch with the classmate she felt closest to, to ask for her support on the day she attended school. They agreed to travel there and return home together. *Identifying* a meaningful goal and working toward it helped Joanne to realize that she also needed to engage in other interventions to address the disordered eating patterns and thoughts about food and weight which, for her, represented a major challenge.

Recovery through Activity

Recovery through Activity (Parkinson, 2014) is an intervention that incorporates aspects of MOHO and combines group work with one-on-one work to reaffirm the long-term benefits of participation in occupations. It is a flexible intervention that has been designed to *facilitate structured exploration* of up to 12 different categories of activity: leisure activities, creative activities, technological activities, physical activities, outdoor activities, faith activities, self-care activities, domestic activities, caring activities, vocational activities, social activities, and community activities. These may be selected and combined in different ways to design client-centered programs capable of meeting the various needs of participants in a range of settings. For instance:

- in an acute hospital setting where group membership is open, the topic might be agreed with the participants each week;
- in a long-term rehabilitation setting, all the topics might be covered in a systematic fashion;
- in the community, it is more likely that the occupational therapists and participants will build a program using a reduced number of topics that have been tailored to meet the participants' needs.

The program recommends a number of MOHO assessments that could be used in conjunction with the intervention, including the OSA, the Role Checklist v2:QP, and an Activity Checklist that has been based on the UK version of the Interest Checklist (Heasman & Salhotra, 2008). The intervention itself is then underpinned by the stages of change identified in the Model of Human Occupation (i.e., exploration, competency, and achievement). The group program focuses on exploration while the one-on-one element is more focused on building competence.

Essentially, the group sessions aim to reaffirm participants' views of themselves as occupational beings—to strengthen their occupational identities by allowing them to explore their interests, values, and beliefs. The group sessions therefore combine **peer support education,** *participation in occupation,* **and facilitation of exploration** as interventions. The occupational therapist provides the *structure* for participants to experience a range of activities, to *validate* their experience, and to *encourage* anticipation of future participation in occupations. (This fits in with stage 4 of the *Remotivation Process*: "Pleasure and Efficacy in Action" (de las Heras et al., 2003)).

The time spent in the one-on-one element takes things a stage further by helping individuals to organize their roles and routines using **occupational consulting and** *MOHO-based skills teaching* as required. The therapists will be working to *identify* specific issues that can facilitate occupational participation and to *negotiate* personal goals, as well as providing *specific feedback, targeted advise, individual coaching,* and, if necessary, *physical support* to access new occupations and environments. In this way they may help participants to address any skill limitations and performance limitations, with the overall aim of increasing occupational participation. (This fits in with stages 5 and 6 of the *Remotivation Process*: "Internalized Sense of Efficacy" and "Living and Telling One's Story" (de las Heras et al., 2003)).

The *Recovery through Activity* handbook ensures the precise application of the intervention and includes 12 sections—one for each category of activity. Each section provides background information about the activities, useful handouts, ideas for facilitating the group, and suggestions for experiential activities.

Conclusion

This chapter presented and discussed a number of MOHO-specific interventions, strategies, and MOHO-based protocols of intervention that have been developed over time responding to people's diverse occupational needs and the settings where they participate in occupations. These methods will form an important component in planning and implementing occupational therapy.

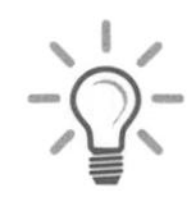

Chapter 14 Review Questions

1. What is the difference between therapeutic strategies and specific interventions?
2. Identify the four premises that sustain the MOHO intervention process.
3. What is the difference between structuring and environmental management?
4. What is the relationship between strategies, specific interventions, and protocols of intervention?
5. Describe the three stages of volitional change in MOHO.
6. On what aspect of MOHO does the Remotivation Process focus?
7. Provide an example of one assessment that may be used to inform the Remotivation Process.

HOMEWORK ASSIGNMENTS

Think of your practice as a professional or student:

1. Identify which specific *interventions* could be used with two people you have observed or worked with.
2. Identify which *strategies* might be most useful in three specific situations experienced during their process of change.
3. Reflect on the needs of the population you work with and consider which MOHO strategies, specific interventions, and protocols of interventions you might use.

thePoint® For additional resources and exercises, visit http://thePoint.lww.com

Key Terms

Achievement (achievement stage of volition): The third and final stage of volition, as described by the Remotivation Process. In this stage, people have reached a higher degree of competence in their skills and they have formed habits that allow them to participate in some new work, leisure activity, or activity of daily living.

Advise: Recommend intervention goals and strategies to the client.

Coach: Instruct, demonstrate, and cue to teach new skills or abilities to clients.

Competency (competency stage of volition): The second stage of volition as defined within the Remotivation Process. In this stage, people focus on practice, consistency, and adequacy in performance.

Encourage: Provide emotional support and reassurance.

Environmental management: The process of structuring or restructuring relevant occupational settings through changing or adapting the physical space and objects, task characteristics, social expectations, and opportunities for participation in occupation.

Evaluation doubling as intervention: The role of MOHO nonstructured and structured evaluation methods on developing self-knowledge, establishing a therapeutic relationship, facilitating problem solving and decision making, goal setting, and planning.

Exploration (exploration stage of volition): The first stage of volition as defined within the Remotivation Process. In this stage, people are not fully committed to their desires and are unsure about their capacities.

Facilitation of exploration: Groups of procedures and strategies that are used to foster desires to investigate environmental and personal aspects, when taking on new opportunities and challenges in different circumstances during the process of occupational change.

Give feedback: Share an overall conceptualization of the client's situation or an understanding of the client's ongoing action.

Identify: Locate and share a range of personal, procedural, and/or environmental factors that can facilitate occupational performance and participation.

MOHO-based protocol of intervention: A set of flexible procedures, which integrate MOHO-specific interventions and strategies into a process of facilitating change, guiding therapists to work successfully with clients who share similar occupational needs.

MOHO-based skills teaching: A progressive process of teaching purposeful actions and strategies that are critical for daily participation.

Negotiate: Engage in give-and-take with the client to achieve a common perspective or agreement about something that the client will or should do in the future.

Occupational competence: This is defined by the actual actions taken to sustain a pattern of participation in occupations that is reflective of one's occupational identity.

Occupational consulting: A private space constructed by the occupational therapist and the person to plan, evaluate, problem solve, and making decisions during the process of change.

Occupational identity: A person's entire construction of who they are and wish to become as an occupational being.

Occupational role development and habit change: Progressive intervention to support exploration, learning, practice, and maintenance of roles and habits.

Occupational self-help groups: Regular meetings that are organized and carried out by people who have similar occupational needs in order to share and give and take support on diverse occupational experiences and to plan and implement significant occupational projects.

Peer support educational groups: Regular meetings planned with participants to learn about occupational topics of common interest, emphasizing clients giving and taking information from one another, and the therapist participating as facilitator of communication and of a shared conceptualization of contributions using MOHO.

Physically support: To use the physical body to support the completion of an occupational form or part of an occupational form when clients cannot or will not use their motor skills or initiative for doing, or to accompany a client somewhere.

Social education: Formal and informal participatory education that shares MOHO pertinent information with clients' relevant social groups of all kinds, to develop their sense of control in facilitating a person's participation in occupations.

Specific interventions: A defined set of procedures and strategies for fostering occupational adaptation.

Structure: Establish parameters for choice and performance by offering clients alternatives, setting limits, and establishing ground rules.

Therapeutic strategy: A therapist's action that influences a client's doing, feeling, and/or thinking to facilitate desired change.

Validate: Convey respect for the client's experience or perspective.

REFERENCES

Deegan, P. (1988). Recovery: The lived experience of rehabilitation. *Psychosocial Rehabilitation Journal, 11*(4), 11–19.

de las Heras de Pablo, C. G. (1999). *Rehabilitación y vida: Teoría y aplicación del modelo de la ocupación humana*. Santiago, Chile: Reencuentros.

de las Heras de Pablo, C. G. (2006). Le processus de remotivation: De la pratique à la théorie et de la théorie à la pratique. *Le Paternaire Journal, 13*(2), 4–11.

de las Heras de Pablo, C. G. (2010). *Modelo de ocupación humana: Teoría e intervención actualizada*. Santiago, Chile: Autora.

de las Heras de Pablo, C. G. (2011). Promotion of occupational participation: Integration of the model of human occupation in practice. *The Israeli Journal of Occupational Therapy, 20*(3), E67–E88.

de las Heras de Pablo, C. G. (2015). *Modelo de ocupación humana*. Madrid, Spain: Editorial Síntesis.

de las Heras de Pablo, C. G, Geist, R., & Kielhofner, G. (1993). *The Volitional Questionnaire (VQ)* [Version 3.0]. Chicago: Model of Human Occupation Clearinghouse, Department of Occupational Therapy, College of Applied Health Sciences, University of Illinois at Chicago.

de las Heras de Pablo, C. G., Llerena, V., & Kielhofner, G. (2003). *Remotivation process: Progressive intervention for individuals with severe volitional challenges: A user's manual*. Chicago: The Model of Human Occupation Clearinghouse, Department of Occupational Therapy, College of Applied Health Sciences, University of Illinois at Chicago.

Dunn, W. (1991). Motivation. In C. H. Royeen (Ed.), *AOTA self-studies series: Neurosciences foundations of human performance*. Bethesda, MD: American Occupational Therapy Association.

Freire, P. (2000). *Pedagogy of the oppressed* (Revised ed.). New York, NY: Continuum International Publishing.

Girardi, A. (2010, May). *Promotion of occupational participation in adolescents of Santiago de Chile' high economic class who undergo a mental illness and occupational privation*. Paper presented at the WFOT Congress, Santiago, Chile.

Heasman, D., & Salhotra, G. (2008). *Interest checklist UK: Guidance notes*. Chicago: University of Illinois at Chicago.

Jonsson, H., Josephsson, S., & Kielhofner, G. (2000). Evolving narratives in the course of retirement: A longitudinal study. *American Journal of Occupational Therapy, 54*(5), 463–470.

Kielhofner, G. (2002). *Model of human occupation: Theory and application* (3rd ed.). Philadelphia, PA: Lippincott Williams & Wilkins.

Kielhofner, G. (2008). *Model of human occupation: Theory and application* (4th ed.). Philadelphia, PA: Lippincott Williams & Wilkins.

Kielhofner, G. (2009). Conceptual foundations of occupational therapy (4th ed.). Philadelphia, PA: F. A. Davis.

Kielhofner, G., Barris, R., & Watts, J. H. (1982). Habits and habits dysfunction: A clinical perspective for psychosocial occupational therapy. *Occupational Therapy in Mental Health, 2*, 1–21.

Kielhofner, G., de las Heras de Pablo, C. G., & Suarez-Balcazar, Y. (2011). Human occupation as a tool for understanding and promoting social justice. In F. Kronenberg, N. Pollard, & D. Sakellariou, *Occupational therapies without borders: Towards an ecology of occupation-based practices* (2nd ed., pp. 269–277). Edinburgh, Scotland: Elsevier/Churchill Livingstone.

Larsson, E. (n.d.). *Participatory education: What and why*. Retrieved from www.ropecon.fi/brap/ch24.pdf

Parkinson, S. (2014). *Recovery through activity: Increasing participation in everyday life*. London, United Kingdom: Speechmark Publishing.

Pépin, G., Guérette, F., Lefebvre, B., & Jacques, P. (2008). Canadian therapists' experiences while implementing the model of human occupation remotivation process. *Occupational Therapy in Health Care, 22*(3), 115–124.

Poletti, L. (2010, June). *"Rumbos", centro de integración comunitaria en Argentina: Promoción de la participación ocupacional*. Paper presented at the WFOT Congress, Santiago, Chile.

Quick, L., Melton, J., Critchley, A., Loveridge, N., & Forsyth, K. (2012, October). *Remotivation process for occupation program*.

Paper presented at the Third Model of Human Occupation Institute, Stockholm, Sweden.

Raber, C., Quinlan, S., Neff, A., & Stephenson, B. (n.d.). A phenomenological study of occupational therapy practitioners using the remotivation process with clients experiencing dementia. *British Journal of Occupational Therapy.* Submitted for publication.

Raber, C., Teitelman, J., Watts, J., & Kielhofner, G. (2010). A phenomenological study of volition in everyday occupations of older people with dementia. *British Journal of Occupational Therapy*, *73*(11), 498–506.

Reilly, M. (1974). *Play as exploratory learning.* Beverley Hills, CA: SAGE.

Scaffa, M., Reitz, M., & Pizzi, M. (2010). *Occupational therapy in the promotion of health and wellness.* Philadelphia, PA: F. A. Davis.

Therapeutic Reasoning Guidelines

Genevieve Pépin and Gary Kielhofner (posthumous)

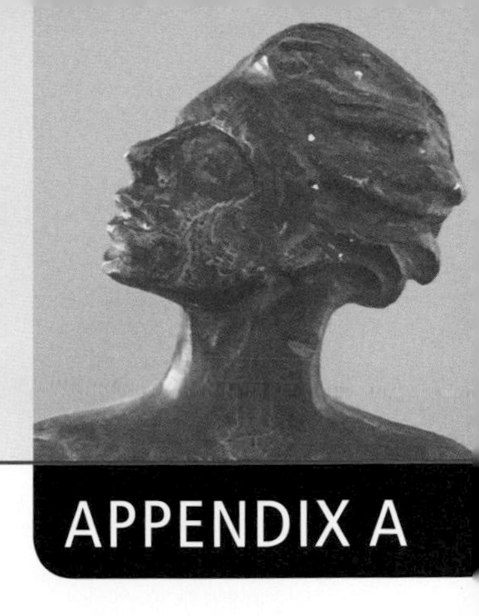

APPENDIX A

Introduction

The Model of Human Occupation (MOHO) is a conceptual model of practice that "*seeks to explain how occupation is motivated, patterned, and performed. By offering explanations of such diverse phenomena, MOHO offers a broad and integrative view of human occupation*" (Kielhofner, 2008, p. 4).

We also know that the dynamic interactions between a person's volition, habituation, performance capacity, and their different environments support occupational performance, participation, and engagement. Our understanding of the dynamics of human occupation also tells us that a shift, even small, in volition, habituation, performance capacity, or the environment can impact these dynamics and lead to new or different occupational patterns and responses. This shift can modify a client's participation in therapy or their engagement in occupations. Clinical intuition and judgment, observations, or results of outcome measures and assessment tools can uncover this shift and help clinicians understand the emergence of a new occupational pattern or a different occupational response. To fully understand what is unfolding in the course of therapy, it is important for clinicians to question the occupational therapy and the therapeutic process.

Therapeutic Reasoning

Therapeutic reasoning describes a process by which therapists use MOHO to understand a client from an occupational perspective, and then apply this understanding to create, deliver, and evaluate a treatment plan (Kielhofner, 2008). When applying the therapeutic reasoning process in occupational therapy, clinical questions therapists might ask themselves include the following:

Why is this client's participation in therapy different?
What has changed?
What is going on from the client's perspective?
How can I better support my client?
How can I promote or enhance occupational engagement?
What needs to be modified and Why?

Some of those questions may emerge because there has been a change in the client's occupational engagement. Others ensure the therapeutic process is reviewed, is client-centered, and evolves as the client progresses.

The therapeutic reasoning guidelines included in this chapter provide guidance to understand the dynamics of human occupation, the changes in participation and engagement in therapy, and new or different occupational patterns and responses. These guidelines aim to help therapists answer clinical questions by asking more specific questions framed around components of MOHO. It provides information to facilitate and promote occupational engagement. The information presented consists of examples to guide your reflection. It is essential that clinicians remain flexible and consider the unique circumstances and characteristics of each client.

When asking clinical questions or when attempting to understand a change in the person's occupational engagement, more precise questions focusing on components of MOHO can help clinicians implement therapeutic reasoning and apply appropriate strategies throughout the course of therapy. Furthermore, framing the questions within MOHO will guide reflective practice and an ongoing decision-making process to better support a client's engaging in therapy (Table A-1).

The following example illustrates how to use MOHO and its different components to help clinical reflection and understand how to better support a client toward enhanced occupational engagement. It also provides guidance on how to analyze a clinical situation that might be problematic or concerning.

Table A-1 Therapeutic Reasoning Table

Clinical Questions	Clinical Questions Framed within MOHO	Components of MOHO
Why is this client's participation in therapy different? What has changed? What is going on from the client's perspective?	• How does the person's volition, habituation, and performance capacity influence the way he/she feels and acts?	• Person: volition, habituation, performance capacity
	• Does this person exhibit the necessary communication/interaction, motor, and process skills to perform what he/she needs and wants to do?	• Performance capacity, skills
	• What is the person's sense of who he/she has been and wishes to become as an occupational being?	• Occupational identity
	• To what extent has this person sustained a pattern of occupational participation over time that reflects his/her values, beliefs, and occupational identity?	• Habituation, roles, occupational competence
	• What impact do the opportunities, resources, constraints, and demands (or lack thereof) have on how this person thinks, feels, and acts?	• Environment
	• Can this person do the occupational forms/tasks that are part of the work, play, and activities of daily living that make up (or should make up) this person's life?	• Performance capacity skills, occupational performance, occupational participation
	• Does this person currently engage in work, play, and activities of daily living that are part of his/her occupational context and that are desired and/or necessary to his/her well-being?	• Habituation, roles, environment
What needs to be modified and why? How can I better support my client? How can I promote or enhance occupational engagement?	Explore and document the different components of MOHO, and provide relevant support to enhance occupational performance. Provide experiences, and modify the environment to enable participation and engagement in occupations	

CASE EXAMPLE: A YOUNG ADULT WITH SPINAL CORD INJURY

Patrick is a 22-year-old man. He lives with his parents and two siblings—Madeline, aged 17, and Luke, aged 14. Patrick studies agronomy and worked part-time at an outdoor store. He was involved in a workplace accident 9 weeks ago and acquired a spinal cord injury. Patrick has complete C6 quadriplegia and is currently an inpatient at a metropolitan specialist rehabilitation service. Patrick is currently mobilizing with a manual wheelchair for short distances over flat surfaces. Patrick and his parents are actively involved in their local community and are grateful for the support they are currently receiving from family and friends. Patrick is still passionate about agronomy. He loves football and surfing, and hanging out with his friends. He has been coaching the junior football team for a few years with one of his best friends. Patrick and his family are open-minded, supportive, and have a very positive attitude toward life.

Patrick's accident has shaken those beliefs and attitudes as he, and his parents and siblings, adjust to a different life. Nonetheless, everybody puts on a brave face and sees Patrick's rehabilitation as a step to something different, although unexpected, trying hard to maintain a positive outlook about the future. However, Patrick is worried about how he will manage by himself, and he knows that his parents, sister, and little brother are also worried. Patrick's involvement in therapy has been consistent, and he has been open with his occupational therapist, Anna, about his feelings and the challenges he faces.

In the last few therapy sessions, Anna has noticed that Patrick seemed distracted and less involved in therapy. He still participates in the different therapeutic activities, but there seems to be something different about him. Anna discussed her impression with the members of the multidisciplinary team. The social worker had also noticed a slight change. The team discussed how such changes were to be expected, but Anna still had the impression that something was not quite right. She wondered how Patrick's variation in his therapeutic engagement would affect rehabilitation outcomes and what she could put into place to better support him. Anna asked herself the following clinical questions: *Why is Patrick's participation in therapy different? What has changed? What is going on for Patrick? How can I better support him? How can I promote or enhance Patrick's occupational engagement? What needs to be modified? Why?* Each of these clinical questions led her to reflect more deeply on the various aspects of MOHO, including how Patrick's volition, habituation, and performance capacity influence the way he feels and acts.

Volition

For example, when considering Patrick's volition, Anna explored Patrick's personal causation. This involved asking him how he felt about and viewed his personal capacity and effectiveness, and how this affected his choices, experiences, interpretation of those experiences, and anticipation about doing things. If Patrick is aware of his capacity (strengths and limitations), is able to choose occupational forms within his capacity, and take on appropriate challenges and responsibilities, and if he has adequate confidence to make decisions about engagement in occupational forms, then these strengths will support Patrick's occupational engagement and positive change. It is important to determine whether Patrick lacks or has limited awareness of his capacity (strengths or limitations). Knowing whether Patrick underestimates or overestimates his abilities will guide Anna's clinical reasoning and support her therapeutic decisions.

If a person underestimates his or her abilities, this can lead to

- overreliance on others;
- avoiding occupational forms commensurate with performance capacity, leading to reduced occupational performance; and
- failing to seek out occupational challenges that would promote learning/growth in skills.

However, if a person overestimates his or her abilities, this can lead to

- taking unnecessary risks by seeking challenges that are higher than one's performance capacity, resulting in poor occupational performance, danger, stress, damage, or injury;
- failing to seek assistance appropriately or make use of needed environmental adaptations;
- feelings of lack of control over occupational performance leading to anxiety (fear of failure) while performing occupations; and
- poor frustration tolerance leading to disengagement with occupational forms.

Once Anna identified whether Patrick underestimated or overestimated certain abilities, she focused on

- enhancing Patrick's understanding of his occupational abilities (strengths and limitations);
- directing Patrick's attention to more accurately note how his strengths and limitations affect his occupational performance;
- developing Patrick's emotional acceptance of limitations and pride in occupational abilities;
- increasing Patrick's ability to choose and do occupations that are consistent with his capacity; and
- building up Patrick's confidence to approach occupational forms that are within his abilities.

Once Anna explored Patrick's personal causation and identified challenges and problems, together they developed strategies to foster changes that would enhance Patrick's occupational engagement and participation. Using the steps of the volitional process, Anna recommended modifications in Patrick's environment that allowed him to take risks safely, explore occupational forms, gradually consolidate his confidence, and strengthen his identity. In doing so, Anna created experiences in which Patrick engaged, and tested his skills and abilities while being supported by his therapist.

As Patrick's experience unfolded, Anna validated his thoughts and feelings concerning his performance capacities and the challenges of engaging in

activities that were difficult and anxiety-provoking, highlighting Patrick's strengths and validating his perceived and actual limitations. Anna provided Patrick with ongoing feedback to support positive reinterpretation of his experience of engaging in occupations. Through these experiences, Anna was able to advise him to engage in occupational forms within his performance capacity to ensure a higher degree of success while sustaining meaning and matching Patrick's interests and values.

Habituation

As Anna continued to reflect on Patrick's occupational engagement within MOHO, she also explored Patrick's habituation. His habits and roles were affected by the accident. How he envisaged his current and future roles was important to understand, because this, too, would have an impact on his engagement in therapy. Collaboratively with Patrick, Anna answered the following questions about his roles:

- **What are Patricks' roles?**
- **What is Patrick's overall pattern of role involvement?**
- **How important is each role to Patrick?**
- **Does Patrick have roles that impact positively on his identity, use of time, and involvement in social groups?**
- **Is Patrick over- or underinvolved in his roles?**
- **Can Patrick meet the obligations of each role?**
- **Are all of Patrick's role requirements, collectively, too few, too demanding, or making conflicting demands on Patrick?**

Answers to these questions guided Anna's ongoing therapeutic decision making and helped her identify the most appropriate interventions to support Patrick's occupational engagement. For example, during one session, Anna focused on increasing Patrick's commitment to assuming specific roles that were necessary and desirable for him. She also worked with Patrick to increase his motivation and ability to become more effective in meeting multiple role expectations through the negotiation of realistic role responsibilities.

As clinicians, we want to know how to enact therapy and what interventions we should be implementing. In this example, Anna will want to structure the therapeutic environment to provide opportunities for Patrick to discuss his roles and their related expectations. Then, she will concentrate on ensuring that the therapeutic environment provides opportunities for Patrick to practice or develop specific skills and engage in the behaviors required by each role. This will allow him to internalize the role script and develop a supportive routine. Anna will continue to recommend and create experiences for Patrick to engage in. Over time, Patrick, with Anna's support, will be able to interpret his experiences and work through what he anticipates when considering his roles and how he can perform each of them. This process will help Patrick continue to make relevant and personalized occupational choices that will support and consolidate his occupational identity and competence.

As Patrick progresses through therapy, Anna's role will take on different forms. She will provide advice and guidance allowing Patrick to make his own choices and decisions. She will advise Patrick to identify different ways of meeting responsibilities and expectations related to his roles. She will also encourage Patrick to make choices to engage in new roles (or old roles in an adapted way—for example, by configuring new responsibilities within each role).

There are other important questions that Anna will need to explore to better support Patrick and encourage him to engage in occupations to the greatest extent possible. Here are some examples of such questions, contextualized within MOHO.

Performance Capacity

- What is the experience of the impairment and its implications for functional adaptation?
- Do any experiences interfere with this person's occupational performance, and how so?
- What are the consequences of sensory, motor, or other capacities for this person's experience of performing occupational forms?
- How do experiences (e.g., pain, fatigue, dizziness, confusion, or altered bodily perceptions) influence this person's occupational performance?
- Does this person have adequate motor/process/communication and interaction skills?

Environment

- Do the spaces in which the person performs his or her occupations represent physical barriers or supports that impact performance?
- Do the objects this person uses support performance?
- Do the spaces and objects constitute a physical environment with adequate resources for doing things this person needs and wishes to do?
- Does the environment provide appropriate occupational forms in which this person can engage?
- Do the occupational forms sufficiently challenge this person and provide a sense of worth?
- Do interactions with others support or inhibit this person's performance?

- Do the social groups of which this person is a member support the assumption of meaningful roles?
- What are the reactions of others in occupational behavior settings to this person's disability?

Conclusion

This section used an example to illustrate how students and occupational therapists should implement therapeutic reasoning. Clinical questions further examined by being framed by MOHO and its components were identified. The reflection and thinking process that should guide therapeutic reasoning and clinical decision making was also illustrated. Therapeutic strategies to foster occupational engagement were suggested. Although questions, thinking processes, and intervention strategies were applied to a specific case study, they can be applied to any clinical situation to guide therapeutic reasoning during occupational therapy practice. It is imperative, however, that students and clinicians remain flexible and attuned to their client's personal circumstances throughout therapy and remember that the information presented here is not prescriptive but provides guidelines to inform therapeutic reasoning.

REFERENCE

Kielhofner, G. (2008). *A model of human occupation: Theory and application* (4th ed.). Philadelphia, PA: Lippincott Williams & Wilkins.

PART III

ASSESSMENTS: COMBINING METHODS OF INFORMATION GATHERING

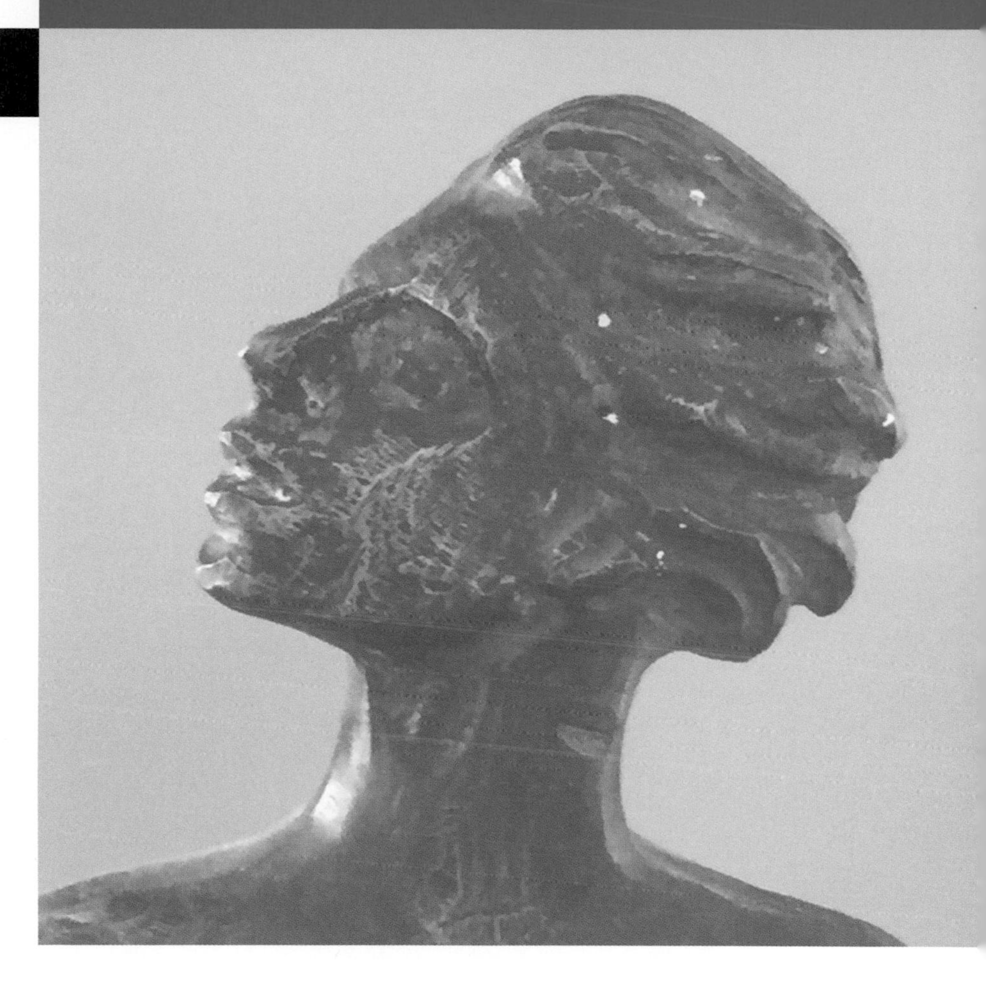

Observational Assessments

Carmen-Gloria de las Heras de Pablo, Susan M. Cahill, Christine Raber, Alice Moody, and Gary Kielhofner (posthumous)

CHAPTER 15

EXPECTED LEARNING OUTCOMES

Upon completion of this chapter, readers will be able to:

1. Understand when to choose an observational assessment.
2. Discriminate between observational assessments.
3. Understand the general procedures of application for observational assessments.

Other than consent from the client to allow them to be observed, observational assessments do not require clients to respond verbally or in writing to questions or to have the capacity to reflect verbally upon their experiences. Within the history of model of human occupation (MOHO), the development of observational assessments began from 1985 to 1987 with the research on the Assessment of Motor and Process Skills (AMPS), the Assessment of Communication and Interaction Skills (ACIS), and the Volitional Questionnaire (VQ).

The objectives behind the AMPS and the ACIS were to (1) capture the construct of occupational performance in the MOHO and (2) gather relevant information about and measure *performance skills,* focusing on *occupational performance* instead of underlying capacities, which can tend to be the main focus in many rehabilitation settings that ascribe to a medical model approach. As we have already learned in this text, MOHO offers a different perspective that focuses upon understanding the strengths, motives, and experience of clients in order to facilitate their maximal engagement and participation within their environments.

Originally, the main reason for developing the VQ was to "give voice" to people who, due to diverse causes, could not verbally express their interests, values, personal causation, and goals, but yet could do it through their behaviors and nonverbal expressions. Since that time, the VQ has been used with both verbal and nonverbal clients as a means to begin and follow up on interactions and/or actual conversations with clients related to the variegated aspects of their volition.

From this time on, ongoing research and practice has focused on developing complete manuals for application and revised versions of the measures, as well as developing corresponding pediatric measures, such as the Pediatric Volitional Questionnaire (PVQ), as a companion to the VQ, and the AMPS school version. In addition, a new observational assessment has been developed recently, the Assessment of Work Performance (AWP). This assessment is designed to focus on a client's work-related skills and how efficiently and appropriately they perform work tasks. The skills are assessed in three domains:

- Motor skills
- Process skills
- Communication and interaction skills

Each observational assessment is unique in its nature, contents, and procedures; however, they share common characteristics that may be desirable to therapists:

- They are not psychologically invasive and can be applied during natural participation in occupation
- Findings are contextualized according to environmental characteristics and their impact on occupational skills or volition
- They offer standardized procedures for observation and for rating a client's actions or volitional behaviors
- They allow for a clear and detailed understanding of peoples' strengths and difficulties, using a rating scale as well as qualitative information, in many cases
- They guide the therapist in terms of detailed therapeutic reasoning, problem solving, and decision making during the intervention process.

Two other MOHO-based assessments, the Model of Human Occupation Screening Tool (MOHOST) and the Short Child Occupational Performance Evaluation (SCOPE), were developed taking into consideration the contents of other MOHO assessments, including the AMPS, ACIS, VQ, and PVQ. Items representing habituation and the environment were also included.

The MOHOST and SCOPE use combined methods to gather information to provide an overall understanding of children, adolescents, and adults' occupational participation. *Observation* is one of their most important methods used.

This chapter describes the main features of **MOHO observational assessments** and illustrates with examples the application procedures, therapist reasoning, analysis of results, and their usefulness in practice. The assessments will be discussed in two sections reflecting work with adults and children.

Application of Observational Assessments with Adults

There are three observational assessments relevant for evaluating the performance skills of adolescents and adults: (1) the AMPS; (2) the ACIS; and (3) the AWP. In addition, therapists can also evaluate older children (more than 6 years), adolescents, and adults' volition through observations by using the VQ.

THE ASSESSMENT OF MOTOR AND PROCESS SKILLS

The AMPS (Fisher & Jones, 2012) is a standardized assessment based on the therapist's observation of a client's performance during activities of daily living (ADLs) and instrumental activities of daily living (IADLs) that would typically occur in the home. The AMPS can be used systematically to measure the quality of 16 motor skills and 20 process skills using a 4-point rating scale, where a score of 4 reflects competent performance and a score of 1 reflects significantly deficient performance. The skills are evaluated simultaneously and in the context of occupational performance. Therapists can use the AMPS to evaluate children as young as 2 years, adolescents, and adults. The AMPS is considered to be free of cultural bias because the task specifications can be modified to allow for cultural variations. The AMPS is appropriate to use with children who present with occupational performance concerns due to developmental, cognitive, or physical conditions.

Administration

The AMPS consists of two scales that separately measure process and motor skills. The two scales are administered simultaneously. This allows for direct evaluation of the interactive nature of motor and process skills such as the use of process skills to compensate for limitations in motor skills. Each item on the two scales is scored with a 4-point rating scale (competent, questionable, ineffective, deficit) that considers the effectiveness, efficiency, and safety of a client's performance. The motor skills scale gathers information on the actions done to move oneself or objects. The process skills scale gathers information on the logical sequencing of actions; selection and appropriate use of tools and materials; and adaptation to problems.

The AMPS takes between 30 and 60 minutes to administer. Prior to administration, the therapist collaborates with the client or caregiver, and, in the case of a pediatric client, the client's family to identify two of the standardized AMPS tasks that the client will perform during the observation. After observing the client's performance during the tasks, the therapist rates the client on motor and process skills. Rating may take from 5 to 20 minutes, depending on the client's performance and the complexity of the task. After the therapist has rated the client's performance in the 16 motor and 20 process skill items, the AMPS scores are entered into a computer software program which is made available to calibrated raters through the Center for Innovative OT Solutions (*www.innovativeotsolutions.com*) and a report is generated. *The results gained from the AMPS can assist the therapist in designing an intervention plan geared at improving the client's occupational performance. The AMPS also determines whether a person has the necessary motor and process skills needed for community living.*

CASE EXAMPLE: AN OLDER ADULT WITH EARLY ALZHEIMER'S DEMENTIA

Judith is a 61-year-old woman who was referred by her general practitioner for assessment of her memory. At the time of referral, she had been working in the kitchen of a local catering company, but had been off work for 4 months because her poor short-term memory was causing difficulties with work performance. She was therefore referred to the Memory Assessment Service for more detailed tests.

An initial cognitive screening assessment was carried out by a Memory Assessment Nurse. This involved taking a detailed history of the presenting factors as well as past and present physical and mental health. The Addenbrooke Cognitive Examination—III (ACE-III) was also administered. Judith scored less than 50/100, which, on the surface, would have suggested a moderate dementia. Her described functional presentation conversely suggested that any memory impairment was only very mild. Occupational Therapy assessment was requested, with the aims of gaining a better understanding of Judith's functional ability to aid diagnosis, and of identifying Judith's

occupational strengths and limitations and how these might relate to her worker role, with a view toward making workplace adjustments.

Initial Occupational Therapy Interview

The therapist met with Judith and her daughter Kate, with whom she shared a home, and interviewed both to get a clearer picture of Judith's volition, past and present routine, plus current roles and functioning. When asked about her memory and any associated functional difficulties, Judith stated that she thought there probably were problems, but turned to her daughter Kate to elaborate on this, seeming unaware of specific details. Kate explained that her mother had been beginning to make mistakes in the kitchen at work, confusing cooked and uncooked foods, which posed serious health and safety concerns within the catering company. When initially taking time off work, Judith had become unwell with pneumonia and was very physically weak. Kate took over the running of Judith's home while she convalesced, and Judith gradually recovered her physical health. Her memory did not appear to improve, nor did she resume performing at her previous level.

Judith appeared uncertain about her current self-efficacy with regard to her daily occupations. As stated above, she had some awareness that her functioning and memory had changed, but did not appear unduly worried by this. When asked how she was feeling about both her memory and the impact of this on her work, Judith replied cheerily that she was "just getting on with things, and that there was nothing she could do about it." Kate agreed that it had seemed odd that her mother was not anxious or worried about her current health. In terms of interests, Judith still very much enjoyed walking and looking after her cat, Sam. She took great pleasure in ironing, and happily carried out ironing both for herself and her daughter. Her initiative appeared to be restricted to these activities and to structured activities with family.

Judith continued to prepare her own breakfast of poached egg made in a saucepan each morning with no apparent difficulty. Kate explained that this was a long-standing part of her routine that she had carried out daily before leaving for work. Judith would take her medications and then feed the cat, but her day appeared to then lack further structure. She would sometimes eat lunch, but equally would sometimes forget to do so if her daughter was not there to prompt her. With prompting, Judith was able to prepare vegetables and wash dishes if asked, but was no longer using the actual oven for cooking. Kate had gradually begun to manage all appointments and finances for her mother. In terms of adaptability, as previously discussed, Judith did not seem particularly bothered by changes to routine or to her health, so did not appear to anticipate or react to change. She had not worked for over 6 months, but still held a position in the catering company, which seemed willing to look at supporting Judith to return to work if an appropriate role and/or adjustments could be made.

Assessment Consideration and Selection

It was agreed that an evaluation of Judith's current occupational strengths and limitations when engaged in familiar occupations would be necessary to better understand the challenges she had been facing in the work environment. In this instance, the following was taken into account when selecting an assessment tool.

- Judith, at the age of 61 years, was young to have a possible memory problem. Therefore, accurate diagnosis would be key in her receiving the right treatment and for both she and her family to be able to plan for her future.
- Judith's functioning appeared incongruent with her low score on the Addenbrooke's Cognitive Examination (ACE-III) (NeuRA, 2012). Occupational therapy assessment would therefore need to capture and evaluate the fine detail of Judith's task performance when carrying out ADLs.
- If she were to be diagnosed with mild cognitive impairment, an assessment that was standardized and repeatable in the future would capture any subtle changes in her functioning over future months.
- Judith would need support to meet with her employer and discuss possible workplace adjustments. A formal assessment report would therefore be required to aid discussion and negotiation.

The AMPS was selected as the main assessment tool to evaluate Judith's ADL performance skills as this is not only standardized, but looks at task performance in fine detail and produces a graphic report of motor and process skill efficacy. The AMPS required Judith to carry out two standardized tasks that she felt familiar with and would present enough of a challenge from the therapist's point of view for an effective assessment to be achieved. She chose the task "Vegetable Preparation" and the task "Ironing Multiple Garments" as these were activities she was already familiar with and confident to carry out. A further session was planned for the assessment to take place.

Once these scores were inputted into the AMPS software, a graphic report was produced showing Judith's overall motor and process ability scores. The therapist then produced a narrative report, interpreting both scores and clinical observations.

Judith's *process ability measure score* suggested that *she had the skills to carry out well-learnt, familiar occupations both safely and independently.*

Both tasks were carefully discussed and clarified prior to Judith starting each. When initiating the vegetable task, she was initially slow to initiate, asking herself out loud what she was going to prepare, and then repeating "potatoes and carrots" out aloud to herself. She searched three cupboards before locating the saucepans that she required, but once all materials and tools were set out and visual, she completed the task with logical sequencing and no pauses or delays. Judith *prepared all of the vegetables that were available however, despite the preparation being for a two-person meal* (what had been discussed and established), suggesting that perhaps she was not at this time able to tailor the amounts required for a later meal/employ logical reasoning and problem solving in this particular aspect. When completing the ironing task that involved ironing three garments, she chose to iron all five that were available, again implying that *she completed the task quite literally based on what was visual.* Again, her sequencing of the ironing was logical and knowledge of the task good.

Once the vegetables were prepared, placed in saucepans, and covered with water, Judith had a *great deal of difficulty finding saucepan lids,* which were out on the worktop in a different area of the kitchen. She searched through her saucepan cupboard several times, before looking elsewhere. It is possible that this delay might have been due to her again trying to problem-solve within her expected routine, *researching in the same places rather than again employing logical reasoning* to widen the search to other places.

Judith was mostly able to retain the agreed task information for both tasks that were familiar to her, but carried these both out *dependent on what was visual as opposed to what had been agreed.* Her overall performance was safe and logical and her work tidy.

Judith's *motor ability score* suggested that she had no difficulty moving herself or objects within her environment. She was observed to bend with only minimal effort to retrieve items from cupboards, plus was able to lift, carry, and set up the ironing board with no apparent difficulty. When peeling vegetables, her grip and dexterity were both good.

Assessment Summary

This assessment demonstrated Judith's ability to carry out well-learned familiar tasks both safely and independently. Her knowledge of both tasks, the tools required, and the necessary sequencing was good; however, she appeared to carry out both tasks quite literally dependent on what was visual as opposed to following the specific agreed plan (preparing all of the available vegetables for a two-person meal and ironing all the available garments). She did demonstrate ability to problem-solve while engaged in familiar occupations; this again appeared to be limited to what she expected within her normal routine, rather than her applying logical reasoning to widen her search for saucepan lids when familiar searches were exhausted. This may begin to explain some of the difficulties she might have been having at work within the catering company if she were basing her actions upon familiar routines and what was immediately visual rather than weighing-up what was needed and adapting the work plan accordingly. For example, if both raw and cooked foods were needing to be prepared and the materials and tools were visual, it is possible that she would dexterously attend to both tasks with great efficiency, but perhaps without utilizing the wider health and safety knowledge that was needed.

If Judith was basing her completion of well-learnt tasks on previous knowledge only, it was deemed likely that she would have some difficulty tackling less familiar/more complex tasks. Additionally, if tools were not immediately visual, or were in unexpected places, this could cause delays to her performance.

Her assessment of performance tied-in with her having a certain amount of ability when prompted, but initiating very little if left to her own devices. Her actual functioning therefore seemed to be better than her ACE-III score of 48 would suggest, but within the confines of what was visual and of familiar knowledge as discussed above.

Application of the AMPS to Judith's Worker Role

Through discussion, it had been ascertained that Judith appeared quite unclear about having a memory problem, and had turned to her daughter on initial interview to explain the impact of this on her occupations. Judith was therefore quite willing to look at whether the catering company could continue to offer her any form of work that would be within her capabilities in order to reestablish her routine.

By now, Judith had been formally diagnosed with early Alzheimer's dementia by the team's consulting psychiatrist.

A meeting was held with Judith and her employer, and the AMPS report discussed (Fig. 15-1). The following points were highlighted. Judith's

Process Skills	"Preparing Vegetables"				"Ironing Multiple Clothes"			
Energy	**1**	**2**	**3**	**4**	**1**	**2**	**3**	**4**
ATTENDS: Maintains focused attention throughout task performance				■				■
Maintains an even and appropriate PACE during task performance		■				■		
Using Knowledge	**1**	**2**	**3**	**4**	**1**	**2**	**3**	**4**
CHOOSES appropriate tools and materials needed for task performance			■					■
USES task objects according to their intended purposes				■				■
HANDLES: knows when and how to stabilize and support task objects				■				■
INQUIRES: asks for needed information				■		■		
HEEDING the goal of the specified task			■			■		
Temporal Organization	**1**	**2**	**3**	**4**	**1**	**2**	**3**	**4**
INITIATES actions or steps of task without hesitation		■				■		
CONTINUING actions through to completion				■				■
Logically SEQUENCES the steps of the tasks		■						■
TERMINATES actions or steps at the appropriate time				■		■		
Space and Objects	**1**	**2**	**3**	**4**	**1**	**2**	**3**	**4**
SEARCHES for/LOCATES tools and materials	■							■
GATHERS tools and materials into the task workforce	■							■
ORGANIZES: Distributes tools and materials in an orderly, logical, and spatially appropriate fashion				■				■
RESTORES: putting away tools and materials or straightening the workplace				■				■
Navigates: maneuvers the hand and body around obstacles				■				■
Adaptation	**1**	**2**	**3**	**4**	**1**	**2**	**3**	**4**
NOTICES/RESPONDS to nonverbal task-related environmental cues				■				■
ACCOMMODATES: modifies own actions to overcome problems		■				■		
ADJUSTS: changes the workspace to overcome problems				■				■
BENEFITS: preventing problems from recurring or persisting		■				■		
Posture	**1**	**2**	**3**	**4**	**1**	**2**	**3**	**4**
STABILIZES the body for balance			■				■	
ALIGNS the body in vertical position				■				■
POSITIONS the body or arms appropriate to task		■						■
Mobility	**1**	**2**	**3**	**4**	**1**	**2**	**3**	**4**
WALKS about the task environment (level surface)				■				■
REACHES for task objects		■					■	
BENDS or rotates the body appropriate to the task				■				■

Continued on next page

FIGURE 15-1 Judith's Strengths and Limitations Observed during the Administration of the AMPS.

Process Skills	"Preparing Vegetables"				"Ironing Multiple Clothes"			
Coordination	1	2	3	4	1	2	3	4
COORDINATES body parts to securely stabilize task objects								■
MANIPULATES task objects		■					■	
FLOWS: executing smooth and fluid arm and hand movements				■				■
Strength and Effort	1	2	3	4	1	2	3	4
MOVES: pushes and pulls task objects over level surfaces or opens and closes doors or drawers				■				■
TRANSPORTS task objects from one place to another				■				■
LIFTS objects used during the task			■				■	
CALIBRATES: regulates the force and extent of movements				■			■	
GRIPS: maintains a secure grasp on task objects				■				■
Energy	1	2	3	4	1	2	3	4
ENDURES for the duration of the task performance				■				■
Maintains an even and appropriate PACE during task performance			■			■		
Key: 4= Competent 3= Questionable 2= Ineffective 1= Deficit								

FIGURE 15-1 *(continued)*

occupational strengths included her good knowledge of familiar, well-learnt tasks, sequencing, and knowing the tools required to carry these out and their uses; her ability to remain focused when carrying out such tasks; her ability to see tasks through to completion; and her ability to compensate for reduced ability to retain all new task information by utilizing visual information. Her occupational limitations included difficulty retaining the finer details of given tasks (e.g., amounts of food to prepare); and her problem-solving skills when engaged in familiar occupations that were visual or part of her normal routine. She was less able to base decisions on logic, or consider issues related to health and safety within the work setting.

Conclusion

In her previous role, Judith had been responsible for preparing a number of different raw foods, using different colored chopping boards according to whether food was raw or cooked, and whether it was meat, fish, dairy, or vegetable. Her ability to select the correct chopping board, change tools, and sterilize work surfaces according to food hygiene rules had become problematic. *Judith's strengths and limitations according to the AMPS assessment enabled her employer* to not only better understand Judith's previous problems, but opened up discussion around the type of tasks she might be able to carry out safely, efficiently, and independently. For example, one accommodation was to prepare fruit or vegetables by using only one chopping board and knife, which would be set up for her. Part of this plan included having one particular workspace available to Judith at all times, with the aim of her work area becoming both routine and familiar to her. For example, if preparing fruit for a fruit salad, vegetables for later cooking or salad ingredients, the exact quantities required should be laid out visually. Another recommendation included having one designated staff member per shift allocated to set Judith up with tools and ingredients. Finally, it was recommended that Judith should initially work mornings, only.

With the above plan in place, Judith was able to return to work in a part-time capacity and reestablish a chunk of her previously familiar routine. Judith was therefore discharged from the Memory Assessment Service following the above assessment and intervention. Her employer was aware, however, that she could be rereferred to the Occupational Therapist again in the future should her needs change and further adaptation become necessary.

THE VOLITIONAL QUESTIONNAIRE

The VQ (de las Heras, Geist, Kielhofner, & Li, 2007) is a valid and reliable observational assessment that can also be useful for monitoring volitional change over time (Alfredsson Agren & Kjellberg, 2008; Li & Kielhofner, 2004). The VQ is appropriate for any individual for whom a self-report assessment of volition is not feasible (e.g., individuals with dementia or brain damage or persons with extreme volitional problems due to environmental stresses or social traumas). The VQ is based on the recognition that, although people may have difficulty formulating goals or expressing their interests and values verbally, they routinely communicate them through actions. Thus, the VQ scale is composed of 14 items that describe behaviors reflecting values, interests, and personal causation. The items are scored using a 4-point rating scale (passive, hesitant, involved, and spontaneous). The rating indicates the extent to which the person readily exhibits volitional behaviors versus the amount of support, encouragement, and structure that is necessary to elicit them.

This assessment also recognizes that a client's motivation may vary in different environments according to how the features of each environment match the client's interests, values, and personal causation. Consequently, clients are observed in at least two different contexts.

Research on the VQ (Li & Kielhofner, 2004) confirmed that the items on the scale are ordered in a particular sequence from less to more volition. This sequence indicates a volitional continuum that begins with basic behaviors such as being able to initiate action and show preferences (exploratory stage of volition). Higher levels of volition are indicated by the client's willingness to try to solve problems or correct mistakes and in the demonstration of pride (competency stage of volition). The highest level of volition is indicated by such behaviors as seeking challenges and new responsibilities (achievement stage of volition). A specific intervention protocol, the Remotivation Process, involves constant use of the VQ to guide intervention and monitor client progress (refer to Chapter 14).

Administration

Occupational therapists administer this assessment by observing and rating people while they engage in work, leisure, or daily living tasks. Because of the nature of the rating scale, the observing therapist can provide support and structure, if it is necessary, to elicit volition. Observation periods ordinarily last approximately 15 to 30 minutes. The scale and the environmental form can be completed in 20 minutes. Because the assessment can be administered as part of a therapy session in which the environment is systematically varied, it can be used efficiently to explore how different environmental factors influence volition.

The main areas to identify in the analysis of the VQ scale and qualitative information are: (1) those factors in the social and physical environment that most affect volition both positively and negatively; (2) how stable or variable volition is across environments; (3) the level of motivation a person typically displays; (4) the kinds of environmental supports that enhance the individual's volition; and (5) the client's personal causation, interests, and values and how they relate. This kind of information allows the therapist to determine the environmental contexts and strategies that will facilitate positive development of the individual's volition and communicate these to others clearly.

MOHO Problem-Solver Case: Using the VQ to Educate Staff in a Dementia Care Unit

Grace is 89. She has lived in the American Midwest in a continuing care retirement community for the past 5 years. She moved to the retirement community approximately 5 years after her husband, with whom she was married for over 30 years, died. Grace was unable to have children. Having a family was important to her, and she talked regularly about the loss she felt with not being able to have children. Grace was a psychiatric nurse for nearly 40 years. She expressed great satisfaction with her work role, and was very proud of the fact that she returned to school in her 40s to obtain a bachelor of science degree in nursing.

While she initiated the move to the retirement community, Grace's adjustment was not easy. She had a great deal of distress, frequently calling and berating her sister, claiming inaccurately that the sister had made Grace move. Initially perplexed by Grace's behavior, the sister slowly began to recognize the signs of cognitive deterioration in Grace. Grace was diagnosed with dementia. Later, it was determined that Grace would benefit from living in the secure assisted living section for residents with memory impairment. She had been on this unit for nearly 1 year when consultation with occupational therapy was requested to assist Grace to better adjust to the unit. She was often isolative, depressed, suspicious, and argumentative with staff. She stayed at her room most of the time. She came to meals with reminders and coaxing and rarely participated in any of the activities on the unit. Grace was independently mobile on unit, using a wheeled walker while being able to walk short distances safely without it. Grace was able to complete all of her self-care with reminders and verbal cues to identify and correct errors.

Just 1 month before the request for occupational therapy consultation, a nurse obtained a 6-week-old kitten for Grace, hoping this would help Grace "take her mind off her troubles."

The VQ was administered during a 30-minute visit in which the therapist visited with Grace and the kitten in Grace's room. By using an environment where Grace was comfortable, the therapist hoped to discover Grace's volitional strengths. It was noted in the VQ and other interactions with Grace that although her verbal skills were better preserved than those of many other residents on the unit, she often repeated herself and retold several recurring stories about her past. These communications provided helpful insights about her values, as the themes in her stories were consistent and focused on the importance of family relationships, independence, and her desire to be her "own person."

On the VQ, all of Grace's involved and spontaneous scores occurred in the context of interacting with her kitten. Her motivation to care for the kitten was strong and spontaneous. For instance, she always brought food from her meals back to the kitten. She worried that the kitten had no food or that it had escaped from her room. She demonstrated motivation to solve problems, and always sought help from the staff when she perceived the kitten needed something that she could not provide. Grace often attempted to care for the kitten's litter box, resulting frequently in a clogged toilet and the box being moved around her room. Nonetheless, this behavior also demonstrated her desire to provide care and her engagement with the kitten. The kitten's spontaneity and playfulness was motivating for Grace, and provided a new reason for her to engage in occupation (i.e., a meaningful occupation). At the same time, even with this meaningful and pleasurable activity, Grace demonstrated a low sense of capacity and efficacy when trying new things, facing own mistakes, and accepting challenges.

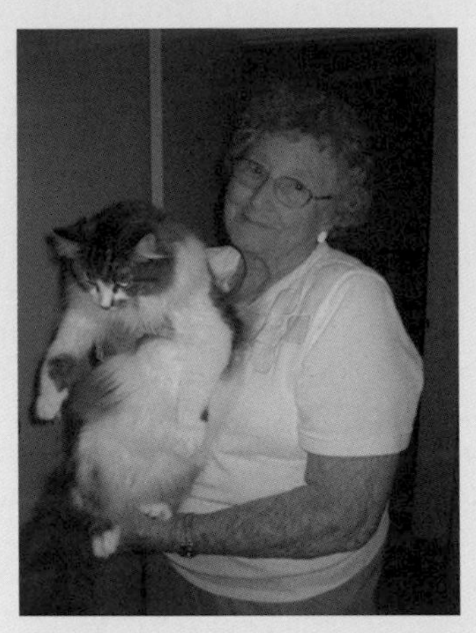

Grace affectionately cuddles with her kitten

Although her sister stated Grace was always well dressed and well made up, and that she loved to be pampered with manicures, Grace said that she did not like "to be fussed over" when the therapist initially offered to give Grace a manicure. The therapist wondered whether this comment indicated a change in her interests. Through using the VQ, it became apparent that Grace's social discomfort drove this comment. As the therapist continued to establish a therapeutic relationship based on empathy and respect toward Grace's values, interests, and decision making, she became more willing to engage in manicures with the therapist.

The exchange between Grace and the therapist during these activities was critical to understand. Recognizing subtle behavioral observations using the VQ ratings can sort out the differences between a client's expressed preferences and her actual willingness to engage in and try new things. Through the VQ and interviews with her sister and staff, the following volitional strengths were noted for Grace: Grace was motivated by her values of independence and for having caring relationships with others. The kitten provided a natural opportunity to exercise these values through developing her caregiver relationship with the kitten. Grace responded well to having her feelings validated in a trusting relationship. Grace's volition was enhanced when the social environment supported her sense of efficacy and honored her values. Grace's volitional weaknesses were seen in her lowered sense of capacity, and her beliefs that she was unable to participate in past interests, as well as her loss of control and sense of despair in coping with the changes in her physical environment. While Grace verbally expressed a lack of attraction to some occupations, these comments were driven by her depression and cognitive impairments and contradicted some things that she still was interested in pursuing. Behavioral observations as captured in the VQ helped identify these remaining interests. When Grace did not feel supported, she became more suspicious and, at times, paranoid. Therefore, she had great difficulty directing and showing interest and investment in doing things, resulting in her isolating herself in her room. The staff often interpreted this behavior as her choice, and if Grace declined encouragement from staff to come out of her room, and join in, staff would leave her alone. The staff's perception was that pushing her made her feel more paranoid.

The therapist shared the findings of the VQ with staff and recommended changing their approach with Grace. Instead of encouraging her to come out of her room, staff was directed to talk with Grace about her major life interests, current and past. They were also guided on how to build trust with Grace more effectively by supporting her sense of efficacy and by honoring her values in their interactions. Staff found that these strategies of interaction proved much more effective in drawing Grace out and in reducing her negative behaviors. Moreover, as the kitten grew, its desire to explore the environment beyond Grace's room created opportunities for Grace to connect more with others and decreased her isolative behavior. Her depression and suspiciousness gradually faded, and Grace began to increase her interactions with residents and staff spontaneously. She appeared to feel more in control of her choices for doing things. Caring for her kitten and visiting remained her valued occupations.

As shown with Grace's story, the VQ is useful not only in terms of understanding important aspects of a client's interests, perceived efficacy, and values (i.e., volition), but in teasing out these volitional aspects by allowing the therapist to attend to what the client is doing and showing nonverbally, rather than to what the client may be saying. Moreover, the VQ may be used to educate professionals from other disciplinary backgrounds to focus more on getting to know clients by observing them nonverbally and by showing clients respect for their volition. The next example demonstrates use of the VQ to enable understanding of the powerful role of a client's environment in terms of influencing volition.

MOHO Problem-Solver Case: Using the VQ to Recognize the Impact of the Therapeutic Milieu (Social Environment) in Dementia Care

Theresa is an 87-year-old widow with dementia who has been residing in an assisted living facility for 5 years. She is a retired nurse who always worked late shifts, and her daily routine still follows these rhythms, preferring to wake late in the morning around 11:00 am. However, at the facility, the breakfast meal is served at 7:00 am, followed by the administration of morning medications. Staff routinely awaken her for both of these activities. When this occurs, she typically goes back to bed and sleeps until 10:30 am. Recently, eating has become of a power struggle between her and most of the staff members, as Theresa refuses to eat meals, especially breakfast and lunch. In this facility, meals are served at designated times in a community dining room. The dining room has seven square tables, accommodating four residents at each table. Linen tablecloths and napkins are used, and meals are served to each resident restaurant style. China dishes and stainless steel flatware are coordinated and contribute to a sense of normalcy for meals. The atmosphere of the dining room is generally calm and soft music is often played, with good overhead lighting. Staff members circulate during meals, assisting with cutting up food, encouraging residents to eat and helping them get started, and stay with, the task of feeding themselves as much as possible. Although staff members employ a range of approaches while working with residents during meals, many take pride in "getting" residents to eat most of their meals, and are usually very task focused while still having a good understanding of food preferences of each resident, such as who likes cream in their coffee and who dislikes soup, and so forth. However, despite these enhancements to the physical environment, staff members often talk to each other while assisting residents, and can be patronizing at times in their approach to encouraging residents to eat.

Theresa has diabetes and requires daily insulin injections and a specific eating routine. According to her family, Theresa historically has enjoyed eating, but on her own terms. Her pattern of eating at home was often skipping breakfast, having a very light lunch (such as cheese, crackers, and fruit), and having a strong preference for sweets and desserts. Because of her diabetes and episodes of hypoglycemia, staff pushed her in each meal to increase her intake, and staff required her to drink a supplement at each meal. Theresa resisted these efforts often, both passively and actively. Her preference to refuse food was seen actively when she said "no," and "I'm not hungry" when coaxed to eat, and passively in her refusal to open her mouth when staff attempted to forcibly coerce her to eat by introducing a spoon into her mouth. At times, Theresa also expressed her preference to not eat by requesting to leave the dining room.

Due to her decreased intake and decline in ability to feed herself, a referral for occupational therapy was initiated to assess Theresa's current ability to feed herself and develop strategies to assist staff in promoting eating in a positive manner. The occupational therapist began by reviewing Theresa's medical record and interviewing staff members who assist Theresa with meals to understand her patterns of eating and to identify potential triggers for her recent decline. One staff member who regularly worked with Theresa during meals reported "You can't fuss over her too much, she doesn't like that." This comment seemed to capture the tension around "getting her to eat," which was experienced negatively by staff and, most importantly, by Theresa. This tension seemed to create a different kind of challenge for staff, namely figuring out how to engage Theresa positively in a way that enhanced her well-being, rather than patronizing her, or demeaning her ability to make choices. The therapist used the VQ to observe one meal with a staff member, and one meal with the therapist. Figures 15-2 and 15-3 show the results of these VQ observations, using Form A (individual observation). The situations in which the VQ was used are described below, highlighting the differences in recognizing and responding to Theresa's volition during two consecutive dinner meals.

Dinner with Staff

Theresa was seated at her usual table, near the window, with two other women who were also residents at the facility. Theresa was pushed back from the edge of the table about one foot, and she was sitting quietly, but bending her knees back and forth so that she was moving forward and backward slightly in her chair, lost in her own thoughts. She was not eating, but her meal had been served. Two staff members, Jane and Sally, were in the dining room, circulating and helping residents with their meals. Sally walked by Theresa's table as she was pouring coffee, and asked Theresa "How's dinner?" glancing at her plate. Theresa turned up her nose and replied "Ehh" and nodded toward her food, which consisted of ground chicken, half a plain baked potato, green beans, a glass of milk, a glass of chocolate supplement shake (which was half finished), a cup of coffee with milk, a glass of water, and a banana. The glasses, cup, and banana were spread out in front of the plate, on a placemat. Jane then came to Theresa's table and served strawberry shortcake to another woman. Theresa looked up at Jane and asked "Can I have some of that?" pointing to the shortcake the woman next to her had begun to eat. Jane nodded, smiled, and said "Sure, let me get your dessert too," and she walked across the room to the dessert cart.

Sally came over to the table, picked up Theresa's spoon, scooped a bite of potatoes and chicken, and moved the spoon within an inch of Theresa's mouth, gruffly saying "You gotta eat . . . you're a diabetic." Sally moved the spoon to touch Theresa's lips, and then Theresa reluctantly opened her mouth and let Sally put the spoon in her mouth. Sally pulled the spoon out, laid it on the table, said "there you go," and turned and walked away from Theresa, going to another table to help someone else to eat. Theresa sat quietly, chewing her bite, swallowed it, and then looked down in her lap. Sally then approached Theresa again, stood over her

Name: Theresa		**Therapist:**				
Age: 87	**Gender:** M F	**Date:**				
Diagnosis: Dementia		**Facility:** Nursing Home				
Meal with Staff Members		**Rating**				**Comments**
Shows curiosity		P	**H**	I	S	*Disengaged from meal unless encouraged by Jane; watched Jane move dishes around and clear her plate away*
Initiates actions/tasks		P	**H**	I	S	*Did not show satisfaction with eating*
Tries new things		**P**	H	I	S	*Did not show satisfaction with eating*
Shows preferences		P	H	I	**S**	*Asked for dessert and showed dislike of dinner meal; asked to leave dining room*
Shows that an activity is special or significant		**P**	H	I	S	*No behaviors indicated that the meal was special or significant*
Stays engaged		**P**	H	I	S	*She did not show emotional connection with eating, despite the constant prompting from Sally and Jane*
Indicates goals		P	H	I	**S**	*Indicated desire to leave dining room and not eating*
Shows pride		**P**	H	I	S	*Did not show satisfaction with eating*
Tries to solve problems		P	H	I	**S**	*Asked Jane to take the dinner plate away, indicating she did not want her dessert plate to sit on top of the dinner plate*
Tries to correct mistakes		**P**	H	I	S	*Passively sat while being fed; momentarily resisted Sally's efforts to feed her*
Pursues an activity to completion/accomplishment		**P**	H	I	S	*Did not finish her meal or supplement shake despite encouragement and being fed by Sally*
Invest additional energy/emotion/attention		**P**	H	I	S	*Required maximum assistance to attend to the activity of eating, even the dessert she requested*
Seeks/accepts additional responsibilities		P	H	I	S	*N/A: No opportunities were given*
Seek/accepts challenges		P	**H**	I	S	*Ate bite of her dessert when it was prepared for her*
Key: (1) P = Passive (2) H = Hesitant (3) I = Involved (4) S = Spontaneous						

FIGURE 15-2 Theresa's Volitional Questionnaire: Meal with Staff Members (Form A).

left side, picked up the spoon and filled it with a bite of potato. Without speaking to Theresa, Sally moved the spoon in front of Theresa's mouth. Looking back at Jane, Sally said loudly, "She gets sugar-free" (referring to the dessert), as she pushed the spoon into Theresa's mouth, not looking at Theresa. Theresa tentatively opened her mouth and took the bite from the spoon.

Jane retrieved the sugar-free strawberry shortcake and brought the dessert to Theresa. Jane began to set the dessert plate at the top right of her plate, and Theresa motioned over the plate, saying "are you going to take this?" Jane asked Theresa "Are you finished?" Theresa said "yes," making a disgusted expression and waving her hand over the plate. Jane picked up Theresa's plate, and pointing to the supplement shake, said, "Then you need to drink your shake." Jane then moved the glass closer to Theresa, repositioned the dessert plate in front of Theresa, speared a bite of the shortcake, and placed the fork on the plate. Theresa nodded, and said "okay," watching Jane as she moved her dishes around. Theresa moved up to the table closer, picked up the shake glass, and took a long sip, setting it

Name: Theresa		**Therapist:**
Age: 87	**Gender:** M F	**Date:**
Diagnosis: Dementia		**Facility:** Nursing Home

Meal with Therapist	Rating				Comments
Shows curiosity	P	**H**	I	S	*Showed curiosity about therapist's joke about being coaxed*
Initiates actions/tasks	P	H	**I**	S	*Readily drank her shake, and took one bite independently, then ate dessert when it was prepared for her on the spoon and placed on the plate*
Tries new things	P	**H**	I	S	*Responded well to the support of having spoon prepared and placed on plate to encourage her to eat cake*
Shows preferences	P	H	I	**S**	*Consistently and spontaneously stated her preferences, and behaviorally showed preference for eating her cake, despite initially verbalizing she wanted to leave the dining room*
Shows that an activity is special or significant	P	**H**	I	S	*Enjoyed eating after the tension of being encouraged to eat was removed*
Stays engaged	P	**H**	I	S	*Stayed engaged with therapist support and then set up to eat dessert*
Indicates goals	P	H	I	**S**	*Stated goals of not eating bites that therapist tried to feed to her, and of wanting to leave, then stay and finish dessert*
Shows pride	P	**H**	I	S	*Small expression of satisfaction when rhythm of eating cake established at the end of interaction*
Tries to solve problems	P	H	**I**	S	*Initiated asking to stay at table to finish dessert when she realized she was being moved away from table*
Tries to correct mistakes	P	H	I	S	*N/A: No mistakes were observed. No indication of mistakes was communicated to Theresa*
Pursues an activity to completion/accomplishment	P	**H**	I	S	*Finished eating cake with supports of preparing each bite and quiet environment*
Invest additional energy/ emotion/attention	P	**H**	I	S	*After moment of humor and being listened to, demonstrated increased attention to eating her dessert*
Seeks/accepts additional responsibilities	P	H	I	S	*N/A: No opportunities were given*
Seek/accepts challenges	P	**H**	I	S	*Accepted to eat with constant support given*
Key: (1) P = Passive (2) H = Hesitant (3) I = Involved (4) S = Spontaneous					

FIGURE 15-3 Theresa's Volitional Questionnaire: Meal with Therapist (Form A).

down again as Jane walked away with the dinner plate. Theresa picked up the fork with a bite of dessert, and ate it, chewing slowly. Then Theresa set her fork down on the plate, and sat quietly.

Sally returned to Theresa's left side, scooped up a bite of the dessert with a spoon, moving the spoon toward Theresa's mouth, without speaking to Theresa. Theresa sat for a moment with her mouth closed, and Sally moved the spoon closer. Then Theresa obediently opened her mouth, and took the bite. Sally put the spoon down, turned and walked away. Jane came to the table again, silently speared another bite of the dessert, and set the fork on Theresa's plate. Jane said to Theresa casually, "How about another bite?" Sally was standing at another table to the left of Theresa, helping another resident eat, and as Jane asked Theresa if she wanted another bite, Sally said to Jane, "Never ask if she wants it, she'll always say no." Jane fed Theresa another bite, and then Theresa asked to go back to her room.

Dinner with the OT

The occupational therapist, Sue, entered the dining room during the evening meal, approached Theresa's table, and pulled up a chair. Sue said, "Hi, Theresa" and Theresa turned to the therapist and, with a look of recognition, said "Hello." Sue sat down in the chair and said to Theresa in a light tone, "Are you still working on your dinner?" Theresa turned up her nose and said "I'm not hungry." Her plate was sitting in front of her, with about one-third of each item eaten. Her meal consisted of ground pork, mashed potatoes, and carrots. Circling the outside of her plate was a glass of strawberry supplement shake, a mug of coffee with milk, and a glass of water. Sue pointed to Theresa's plate and asked "how about another bite?" Theresa shook her head, held out her hand, waving it over the plate, and said "no." With a smile, Sue scooped up some mashed potatoes on her spoon, held up the spoon, and asked again "Try another bite?" Theresa shook her head, pulled back, and said "I'm just not hungry," and she looked at Sue plaintively. Sue put the spoon down and said slowly, "I understand." They sat for a while, and Sue asked Theresa some general questions about her past work as a nurse. Sue then said, "You know, you need to eat . . . Since you have diabetes, if you don't eat, your sugar will be low. And that makes you feel sick." Theresa looked at Sue with a resigned look, and said "But I'm just not hungry." Sue nodded, then suggested to Theresa, "Look at it like a job . . . something you have to do. I bet you needed to encourage your patients to eat when you were a nurse." Theresa shrugged, gave a small smile, and said "I guess." Sue held the spoon of mashed potatoes up over the plate again, and asked "Another bite?" Theresa said "no" and Sue set the spoon of mashed potatoes back on Theresa's plate.

A staff member brought Theresa a small plate of chocolate cake, and Theresa groaned as she saw it being placed on the table. Sue commented, "That looks good." Theresa shook her head again and said emphatically "but I'm not hungry!" Sue nodded, waited for a minute, and then moved the dinner plate off the table. Sue then quietly placed the dessert in front of Theresa and asked, "Want to try your dessert instead?" Noticing that her spoon still had mashed potatoes on it, Sue said, "let me get you a clean spoon" and Theresa nodded at the therapist. Sue stood up and walked over to the shelves where the silverware was located, and retrieved a clean spoon. Sue returned to the table, scooped up a bite of cake, and held it up, saying "Try a bite. It looks good." Theresa made a face at the therapist, keeping her mouth closed. Sue smiled and joked "you never knew you had so many mothers, did you?" Theresa looked at Sue with a confused expression and said "What?" Sue repeated the comment a little louder, looking directly at Theresa, and then Theresa laughed and smiled at the therapist. Sue set the spoon with cake on the dessert plate, and waited. After a moment, Theresa picked up the spoon, and ate the bite. Sue sat quietly with Theresa, and prepared another bite, and set it on the plate, with the spoon angled toward her.

Theresa ate the bite, sighed, and said "I just want to go to my room." Sue pointed to the strawberry shake and said, "If you don't want to eat more, can you finish your shake?" Theresa nodded, picked up the glass, and began sipping it, taking long draws. Sue asked "do you still want to go to your room?" and Theresa said "yes." Sue stood up, went behind Theresa, and began to pull her wheelchair back from the table. Theresa looked up at Sue, confused, and asked "Where are we going?" Sue calmly replied "To your room. I thought you wanted to go?" Theresa shook her head and said "no, I want to finish that" and she pointed to her dessert. Sue said "I'm sorry, I thought you wanted to go. No problem." Sue returned Theresa's wheelchair to the table, and sat down beside her. Sue silently scooped another bite of the dessert, and set the fork on Theresa's plate. Within another minute, Theresa picked up the fork and ate the bite herself, chewing it with enjoyment. Theresa picked up the spoon, scooped a bite up, and ate it, setting the spoon back on the plate. Sue waited, and when Theresa did not initiate taking another bite, she fixed the rest of the cake in the same fashion as before, and Theresa ate in silence, appearing to enjoy the dessert and quiet companionship.

For Theresa, the presence of others while she eats is both a challenge and a support for her volition for eating. Without the support of others, Theresa would have challenges with nutrition. Yet, eating was an activity fraught with many tensions. Using the results of the VQ, the occupational therapist worked with Theresa and staff members, noting that the key to Theresa having an enjoyable meal, while eating a sufficient amount for her health, was to consider her by talking about other things than eating, asking her about her preferences with genuine care, listening to her verbal preferences, and also recognizing her behavioral expressions of preferences. The therapist provided training and worked with staff to help them identify and practice consistent positive responses to support Theresa's observed preferences and abilities, while encouraging health goals of eating enough to maintain her blood sugar at an acceptable level. This paradigm shift requires a greater focus on the relationship with Theresa rather than on the task of eating, which presented a challenge for staff members who derived pride from ensuring residents ate a certain amount of food. With time and coaching, staff members were better able to distinguish her preferences when verbalizations did not match her behaviors, and to determine and use volitional supports that engaged Theresa positively. Through use of these strategies, Theresa's choices and preferences were honored and eating meals became more satisfying. By teaching staff about the importance of volition and the impact of the social environment, the tensions around Theresa's eating were lessened for everyone.

THE ASSESSMENT OF WORK PERFORMANCE

The AWP was originally developed in Sweden with the goal to have an observational assessment based on MOHO, which could be sensitive to assess work performance for diverse populations. The AWP can be used to assess the working skills of individuals with various kinds of work-related problems. As with other MOHO assessments, this instrument is not limited to any particular diagnosis or impairment. The AWP does not target any special tasks or contexts and can be used in various work assessment settings and with work activities performed in actual employment situations/settings, situations where structured work tasks are provided to clients (e.g., work therapy programs, sheltered workshops, work training environments) and in simulated work environments (Sandqvist, Lee, & Kielhofner, 2010).

The purpose of the AWP is to provide information on how efficiently and appropriately the client performs a work activity, assessing three skill domains: motor skills, process skills, and communication and interaction skills. These three domains contain 14 skill items: 5 in the domain of motor skills, 5 in the domain of process skills, and 4 in the domain of communication and interaction skills. Each skill item considers a subgroup of skills which are based on the configuration and content of the AMPS and the ACIS reviewed in this chapter. The authors have organized and redefined some skills to fit them with work contexts and the goals of this new assessment. The instrument has evidence of face validity, content validity, construct validity, and clinical utility (Sandqvist et al., 2010). The instrument is currently used by a large number of assessors working in a variety of work rehabilitation settings which attests to its value in work evaluation. The administration of the AWP is a flexible one in that it considers the unique conditions of workers to adjust the time of evaluation and the involvement of the therapist (or not) as a participant-observer in doing the work task. Moreover, the person assessed is allowed to use any kind of assistive technology or device (e.g., magnification programs for computers or a large print keyboard). Adaptations and adjustments already made before the assessment are considered part of the work situation. Therapists take notes during the entire time of observation, which then serve as data collected for rating the different skill domains. The 14 skills are rated on a 4-point ordinal rating scale, where 1 is the lowest rating (incompetent performance) and 4 is the highest rating (competent performance; Fig. 15-4).

The AWP is typically used in combination with the Worker Role Interview (WRI) and the Work Environment Impact Scale (WEIS) providing complementary, meaningful, and useful information for facilitating the efficiency and efficacy of a person's working role. Chapter 24 contains more detailed information and examples of the use of the AWP and other MOHO work assessments.

Observational Assessments with Children

Therapists can use three of the observational assessment tools to evaluate children's performance skills: (1) the AMPS; (2) the School AMPS (Fisher, Bryze, Hume, & Griswold, 2007); and (3) the ACIS (Forsyth, Salamy, Simon, & Kielhofner, 1998). Therapists can also evaluate children's volition through observations by using the PVQ (Basú, Kafkes, Geitz, & Kielhofner, 2002) for children up to 6 years of age, and the VQ for children older than 6 years of age. The following case examples illustrate the use of these various observational assessments.

Skills	Motor Skills					Process Skills					Communication and Interaction Skills			
	Posture	Mobility	Coordination	Strength	Physical energy	Mental energy	Knowledge	Temporal organization	Organization of space and objects	Adaptation	Physicality	Language	Relations	Information exchange
Ratings	4	4	4	4	4	4	4	4	4	4	4	4	4	4
	(3)	(3)	3	3	(3)	3	3	(3)	3	3	3	(3)	3	(3)
	2	2	(2)	(2)	2	(2)	(2)	2	2	2	(2)	2	(2)	2
	1	1	1	1	1	1	1	1	(1)	(1)	1	1	1	1
	LI	LI	LI	LI	LI	LI	LI	LI	LI	LI	LI	LI	LI	LI
	NR	NR	NR	NR	NR	NR	NR	NR	NR	NR	NR	NR	NR	NR

Key: **4= Competent performance 3= Limited performance 2= Questionable performance 1= Incompetent performance LI= Lack of information NR= Not relevant or N/A.**

FIGURE 15-4 Excerpt from Sample of AWP Summary Form (From Sandqvist, Lee, & Kielhofner, 2010, p. 8).

MOHO Problem-Solver: Using the AMPS with a Preschool-Aged Child

Maggie is a 4 year old who was referred to occupational therapy due to difficulty with basic age-appropriate self-care skills. It is suspected that Maggie has a developmental delay. Maggie lives in a third floor apartment with her two parents and her pet cat. Maggie's mother reportedly lays out Maggie's clothes each evening and gets her dressed each day. Maggie's mother also bathes Maggie and brushes her teeth. Maggie's mother identified that she has difficulty manipulating small tools like puzzle pieces, crayons, her toothbrush, and her hairbrush. Maggie is also reported to have difficulty with completing routine tasks (e.g., toothbrushing) completely and in a logical order.

The occupational therapist's initial assessment plan included the use of a norm-referenced, standardized tool focusing on fine motor and gross motor skills. The results of the evaluation suggested that Maggie did have a delay in fine motor skills. The occupational therapist designed intervention activities such as playing with a peg-board and lacing cards in an attempt to increase Maggie's fine motor skills. After four weekly intervention sessions, the occupational therapist and Maggie's mom were both unsatisfied with Maggie's progress. After discussing Maggie's progress with her mother, the occupational therapist decided to complete another evaluation with a new assessment tool (the AMPS). The occupational therapist knew that this tool would be helpful in identifying Maggie's strengths and areas of need with performing ADLs that were valued by her family.

The evaluation took place in Maggie's home, and the occupational therapist observed Maggie brush her teeth and put on her shoes and socks. The AMPS helped to identify the motor and process skills that Maggie performed competently and those that she had difficulty performing. Maggie demonstrated ineffective performance with the following skills:

- *Aligning* to complete the task by increased propping on bathroom vanity
- *Positioning* to complete the task by long reaches and awkward arm positions
- *Manipulating* to complete the task by difficulty opening the toothpaste and fastening her shoes
- *Coordinating* the two sides of her body as to successfully complete the tasks

- *Continuing* to brush her teeth before rinsing the sink
- *Sequencing* the order of the tasks in a logical fashion
- *Terminating* the tasks by stopping performance before the tasks were completed
- *Noticing and responding* to nonverbal and task-related cues
- *Accommodating* to overcome problems
- *Benefiting* from experience to prevent future difficulties

After interpreting the results of the AMPS, the occupational therapist could tell that focusing on fine motor development would not help Maggie to complete self-care tasks more effectively or efficiently. The AMPS provided the occupational therapy with specific skills on which to focus intervention.

This case illustrated how the AMPS may be used as an observational assessment to identify a child's difficulties with motor and process skills at a granular occupational level. Integrated with detailed assessments of the other occupational dimensions of MOHO, these details allow for more specific treatment planning and therapeutic intervention.

THE SCHOOL ASSESSMENT OF MOTOR AND PROCESS SKILLS

The School AMPS (Fisher et al., 2007) is a standardized assessment based on the therapist's observation of the quality of the child's performance during typical school tasks. The School AMPS can be used to simultaneously measure the quality of 16 motor skills and 20 process skills using the AMPS' 4-point rating scale. Therapists can use the School AMPS to evaluate children between the ages of 3 and 15 years with and at-risk for school-related performance difficulties. This tool is administered in the child's typical classroom environment with the child's teacher, and with at least four classmates. The School AMPS can be readministered over time to assess the child's progress, which makes it particularly useful for the educational team. Prior to administration, the therapist collaborates with the child's teacher to identify two of the standardized AMPS tasks during which the therapist will observe and rate the quality of the child's performance. The results gained from the School AMPS can assist the therapist in designing an intervention plan geared at improving the child's occupational performance at school. The results can also serve as a basis for providing education and consultation to school teams.

THE ASSESSMENT OF COMMUNICATION AND INTERACTION SKILLS

The ACIS (Forsyth et al., 1998) is a valid and reliable formal observation tool that is focused on gaining information to determine a client's strengths and weaknesses in interacting and communicating with others in the course of daily occupations (Forsyth, Lai, & Kielhofner, 1998). Like the other observation-based tools previously discussed, the ACIS helps the therapist to discover the client's strengths and weaknesses as they relate to communication and interaction.

The ACIS is appropriate to use with children above 3 years of age, adolescents, and adults. The ACIS observations are carried out in varied social contexts that are meaningful and relevant to the clients' lives. The group context can range from a dyadic interaction to participation in a large group, and a wide range of social contexts can be used for observation. Because social situations cannot be standardized with the same precision as solitary occupational forms (such as those used in the AMPS), the ACIS does not adjust scores for the type of social group or task in which the person is observed. Thus, therapists who use the ACIS must be culturally and socially competent so that they are able to assign accurate ratings based on the social interactions observed.

The ACIS consists of 20 skill items that are divided into three domains: physicality, information exchange, and relations. The therapist rates the client using the ACIS on a 4-point scale (competent, questionable, ineffective, and deficit) and considers the impact that the skills have on the progression of the social interaction, the impact on other persons with whom the client interacts, and the impact on the completion of a common task or activity.

Administration

Prior to administration, an interview should be conducted with the client or a caregiver in order to select the occupational contexts that will be the focus of the observation. After the interview, the therapist completes the observation, rating, and interpretation.

The total administration time for the ACIS varies from 20 to 60 minutes. Observation time ranges from 15 to 45 minutes. The rating is completed after conclusion of the session. Rating time ranges from 5 to 20 minutes depending on the amount of qualitative comments the therapist wishes to enter into the form. The ACIS can be used to generate a profile of strengths and weaknesses and qualitative details about any of the client's problems. This profile is the most important source of information for deciding what skills to target for change. In addition, the qualitative information gained in the course of administering the ACIS is often helpful for understanding why a particular client is having difficulty with some communication/interaction skills. A final use of the ACIS is to identify social environments that have the most positive impact on the client's communication and interaction. Such information can be useful in deciding a program of enhancing communication interaction skills in relevant social settings.

MOHO Problem-Solver Case: Application of the ACIS with a School-Aged Child

Ethan is an 8-year-old student in a segregated school for children with significant social and emotional disabilities. Two of Ethan's teachers report that he has trouble interacting with adults and fellow classmates, and they believe this is due to his difficulties speaking. Ethan particularly seems to struggle when he perceives the task demands to be greater than his skill level, which is particularly pronounced in physical education. Ethan can generally follow along with the routine of practicing new skills. When learning new skills, the physical education teacher will generally do a demonstration in front of the entire class and then ask for individual students, who already have some proficiency with the skill, to act as another model. Then, the class breaks up and each student goes to his or her own area of the gym to practice the skill individually while the teacher walks around and provides feedback. Ethan struggles with bilateral coordination and is often slow to master the new skills that are presented in physical education. He has previously been heard saying, "My dad says sports are stupid. Why do I have to do this stuff?" Often, before he has experienced a sense of mastery, the physical education introduces a game where students need to demonstrate their proficiency with the different skills. Ethan has a great deal of difficulty with social interactions during group sports that involve ball skills (e.g., basketball, soccer, and volleyball). For example, when Ethan feels pressed by time or that another student has committed a foul or stolen the ball from him, Ethan will often raise his voice, confront the other student using inappropriate language, and gesture like he is going to hit him or her. When an adult intervenes, Ethan generally continues to have difficulty controlling the volume of his voice and accepting the adult's redirections.

Despite these challenges, Ethan's speech and language pathologist believes that Ethan has made a great deal of progress on his speech goals. The occupational therapist mentioned at a team meeting that there might be a way to evaluate Ethan's difficulties with social interactions without focusing on speech production. The team encourages the occupational therapist to complete an observation. The therapist gets ready to schedule the observation and realizes that, without an occupation-focused framing of social interaction, the observation will be difficult to complete. The therapist researches various assessments and decides to complete the ACIS.

The therapist interviews Ethan's teachers prior to ACIS administration and they determine that Ethan should be observed during noncompetitive social situations that involve group effort, rather than individual effort. The therapist and the teacher agree that Ethan will be observed during classroom group work and during physical education class. During the first observation, Ethan is observed in math class where students are divided into groups of four to practice math flash cards. Each student takes turns holding the deck of flashcards and quizzing the other students. Ethan knows his multiplication facts and enjoys playing the flashcard game. Ethan likes quizzing his peers and taking his turn to answer the questions. When Ethan is quizzing his peers and they do not know an answer, Ethan tries to give them a clue and allows them to make another guess before providing the correct answer. Ethan provides high-fives to his classmates when they get an answer correct and is heard providing positive verbal feedback (e.g., "Nice job"). When Ethan gets a question incorrect, which is infrequently, he snaps his fingers and says, "I'm going to practice that one with my dad at home."

During the second observation, Ethan is observed in physical education class during the volleyball unit. The students are divided into two teams, and each team member rotates through the different positions on the floor. When it is Ethan's turn to serve the ball, his classmates cheer him on. Ethan fails at his first attempt to serve the ball over the net and is given a second chance by the physical education teacher. When Ethan's teammates begin cheering again, Ethan slams the volleyball down on the court and runs up to one of the students that was cheering the loudest. Ethan makes a motion like he is going to strangle the student and then proceeds to move closer to the student and wave his arms around while yelling curse words loudly. When the teacher attempts to redirect him by placing a hand on his shoulder, Ethan does not make eye contact and harshly brushes the teacher's hand off of his shoulder. Ethan is told to take a different position on the floor. During the rest of the game, Ethan does not rotate to a new position unless he is given multiple redirections. When a teammate calls to him for an assist to get the ball over the net, Ethan turns away from the student and does not attempt to make contact with the ball. When a ball comes toward Ethan, he attempts to get it over the next but does not ask for similar assistance. At the end of the game, Ethan does not line up with the rest of his teammates to shake hands with the opposing team nor does he join his team's schedule.

After the observations, the occupational therapist determines that Ethan is more effectively able to use communication and interaction skills during classroom group work than during athletics. During classroom group work, Ethan is able to competently exchange information, engage in appropriate relations, and maintain appropriate physicality (e.g., contacting, gazing, gesturing, orientating, and posturing). However, in physical education, Ethan is ineffective with the following communication and interaction skills:

- Gesturing
- Maneuvering
- Orienting
- Posturing
- Articulating
- Asking
- Modulating
- Collaborating
- Conforming
- Focusing
- Relating
- Respecting

The therapist presents the findings from the ACIS to Ethan's team and they determine that Ethan would benefit from joining a social skills group. In addition, the occupational therapist plans to consult with the physical education teacher regarding how the environment could be modified to better support the communication and interaction skills of Ethan and his classmates.

This example illustrates how the ACIS may be used to more precisely identify the nature of a child's communication difficulties. When first working with Ethan, it was unclear whether his central difficulty was one of speech production or one more social in nature, involving communication and interaction skills. The ACIS helped to clarify that therapy intervention needed to focus on the latter of the two issues under consideration.

THE PEDIATRIC VOLITIONAL QUESTIONNAIRE

The PVQ (Basú et al., 2002) is an observational assessment that is similar to the VQ and intends to capture a younger child's volition and the environmental impact on it. The PVQ is appropriate to use with children between the ages of 2 and 6. However, it may be used with older children and adolescents that demonstrate significant developmental delays. The assessment has shown to be valid and reliable (Anderson, Kielhofner, & Lai, 2005) and it can also be used to measure progress of volition over time (Taylor et al., 2010).

The PVQ consists of 14 items that are plotted along a continuum of volitional development ranging from exploration to competency to achievement. The PVQ items parallel many of those on the VQ, but the items are designed to be developmentally appropriate to younger children. The items are rated using the same scale as used for the VQ.

Administration

Prior to administration, the therapist selects the environments that will be relevant for observing the child. Selecting different environments allows the therapist to determine how environmental factors influence the child's volition. Therapists may opt to observe the child in natural environments, such as a child's home, school, local public playground, or in different clinical environments, such as an OT clinic. It is recommended that the therapist observe the child for at least 15 minutes in each environment, with most observations ranging between 15 and 30 minutes.

The PVQ follows the same procedures of administration, rating, analysis than the VQ, including filling out the environmental forms and summary of observations. The PVQ ratings and qualitative information can be used in designing treatment programs and interventions as well as for providing feedback and suggestions to parents, teachers, or other caregivers.

CASE EXAMPLE: USING THE PVQ WITH A SCHOOL-AGED CHILD

Michael is a 6-year-old boy who likes cars, going to the movies, and playing with his dog, "Pal." Michael has four older brothers and one younger sister. He lives with his siblings and parents in a single-family home in a suburban community. Michael attends full-day kindergarten at his local elementary school. He has been receiving occupational therapy services since he was 6 months old due to occupational performance difficulties related to his diagnosis of Down's syndrome. Michael wears glasses and generally communicates by using sentences that are two-to-four words in length. Michael is sometimes difficult to understand, particularly when he is excited or upset. Michael is able to use a spoon and a fork, undress himself, and color simple shapes. He is making good progress using his two hands together to snip paper with scissors and put on his shoes. He enjoys going to kindergarten and can name several friends. Michael's siblings all play baseball and he was recently enrolled in a park district tee-ball program. Initially, Michael was excited for the opportunity to play ball like his older siblings. However, recently, Michael has begun throwing himself on the floor and crying when he learns that it is time to go to tee-ball. It generally takes 10 minutes for Michael's dad to calm him down enough to get him in the car and take him to tee-ball.

Rationale for Using the PVQ

Michael's dad does not understand why Michael does not want to go to tee-ball, since he enjoys watching his siblings play baseball and often wears his baseball glove at home. Michael's dad shares his concern with the occupational therapist. The occupational therapist determines that more information is needed in order to develop strategies that could facilitate Michael's participation in tee-ball. The occupational therapist was especially curious to learn more about Michael's participation in other environments that potentially pose challenges to him. The occupational therapist decided to complete the PVQ to gain insight into Michael's volition and to better understand aspects of the environment that influence Michael's volition.

Administration of the PVQ

The occupational therapist made arrangements to visit Michael's classroom under the assumption that he may encounter situations that pose a challenge in his kindergarten program. The occupational therapist consulted with Michael's teacher and learned that the activities included during more complex and physically engaging activities (such as Center Time) sometimes posed a challenge to Michael, as well as to several other students. The occupational therapist also consulted with Michael's dad and arranged a time to observe Michael during tee-ball.

Center Time Observation

The first observation took place in Michael's kindergarten classroom and lasted 20 minutes. Michael's teacher, a student teacher, and 19 other students were present during the observation. The students sat in child-sized tables and chairs, rather than desks. Each table had four students. Michael knew the students at his table well. The teacher announced that center time was about to begin and explained that the students at each table were a group and that each group would rotate together to the different centers. The students would rotate when the teacher rang a bell. The different centers for the day included the art center, the reading center, the math center, the science center, and the listening center. Each of the centers included a written checklist with picture cues and was included with the intention that the students would be fairly independent with completing the task at each center. The art center activity consisted of the students using a model to replicate an outdoor scene with construction of paper shapes. Some of the shapes used to make the scene were precut. However, one of the shapes required the students to cut a piece of paper in half. Students were also required to use a glue stick to adhere the shapes to a larger piece of paper. The reading center activity involved the students reading sight words out aloud to each other and to the teacher. The math center activity involved the students counting small colored blocks and graphing the number of blocks using crayons on a premade worksheet. The science center activity involved watching a frog in an aquarium and drawing it with the appropriate number of body parts. The listening center activity involved listening to a story through headphones and following along in a story book. For the purpose of the observation, the occupational therapist observed Michael during transitions to two centers, as well as during the art and math centers.

When the first bell rang, Michael clapped his hands, smiled, and walked with his group over to the art center. One of the students read the checklist out aloud to the rest of the group and pointed out each picture cue. The three other students picked up their scissors and began cutting a green piece of paper in half. Michael smiled and watched the students cut until one of his classmates cued him to get started. Michael then picked up the scissors and began snipping with a look of concentration on his face. Michael and another student were unable to cut the paper in half. However, Michael did not appear deterred. Rather, when Michael encountered this difficulty, he turned to see what his peer was doing. Michael watched the other student who had difficulty cutting his paper in half and without hesitation, Michael followed suit. Michael then immediately picked up the glue stick and began to put glue on half of the green piece of paper. The rest of the students completed this step as well. Once everyone had glued the green piece of paper, another student asked the group what was next. Michael gestured to the checklist and a student read the next direction out aloud. Michael clapped his hands and smiled and then picked up the next shape and began gluing it on to his piece of paper. Michael completed the rest of the art project in a similar fashion. Two out of the eight shapes that Michael glued on the paper matched the model. When the bell rang to go to the next station, one of the students gave Michael a high-five. Michael smiled at the student and laughed. Then, Michael continued smiling and laughing and high-fived the other two students. Michael laughed to himself while he walked with his group to the math station and pointed at the checklist. Another student read the checklist instructions out aloud and pointed to the picture cues. Michael quickly picked up the baggies of the colored blocks, smiled, and put one on his head. The students laughed. Then, Michael looked at each of the bags and took the one with the green blocks for himself. Michael then gave a bag to each of the students. As Michael gave the baggies to the students, he smiled and patted each of their hands. Another student passed out the graphing worksheets. Michael accepted his graphing worksheet, smiled, and signed, "thank you." Michael opened his baggie and dumped out his blocks immediately and began constructing a face (i.e., two blocks for eyes, one block for a nose, and four blocks for a mouth). Then, he watched with concentration the student sitting next to him. The student said, "I'm going to find all of the red ones first and put them in a pile." Michael intently watched the student for approximately another 30 seconds and then began putting the red blocks in a pile. The other student asked the group, "Do we sort them all first or fill out the graph after the red ones?" The two other students gave their opinions and one of the students asked Michael what he thought. Michael laughed and smiled and said, "Sort." The three other students agreed to sort the rest of the blocks before filling out the worksheet. Michael clapped when he saw that his peers were following his direction. When the teacher's bell rang, the other students in Michael's group were filling out their worksheets and Michael was still intently sorting his blocks. The other students began putting their blocks back in their baggies. When Michael heard the group chattering about putting their blocks away, he looked up, smiled, and then followed suit. Once all of the blocks were in his baggie, Michael laughed and initiated a high-five with another classmate and the observation concluded.

Tee-Ball Observation

The second observation took place at tee-ball. The occupational therapist observed Michael get out of his family's car and walk with his dad over to the tee-ball field. Michael's dad led him to the tee-ball field and Michael walked with his head down. The coach greeted Michael warmly and instructed him to line up for stretching and calisthenics. Michael smiled and waved hello and put his head back down. Five other children were already on the field. They were talking and playing a modified game of tag. Michael walked over to the group after more coaxing from the coach. Michael kept his head down and none of the children acknowledged him. Within approximately one minute of Michael's arrival, the coach blew his whistle and began to call out exercises and stretches. The coach's whistle appeared to startle Michael. The coach called out jumping jacks and the five other children began doing jumping jacks and counting out aloud. Michael picked up his head and observed the children jumping; however, the children had completed nine jumping jacks before Michael began jumping and moving his arms, approximating a jumping jack. The other children abruptly stopped performing jumping jacks after they counted to 10. Michael continued to jump and move his arms about. The coach blew his whistle and said, "Michael, stop. We're moving on." Michael appeared frustrated when the coach provided him with that redirection and let out an audible sigh. The coach then called out arm circles. The other children began performing arm circles and counting. This time, Michael smiled and began moving his arms around after the other children's third repetition. The children abruptly stopped again once they had counted to 10. Michael smiled and continued to move his arms around and the coach again blew his whistle and corrected Michael. Michael appeared startled by the coach's whistle. Michael again let out an audible sign, and this time he stamped his right foot and crossed his arms. Michael and the other children completed several other exercises and stretches in a similar fashion before the coach blew his whistle again and then started calling out positions on the baseball diamond. When the coach told Michael to go to third base, he looked down at the ground and did not move. The coach blew his whistle again and repeated the instruction. Michael, startled at the sound of the whistle, then made an audible sigh before walking reluctantly to first base. The child that was at first base pushed Michael and Michael started crying. The coach walked over, said something inaudible to the occupational therapist, took Michael's hand, and walked him over to third base. Michael continued to cry and walked with the coach with his head down. Michael sat down on the top of third base and continued to cry for approximately 2 minutes. After approximately 2 minutes, Michael was no longer crying. However, he remained seated and began playing with a shoe lace. Michael did not attend to the game that was being played on the field. The observation concluded (Fig. 15-5).

After the two observations, the occupational therapist shared the findings from the PVQ with Michael's parents. The occupational therapist noted that Michael struggled more with volition during tee-ball than he did during center time and suggested that a lack of volition was impacting his participation during tee-ball. The occupational therapist noted two key differences between the observations: (1) external structure and (2) the use of peer supports.

PEDIATRIC VOLITIONAL QUESTIONNAIRE (PVQ) (Form B)

	Shows curiosity	Initiates actions	Task directed	Shows preferences	Tries new things	Stays engaged	Expresses mastery pleasure	Tries to solve problems	Tries to produce effects	Practices skill	Seeks challenges	Modifies environment	Pursues activity to completion	Uses imagination
Session 1				**Date: 4/24/15**							**Setting: Classroom Center Time**			
	S	**S**	**S**	**S**	S	**S**	S	S	S	**S**	S	**S**	S	**S**
	I	I	I	I	**I**	I	**I**	**I**	**I**	I	**I**	I	**I**	I
	H	H	H	H	H	H	H	H	H	H	H	H	H	H
	P	P	P	P	P	P	P	P	P	P	P	P	P	P
Session 2				**Date: 4/26/15**									**Setting: Tee-ball**	
	S	S	S	S	S	S	S	S	S	S	S	S	S	S
	I	**I**	I	I	I	I	I	I	I	I	I	I	I	I
	H	**H**	H	H	**H**	**H**	H	H	**H**	**H**	H	H	H	H
	P	P	P	**P**	P	P	**P**	**P**	P	P	**P**	**P**	**P**	**P**

Key: **P=Passive** **H=Hesitant** **I=Involved** **S=Spontaneous**

Strengths: Task directed in both settings, shows curiosity, initiates actions, shows preferences, stays engaged, practices skill, modifies environment, and shows imagination during center time.

Needs Support: Michael received a rating of passive for showing preferences, expressing mastery pleasure, trying to solve problems, seeking challenges, modifying environment, showing imagination, and pursuing activity to completion during tee-ball.

Other Notes: Michael appears to benefit from peer supports.

FIGURE 15-5 Michael's PVQ Ratings and Summary.

First, the teacher constructed center time in a way that provided the students with external structure and supported Michael's demonstration of volition. The use of a bell to signal transitions, the establishment of groups, and the inclusion of a written checklist with picture cues were all factors that likely influenced Michael's volition. Second, the other students in Michael's center time group supported his volition when they read the directions out aloud, pointed out picture cues, asked for his opinion, and gave him high-fives. This structure and the inclusion of positive peer supports provided Michael with an opportunity to feel good about his performance, which helped to foster his personal causation.

The occupational therapist concluded that Michael would benefit from a peer buddy during tee-ball so that he could follow a model and feel more efficacious about his performance. The peer buddy could also greet Michael when his dad dropped him and off. The peer buddy could also bring him to the stretching area. The occupational therapist recommended ways to provide more external structure to tee-ball. For example, rather than lining up for exercises, the occupational therapist recommended that the coach arrange the children in a circle so that Michael could look directly across the circle and follow the actions of a peer. The occupational therapist also suggested that the coach allow just a few seconds more of additional transition time before starting the next exercise in order to give Michael the chance to catch up and switch gears. The occupational therapist also recommended the use of additional visual supports (e.g., color coding the bases) to cue Michael, as well as the other children, to their positions on the field.

As this case illustrates, the PVQ framed the occupational therapist's observations and allowed for a richer understanding of Michael's participation during circle time and tee-ball. By using this assessment, the occupational therapist helped Michael's dad understand why he was hesitant to participate in tee-ball, which was connected directly to one of the family's highly valued occupations.

Conclusion

This chapter described a range of MOHO assessments that use observation as a means of collecting information about clients. Four assessments provide important information about clients' motor, process, and communication/interaction skills. The two volitional assessments provide information about the client's motivation. All assessments use rating scales to record the observations and allow qualitative information to be gathered as well. Each of the assessments also takes into consideration the effects of the environment on the observed skill or volition.

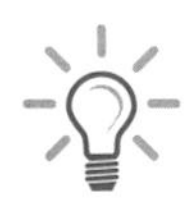

Chapter 15 Review Questions

1. What are the observational assessments that are developed explicitly to be administered by others than the occupational therapist?
2. What is the difference between the scales of the AMPS and the ACIS versus the ones of the VQ and the PVQ?
3. What is the difference between the AMPS, ACIS, and AWP?

HOMEWORK ASSIGNMENTS

1. Think of a child or adult you know well in your practice. (A) Select one or more observational assessment that could meet his or her needs and give arguments about why you chose it. (B) Think of which environmental contexts would be appropriate for its administration with this unique person.
2. Reflect on differences on ratings of both VQ forms of Theresa. Look at the forms first, and then get back to the comments that the therapist makes.
3. Describe the involvement of the occupational therapist when administering the AMPS, the ACIS, and the VQ or PVQ.

Key Term

MOHO observational assessments: Assessments that use systematic observation as the method to gather information about performance, volition, and environmental impact.

REFERENCES

Alfredsson Agren, K., & Kjellberg, A. (2008). Utilization and content validity of the Swedish version of the Volitional Questionnaire. *Occupational Therapy in Health Care, 22*(2–3), 163–176.

Anderson, S., Kielhofner, G., & Lai, J. S. (2005). An examination of the measurement properties of the Pediatric Volitional Questionnaire. *Physical and Occupational Therapy in Pediatrics*, 25, 39–57.

Basú, S., Kafkes, A., Geist, R., & Kielhofner, G. (2002). *The pediatric volitional questionnaire: A user's manual* [Version 2.0]. Chicago: The Model of Human Occupation Clearinghouse, Department of Occupational Therapy, College of Applied Health Sciences, University of Illinois at Chicago.

de las Heras, C. G., Geist, R., Kielhofner, G., & Li, Y. (2007). *The Volitional Questionnaire (VQ)* [Version 4.1]. Chicago: Model of Human Occupation Clearinghouse, Department of Occupational Therapy, College of Applied Health Sciences, University of Illinois at Chicago.

Fisher, A. G., Bryze, K., Hume, V., & Griswold, L. A. (2007). *School AMPS: School version of the assessment of motor and process skills* (2nd ed.). Ft. Collins, CO: Three Star Press.

Fisher, A. G., & Jones, K. B. (2012). *Assessment of motor and process skills: Vol. 1: Development, standardization, and administration manual* (Revised 7th ed.). Fort Collins, CO: Three Star Press.

Forsyth, K., Lai, J., & Kielhofner, G. (1998). The Assessment of Communication and Interaction Skills (ACIS): Measurement properties. *British Journal of Occupational Therapy, 62*(2), 69–74.

Forsyth, K., Salamy, M., Simon, S., & Kielhofner, G. (1998). *The assessment of communication and interaction skills* [Version 4.0]. Chicago: Model of Human Occupation Clearinghouse, Department of Occupational Therapy, College of Applied Health Sciences, University of Illinois at Chicago.

Li, Y., & Kielhofner, G. (2004). Psychometric properties of the Volitional Questionnaire. *The Israel Journal of Occupational Therapy, 13*(3), E85–E98.

NeuRA. (2012). *Addenbrooke's cognitive examination*. New South Wales, Australia: Author.

Sandqvist, J., Lee, J., & Kielhofner, G. (2010). *Assessment of Work Performance (AWP): A user's manual* [Version 1.0]. Chicago: Model of Human Occupation Clearinghouse, Department of Occupational Therapy, College of Applied Health Sciences, University of Illinois at Chicago.

Taylor, R. R., Kielhofner, G., Smith, C., Butler, S., Cahill, S. M., Ciukaj, M. D., et al. (2010). Volitional change in children with autism: A single-case design study of the impact of hippotherapy on motivation. *Occupational Therapy in Mental Health, 25*(2), 192–200.

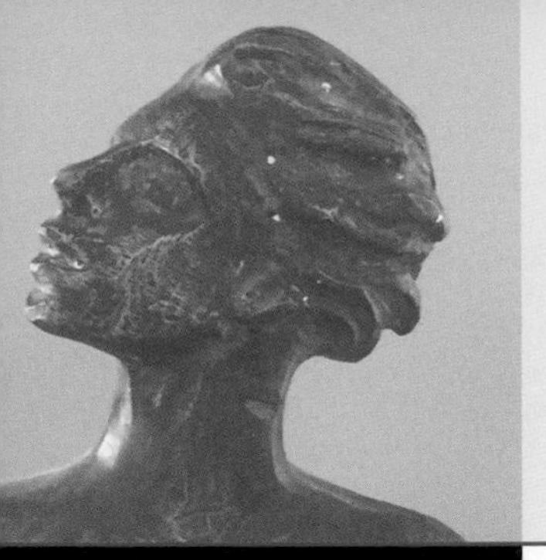

Self-Reports: Eliciting Clients' Perspectives

Jessica Kramer, Kirsty Forsyth, Patricia Lavedure, Patricia J. Scott, Rebecca Shute, Donald Maciver, Marjon ten Velden, Meghan Suman, Hiromi Nakamura-Thomas, Takashi Yamada, Riitta Keponen, Ay-Woan Pan, and Gary Kielhofner (posthumous)

CHAPTER 16

EXPECTED LEARNING OUTCOMES

Upon completion of this chapter, readers will be able to:

1. Identify self-reports appropriate for clients across the life course, from childhood to older adulthood.
2. Identify the model of human occupation (MOHO) concepts assessed by a variety of self-reports.
3. Describe administrative procedures for self-report assessments.
4. Understand how a self-report assessment can be used to identify client-centered goals and plan occupational therapy intervention.

Self-Report Assessments

Clients are experts on their own lives. Self-reports based on the model of human occupation (MOHO) capture this expertise and allow clients of all ages to share information about themselves, their life circumstances, and their environments. Occupational therapists can use this information to identify client-centered goals and to design interventions that address a client's unique needs in the areas of volition, habituation, skills, and the environment.

The use of self-report assessments has several benefits. First, the act of thinking about and responding to a self-report provides clients with the opportunity to reflect on their abilities and needs, which can lead to more effective problem-solving and planning during intervention. Second, the use of a self-report demonstrates a value for client-centered occupational therapy and conveys respect for a client's perspective and experiences. Third, the information gathered during self-reports can provide therapists with a deeper understanding of a client's circumstances and may reveal new knowledge that is essential for successful intervention or that helps resolve a clinical challenge (Kramer et al., 2012).

MOHO has a variety of self-reports appropriate for clients of all ages to share their perspectives and participate in intervention planning. MOHO self-reports may also be used with clients with different diagnoses. Some self-reports, such as the Interest Checklist (Kielhofner & Neville, 1983) or Role Checklist (Oakley, Kielhofner, & Barris, 1985), are shorter and ask about concrete activities, and can be completed by clients with more significant cognitive and communication impairments who are able to communicate basic interests and preferences. Other self-reports include more complex questions and rating responses, such as the Occupational Self-Assessment (Baron, Kielfhofner, Iyenger, Goldhammer, & Wolenski, 2006) and require clients to recall a greater range of experiences and use abstract reasoning to match their personal experiences with different rating categories. To determine whether a self-report is appropriate for a client, therapists should consider the match between a client's motor, process, and communication/interaction skills and the self-report questions, rating scales, and other features. Table 16-1 summarizes the age group that may be appropriate for each self-report and the MOHO concepts assessed by each self-report. This chapter will review the basic information about each self-report and provide a few in-depth examples of self-report administration with clients.

ADMINISTERING SELF-REPORTS FOR OPTIMAL INFORMATION

The MOHO self-report assessments are designed to be user friendly, and much focus has been placed on the clarity of language, directions, and form design during the development of these assessments. The goal has been to make the self-reports easy to use across a variety of intervention contexts for clients with a range of abilities and needs. Although these assessments are ordinarily administered as forms to be filled out independently by the client, therapists do administer them in different ways

Table 16-1 Summary of MOHO Self-report Assessments

	Age				MOHO Concepts Assessed			
	Children	*Adolescents/ Young Adults*	*Adults*	*Older Adults*	*Volition*	*Habituation*	*Skills*	*Environment*
ACHIEVE Assessment	X	X			X	X	X	X
CIRCLE Assessment	X	X			X	X	X	X
Child Occupational Self-assessment (COSA)	X	X			X	X	X	
Making it Clear				X	X	X		X
Modified Interest Checklist		X	X	X	X			
Occupational Self-Assessment (OSA)		X	X	X	X	X	X	X
Occupational Questionnaire and Activity Record								
Pediatric Interest Profiles	X	X			X			
Role Checklist Version 3: Performance and Satisfaction		X	X	X		X		

to accommodate needs of clients. For example, they are sometimes given verbally when clients have difficulty reading and/or writing. Some self-reports, such as the Child Occupation Self-Assessment (Kramer et al., 2014) and Pediatric Interest Profiles (Henry, 2000), include images to help younger children or adolescents with cognitive impairments understand the questions and rating scales. It can also be appropriate to administer self-report assessments as part of a group planning or problem-solving exercise, as long as individual clients are assured they can choose to keep their answers private from the group.

When completing a self-report, therapists should assure clients that there are no right or wrong answers, and that the information shared will help therapy meet the client's needs. Box 16-1 includes an example script to describe the purpose

Box 16-1: A therapist explaining a self-report to a client

I'm your occupational therapist, and I can help you be better at all the things you do each day—taking care of yourself, your family, and your home; working at your job (if you have one); doing things in your neighborhood; and having fun. We can make sure occupational therapy helps you by finding out how you feel about different activities.

To do that, you are going to answer some questions about yourself using this form. There are no right or wrong answers. You can fill this out by yourself, and when you are done we can talk about it. Or, if you would like, I can stay here to help you.

I want to know what you think about doing these different activities. Don't worry about what other people think about you, like your parent/caregiver or your doctor/teacher, just answer for yourself. Remember, everyone has problems doing some activities and is good at others, and that's ok. We can work together to help you get better at the things that are most important to you.

of a self-report to a client. When using self-reports with all clients, therapists should always discuss the client's answers in order to clarify what the client was thinking about. It is often useful to discuss the questions given the highest and the lowest rating. For clients who have difficulty with memory and attention, such as younger children, adults with intellectual disabilities, or older adults with dementia, therapists may gather better information by discussing a client's answer to each question as it is answered rather than waiting until the entire assessment is completed. Therapists may also want to monitor a client when they are completing a self-report. Clients who change their pace of response (answer each question more quickly or more slowly) may be losing attention and may need to take a break. Clients who show "thinking" actions (hand to chin, furrowing their brow) or who change their answers may need help understanding the question or selecting the response that best matches what they are thinking. Therapists should refer to each self-report assessment manual for more specific directions on administering the different MOHO self-reports.

Modified Interest Checklist

The Modified Interest Checklist is a leisure interest inventory appropriate for adolescents, adults, and older adults (Kielhofner & Neville, 1983). As shown in Figure 16-1, clients indicate their level of interest in each of the items over the past 10 years and the past 1 year. Further, clients indicate whether they actively participate in and would like to pursue each potential interest in the future. This checklist is interpreted by examining each client's unique pattern of interests and determining whether a client: (1) does not have sufficient interests to support occupational adaptation, (2) is unable to enact interests because of disability or the environment, or (3) requires support to continue or begin participation in valued activities. Therapists and researchers have also made numerous modifications to the Interest Checklist to reflect local customs and cultures. One example is a British Activity Checklist that utilizes a modified rating scale and an alternative method of interpreting results. Another example is the Japanese Elderly Version of the Interest Checklist (Yamada, Ishii, & Nagatani, 2002) that is illustrated in the Akira case.

	What has been your level of interest?						Do you currently participate in this activity?		Would you like to pursue this in the future?	
	In the past ten years			In the past year						
Activity:	Strong	Some	No	Strong	Some	No	Yes	No	Yes	No
Gardening/Yardwork										
Sewing/Needlework										
Playing cards										
Foreign languages										
Church activities										
Radio										
Walking										
Car repair										
Writing										
Dancing										
Golf										
Football										
Listening to popular music										

FIGURE 16-1 Format of the Modified Interest Checklist.

MOHO Problem-Solver: Using the Interest Checklist Japanese Elderly Version (ICJEV) to Engage a Client with Dementia

Akira is a married elderly man and is currently living in a nursing care facility in Tokyo, Japan, because of onset of dementia. Upon moving to the nursing care facility, he seemed depressed and refused to leave his room. Nursing staff were unable to engage Akira in group activities like music group. Akira's occupational therapist used the Japanese Elderly Version of the Interest Checklist (ICJEV) to identify interests that could help Akira participate in the facility.

Using the ICJEV, Akira indicated two strong interests: "Gardening/Vegetables" and "Taking care of pets or animals." He explained to the therapist that he used to have a small yard and grew vegetables for many years. He also had a dog and said: "somehow my dog understands me." However, he could not bring his dog into the nursing care facility, and he expressed his frustration with his new living situation by saying: "I had to give up my yard and dog." He also indicated casual interest for "Listening to music" and "Singing," but he preferred listening to his favorite singers on his small radio while gardening.

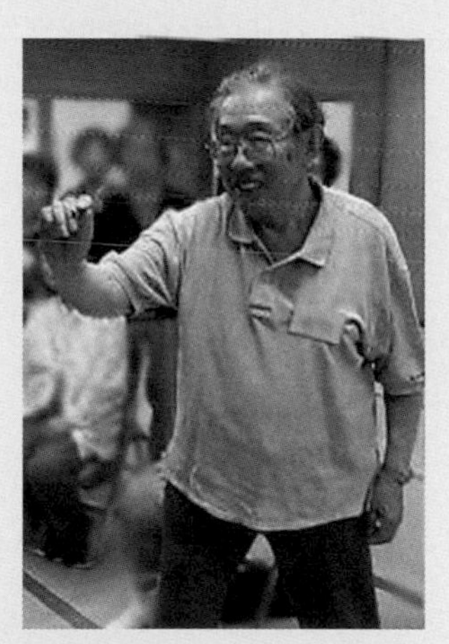

Akira explores new interests, here a game of darts, along with other residents in the nursing care facility

Akira's responses on the ICJEV (Fig. 16-2) confirmed that the new environment, the nursing care facility, did not provide Akira the opportunity to participate in his preferred interests. The occupational therapist sought to provide Akira with opportunities to continue his previous interests in his new living situation. The occupational therapist asked Akira to teach her how to grow vegetables. Akira told the occupational therapist that he would like to grow baby tomatoes, and they worked together to prepare planters in a hallway of the facility. Akira began leaving his room to water the planters. When his tomatoes started blooming, Akira noted on his notebook how many flowers bloomed, and when people passed by in the hallway, he would get their attention by pointing to the growing fruit. Akira still refused to join group programs, but he liked growing his tomatoes. Akira and his occupational therapist began making a plan to expand his activity of growing vegetables and supply fresh produce for the cooking group.

Occupational Self-Assessment and Child Occupational Self-Assessment

The Occupational Self-Assessment (OSA; Baron et al., 2006) and the Child Occupational Self-Assessment (COSA; Kramer et al., 2014) are designed to assess clients' occupational competence for everyday occupations. These self-reports also allow clients to indicate values and to set priorities for therapy. Large gaps between occupational competence and values may identify clients at risk for poor occupational adaptation; clients who report high values but low competence for an occupation will require intervention to maintain or regain occupational adaptation. The OSA and COSA are also designed to be outcomes measures that capture self-reported client change. To be used as outcomes measures, the OSA and COSA are administered at the beginning and at the end of therapy.

The OSA and COSA ask about a range of occupations including self-care activities, social interactions with others, and participating in interests. Each self-report also includes age-specific occupations. For example, the OSA includes money management, taking care of one's home, and working at a job. The COSA includes schoolwork, getting along with classmates, and following rules. These occupations can also be aligned with major MOHO concepts, such as volition (participating in interests), habitation (meeting role expectations), and skills (ability to perform specific tasks), to build a client's occupational profile.

On both self-reports, after reading each question about an occupation, clients rate how well he or she performs the occupation using a four-point scale. Clients also rate the importance of each occupation using a

Occupational Forms	Interest		
	Strong	Casual	No
1. Gardening/Growing vegetables	✘		
2. Sewing			✘
3. Radio			✘
4. Going for a walk			✘
5. Haiku/Senryu (Japanese poetry)			✘
6. Dancing			✘
7. Listening to music		✘	
8. Singing		✘	
9. Taking care of pets or animals	✘		
10. Lectures			✘
11. TV/Movies			✘
12. Visiting acquaintances			✘
13. Reading			✘
14. Traveling			✘
15. Enkai (Japanese style parties)			✘
16. Sumo			✘
17. Dusting/Laundry			✘
18. Politics			✘
19. Clubs for women/elderly people			✘
20. Clothes/Hair style/Makeup			✘
21. Picking wild plants			✘
22. Socialization with the opposite sex			✘
23. Driving			✘
24. Gate ball (Japanese croquet)			✘
25. Cooking			✘
26. Collection			✘
27. Fishing			✘
28. Shopping			✘
29. Ground golf (Japanese style par three hole)			✘
Other special interests: (none indicated)			

FIGURE 16-2 Akira's Responses on the ICJEV.

four-point scale. When completing the OSA, once clients have completed the ratings, the client selects and ranks by priority the specific everyday activities to address during therapy. Some clients independently determine their priorities for change and then discuss them with the therapist. Other clients, who need or wish more structure, do this with the therapist while reviewing their responses to the OSA. The OSA also includes a form in which the therapist and client together may formally record and review therapy goals and strategies. The OSA manual also includes a scoring form for each rating scale, competence, and importance, which allows one to generate a client measure or score that can be used to track changes in competence or values over time, as demonstrated in the Sinikka case.

The COSA is similar to the OSA but uses age-appropriate rating scales. To maximize the accessibility of the self-report for as many children and youth as possible, three versions of the COSA rating form are available: A youth rating form with symbols, a youth rating form without symbols, and a card sort option that also uses symbols. Symbols are used to help youth understand the meaning of each response category: Sad and happy faces are used to depict the competence scales, and stars are used to depict the importance scale. After responding to the COSA items, children have an opportunity to talk about any additional concerns and strengths that were not addressed in the COSA items by responding to a series of open-ended follow-up questions. The COSA form does not include a third step for selecting areas of priorities for change. Instead, the therapist structures the process, helping the child review the items, identify occupations with the largest gap between competence and importance ratings, and select priorities for change.

Both the OSA and the COSA demonstrate strong psychometric properties, and have been validated with large, international client populations. The OSA items coalesce to represent a valid construct of occupational competence and values (internal validity), and the meaning of the constructs remained stable over a series of three studies with international clients (Kielhofner, Forsyth, Kramer, & Iyenger, 2009). The OSA also has good stability over time, making it an appropriate outcome measure (Kielhofner, Dobria, Forsyth, & Kramer, 2010). The COSA items also measure the two constructs of competence and value (internal validity) when used with an international sample of youth ages 7 to 18 years with a variety of disabilities and diagnoses (Kramer, Kielhofner, & Smith, 2010). One study suggests that while most youth use the four-point rating scales appropriately, youth who are younger or who have an intellectual disability may have difficulty using the rating scales (Kramer, Smith, & Kielhofner, 2009). Studies in both the United States and the Netherlands confirm that the COSA items ask about activities that are relevant and important to youth (Kramer, 2011; O'Brien et al., 2009; ten Velden, Couldrick, Kinébanian, & Sadlo, 2013).

MOHO Problem-Solver: Using the OSA with an Adult with Complex Regional Pain Syndrome to Increase her Volition

Sinikka is a 30-year-old catering worker who lives in Helsinki. She has had complex regional pain syndrome for the past 2.5 years, since she experienced a workplace accident in which she sustained an electrical shock from a food processor to her right, dominant hand. Sinikka had sought a variety of interventions to no avail. These included undergoing previous occupational therapy that emphasized assessment of her hand function and learning to use a wrist support.

Sinikka recently began a pain rehabilitation program that consists of group treatment followed by outpatient, individualized therapy. Sinikka is anxious about her condition and symptoms and angry about the lack of efficacy of the previous care she received. She indicates that she feels like her hand and arm are living a life of their own, over which she has little control. To maintain some measure of control, she has organized a structured daily routine aimed at minimizing her chronic pain. For example, at home she uses electronic equipment to reduce work demands, spaces her workload, and uses her left hand whenever possible. She frequently wakes up during the nighttime because of pain. When she tries activities that are not part of her current routine, she is hesitant, fearful of evoking pain, and has difficulty making decisions. Sinikka expressed doubt over whether therapy would be able to help her in the long run.

The therapist introduced the OSA to Sinikka as a means of giving her an opportunity to take more control over the therapeutic process. Sinikka indicated that the chronic pain had made many negative changes in her ability to do things she valued. These included difficulties in her roles as daughter-in-law, spouse, sister, home maintainer, caregiver, and worker. She explained that before her injury, she saw herself as a woman who was able to do anything she undertook and was recognized by others as resourceful and self-reliant. Now even the people closest to her could not comprehend her situation. She had very high standards for her performance, and the problems of pain and inability to use her dominant hand effectively left her feeling ineffective and helpless at times. Yet Sinikka refused to ask others for help.

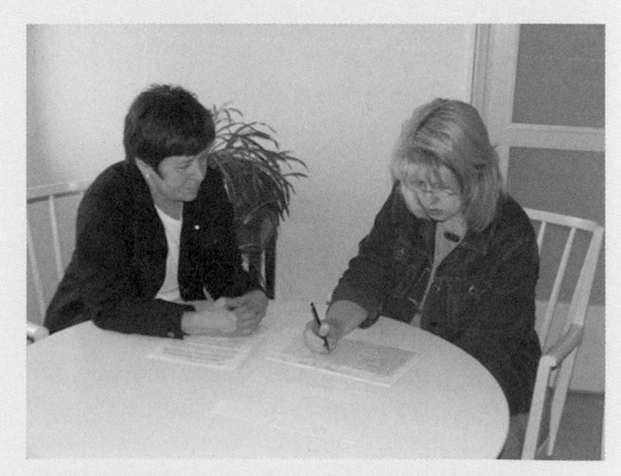

Sinikka contemplates her current life circumstances while completing the OSA

During the next therapy session, Sinikka told the therapist that doing the OSA had a profound effect on her. She told the therapist that she had started to think about what she really wanted in her life and what kind of options she would have in the future. At this point, she decided to choose the following priorities from the OSA statements to work on in therapy:

- Being involved as a student, worker, volunteer, and/or family member
- Handling my responsibilities
- Making decisions based on what I think is important

Consequently, therapy sessions were organized to address these as goals. The therapist supported Sinikka to choose occupational forms/tasks for therapy that were linked to her roles and habits. For example, she resumed cooking, because this was an important part of her homemaker role, and she completed some bookkeeping for her husband's business to reengage in the worker role. First, the therapist supported Sinikka to complete these occupations in therapy and to problem-solve needed adaptations to reduce pain and fatigue. Then Sinikka carried them out at home independently. For example, Sinikka had to drive her car to come to therapy. This was hard because the rough road near her house made driving a challenge and precipitated pain. The therapist and Sinikka discussed the potential benefits of an armrest, wondering whether the support would reduce pain. Sinikka decided to rent a car with an armrest from a dealer and experienced less pain. She then sold her old car and purchased a new one. She managed to get her personal insurance to pay for aids she found useful in kitchen tasks as well as for a movable armrest for the computer she used at home.

With each successful experience, Sinikka's personal causation developed: She became a better judge of her capacity to meet responsibilities, and her self-efficacy increased each time she successfully problem-solved a task that produced pain. A few months after therapy ended, the therapist received an e-mail message from Sinikka. Her increased personal causation enabled her to take a risk and apply for several jobs, and she successfully secured a work-training position in a high-class hotel.

MOHO Problem-Solver: Using the COSA over Time to Increase Participation in Daily Routines with a Medically Complex Hospital Inpatient

Kerri was 11 years old and had Klippel Trenaunay Weber Syndrome, which is characterized by varicose veins, arteriovenous malformation, and bone and soft tissue hypertrophy. In Kerri's case, this syndrome caused multiple hemangiomas on her body, excessive bleeding, and pain. Owing to uncontrolled bleeding, she was transferred to a pediatric intensive care unit (PICU) and on bed rest for 32 days prior to referral to occupational therapy because of concerns about depression and deconditioning. The occupational therapist learned that Kerri refused to speak to the doctors and would not help with the bed mobility needed to complete hygiene and change her bandages. The physical therapist reported that Kerri consistently refused therapy.

At first, Kerri was reluctant to speak with the occupational therapist. The therapist explained that she wanted to learn more about what was important to Kerri by having her complete the COSA (Fig. 16-3). Kerri made general statements such as "I don't like it when the people bother me" and "I feel tired," but still was willing to answer "some" of the questions on the COSA. Kerri took her time and thoughtfully filled out the COSA. When she was done, the therapist first discussed Kerri's strengths. Kerri identified herself as being really good at doing things with her family, keeping her mind on what she was doing, and taking care of her things. Kerri shared that she felt successful with her family because they listened to her and because she helped decide what activities they would do together. Kerri shared that she felt she was able to keep her mind on what she was doing because she was "smart" and "good at figuring things out." Kerri also told the therapist that she needed to be good at taking care of her things in the hospital because if someone moved one of her possessions, she might not be able to reach it, and if something was lost, she was not able to look for it. On the COSA qualitative follow-up questions, she wrote "watching TV" was her only leisure activity. Additional things she felt she was good at included art and playing with animals, although she had not done either of those activities during her hospital stay.

Myself	I have a big problem doing this	I have a little problem doing this	I do this ok	I am really good at doing this	Not really important to me	Important to me	Really important to me	Most important of all to me
Keep my body clean	☹☹	☹	☺	☺☺	☆	☆☆	☆☆☆	☆☆☆☆
Dress myself	☹☹	☹	☺	☺☺	☆	☆☆	☆☆☆	☆☆☆☆
Eat my meals without any help	☹☹	☹	☺	☺☺	☆	☆☆	☆☆☆	☆☆☆☆
Buy something myself	☹☹	☹	☺	☺☺	☆	☆☆	☆☆☆	☆☆☆☆
Get my chores done	☹☹	☹	☺	☺☺	☆	☆☆	☆☆☆	☆☆☆☆

FIGURE 16-3 Sample Portion from the COSA.

Next, they discussed the COSA questions that Kerri identified as being important and difficult to complete. Kerri reported that she had a big problem with three important activities: dressing, making her body to do what she wanted it to do, and getting around from one place to another. Kerri stated that dressing was a problem because it hurt when the nurses moved her body around. She reported that pain also limited her ability to get her body to do what she wanted. Kerri explained that she was unable to do things with her friends because they were all several hours away from her hometown, and because phone calls from the hospital were too expensive. Kerri was unable to get out of bed owing to her order for mandatory bedrest, but she reported difficulty with bed mobility such as rolling onto her side to reach an item on her nightstand.

The occupational therapist felt that using Kerri's answers on the COSA to create her goals for therapy could improve her feelings of self-efficacy, and motivate her to participate in daily self-care and leisure routines. Kerri worked with the therapist to develop the following goals:

1. Kerri will identify three leisure activities she can participate in while maintaining her movement precautions.
2. Kerri will participate in an upper-extremity exercise program four to five times per week to improve independence in bed mobility.
3. Kerri will don a pull-over shirt with moderate assistance while seated in bed without too much pain.

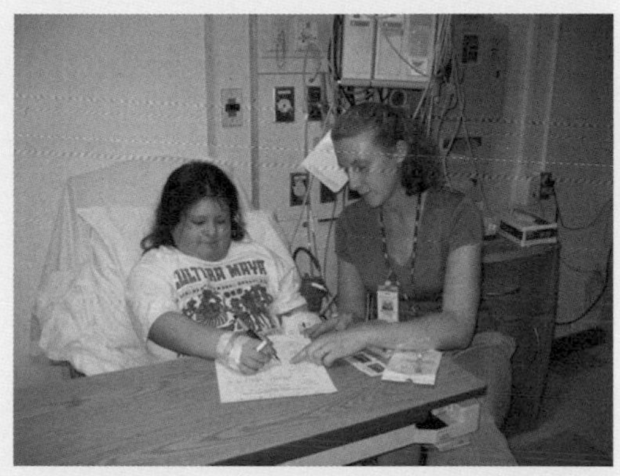

Kerri completes a follow-up COSA to identify goals for intervention

Kerri and the OT made a "Rehab Plan" and posted it in her room so she and the therapist would know what activities they would do during each session to meet her goals. Although Kerri was resistant to exercise at first, the therapist explained how strengthening her arms would help her perform her own bed mobility so the nurses would not have to lift her and roll her. Kerri and the occupational therapist worked together to find ways to make exercise fun, such as combining it with art activities (e.g., painting while wearing wrist weights). With time, Kerri became independent in her exercise program and was able to roll to and from side lying independently and with reduced pain. She also started drawing daily and contributing pictures for the hospital newsletter. With her improved strength and endurance, she demonstrated an improved tolerance for engaging in daily self-care routines. Over the next 2 months, Kerri's health improved, and her bed rest order was cancelled. However, Kerri again began to refuse intervention and did not want to complete her self-care out of bed.

Kerri and the OT decided to complete the COSA for a second time. Kerri's responses showed that she still perceived herself as having a problem with dressing, making her body do what she wanted it to do, and getting around from one place to another, but no longer identified these as big problems. She also identified two new problem areas, which were finishing what she was doing without getting tired too soon and doing things with friends. Kerri explained to the occupational therapist that she was still afraid of being in pain if she tried to dress herself, and that she was scared to transfer out of the wheelchair because it was painful. She only wanted her parents to transfer her because she felt her mom and dad would be gentler than the nurses. Kerri agreed to transfer with her parents in order to get out of bed. Based on her responses, Kerri and the occupational therapist worked together to establish new goals as follows:

1. Kerri will spend time up in her wheelchair at least 5 days each week.
2. Kerri will participate in three social activities with teenagers each week.
3. Kerri will complete upper-body dressing independently at least 4 days each week.

Kerri and the occupational therapist again came up with strategies to meet her goals. The therapist showed how Kerri could use skills she reported as strengths on the COSA, especially making others understand her ideas and working on something even when it becomes hard to achieve her goals. They agreed that the occupational therapist should see how Kerri's parents are transferring her, and they work together to identify what strategies nursing staff could use to make it less painful. Kerri also agreed to tell her parents and the therapist which parts of the transfer were painful, so they were able to make the transfer more tolerable. The occupational therapist also suggested that Kerri meet some new people by participating in social activities with other teenagers in the hospital. Kerri was reluctant at first, but she agreed to try participating in social activities for 1 week. Finally, Kerri and the occupational therapist agreed to try several techniques for dressing and that Kerri could choose which one she liked the best. To help Kerri choose a technique, they decided to keep track of how tiring each technique was, how long the technique took, and the amount of pain it caused.

Kerri remained hospitalized in the PICU for a total of 112 days before she was stable enough to be transferred to an inpatient rehab facility closer to her home. By the time of discharge, she was able to transfer to her wheelchair with minimal assistance and complete her upper-body dressing with assistance only for setup. Kerri even formed friendships with two other clients her age in the hospital that she kept in touch with after discharge.

As these two cases illustrate, the OSA and COSA give clients a voice about their own problems, strengths, and desires. The instruments also begin a process that can empower and enable clients to achieve more control over their situations and over the objectives and courses of their therapy. Finally, as the case of Kerri illustrates, the instruments can serve as a concrete means to demonstrate change achieved in therapy. This is helpful not only to document change but also for clients to concretely see and be reinforced by the changes they accomplish.

Occupational Questionnaire and the NIH Activity Record

The NIH Activity Record (ACTRE) (Furst, Gerber, Smith, Fisher, & Shulman, 1987; Gerber & Furst, 1992) and the Occupational Questionnaire (OQ; Smith, Kielhofner, & Watts, 1986) are self-report forms that ask the client to indicate what activity he or she engages in over the course of a weekday and weekend day. The OQ and ACTRE are appropriate for use with adolescents and adults.

The OQ allows clients to report what they are doing during each half-hour waking period of their day and then indicate whether the activity is work, leisure, daily living task, or rest; enjoyment; importance; and quality of performance. These latter questions reveal the personal causation, interest, and value experienced in the activity.

The ACTRE, developed for use with persons who have physical disabilities, asks additional questions pertaining to pain, fatigue, difficulty of performance, and whether one rests during the activity (Fig. 16-1). Consequently, in addition to the information provided by the OQ, the ACTRE provides detailed information about how a disability influences performance of everyday activities (e.g., it asks about the level of energy required, the amount of pain and fatigue experienced, and whether rest was taken during the activity).

Although both forms are designed to be used as self-reports, they can be administered as semistructured interviews. Clients can complete either assessment in two ways: as a time-use diary of a specific day or to describe a typical day. Each of these methods has its advantages (e.g., diaries tend to be more accurate if completed during the course of a day but may reflect an unusual day). Actual use depends on the purpose and circumstances of therapy. Ordinarily, therapists minimally ask clients to report on a weekday and a weekend day, but this also depends on the circumstances in which the instruments are being used.

In addition to providing details about a client's use and experience of time, these instruments potentially give the occupational therapist important information about the following kinds of problems:

- Particularly troublesome times or activities in the daily schedule
- Disorganization in the person's use of time
- Lack of balance in time use
- Problems such as a low occupational competence, a lack of interest, or a lack of value in daily activities

The instruments can be used to produce scores that represent the amount of value, interest, personal causation, pain, and fatigue experienced in a day. In addition to the possibility of generating such numbers from the instruments, the results of the instruments can be graphically portrayed for or by the client. For example, the time spent in any area (e.g., work, play, or rest) can be portrayed as the portion of the day devoted to each of these life spaces, the portion spent doing things not valued, and so on. This can be done as an individual or group exercise. It provides clients a new way to examine their patterns of doing things and identify changes they would like to make.

MOHO Problem-Solver: Encouraging Self-Reflection in a Client with Mental Illness

Lin is a 25-year-old man who lived in Taipei. He was diagnosed as having obsessive-compulsive disorder with a suspected schizoid personality. Lin was admitted to a psychiatric ward owing to compulsive behaviors he exhibited since college. Lin spent a great amount of time washing himself, washing his hands, and folding his clothes. However, he was able to graduate with a Bachelor's degree in accounting. After graduation, he enlisted in the Taiwanese army. However, he was disciplined for spending too much time washing himself and his hands and was eventually dismissed. Since that time, he has been living alone in an apartment in Taipei, relatively isolated from others and without employment. He was referred to occupational therapy, although Lin insisted he was satisfied with his daily routines and did not require assistance. The occupational therapist asked Lin to complete the OQ. Lin was very serious about filling out the questionnaire and took a great deal of time deciding how to respond, making several corrections.

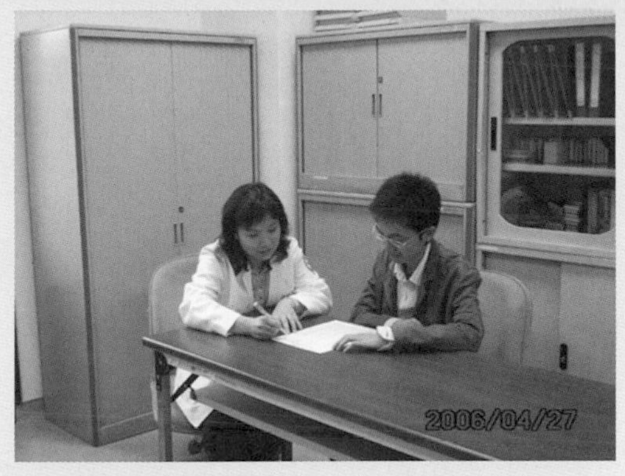

The occupational therapist shows Mr. Lin how to complete the OQ

The OQ (Fig. 16-4) highlighted that Lin spent about 10.5 hours in mainly passive and solitary leisure things, 3.5 hours in activities of daily living, and 4 hours doing work-related things. The only thing Lin indicated doing very well was eating meals, which, along with sleep, were the only things that he rated as extremely important. Similarly, these and mainly passive leisure things were what he indicated liking most. Although he did not see himself as having a problem doing anything, or find anything he did to be a waste of time or distasteful, he also did not indicate that he valued or derived a high level of competence or enjoyment from anything productive. Lin found the information derived from the OQ to be very revealing. It made him more aware of features of his daily routine. He realized that his routine "just sort of happened." Moreover, he indicated that it was a sad thing that the highlight of his day was when he ate meals. Thus, he was very motivated to improve his life by incorporating more goal-directed and meaningful activities into his daily schedule.

Because his length of hospital stay was anticipated to be only a few days, Lin and his therapist decided to focus on goals and plans that he could work on after discharge. To reduce the time spent in self-care and leisure activities, he systematically examined each activity he did in the course of the day, and identified alternative activities he could complete at home or in the community. This planning process helped Lin prepare for a successful discharge home.

Time	Typical Activities	Question 1 I consider this activity to be: W: Work D: Daily living task R: Recreation RT: Rest	Question 2 I think that I do this: VW: Very well W: Well AA: About average P: Poorly VP: Very poorly	Question 3 For me this activity is: EI: Extremely important I: Important TL: Take it or leave it RN: Rather not do it TW: Total waste of time	Question 4 How much do you enjoy this activity? LVM: Like it much L: Like it NLD: Neither like nor dislike D: Dislike it SD: Strongly dislike
06:30-07:00	Sleep	W D R **RT**	VW **W** AA P VP	**EI** I TL RN TW	**LVM** L NLD D SD
07:00-07:30	Breakfast	W **D** R RT	**VW** W AA P VP	**EI** I TL RN TW	**LVM** L NLD D SD
07:30-08:00	Computer	**W** D R RT	VW **W** AA P VP	EI **I** TL RN TW	**LVM** L NLD D SD
08:00-08:30	Computer	**W** D R RT	VW **W** AA P VP	EI **I** TL RN TW	**LVM** L NLD D SD
08:30-09:00	Read Newspaper	**W** D R RT	VW **W** AA P VP	EI **I** TL RN TW	**LVM** L NLD D SD
09:00-09:30	Reading	**W** D R RT	VW **W** AA P VP	EI **I** TL RN TW	**LVM** L NLD D SD
09:30-10:00	Reading	**W** D R RT	VW **W** AA P VP	EI **I** TL RN TW	**LVM** L NLD D SD
10:00-10:30	Listen to Music	**W** D R RT	VW **W** AA P VP	EI **I** TL RN TW	**LVM** L NLD D SD
10:30-11:00	Music	**W** D R RT	VW **W** AA P VP	EI **I** TL RN TW	**LVM** L NLD D SD
11:00-11:30	Music	**W** D R RT	VW **W** AA P VP	EI **I** TL RN TW	**LVM** L NLD D SD
11:30-12:00	Lunch	W **D** R RT	**VW** W AA P VP	**EI** I TL RN TW	**LVM** L NLD D SD
12:00-12:30	Lunch	W **D** R RT	**VW** W AA P VP	**EI** I TL RN TW	**LVM** L NLD D SD
12:30-01:00	Computer	W D **R** RT	VW **W** AA P VP	EI I **TL** RN TW	LVM L **NLD** D SD
01:00-01:30	Computer	W D **R** RT	VW **W** AA P VP	EI I **TL** RN TW	LVM L **NLD** D SD
01:30-02:00	Go to Library	W D **R** RT	VW **W** AA P VP	EI I **TL** RN TW	LVM L **NLD** D SD
02:00-02:30	Library	W D **R** RT	VW **W** AA P VP	EI I **TL** RN TW	LVM L **NLD** D SD
02:30-03:00	Exercise	W D **R** RT	VW **W** AA P VP	EI I **TL** RN TW	LVM L **NLD** D SD
03:00-03:30	Exercise	W D **R** RT	VW **W** AA P VP	EI I **TL** RN TW	LVM L **NLD** D SD
03:30-04:00	Play ball	W D **R** RT	VW **W** AA P VP	EI I **TL** RN TW	LVM L **NLD** D SD
04:00-04:30	Play ball	W D **R** RT	VW **W** AA P VP	EI I **TL** RN TW	LVM L **NLD** D SD
04:30-05:00	Play ball	W D **R** RT	VW **W** AA P VP	EI I **TL** RN TW	LVM L **NLD** D SD
05:00-05:30	Dinner	W **D** R RT	**VW** W AA P VP	**EI** I TL RN TW	**LVM** L NLD D SD
05:30-06:00	Dinner	W **D** R RT	**VW** W AA P VP	**EI** I TL RN TW	**LVM** L NLD D SD

FIGURE 16-4 Lin's Responses on the Occupational Questionnaire.

Time	Typical Activities	Question 1 I consider this activity to be: W: Work D: Daily living task R: Recreation RT: Rest	Question 2 I think that I do this: VW: Very well W: Well AA: About average P: Poorly VP: Very poorly	Question 3 For me this activity is: EI: Extremely important I: Important TL: Take it or leave it RN: Rather not do it TW: Total waste of time	Question 4 How much do you enjoy this activity? LVM: Like it much L: Like it NLD: Neither like nor dislike D: Dislike it SD: Strongly dislike
06:00-06:30	Watching	W D **R** RT	VW **W** AA P VP	EI I TL **RN** TW	LVM **L** NLD D SD
06:30-07:00	TV	W D **R** RT	VW **W** AA P VP	EI I TL **RN** TW	LVM **L** NLD D SD
07:00-07:30	&	W D **R** RT	VW **W** AA P VP	EI I TL **RN** TW	LVM **L** NLD D SD
07:30-08:00	Phone	W D **R** RT	VW **W** AA P VP	EI I TL **RN** TW	LVM **L** NLD D SD
08:00-08:30	Call to	W D **R** RT	VW **W** AA P VP	EI I TL **RN** TW	LVM **L** NLD D SD
08:30-09:00	Friend	W D **R** RT	VW **W** AA P VP	EI I TL **RN** TW	LVM **L** NLD D SD
09:00-09:30	Bathing	W D **R** RT	VW **W** AA P VP	EI I TL **RN** TW	LVM **L** NLD D SD
09:30-10:00	Bathing	W D **R** RT	VW **W** AA P VP	EI I TL **RN** TW	LVM **L** NLD D SD
10:00-10:30	Bathing	W D **R** RT	VW **W** AA P VP	EI I TL **RN** TW	LVM **L** NLD D SD
10:30-11:00	Clean up room	W D **R** RT	VW **W** AA P VP	EI I TL **RN** TW	LVM **L** NLD D SD
11:00-11:30	Clean up room	W D **R** RT	VW **W** AA P VP	EI I TL **RN** TW	LVM **L** NLD D SD
11:30-12:00	Clean up room	W D **R** RT	VW **W** AA P VP	EI I TL **RN** TW	LVM **L** NLD D SD
12:00-12:30	Go to sleep	W D R **RT**	VW **W** AA P VP	**EI** I TL RN TW	**LVM** L NLD D SD

FIGURE 16-4 *(continued)*

The Pediatric Interest Profiles

The Pediatric Interest Profiles (PIP; Henry, 2000) are three age-appropriate profiles of play and leisure interests and participation that can be used with children and adolescents. The three profiles are as follows:

- Kid Play Profile, which is designed for use with children from 6 to 9 years of age
- The Preteen Play Profile, which is for children from the ages of 9 to 12 years
- Adolescent Leisure Interest Profile, which can be used with adolescents from 12 to 21 years of age

The items, the questions about them, and the response formats of each version of the PIP have been designed to be appropriate for and easily understood by clients within the targeted age range.

In the Kid Play Profile, the child answers up to three questions about each of 50 activity items. For each activity item, the child is asked, "Do you do this activity?" If the answer is yes, the child is also asked, "Do you like this activity?" and "Whom do you do this activity with?" The child answers the questions by circling or coloring in a response. As shown in Figure 16-5, stick-figure drawings are used to depict each item. Simple drawings also depict the response options. The Kid Play Profile activity items are grouped into eight categories: sports activities, outside activities, summer activities, winter activities, indoor activities, creative activities, lessons/classes, and socializing.

In the Preteen Play Profile, the child answers up to five questions about each of 59 activity items. For each activity item, the child is asked, "Do you do this activity?" If the answer is yes, the child is also asked about the frequency of participation, enjoyment, sense of competence, and social interactions during the activity. As with the Kid Play Profile, stick-figure drawings are used to depict each activity. The Preteen Play Profile activity items are grouped into eight categories: sports activities, outside activities, summer activities, winter activities, indoor activities, creative activities, lessons/classes, and socializing.

In the Adolescent Leisure Interest Profile, the adolescent answers up to five questions about each of 83 activity items. For each activity item, the adolescent is asked, "How interested are you in this activity?" and "How often do you do this activity?" If the adolescent does the activity, he or she is also asked about sense of competence, enjoyment, and social interactions during the activity. No drawings are used in the adolescent profile. The Adolescent Leisure Interest Profile activity items are grouped into eight categories: sports activities, outside activities, exercise activities, relaxation activities, intellectual activities, creative activities, socializing, and club/community organizations.

Therapists can use the information gathered with the PIP to identify children or adolescents who may be at risk for play-related problems and/or who have a limited repertoire of play activities. The PIP can also

Kid Play Profile

Outdoor Activities	Do You Do This Activity?	Do You Like This Activity?	Who Do You Do This Activity With?
4. Play Catch	Yes No	A Lot A Little Not at All	By Myself With Friends With a Grown-Up
5. Ride a Bike	Yes No	A Lot A Little Not at All	By Myself With Friends With a Grown-Up

FIGURE 16-5 Sample Items from the Kid Play Profile.

be used to identify specific play activities that are of interest to an individual child or adolescent to engage the child in therapeutic or educational interventions. Research demonstrates that all three questionnaires can be used in a reliable manner by the targeted age group (Budd et al., 1997; Henry, 1998, 2000).

Moho Problem-Solver: Using Play Interests to Encourage Social Interactions in a Young Child with Behavioral Difficulties

Jerome was 6 years old and attended first grade at an urban, public elementary school in Maryland.

Jerome had trouble attending in class, was often disruptive because he could not sit still, and was falling further behind in developing reading-readiness skills. He was having difficulty with handwriting and other fine motor tasks. Although his teacher was very supportive and patient, she was beginning to feel frustrated with her ability to manage his behavior in the classroom and worried about his ability to keep up with the pace of classroom activities. He interacted only minimally with classmates, and on the playground spent most of his time on the swings or running in circles.

The occupational therapist administered the Kid Play Profile to better understand Jerome's play interests. Jerome was able to complete the Kid Play Profile with considerable assistance from the occupational therapist. His responses on the Kid Play Profile indicate that he primarily enjoyed outdoor, gross motor activities, and playing "superheroes." However, he reported his older brother "doesn't always like to do stuff with me" and could only name one boy in his class with whom he plays during recess. When asked whether he has any other friends, he stated, "Well, they don't really like me." The occupational therapist enrolled Jerome to the Friendship Group, jointly run by herself and the school psychologist. The goals of this group are to help referred children develop appropriate social interaction skills in the context of structured dyadic play with one other child. The play activities used in the group require cooperation, turn-taking, and negotiation. The group teaches skills in communication and self-regulation. The occupational therapist suggested a "superhero" theme on Jerome's first day in order to capture his interest and provide motivation for engagement. The first session was a success, with Jerome and another peer playing "superhero" for 10 minutes with support from the therapist. Jerome was able to engage in pretend play with the peer, and with structured cues from the therapist, negotiated a disagreement about "good guy" and "bad guy" roles. At the end of the session, Jerome and the peer exclaimed, "That was fun!"

The Role Checklist Version 3: Performance and Satisfaction

The original Role Checklist (Oakley, Kielhofner, Barris, & Reichler, 1986) was developed to obtain information on clients' perceptions of their participation in roles throughout their life and on the value they place on those roles. The checklist can be used with adolescents or adults. The client considers each of 10 occupational roles described on the checklist. In part one, clients check those roles they have performed in the past, are currently performing, and/or plan to perform in the future. For example, if a client volunteered in the past, does not volunteer at present, but anticipates volunteering in the future, he or she would check the role "Volunteer" in both the past and future columns. In part two of the checklist, the client rates each role as to whether he or she finds it not at all valuable, somewhat valuable, or very valuable. Brief definitions of each role are provided, followed by examples of that particular role. For example, being a family member is defined as doing something with a family member such as a child, parent, spouse, or other relative at least once a week. In this way, when persons indicate they are in a role, it also means that the role influences what the person does. The Role Checklist is available for free from the MOHO clearinghouse.

In 2015, Scott modified the Role Checklist, thus creating Version 3. The modified version focuses on current satisfaction with performance of the same 10 roles as well as the desire (or not) to perform the rest of the roles on the checklist. The responses on the Role Checklist v3 provide the therapist with areas needing improvement in the short term, as clients rate their satisfaction with performance on a four-point scale from very dissatisfied to very satisfied. In addition, the Role Checklist v3 will indicate to the therapist whether the client is satisfied waiting for future opportunities for role engagement or whether they would prefer to engage currently. For example, an occupational therapy student during her coursework completes the Role Checklist v3 during class. In the future, she wants very much to be a parent and checks satisfied waiting for future performance. She first wants to complete school, pass her exam, obtain licensure, and work as an occupational therapist for a period. Ten years later, this same student may indicate she wants to be performing the role now; thus her response on the Role Checklist v3 would change. In this way, the Role Checklist v3 enables the therapist to track change over time. Scott encourages electronic administration of the Role Checklist v3 whenever possible to create the opportunity to follow up and measure client progress and treatment outcomes (Scott, McFadden, Yates, Baker, & McSoley, 2014). In general, the Role Checklist identifies the roles a client currently engages in, and identifies desired future roles: volition and habituation. Version 3 adds a measure of performance capacity through the client perspective on current performance and desired future role engagement. Thus, the results provide the opportunity for the therapist and client to engage in a conversation to identify current and desired habits, skills, and routines that must be addressed during therapy to support successful participation in valued roles.

Construct validity and sensitivity of the Role Checklist v2 has been verified by Bonsaksen et al. 2015. Concurrent validity between occupational circumstances assessment interview and rating scale (OCAIRS) and the RC v2: was found at $r\,(18) = 0.63$, $p < 0.01$ (Cacich, Fulk, Michel, Whiffen, & Scott, 2015). Because the RC v3 contains the same 10 roles as v2, it is assumed v3 maintains the same level of concurrent validity with the OCAIRS. Cross-cultural validity studies are currently in progress as is a scoring system. The website www.rolechecklist.com continually updates progress on the instrument.

MOHO Problem-Solver: Maintaining Role Involvement in a Single Mother Recovering From a Liver Transplant

Mary is a 58-year-old English teacher and the mother of three teenage children. One month ago, she received a liver transplant for a cirrhotic liver due to primary sclerosing cholangitis. Mary completed the Role Checklist v3 during a routine follow-up appointment in the postsurgical transplant clinic.

Mary's pattern of role identification, satisfaction with current performance, and feelings about her desired future reflects her view that 1 month post transplant, she has minimal role involvement and is dissatisfied with her performance in three of the four roles she is currently engaged with. Her expectations pre transplant were that by 1 month she would be taking care of her children again and actively maintaining her home. Instead, she spends most of the day resting, and her energy is consumed with traveling back and forth to the posttransplant clinic. Neither Mary nor her children expected this. The occupational therapist could see that Mary had unrealistic expectations about the length of time it takes to recover. The therapist and Mary worked on body mechanics to help her cope with the large healing abdominal wound, work simplification and energy conservation techniques, and create an active plan for her children to complete regularly assigned chores around the house. In this way, Mary felt more in control of her household as she slowly worked toward being able to regain the strength to perform the caregiving and home maintainer roles she values. At her next visit, Mary reported feeling more in control and less of a burden to her children. On the Role Checklist v3, Mary indicated she was satisfied waiting a bit longer to resume all the desired future roles except going to church. This is something she would like to do now. The occupational therapist discussed how it was still too early to attend services where there would be a large number of people, and the risk of catching a cold was high given her highly immunosuppressed state. Mary had also been told it would be another month before she was cleared to drive. The occupational therapist provided Mary with a link to complete the Role Checklist v3 in 6 weeks. After 6 weeks, the therapist could see that Mary's satisfaction with her performance in Caregiver and Home Maintainer had improved and Religious Participant had moved into the current column on part one. The therapist sent Mary an e-mail asking her to complete the Role Checklist v3 again electronically in 6 more weeks and contact the therapist if she had any concerns in the meanwhile.

MOHO-Based Self-Reports Emerging in Practice

Three MOHO based self-report assessments (ACHIEVE, CIRCLE, and Making It Clear) have emerged recently in practice in response to contextual practice demands and new opportunities for occupational therapy to emerge as leaders in nontraditional health care settings. These self-reports were designed to facilitate communication with other disciplines, community partners, and/or clients to address occupational needs and plan intervention guided by MOHO theory. These self-reports also have corresponding decision-making manuals to guide intervention planning based on self-report responses.

ACHIEVE Assessment

The ACHIEVE Assessment (ACHIEVE Alliance, 2014) was designed to gather information prior to initial clinical contact about children's occupational participation at home, school, and in the community. The ACHIEVE is completed by a child's parent and teacher, making it appropriate for children with a range of abilities and needs aged 5 to 18 years who may or may not be able to complete a self-report. The ACHIEVE Assessment includes a separate parent and a teacher questionnaire (Figs. 16-6 & 16-7), allowing the therapist to gather comprehensive information about a child's occupational strengths and challenges across contexts in order to formulate an occupational profile. Therapists send the questionnaire forms to parents and teachers when they first receive referrals to their service for children.

The ACHIEVE Assessment adopts a user-friendly approach to gather information about the personal (volition, habitation, and skills) and environmental factors that influence a child's occupational participation. The ACHIEVE Assessment first asks respondents to indicate *what* activities the young person is able to do (occupational participation) within a range of environments (e.g., able to manage their clothing). Next, respondents answer a series of questions aligned with MOHO personal and environmental factors to provide information about *why* he/she may experience success or

LIFE SKILLS THAT RELATE TO NURSERY/SCHOOL

	None of the time	Some of the time	Most of the time	All of the time
a. Your pupil is able to clean him/herself after they've been to the toilet or manage their own personal hygiene (e.g., washing hands)	1	2	3	4
b. Your pupil is able to manage their clothing (e.g., managing their outdoor clothing when going to the playground, taking off a cardigan when they feel warm, managing their shoelaces)	1	2	3	4
c. Your pupil is able to manage their own snacks/lunch in school (e.g., use a fork and a knife, open snack/drink containers)	1	2	3	4
d. Your pupil is able to clean up effectively after an activity (e.g., wash paint brushes, tidy away an art activity, wash down table)	1	2	3	4
e. Your pupil is able to get prepared for nursery/school in the morning (e.g., when they arrive at nursery/school, their bag is organized, remembered P.E. kit, completed homework)	1	2	3	4
f. Your pupil is able to move from one activity to another effectively (e.g., settle after play time, moving from play/P.E. to an activity that requires quiet listening and attention)	1	2	3	4

Additional comments: ______________________________

____

____

FIGURE 16-6 Sample "WHY" Items from the ACHIEVE Teacher Questionnaire ACHIEVE Assessment.

SUMMARY SCORES SHEET—Standard Version

Name: ______________________ | Date of birth: ______________ | Age: ________(years) ________(months)

CHI Number: ______________________ | Clinician(s) scoring: ______________________

Scale: 1—None of the time | 2—Some of the time | 3—Most of the time | 4—All of the time

		Parent questionnaire		Education questionnaire	
Home activities / life skills relating to school	PARENTAL OBSERVATION OF ACTIVITY FREQUENCY—WHAT?	1 2 3 4	a. Able to clean after toileting	1 2 3 4	EDUCATION OBSERVATION OF ACTIVITY FREQUENCY—WHAT?
		1 2 3 4	b. Able to manage their clothing	1 2 3 4	
		1 2 3 4	c. Able to help with/manage snacks	1 2 3 4	
		1 2 3 4	d. Able to help with/clearn up effectively	1 2 3 4	
		1 2 3 4	e. Able to get prepared for nursery/school	1 2 3 4	
		1 2 3 4	f. Able to move from one activity to another	1 2 3 4	
Nursery / school activities		1 2 3 4	a. Able to use learning materials	1 2 3 4	
		1 2 3 4	b. Able to make effective shapes/letters/writing	1 2 3 4	
		1 2 3 4	c. Able to engage in sports/leisure	1 2 3 4	
		1 2 3 4	d. Able to engage in curriculum	1 2 3 4	
		1 2 3 4	e. Able to clean after toilet at school	1 2 3 4	
		1 2 3 4	f. Able to get dressed after P.E./Gym	1 2 3 4	
Community activities		1 2 3 4	a. Able to use learning materials	1 2 3 4	
		1 2 3 4	b. Able to make effective shapes/letters/writing	1 2 3 4	
		1 2 3 4	c. Able to engage in sports/leisure	1 2 3 4	
		1 2 3 4	d. Able to engage in curriculum	1 2 3 4	
		1 2 3 4	e. Able to clean after toilet at school	1 2 3 4	
		1 2 3 4	f. Able to get dressed after P.E./Gym	1 2 3 4	
Routine and role	PARENTAL OBSERVATION OF CHILD CHARACTERISTICS—WHY?	1 2 3 4	a. Organises routines	1 2 3 4	EDUCATIONAL OBSERVATION OF CHILD CHARACTERISTICS—WHY?
		1 2 3 4	b. Copes with change in routine	1 2 3 4	
		1 2 3 4	c. Copes with a variety of activities	1 2 3 4	
		1 2 3 4	d. Understands their responsibilities	1 2 3 4	
		1 2 3 4	e. Understands their responsibilities	1 2 3 4	
		1 2 3 4	f. Manages multiple responsibilities	1 2 3 4	
Confidence		1 2 3 4	a. Confident in their abilities	1 2 3 4	
		1 2 3 4	b. Enjoys nursery/school activities	1 2 3 4	
		1 2 3 4	c. Satisfied with performance in activities	1 2 3 4	
		1 2 3 4	d. Identifies what he/she wants to get better at	1 2 3 4	
		1 2 3 4	e. Keeps trying despite challenges	1 2 3 4	
Social skills		1 2 3 4	a. Plays well with others	1 2 3 4	
		1 2 3 4	b. Chatty/sociable and talks with friends	1 2 3 4	
		1 2 3 4	c. Speaks clear when with others	1 2 3 4	
		1 2 3 4	d. Understands others' feelings	1 2 3 4	
		1 2 3 4	e. Can ask for the support he/she needs	1 2 3 4	
Organizational skills		1 2 3 4	a. Organizes and uses objects for activities	1 2 3 4	
		1 2 3 4	b. Maintains concentration during activities	1 2 3 4	
		1 2 3 4	c. Works out problems if stuck on a task	1 2 3 4	
		1 2 3 4	d. Follows through instructions for activities	1 2 3 4	
		1 2 3 4	e. Does the steps of an activity in the right order	1 2 3 4	
Physical skills		1 2 3 4	a. Completes activities without being clumsy	1 2 3 4	
		1 2 3 4	b. Completes activities without losing balance	1 2 3 4	
		1 2 3 4	c. Grips objects effectively when doing activities	1 2 3 4	
		1 2 3 4	d. Physical dexterity to complete activities	1 2 3 4	
		1 2 3 4	e. Completes activities without physical fatigue	1 2 3 4	
Environment		1 2 3 4	a. Can navigate around physical environment	1 2 3 4	
		1 2 3 4	b. Environment has opportunities	1 2 3 4	
		1 2 3 4	c. Access to the things to help them take part	1 2 3 4	
		1 2 3 4	d. Staff/family available for support	1 2 3 4	
		1 2 3 4	e. Environment supports activities	1 2 3 4	
		1 2 3 4	f. Does activities in usual/accepted way	1 2 3 4	

FIGURE 16-7 ACHIEVE Assessment Summary Scores Sheet.

MOHO Problem-Solver: Understanding a Child's Occupational Performance Across Contexts

Alan lives at home with his two parents and his brother. Alan has been referred for a specialist assessment by his elementary school teacher who was concerned about his motor skills and handwriting. Alan is a 7-year-old boy who is a third grader in elementary school. He is described by his family as a lovable, endearing boy. Conversely, his school teacher describes him as chaotic, disorganized, and worried. These issues have been long standing, and the strategies tried within the school have not been helpful and challenges persist. There is a concern that if the issues are not resolved, Alan will not be able to keep up with his class peers. The ACHIEVE Assessment was chosen to answer the question *"how and why does Alan's occupational performance vary in different environments?"* This assessment was administered by mail and was completed by Alan's mother and by Alan's teacher. The therapist then compiled the information before the initial visit and reviewed the findings with the team during the clinic review.

On review of the ACHIEVE Assessment, Alan had many areas of strength including home and community activities; he is able to get dressed/undressed, able to ride a bike, and able to take part in social events. Alan's teacher reports Alan enjoys Math and Physical Education (PE). Alan also had appropriate social skills and mostly understood his responsibilities at home and school. Reponses from the parents and teachers also confirmed Alan had routines at home and school that facilitated his participation, and a supportive school and home environment matched to his abilities and skills.

Comparing teacher and parent ACHIEVE Assessments, Alan performs more consistently in activities at home and in the community rather than at school. He did not have any areas of challenge at home. However, he was reported by the teachers in the classroom to have challenges using learning materials effectively (e.g., pens, pencils, crayons, rules, glue sticks, scissors) and being able to make effective shapes/letters and writing within a school context. Alan's teacher also reported he has challenges navigating around his physical school environment and challenges in general coordination. The impact on Alan's confidence in school was noticeable in the classroom (i.e., having confidence in abilities, enjoyment, or having satisfaction in school activities, and not trying despite challenges). When reviewing these results in the clinical review, Alan's mother shared that she wanted Alan to write with less effort and improve his confidence. Alan's teacher wanted Alan to be less clumsy, less distractible, and for his writing to be less laborious. To ensure Alan provided input to the goal-setting process, the therapist also asked Alan how he was feeling about school. He stated, *"Writing is not my thing"* and wanted to be able to keep up with his friends and not feel panicky about being the last in class.

This process identified that the main area to target in therapy was improvement in use of learning materials through developing confidence for tasks completed within the classroom. The joint measurable goal shared between therapy and education was therefore *"Within 8 weeks, Alan will be able to confidently use learning materials (such as scissors, writing utensils) through organizing objects and maintaining concentration within his classroom independently."* The therapist used the ACHIEVE Assessment framework and MOHO concepts to create a common language and discuss strategies that Alan could use to improve his organizational skills and concentration in the classroom. For example, his mother shared at home he was encouraged to direct his own management of chores—the team decided to implement similar self-directed strategies at school.

Four weeks later, Alan was observed using self-monitoring strategies such as checking off each step of the written directions for classroom activities. The teacher reflected that Alan was more "organized" in the classroom, and was able to more independently locate the learning materials he needed to complete his class work. Most importantly, Alan stated he felt less panicked when writing, and he proudly showed his workstation to the therapists as his space. The ACHIEVE Assessment allowed the team to identify Alan's strengths and the priority issues to address in therapy and set alan on a path to increased success at school.

challenges in some areas of activity (e.g., maintains concentration throughout activities). These ratings are understood to reflect the parent or education professional's expectations of what activities the young person should be able to engage in given his/her age, level of impairment (if applicable), prior life experiences, societal expectations, and environmental context. The practitioner can therefore consider whether the young person is able to achieve the kind of participation in life that fits with his/her desires and what his/her environment (e.g., family, school) expects.

To interpret assessment results, the therapist transfers the parent and teacher ratings to a summary form. The form illustrates a visual pattern of all ratings obtained across all items, thus facilitating comparison and contrast of two important perspectives across different settings. Similarities and differences are identified, and MOHO theory is used to understand and explain potential reasons for occupational challenges in various settings and to build an initial understanding of the client's strengths and needs. Other assessments, including child self-reports, can be used to gather additional information as needed to build a robust occupational profile. The parent and teacher perspectives, along with other assessment results, are then used to engage in collaborative goal setting with the full team.

CIRCLE Assessment

A series of two self-reports, CIRCLE Inclusive Classroom Scale (CICS) and the CIRCLE Participation Scale (CPS), are designed for independent use by teaching professionals providing education and support to students with disabilities under a consultative occupational therapy model. Both assessments come as part of one manual, called *Inclusive Working and Collaborative Working: Teachers Ideas in Practice* (CIRCLE Collaboration, 2015). Occupational therapists can consult with teachers and other educational professionals to use the CIRCLE tools and related intervention strategies to foster an inclusive environment and the participation of children with disabilities. The CIRCLE self-report assessments support nonoccupational therapists to implement MOHO best practices, and the manual also includes detailed information on supports and strategies for the teacher to try in class.

The CICS tool (Fig. 16-8) assesses *environmental* factors in the classroom in four areas based on MOHO conceptualization of the environment: the physical environment, the social environment, and structures and routines within the environment. The CICS also includes a set of reflective questions that help users when considering the quality of the classroom

Adequacy of space	4	Exemplary availability of different areas and seating for meeting needs
	3	Variety of areas and seating available when needed, available spaces match requirements
	2	Constraints of available space, some needs not met by spaces or seating
	1	Spaces not matching needs, overcrowded, required spaces or seating not available
Sensory space	4	Excellent sensory conditions, temperature pleasant, lighting and/or noise levels optimized for sensory preferences
	3	Comfortable sensory conditions, temperature, light and/or noise levels adjustable
	2	Some challenges with sensory conditions, variable ability to adjust these, e.g., unwanted noise
	1	Hot/stifling or too cold, noisy, poor lighting, cannot adjust sensory conditions
Activity demands	4	Activities promote exceptional challenge and enjoyment
	3	Activities appropriate to allow for "just right challenge"
	2	Activity demands are somewhat high/low, some boredom/stress
	1	Activity demands too high/too low, causing boredom/stress
Rules and boundaries	4	Exceptionally clear expectations/rules/rewards/sanctions provided in a variety of formats and consistently applied
	3	Expectations/rules/rewards/sanctions provided in a variety of formats and consistently applied
	2	Challenges with expectations/rules/rewards/sanctions, some learner disengagement or anxiety
	1	Expectations/rules/rewards/sanctions unclear, learners disengaged or anxious

FIGURE 16-8 Sample Items from CIRCLE Inclusive Classroom Scale (CICS).

environment. Scoring is based on observation of the classroom context over a period of time. The CICS can be completed by one individual, or by colleagues working together.

The CPS tool (Fig. 16-9) assesses a child's *inclusion* and participation in a classroom, and the personal and environmental factors impacting the child's participation. The CPS consists of items representing the child's environment, routines, motivation, motor skills, process skills, and communication and interaction skills. The scale is designed to record whether the personal or environmental factor supports or interferes with a child's participation in school life. The tool also records the frequency with which it applies to the student. The tool allows the teacher to gain an overview of the child's performance and to capture the child's relative strengths and weaknesses in the school and classroom context. Scoring is based on a teacher's individual observation of the child in the classroom context.

After teachers score the CICS and CPS, the manual contains specific suggestions for implementing strategies that address areas of need identified in the assessment scores. For example, the manual contains strategies for improving fine motor skills or self-efficacy. If the educator is still struggling after applying CIRCLE strategies, then they will refer for specialist support from an occupational therapist. The occupational therapist can also oversee the teacher's

Moho Problem-Solver Cases: Using an OT Consultative Model in Primary Education to Support Classroom Participation

Sabina is a 7-year-old girl who attends a small rural school, and her class includes 20 other children. Sabina's teachers were worried about her level of disorganization in school and inability to keep up with other children; they have queried possible developmental delay and contacted an occupational therapist for help. The occupational therapist, working to a consultative model, recommended that the teacher complete her own assessment of Sabina using the CIRCLE tools to identify and implement classroom support strategies.

The teacher observed the classroom over the course of a day, making notes on her CIRCLE Inclusive Classroom Scale (CICS) classroom observation form. On completion of the scale, it was noted that there were no barriers in the physical environment: There were no hazards, children could move around easily, and the classroom and corridor spaces were organized and uncluttered. No issues were noted with the sensory qualities of the space, and some visual supports were present (e.g., child's name and icon above jacket peg, and child's name and icon on book return tray). Objects were appropriately placed, suitable, and accessible. In examining the social environment, adults were found to be supportive and learner-centered; however, it was noted that most guidance was provided verbally, which Sabina found difficult to follow. The teacher also noted that Sabina was isolated from other children and did not interact with others in comparison to her peers, especially at break time. In examining structures and routines, activity demands placed on Sabina were high, as she appeared to struggle keeping up. The appeal of activities offered in class was scored very positively, with activities offered to learners showing variety and tailoring to different interests and cultures. The routines used in class were good, with high levels of consistency and structure. However, Sabina was seen to be distressed at the start of the day when she was expected to take her coat off and hang it on the correct peg, change into her indoor shoes, put her lunch box on the trolley, return her book to the correct tray, and then find her seat in the classroom. She often became muddled doing this and puts her things in the wrong place, and became upset. It was noted that the teacher did not have time to support Sabina individually in the morning.

The teacher also used the CIRCLE Participation Scale (CPS) questionnaire to assess the personal and environment factors impacting Sabina's participation. The teacher identified strengths in several areas of motivation, including working toward specific goals with support, showing curiosity, willingly engaging in activities, and showing enthusiasm for activities at school. No issues were noted with Sabina's fine motor skills—she was able to manipulate small objects and use both her hands at the same time with ease, and Sabina's gross motor skills also appeared normal to the teacher. The teacher did identify that Sabina found it hard to follow instructions, or to remember what she had been asked to do. Sabina also needed prompts to remind her of what she was supposed to be doing and where she was supposed to be. Sabina was aware of school routines, but found it difficult to move between tasks, activities, and/or classes during school day and did not cope well with changes to routine or patterns. Sabina's desk was often untidy, and she rarely had a pencil and frequently lost things. Sabina was not involved in many extra roles/activities in school (e.g., clubs, or after school), and the social environment was again highlighted because of Sabina's relative isolation from other children and the ineffectiveness of verbal prompting from teaching staff. Other issues noted were problems with choosing tools and materials, remembering items needed for the day, and completing tasks in correct sequence.

Once Sabina's teacher had completed her assessments, the occupational therapist met with her to discuss the results. The information gathered helped the teacher and the occupational therapist identify the areas of greatest need to be addressed in intervention. The therapist, drawing guidance from the MOHO resource "CIRCLE Therapy Manual: Occupational Therapy" (Forsyth, 2010), recommended that the teacher focused further on building social skills and habits. Sabina's teacher shared: "*Sabina found the start of the day overwhelming. I have tried to make it more manageable by organizing a 'planning buddy.' This is an older learner who helps her change her shoes and organize herself with the other tasks. I have introduced a visual timetable with photographs of the things she has to do, which she ticks off as she completes them. She is much happier and more settled in the class but continues to require this ongoing support at the moment.*" The teacher had also worked with Sabina's parents to make sure she was as organized as possible at home to prepare for school: "*We introduced a checklist and timetable in her bag and on her bedroom wall.*" The occupational therapist also recommended setting up a small group project where Sabina was given the role of a "project manager" in charge of the central desk tidies in the class, and to set up other opportunities for Sabina to interact more with her classmates. A review meeting was set for 3 months where they would again discuss Sabina's process. The therapist recommended use of the CPS and the CICS again at that time to monitor any change and adjust strategies as needed.

reevaluation of the child using the CICS and CPS to measure the impact of the strategies on student performance and participation.

Making It Clear

The Making It Clear (MiC) (Making it Clear Collaborative, 2015) self-reported measure was created to assess an older person's perception of their level of resilience. The self-report is associated with a MOHO-based prevention program that enables older adults to live well within their communities by capitalizing upon and building resilience. The MiC measure and prevention program proposes that resilience is supported by environmental factors such as social support, community safety, resources such as housing and income, and the opportunity to participate in meaningful activities. Person factors also contribute to resilience, including personal causation, values, interests, habits, and roles.

The MiC assesses resilience by examining factors at the personal (30 items) and community (16 items) level that are aligned with MOHO concepts (e.g., volition, environment) as well as participation in essential activities (e.g., work, leisure, self-care). The items are grouped into four subscales that use everyday language:

- How you connect with your friends, family, and neighborhood
- How you find and use resources and services to meet your everyday needs
- How you live your life and what you believe is important
- What you think about yourself and the way you do things

Each MiC item is presented as a statement, for example, "I have family who support me," which is rated from strongly disagree (1) to strongly agree (4).

The MiC is designed to be administered by nonprofessional staff or volunteer associated with community-based aging service providers under the supervision of an occupational therapist. As needed, occupational therapists can also complete the form directly. There is a short form (six questions) that can be used as a screen to determine whether there is a potential need that could be met by the MiC program. If the screening leads to a referral to the MiC program, the long form is then used to find out more detail about the person (Fig. 16-10). The administrator reviews the responses to identify areas of resilience and need-based item and subscale scores. The MiC manual provides a guide to help identify appropriate goals, and the therapist or staff partners with the older adults to build upon areas of resilience to strengthen areas of need and achieve goals.

Learning Environments: Social				
a. Peers include learner in class activities	1	2	3	4
b. Peers include learner in play/recreation activities	1	2	3	4
c. Relevant school staff recognize and understand learners' needs	1	2	3	4
d. Relevant school staff proactively provide support to meet learners' needs	1	2	3	4
e. Family circumstances allow learner to participate fully at school	1	2	3	4
Structures and Routines				
a. Learner is aware of and adheres to normal school routines	1	2	3	4
b. Learner is able to move between tasks, activities, and/or classes during school day	1	2	3	4
c. Learner copes well with changes to routine or patterns	1	2	3	4
d. Learner meets relevant school staff expectations	1	2	3	4
e. Learner is involved in extra roles/activities in school (e.g. clubs, or after school)	1	2	3	4
Motivation				
a. Learner is aware of own skills and abilities	1	2	3	4
b. Learner seeks challenges or new activities and is optimistic about success	1	2	3	4
c. Learner shows curiosity and willingly engages in activities	1	2	3	4
d. Learner shows enthusiasm for activities at school	1	2	3	4
e. Learner shows pride in their achievements	1	2	3	4

FIGURE 16-9 CPS Form Sample Items from the CIRCLE Participation Scale (CPS).

MOHO Problem-Solver: Fostering Resilience by Increasing Self-Efficacy in an Older Adult with Depression

Gordon is a 70-year-old man who lives alone and has become increasingly isolated after quitting his job to care for ill family members who recently passed away. Gordon is also an accomplished musician and previously played in bands but stopped playing owing to health concerns. Since the beginning of this year, he has been free of his caring role but has been struggling with mental health problems, specifically depression. Gordon feels that the loss of his job, his family, and many friends in quick succession led him to lose his confidence; "I just started bursting out into tears . . . it was whole series of events. From being this super-confident chartered accountant, but my confidence just vanished. It was one thing after another."

Gordon's physician referred Gordon to his community older adult services. A liaison from the agency visited Gordon and provided him with the MiC questionnaire. Gordon said he felt "a wee bit pathetic" after filling in the questionnaire because he had scored low on the majority of questions (mostly 1 and 2s). Gordon and the liaison, Fraser, could not identify just one activity that would help to resolve some of Gordon's problems; so they agreed to work incrementally, with the first focus to increase Gordon's self-efficacy.

On the questionnaire, Gordon identified that he enjoyed walking. Gathering this information from the MiC began a series of actions that began to increase his self-efficacy. The liaison, Fraser, introduced him to a local walking group. After a few sessions, Gordon found that the rest of the group were older than him and did not walk at a pace he found challenging. Gordon and Fraser then brainstormed other options, and Gordon agreed that he could regularly go to the gym. He walked to the gym every day and spent time on the treadmills and cycling machines. Gordon had found that he really enjoyed this new part of his daily routine.

When Gordon filled in a MiC questionnaire a second time 6 months after his initial referral to the agency, his score had gone from 35 to 64. His scores had moved from 1s and 2s (disagreeing) to mostly 3s and 4s (agreeing). The only items Gordon continued to strongly disagree with were related to family, and accepting whatever life throws at him. He is keen to get back to work or consistent volunteering, but has found making the first step overwhelming. However, he had sufficient self-efficacy to take the first step of providing resumes to several small local business and part-time jobs at a regional grocery store. As Gordon shared: "It's motivation, I can do all these things . . . it's just finding the motivation to do it."

	Strongly disagree	Disagree	Agree	Strongly agree
a. I can always present myself in the way I want to (e.g., putting on my makeup, wearing a shirt and tie)	1	2	3	4
b. I have no problems taking care of the place where I live (e.g., vacuuming, changing bedsheets)	1	2	3	4
c. I can take part in the leisure activities that I want (e.g., sports, hobbies)	1	2	3	4
d. I can take part in the social activities that I want (e.g., meeting friends, family events)	1	2	3	4
e. I can find and use the community services I need (e.g., voluntary agencies, carer support, social work services)	1	2	3	4
f. I can find and use the learning/training resources that I want (e.g., library services, further education, interest groups)	1	2	3	4
1. I have additional roles in my community/ society (e.g., volunteer/unpaid work, member of an organization)	1	2	3	4
2. I am part of a circle of friends (e.g., socially involved with friends, neighbors and/or support groups)	1	2	3	4
3. I have no problems getting around my home and neighborhood (e.g., getting up and down stairs, reaching cupboards, getting to the shops)	1	2	3	4
4. I live in safe and suitable housing	1	2	3	4
5. My circle of friends helps me get through life's demands	1	2	3	4

FIGURE 16-10 Sample Items from Making It Clear.

CASE STUDY: USING COMPLIMENTARY SELF-REPORTS TO BUILD AN OCCUPATIONAL PROFILE AND AN EFFECTIVE ENVIRONMENTALLY FOCUSED INTERVENTION PLAN FOR AN ELEMENTARY SCHOOL STUDENT WITH DEVELOPMENTAL COORDINATION DISORDER

The occupational therapist and the teacher quickly consulted in the hallway between classes about their previous unsuccessful attempts to meet the needs of the third grader, Aashi. After years of individualized education and related services, including occupational therapy, Asahi's academic performance, social skills, and motivation were decreasing instead of improving. A sweet and gentle girl, the occupational therapist and the teacher knew they needed to try a different way of understanding and addressing Aashi's needs to ensure her success.

Aashi's story began at 18 months, when she was diagnosed with global developmental delay and began receiving EI services. Services focused on supporting Aashi's participation in her family's busy life and their management of her development needs in the context of their rich Indian heritage. Aashi's parents worked hard to support her interaction with them and her two older and very active brothers throughout her infancy and toddlerhood. At 3 years old, Aashi was found eligible to receive special education services on the basis of developmental delays in cognitive, motor, and language skills and a new diagnosis of Developmental Coordination Disorder (DCD). Although she made steady gains during preschool and early school years in her cognitive and language skill development with the support of occupational therapy and other services, Aashi made only incremental gains in her motor skills. She frequently suffered bruises from bumps and falls; she had difficulty managing her self-care needs; learning to ride her bike and playing ball games with her peers were challenging; and she had difficulty managing school tools and manipulative tasks.

Aashi's occupational therapy services were focused on the development of handwriting and on building the skills necessary to manage dressing routines and clothing closures independently at school. In addition, support was provided in the classroom to modify worksheets for the reduction of written work. Throughout the school year, Aashi became increasingly frustrated with the completion of school work tasks and was notably more avoidant of fine motor activities. She was frequently fatigued, and her weariness began to impact her attention and engagement in learning tasks that she had previously come to enjoy.

In addition, Aashi was struggling socially both at home and school. Other classmates, who in previous school years often took her under their wings and found natural ways to scaffold her participation, now ran swiftly away from her halting gait and excluded her from their games of jump rope, which Aashi was unable to play. Aashi began to isolate herself on the playground, even at times misbehaving to avoid recess. Aashi's parents shared their frustration with her limited engagement in home responsibilities, including home work, and family, social, and cultural activities. They worried about her limited social engagement and shared that she had not yet had an opportunity to join a friend at her house for a play date. They began to notice an increasing gap between the social engagement and belonging of their daughter and her siblings and cousins without disabilities.

To prepare for the upcoming educational planning meeting, the occupational therapist and teacher decided to undertake a comprehensive assessment of Aashi using several MOHO self-reports: The CIRCLE assessment would be completed by the teacher, and the occupational therapist would support Aashi to complete the COSA. Gathering assessment data from parents, the teacher, and Aashi would allow the occupational therapist to gain an in-depth understanding of Aashi's occupational strengths and needs and to potentially identify a more effective approach to meeting her educational needs.

The CICS identified that the classroom teacher was effectively modifying the physical environment to meet Aashi's motor needs; for example, she used a chair with a table instead of an attached desk to make it easier for her to transition from sit to stand and to use a variety of body postures to support her writing. The school team also effectively differentiated instruction (e.g., activity demands) to reduce Aashi's fatigue and frustration; for example, they gave Aashi shorter assignments and would allow a peer to help her complete tasks involving fine motor skills such as extended writing or cutting. However, the ratings on the CIRCLE Participation Scale (CPS) helped the teacher realize the assistance of other students did not create an optimal social environment; instead of seeing Aashi as a peer, students began to view her as someone who needed their help to complete classwork. In addition, this further decreased Aashi's self-efficacy for both classroom tasks as well as social interactions. A lack of resources in the classroom, including computers and other technology, restricted Aashi's ability to complete writing tasks more independently and effectively.

The occupational therapist administered the card sort version of the COSA Competence and the Values scales on two separate days to reduce fatigue. Aashi placed each card into one of four containers that were labeled with the images from the rating scales. In class, however, she saw herself as competent in getting her work done on time; she worried about the shortened class assignments and shared that she wanted to complete more of the work on her own, like her classmates. She reported that she lacked the ability to do the things that she wanted to do, such as "...playing chase and jump rope on the playground" and difficulty making friends and playing with her peers on the playground. She shared, "I wish I had more friends." Aashi indicated that at home she was unable to manage her Barbie doll clothing independently; so she did not play with her cousins when they came to play. This further contributed to her feelings of inadequacy as a family member, and she reported feeling "sad" from time to time. At the end of the COSA, the therapist asked Aashi to share her greatest wish as a way to identify a therapy goal. Aashi exclaimed, "I just wish I could jump rope!"

The results of the assessment indicated that Aashi did not see herself as successful in the roles of student, peer, and family member because of her challenging motor needs. Aashi's rope jumping request was aimed not at learning the motor skill but at helping her find ways to support her understanding of the differences between the motor performance of her and her peers; build positive feelings about her capacities; and establish a positive and productive role and a sense of belonging in her home and school community.

Children with disabilities are often encumbered by barriers that impede their participation in occupations of choice and obstruct their interactions with others. The results of Aashi's assessment using the ACHIEVE tools and the COSA shifted the focus of Aashi's intervention from improving her motor performance and reducing the physical barriers to her participation to reducing her social isolation and increasing opportunities for successful engagement in occupations of interest and value. Aashi's teacher, parents, and occupational therapist collaborated to identify the following educational goals:

- Initiate and sustain social interactions with peers during recess
- Use a computer to complete class assignments that are the same length as peers.

Aashi worked with the occupational therapist to identify activities that she could be successful with on the playground, and, with the help of the classroom and physical education teachers, her classmates were taught games that she could access. Aashi and her peers developed several games with the jump rope in which she could be successful. Aashi discovered a hidden strength in her ability to learn and recite the cadence songs and counts while her friends jumped along.

The teacher and occupational therapist worked to obtain a laptop with an adapted keyboard for Aashi to use at her desk. Although she was slow with her typing and made many key errors, she was excited to complete her work independently and showed less fatigue with typing. She also started to learn how to use autocomplete text features to improve the accuracy and speed of her writing.

As she grew successful, her classroom teacher noted that Aashi was growing increasingly confident in the classroom and took on new roles as desk helper, librarian, and line leader.

The following fall, progress data collected showed that although the therapist had not directly targeted Aashi's fine motor skills, she was managing clothing closures more independently and improved her ability to use the keyboard for lengthier written language assignments. As the barriers influencing her ability to participate successfully in occupations of choice and her ability to fulfill occupational roles in the classroom and on the playground increased, her performance capacities increased across all contexts. Aashi found her value in her transformed identity as a competent student and friend. She was empowered to construct a new identity of herself—an identity as a healthful, capable, and relational being.

Conclusion: Self-report Assessments in Perspective

This chapter presented self-report assessments and illustrated how gathering information directly from clients can allow therapists to solve clinical challenges and engage clients in meaningful occupations. The cases demonstrate that clients of various ages and in various contexts can use self-report assessments with support to identify concerns and participate in intervention planning. Written responses on self-report forms and subsequent discussions between the therapist and client provide insights into the client's needs and goals, and provide an opportunity for the

Talking with Clients: Assessments that Collect Information through Interviews

Helena Hemmingsson, Kirsty Forsyth, Lena Haglund, Riitta Keponen, Elin Ekbladh, and Gary Kielhofner (posthumous)

CHAPTER 17

EXPECTED LEARNING OUTCOMES

Upon completion of this chapter, readers will be able to:

1. Identify different types of model of human occupation (MOHO) assessments that are administered via interview format, and to recognize the focus of each assessment.
2. Choose the appropriate MOHO interview assessment depending on the client and the situation.
3. Understand how occupational participation can be assessed and described according to the concepts of MOHO.
4. Understand the function of rating scales and how to use the results of MOHO interview assessments to plan individually targeted interventions.

Whether formal or informal, client interviews provide a large portion of the information through which therapists come to know their clients (Fig. 17-1). Five assessments that use interviews have been developed for use with the model of human occupation (MOHO):

- Occupational Circumstances Assessment—Interview and Rating Scale
- Occupational Performance History Interview—Second Version
- School Setting Interview
- Worker Role Interview (see also Chapter 24)
- Work Environment Impact Scale (see also Chapter 24)

Each of these assessments has a distinct format and purpose. The Occupational Circumstances Assessment—Interview and Rating Scale (OCAIRS) focuses primarily on the client's current occupational participation. The Occupational Performance History Interview—Second Version (OPHI-II) is a life history interview. The School Setting Interview (SSI) is designed to assess school environment impact and identify the need for accommodations for students with disabilities. The Worker Role Interview (WRI) is designed for use with injured or disabled workers. The Work Environment Impact Scale (WEIS) was developed to examine the impact of the work environment on the worker.

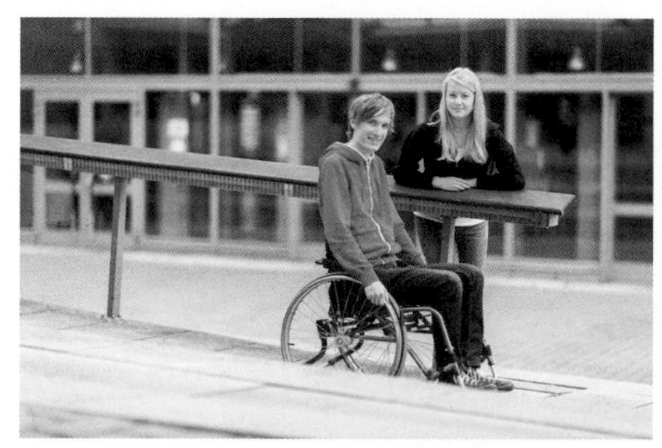

FIGURE 17-1 An Occupational Therapy Interview.

These assessments all share some common features. Each has a semistructured interview that the therapist adapts to fit the unique circumstances of each client. After the interview is conducted, the therapist must have some means of analyzing the information. Each assessment has a rating scale or checklist that, when completed, represents what was learned in the interview. Each of these assessments also has a means of recording qualitative information gathered during the interview. This chapter focuses on OCAIRS, OPHI-II, and SSI as a full description of WRI, and WEIS is provided in Chapter 24 that concerns work rehabilitation.

Occupational Circumstances Assessment—Interview and Rating Scale

The OCAIRS (Forsyth et al., 2005) is based on the Occupational Case Analysis Interview and Rating Scale (Kaplan, 1984; Kaplan & Kielhofner, 1989). The OCAIRS provides a structure for gathering, analyzing, and reporting data on the extent and nature of an individual's occupational participation. The OCAIRS is designed to be relevant to adolescent and adult clients with a wide range of backgrounds and impairments. OCAIRS is one of the first assessments developed in relation to MOHO, and even if the assessment has been used for many years, the scientific standard and its usability continue to be investigated (Haglund & Forsyth, 2013).

ADMINISTRATION

The OCAIRS manual provides information on conducting the interview and completing the scale (Forsyth et al., 2005). The OCAIRS consists of a semistructured interview that can be adapted to each unique client. The assessment manual details interview formats for mental health, forensic, and physical rehabilitation practice contexts. After conducting one of these interviews, the therapist completes a rating scale and records comments regarding the client's occupational participation. The interview averages 20 to 30 minutes, and completion of the scale with comments takes between 5 and 20 minutes, depending on the occupational therapist's familiarity with the assessment and the level of detail in the comment sections.

The rating scale is completed by checking off criteria that best describe the client and then using them as a guide to selecting the appropriate rating. A sample item is shown in Figure 17-2. The rating scale provides a profile of strengths and weaknesses affecting the clients' occupational participation, in addition to generating a measure of the clients' occupational participation, which is useful for therapy and discharge planning.

CASE EXAMPLE: USING THE OCAIRS TO GUIDE INTERVENTION AND DISCHARGE PLANNING FOR A YOUNG ADULT WITH MENTAL ILLNESS

At the age of 23, Olaf was hospitalized for the first time in an acute psychiatric ward. His older sister, younger brother, and parents (who are professors) live in the same town in Sweden. Olaf had moved to his own apartment 2 years earlier when he began

Interests	
F	☐ Participates in many interests regularly outside of work ☐ High level of interest in primary occupation ☐ High level of satisfaction with level of participation in an interest(s)
A	☐ Participates in few, but clearly expressed, interests regularly outside of work ☐ Some interest in primary occupation ☐ Some satisfaction with level of participation in an interest(s)
I	☐ Few and vaguely defined interests outside of work, no regular participation ☐ Very little interest in primary occupation ☐ Very little satisfaction with level of participation in an interest(s)
R	☐ Does not participate in any identified interests outside of work ☐ No interest in primary occupation ☐ Dissatisfaction with level of participation

Key: **F** = Facilitates: Facilitates Participation in Occupation
A = Allows: Allows Participation in Occupation
I = Inhibits: Inhibits Participation in Occupation
R = Restricts: Restricts Participation in Occupation

FIGURE 17-2 Sample Item (Interests) from the OCAIRS.

studying nursing at the local university. When he was younger, Olaf always had many friends. However, in the past 4 years he had been very isolated, spending most of his time studying. For 6 months, Olaf had increasing difficulty keeping up with his studies. Most recently, he complained of hearing a voice that told him to hurt himself because he was not good enough for this world.

The occupational therapist used the OCAIRS to gather information about Olaf's occupational participation to help with planning during his anticipated 4-week hospitalization. Olaf was quite confused about what was happening to him. Several times during the interview, he asked, "Do you think I'm schizophrenic?" Despite his confusion and fear, he was able to participate effectively in the interview. Olaf's scores on the OCAIRS are shown in Figure 17-3. The following qualitative information was also gathered during the interview.

When asked about his interests, Olaf noted that he used to like to listen to hard rock music, study, and read science literature, but he had not been able to do these things for some time. He did have some goals. In particular, he wanted to resume his studies. After finishing the nursing program, he wanted to enroll in management courses at the university and then start his own business. He said that it was very important for him to be smart and successful.

In contrast to his goal of resuming study, Olaf's sense of personal causation was extremely low. He felt very much out of control. He feared that the voice he heard would control him. Although he felt compelled to return to his studies, he did not see how he could possibly succeed. Olaf indicated that he was no longer able to do anything well, and he could not point out any skills of which he was proud. He complained that he could not plan or organize his behavior to accomplish even everyday activities.

Olaf was previously able to maintain a daily routine as follows: He attended the university in the morning and studied in the evening. He carried out his routine alone, remaining isolated during the weekend. He disliked cooking; so he mostly ate at the university canteen or a local restaurant. He noted that each day had been more or less the same for him for the past 4 years. He indicated, "I'm not a sociable person anymore." During the previous 6 months, Olaf had difficulty completing daily routines and concentrating on tasks. In the 3 weeks before being hospitalized, he remained in his flat alone, drinking tea and eating sandwiches, ignoring everything else including his personal hygiene.

Olaf described actively avoiding other people, noting that he was very shy and felt uncomfortable initiating conversation. When asked about important people in his life, he hesitated and then finally mentioned his sister. He recalled that he had a girlfriend some years before. However, at the time, there was no person whom he considered a significant support. Although Olaf recalled a happy family life during childhood and adolescence, he felt that he no longer had anything to say to his parents. He admitted feeling very lonely and longed for more social contact.

Olaf liked his flat and very much wanted to return to it. He received a substantial amount of money from his grandmother when he bought his flat so he could furnish it the way he wanted. The flat is in the central part of the town, a location that he liked.

The interview helped the occupational therapist identify Olaf's strengths and weaknesses, as shown in Figure 17-3. Although many aspects of his occupational life were quite eroded, his long-term

	Facilitates	Allows	Inhibits	Restricts
Roles			✘	
Habits				✘
Personal causation				✘
Values			✘	
Interests		✘		
Skills			✘	
Short-term goals			✘	
Long-term goals		✘		
Interpretation of past experiences		✘		
Physical environment		✘		
Social environment			✘	
Readiness for change	✘			

FIGURE 17-3 Olaf's Ratings on the OCAIRS.

goals and his physical environment were strong points. It was apparent during the interview that Olaf's greatest priorities were to

- engage in his studies again;
- take part in some social occupations; and
- move back to his flat as soon as possible.

The OCAIRS also provided a structured way of helping the therapist start to plan Olaf's intervention. She planned to address his volitional status through structured graded occupations. Information about Olaf's occupational lifestyle gained from the OCAIRS was used to select the specific occupational forms used in intervention. These were things he indicated an interest in and that related to his long-term goals.

The occupational therapist, for example, suggested, "*Olaf, how about following me to the occupational therapy department. I can show you our facility and maybe you and I can do some computer work trying to identify short science stories, one to two pages? Stories that we may print and read together?* Olaf directly answered, "*I do not think so; I do not know your computer at the department.*" The occupational therapist said, "*Yes you are right, you do not know our computer but we shall do it together, and I know the computer.*"

She also chose occupational forms that were within his skill level so that he could experience success and thereby begin to rebuild personal causation. Given that Olaf felt he could not do anything, the therapist routinely provided Olaf with concrete feedback aimed at shaping his experience of doing things. Therefore, whenever he completed an occupational form, the therapist took time to review what he had accomplished and highlighted his strengths. She also carefully pointed out how his successes in therapy related to his long-term aims. "*Olaf, you have now been at the hospital seven days, and you have started to use our own computer frequently. You are searching and listening to music you like. This is really different compared to what you were doing for weeks at home before you came to the hospital,*" she concluded.

As Olaf gained some confidence, the therapist and he started to work together on his goal of returning to independent living in his own flat. He began by taking increased responsibility for self-care and care of his immediate environment. Because Olaf stated he was having difficulties maintaining a daily routine and completing his homemaker tasks, they developed a routine that included some of these tasks in the inpatient setting. This included making the bed, keeping track of his things in the room, and dusting and sweeping his room daily. Olaf followed this routine and reviewed it twice a week with the therapist. As he approached time for discharge, the therapist accompanied Olaf to his apartment several times to identify and practice homemaking tasks. "*Olaf, what are the most important things, from your point of view, to manage, in order to stay at home by yourself?*" the occupational therapist asked. "*Can you list the tasks?*" Olaf mentioned going shopping, making an easy supper, washing the dishes, cleaning, and washing up. "*And which of them do you want to start to work on tomorrow when we go to your flat?*" "*I want to do some shopping and make lunch. I am longing for a taco pizza,*" he said.

Finally, Olaf was enrolled in several inpatient groups to increase his level of social interaction. Although he remained quiet, his level of skill became adequate for social interaction once he regained some of his confidence in interacting with others.

The OCAIRS was also useful in planning for Olaf's discharge. His level of functioning was still not consistent with the demands of returning to university studies. However, given the importance of Olaf being involved in studies, the therapist arranged for him to attend a supported educational facility for persons with psychosocial impairments. She worked with him to make choices for courses, focusing on those related to his long-term goals. She also helped Olaf plan a daily routine to accommodate attending the courses. Because of his poor sense of efficacy, she accompanied him to the school to sign up for the first day of classes. She also guided him to identify some groups at the school that he could join to have social contact. The therapist continued to make home visits with Olaf in his apartment after discharge to monitor the routine they had planned together so that he could manage his self-care and maintain the apartment.

In sum, the OCAIRS provided the therapist with information to gain an understanding of Olaf's occupational life, the challenges he faced, and his goals for the future. This information helped in identifying therapeutic goals and strategies and ensured that therapy addressed what mattered to Olaf.

OCCUPATIONAL PERFORMANCE HISTORY INTERVIEW—SECOND VERSION

As a historical interview, the Occupational Performance History Interview—Second Version (OPHI-II) (Kielhofner et al., 2004) gathers information about a client's past and present occupational adaptation. The OPHI-II is a three-part assessment that includes

- a semistructured interview that explores a client's occupational life history;
- rating scales that provide a measure of the client's occupational identity, occupational competence, and the impact of the client's occupational behavior settings; and
- a life history narrative designed to capture salient qualitative features of the occupational life history.

It is designed to give the interviewer a means of understanding the way a client perceives her or his life to be unfolding. The OPHI-II may be used with adolescents and adults who have a range of impairments.

As a semistructured interview, the OPHI-II provides a framework and recommended questions for conducting the interview to ensure that the necessary information is obtained. At the same time, the semistructured nature of the interview allows the interviewer and respondent to digress from the structure and recommended questions so that additional questions about a related area and/or deeper questions about a particular topic may be asked. At the same time, the semistructured nature of the interview allows the interviewer to skip questions that are not pertinent for a particular client or clinical situation. The interview is organized into the following thematic areas:

- Activity/occupational choices,
- Critical life events,
- Daily routine,
- Occupational roles, and
- Occupational behavior settings.

Within each of these thematic areas, a possible sequence of interview questions is provided. The interview is designed to be very flexible so that therapists can cover the areas in any sequence or move back and forth between them.

The second part of the OPHI-II is composed of the following three rating scales:

- Occupational identity scale
- Occupational competence scale
- Occupational behavior settings scale

The three scales provide a means of converting the information gathered in the interview into three measures. The occupational identity scale measures the degree to which persons have values, interests, and confidence; see themselves in various occupational roles; and hold an image of the kind of life they want. The occupational competence scale measures the degree to which a person is able to sustain a pattern of occupational participation that is productive and satisfying. The occupational behavior settings scale measures the impact of the environment on the client's occupational life. A key form has been developed for these three scales that allows interval measures to be derived from the ordinal ratings made on the scale (Kielhofner, Dobria, Forsyth, & Basu, 2005).

ADMINISTRATION

The OPHI-II is presented in a detailed manual designed to allow the therapist to learn by reading how to administer the assessment. It includes detailed guidelines for conducting the interview and provides several resources for supporting the interview process. It also gives detailed instructions and examples for completing the rating scales and life history narrative.

The therapist begins by conducting the interview, which, in its entirety, takes approximately 45 to 60 minutes to complete. Although the OPHI-II is designed to be completed as a single interview, therapists may conduct the interview in more than one part, or may decide to administer only one part for an interview of a much shorter duration. Following the interview, the therapist scores the three rating scales consisting of a total of 29 items. The therapist rates each item with a four-point rating that indicates the client's level of occupational adaptation/environmental impact. The rating is completed by first noting criteria that describe the client for each item and then selecting the corresponding rating, as shown in Figure 17-4. Each of the three scales provides a profile of strengths and weaknesses related to identity, competence, and environmental impact, which is useful to planning therapy. As with other assessments, a measure may be calculated for each scale by computer. Paper-and-pencil methods of generating measures from each scale have been developed.

Finally, the therapist completes the life history narrative form that is used to report qualitative information from the interview. As part of this process, the therapist graphically plots the client's life story, thereby indicating the narrative slope, as discussed in Chapter 9. This allows the therapist to develop an appreciation of the plot of the occupational narrative underlying the client's identity and competence.

MOHO Problem-Solver: An Overfunctioning Older Adult

Ellen is a 70-year-old widow who has fallen twice within the past 6 months and has fractured both her hips. She referred to herself as a "pro bone cracker" when she told the story of her second accident. Luckily, it was the day for the home care people to conduct their daily visit to help her with cleaning her apartment. She had a wrist alarm, but it was

Item	Rating criteria
☐	Has personal goals and projects
☐	Goals/personal projects challenge/extend/require effort
☐	Feels energized/excited about future goals/personal projects
☐	Goals/personal projects fit strengths/limitations
☐	Enough desire for future to overcome doubt/challenges
☐	Motivated to work on goals/personal projects
☐	Goals/anticipated projects under/overestimate abilities
☐	Not very motivated to work on goals/personal projects
☒	Difficulty thinking about goals/personal projects/future
☒	Limited commitment/excitement/motivation
☐	Cannot identify goals/personal projects
☐	Personal goals/desired projects are unattainable given abilities
☐	Goals bear little/no relationship to strengths/limitations
☐	Lacks commitment or motivation to the future
☐	Unmotivated due to conflicting/excessive goals/personal projects

Key: **4** = Exceptionally competent occupational functioning
3 = Appropriate satisfactory occupational functioning
2 = Some occupational dysfunction
1 = Extremely occupationally dysfunctional

FIGURE 17-4 An Example of Scoring the OPHI-II Scale: Criteria Are Checked and the Rating Indicated by the Criteria Selected.

not working, so she lay on the floor waiting for 4 hours in pain and unable to move. She was then rushed to the hospital and had a hip replacement surgery, which was the only option in view of the damage that was done. Ellen's injuries were complicated by a 10-year history of osteoarthritis and chaotic changes in blood pressure, which cause dizziness. Ellen reported how her blood pressure "flew her on the floor" the morning of her accident.

After her first accident, Ellen was taught to stand without weight bearing on the leg with the replacement, walk with crutches, and dress using a reacher and a long-handled shoehorn. Staff had not noticed her comments about having cleaned her house, attended her friend's grandson's soccer game, and gone running before her first fall. Staff had not paid attention to another inference she made about feeling overworked, finding her home care staff to be "a little lazy."

After her second accident, staff noticed that, unlike after her first accident, Ellen was sleeping a lot and preferred to stay in her bed. Compared with her previous hospitalization 6 months ago, it seemed that this time, discharging her would not be as straightforward. The occupational therapist went through the precautions Ellen should follow owing to the artificial hip and the assistive devices she would need in order to be able to use the bathroom until she recovered muscle strength in the muscles around her hip. She also got a rail attached to her bed for more secure rising out of the bed. Ellen told the occupational therapist that she was afraid she was now going to be "really disabled." Besides the usual intervention, the occupational therapist convinced both the team and Ellen to begin visiting a local day center for the elderly after she had returned home. The aims included finding her footing and getting support for returning to her previously active lifestyle. The occupational therapist got permission to contact her colleague at the day center and informed her of her concerns about Ellen's fears of "being stuck and unable to move herself."

At the day center, the occupational therapist assessed Ellen in order to help her plan her weekly program. The therapist decided to find out more about Ellen's occupational history by inviting her to participate in an OPHI-II interview. One of the results of this interview is the three rating scales shown in Figure 17-5.

Ellen enjoyed the interview, but the most powerful effect on her was made by the narrative that the occupational therapist had written based on the interview and then shared with her. She could not believe how well it described who she was and how her life had unfolded.

Ellen grew up in a family with modest income and three brothers. She was close to her mother and used to help her with many chores. She married young and had a successful marriage. She was pleased that her son and daughter had found careers and that her daughter had given her a grandchild. She has kept in touch with her children for the last 20 years, because of living 200 km apart, being a mother and a grandmother was not a role that would fill her days. At the age of 50, she had moved back to the city where her husband had grown up. Her husband had retired, and he wanted to return to a familiar town. This enabled both of them to better assist his 90-year-old mother.

Two years after the move, Ellen's mother-in-law passed on, and so did her husband not long after. This was a very difficult change in her life. She was able to find comfort in working on her small vegetable plot. She also grew beautiful flowers, and her grandchildren told her that her potatoes were the best. When Ellen was young, her mother used to love to grow a lot of things and got help from her. In those days, especially during the wartime, it had been a necessary provision of food for the family. Ellen was 6 years old when the war ended, so she knew how her mother had to manage with help from her brothers while her father was at the frontier.

As Ellen neared her 60th birthday, her hips and right knee became a problem. The orthopedic surgeon was famous for treating athletes, and he strongly advised her to take up running in order to keep her muscles strong. This became important for her, and she joked with her family and friends that it is never too late to become a marathon runner. She advanced and kept a training diary to show the doctor her progress. She was able to run 10 to 15 km runs several times a week. Ellen explained, "I used to love walking when I was young, and in those days we used to have to walk or ski 3 km and back from school. I did not mind at all. Ever since I can remember, being on the go has been a way of life for me."

The condition of her hips got worse, but she did not want to give up her lifestyle. To manage the gardening even though she was not able to kneel down, she lay in the garden in order to take care of the plants and weeds, but eventually had to let it go. She was able to do some running until she had the first fall and the fracture.

At the time of having to give up gardening, her best friend moved to a serviced apartment block designed for the elderly. Because her hips had gotten worse, Ellen decided to follow her friend's example. After returning home from the hospital for the first time, she found it had been a good decision to move. Now it was possible for her to get some help when needed from the home help service at the housing complex. She also emphasized that there were paved routes outside the block, and she gained her mobility quickly by taking walks nearby. "There is a hill nearby which I could not climb anymore, but I took a route around it and was able to go back down the hill. Now with this replacement and the other one not perfect either, I do not know if I can do any walks anymore."

At the day care center, the interview and writing the narrative were important turning points in planning a weekly program with Ellen. Usually, the newcomers were automatically introduced to such group activities as planning of outings and parties or to several handcraft activities. Ellen was not very sociable and did not prefer to join the bigger group. Through the narrative, the occupational therapist was able to see Ellen's occupational history and her occupational adaptation during the previously difficult times in her life. She understood that Ellen previously valued growing plants and being a runner. For her, it was also important to be able to make decisions. It seemed that at the moment, Ellen felt quite helpless about not being able to build up a routine that would be a continuation of who she felt she was, because of the recent accident that limited her mobility.

Through rating the interview and sharing the narrative, both the therapist and Ellen herself were able to see that being physically fit and active, independent in her decisions,

OPHI-II CLINICAL SUMMARY REPORT FORM

Client: Ellen Age: 70 Diagnosis: Total hip replacement Date of assessment: ______

Therapist: ______ Therapist signature: ______

Ratings key: 1 = Extreme occupational functioning problems; **2** = Some occupational functioning problems; **3** = Appropriate satisfactory occupational functioning; **4** = Exceptionally competent occupational functioning

Occupational Identity Scale	1	2	3	4
Has personal goals and projects		X		
Identifies a desired occupational lifestyle		X		
Expects success		X		
Accepts responsibility			X	
Appraises abilities and limitations		X		
Has commitments and values		X		
Recognizes identity and obligations			X	
Has interests		X		
Felt effective (past)				X
Found meaning and satisfaction in lifestyle (past)				X
Made occupational choices (past)				X

Occupational Competence Scale	1	2	3	4
Maintains satisfying lifestyle		X		
Fulfills role expectations	X			
Works toward goals		X		
Meets personal performance standards		X		
Organizes time for responsibilities			X	
Participates in interests	X			
Fulfilled roles (past)				X
Maintained habits (past)				X
Achieved satisfaction (past)			X	

Occupational Settings (Environment) Scale	1	2	3	4
Home life occupational forms			X	
Major productive role occupational forms		X		
Leisure occupational forms		X		
Home life social group			X	
Major productive role social group			X	
Leisure social group			X	
Home life spaces, objects, and resources				X
Major productive role spaces, objects, and resources			X	
Leisure spaces, objects, and resources			X	

Occupational Identity Scale
OPHI-II Key form results
Client Measure: 49
Standard error: 4

Occupational Competence Scale
OPHI-II Key form results
Client Measure: 49
Standard error: 4

Occupational Settings (Environment) Scale
OPHI-II Key form results
Client Measure: 55
Standard error: 5

Analysis/plan: Does not see how to manage like before. Plan is to engage Ellen in previously valued interests;
1) Walking outdoor with a rollator (accompanied with staff member)
2) Group activity; green care → laiter planting on own balcony with friends and granddaughter's help → aim is to build up confidence and assist return to more active life style.

FIGURE 17-5 Summary of Ellen's Scores on the OPHI-II.

and a skillful gardener had been the most important parts of who she was. The therapist and Ellen also drew a narrative slope, shown in Figure 17-6. This helped them to discuss how she had managed when it had been difficult, what had been most valuable and enjoyable for her, and what she envisioned for the future. Also important was how and with whom she would make the future happen.

The next important development in Ellen's recovery was the fact that she shared the narrative with her granddaughter, her friend, and the staff of the center. Ten months earlier, her granddaughter had moved to the city to begin her studies at the university. With the occupational therapist, the staff of the day care center, and her granddaughter, she began her daily walks. She got a walker, and it had a seat adjustable to a suitable height so she could walk for short distances and take a rest using the seat of her walker.

One of the first things Ellen and her best friend did at the center was to attend a green care program. Participants planned, planted, and took care of plants. They also got her granddaughter involved. The future plan was that she would help to set growing bags or boxes on a long, raised bench on Ellen's balcony. The three of them were looking forward to sharing the enjoyment of tasting the first crop of vegetables, including some potatoes.

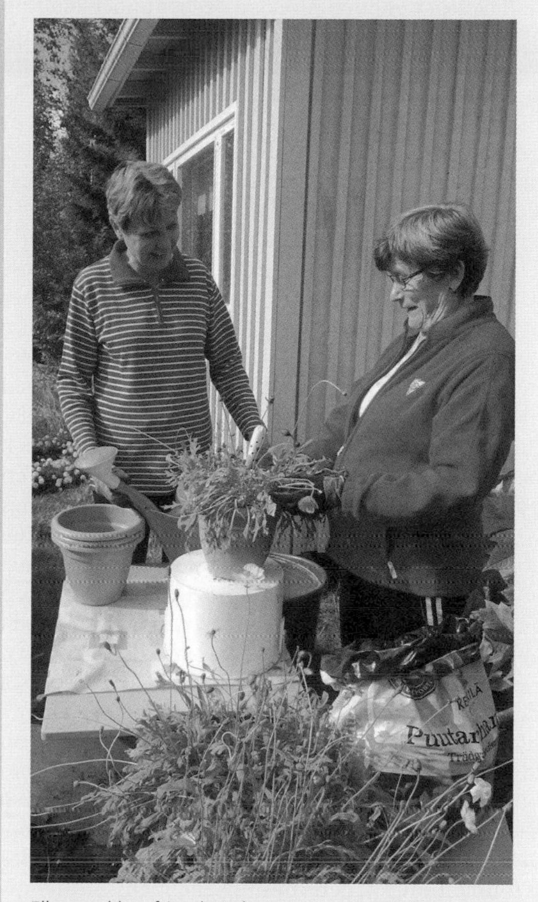

Ellen and her friend at the green care program

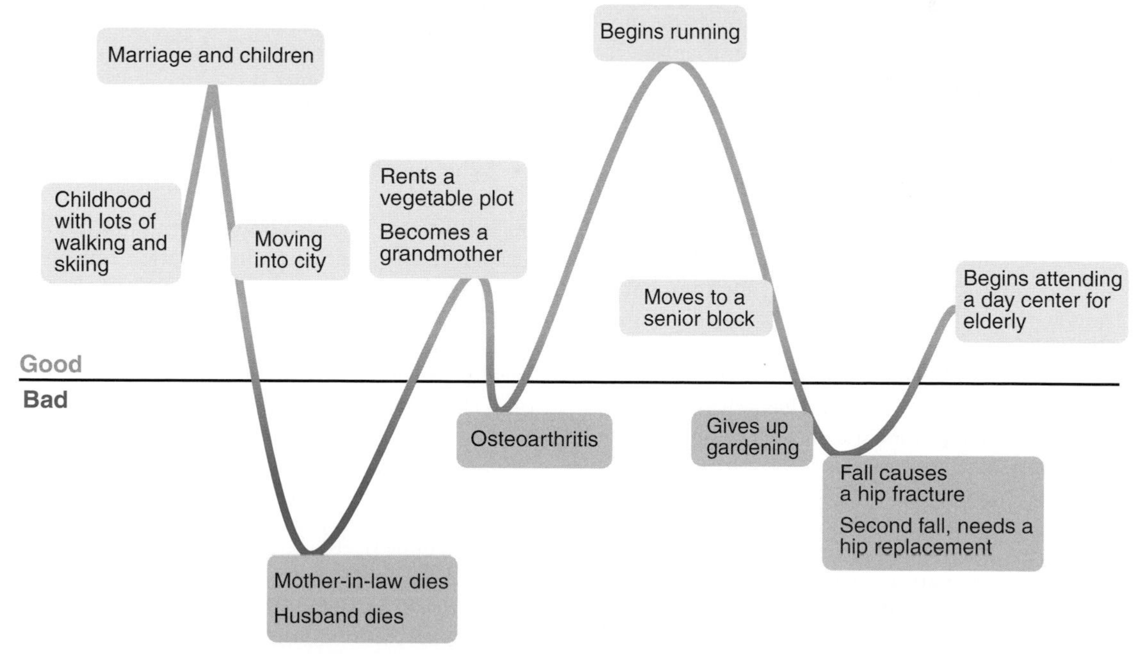

FIGURE 17-6 Ellens's Narrative Slope.

The story of Ellen reveals a deeper understanding of how her newly acquired impairments affected her sense of herself, and how, at first, she felt like a failure and called herself "a bone cracker." In her narrative, she revealed a central metaphor involving a lack of momentum. She felt like she was stuck and unable to move. She described this with a metaphoric expression: "It feels like I am floating in the water in a very small pond, and I am not able to move myself at all." This is quite the opposite of her previous success with becoming a long-distance runner to address her osteoarthritis. The strategy she had in her life before her second hip fracture was one of momentum: mowing, walking, or running, to the extent that it seemed like a matter of life or death for her. In Ellen's story, this was the thing that needed fixing—getting back her mobility. Participation in occupations driven by occupational identity and one's inherent values is necessary for a person to build up occupational competence and gain a positive sense of occupational adaptation. Without the OPHI-II interview, Ellen and the occupational therapist could not have been able to plan as effective a way toward Ellen's recovery.

As this case illustrates, the OPHI-II provides a detailed chronicle of the salient features of a client's life and the impact of events and environment on identity and competence. It also provides insight into how the client interprets his or her life by evoking the client's occupational narrative. This information, as illustrated through the previous case, provides a foundation for determining the focus of therapy and negotiating its meaning with the client. In this regard, the OPHI-II is a powerful tool to ensure that therapy is client centered. More specifically, it can allow therapy to address and effectively become part of the lives clients want to craft for themselves.

THE SCHOOL SETTING INTERVIEW

The SSI version 3.1 (Hemmingsson, Egilson, Lidström, & Kielhofner, 2014) is a semistructured interview designed to assess the impact of the school environment on the student. The SSI uses MOHO's conceptualization of the social and physical environment as a framework for the assessment.

The SSI is used to assess the student–environment fit to identify the need for school setting accommodations for students with disabilities. It is a client-centered interview that examines the student's interaction with the physical and social environments at school. It includes 16 items of everyday school activities that make up a student's participation in school and together address the content areas of write, read, speak, remember things, do mathematics, do homework, take exams, participate in sport activities, participate in practical subjects, participate in the classroom, participate in social activities during breaks, participate in practical activities during breaks, go on field trips, get assistance, access the school, and interact with the staff. The SSI is intended for students who are able to communicate adequately to discuss their experiences. This assessment is administered as a collaborative discussion that examines the student's performance with a specific focus on how the school setting influences the student. Although it was originally designed for students who had physical impairments, based on research (Egilson & Hemmingsson, 2009) and clinical practice, the SSI version 3.1 is updated to include students who have emotional, developmental, and behavioral impairments.

The SSI considers the student's occupational performance in all aspects of the school environment, such as the classroom, playground, toilets, lockers, gymnasium, corridors, and field trips. In addition to determining whether accommodations are necessary, the therapist gains a qualitative understanding of the student's experiences. Furthermore, the SSI guides the therapist to discuss with the students how they want to manage in school. The SSI empowers students to collaborate with the therapist in determining the types of accommodations they may need. It reflects the assumption that determining the student's preferences, values, needs, and interests is crucial to successful physical and social accommodations in the school setting.

ADMINISTRATION

Before beginning the interview, the therapist explains to the student that the SSI is not designed to identify the student's weaknesses, but instead to make sure the school is doing its best to assist the student to do well. In conducting the interview, the therapist explores each of the 16 items, asking the student the following:

- How he or she has functioned and currently functions in the area
- Whether the student perceives a need for accommodation to perform in the area
- Whether the student currently has an accommodation in this area

The SSI interview takes about 40 minutes, and the therapist records necessary information during the interview. A form allows identification of whether there are accommodation needs in each area and whether they are partly or fully met. Another form allows recording of accommodation recommendations. This form indicates recommended changes to be made in the physical and social environment. It also records who will be responsible for each accommodation and how it will be implemented.

To give the therapist and other professionals a quick overview of the student–environment fit and to track changes, a summary form is provided. After the interview, the therapist indicates the extent of the student's accommodations, needs, and unmet needs on each item using a four-point rating scale.

CASE STUDY: A HIGH SCHOOL STUDENT WITH MUSCULAR DYSTROPHY

The principal of a high school in a Stockholm suburb invited the school occupational therapist to a routine planning meeting concerning Thomas, a first-year high school student. Thomas' parents; the school nurse; a special education teacher; and his language, physical education, and math teachers were also invited to attend. The therapist had known Thomas and his family for nearly 10 years.

At the age of 4, Thomas was diagnosed with muscular dystrophy. He always attended a regular school, and most things went well. Throughout primary school, he had a couple of good friends in his class. He also had a teacher who was empathic, flexible, and adept at including Thomas in class activities with the other children. The therapist had previously worked with Thomas and occasionally consulted with Thomas' mother by telephone.

Thomas' mother called the therapist, indicating that Thomas had asked her to make the call. The mother said that, as far as she knew, everything was going fine with Thomas in his new school. Thomas then took the telephone and explained that he had heard of the upcoming meeting from his mother. As far as Thomas knew, he was not invited, and none of the teachers had spoken to him about it. He wanted to know what the meeting was about. The therapist explained that she understood the meeting to be a routine review meeting to ensure Thomas was doing fine. When the therapist asked Thomas how he liked the new school, he responded, "It's okay, I suppose." Thomas' tone suggested otherwise, so the therapist made an appointment to meet Thomas after school that week.

The therapist then called the principal back to ask if there was some special preparation that he wanted her to do before the meeting. He explained again that it was a routine meeting. The principal was not aware of any problems. Thomas appeared to be doing fine and had not complained of anything. He expected the meeting to affirm that Thomas was performing well and adjusting to the new school.

Thomas' school was big and rather traditional, having been built at the beginning of the 20th century. When the therapist arrived for the appointment, Thomas was waiting at the entrance and appeared to be the only student present. He explained that it was the day of a sports outing. Thomas was not capable of going along, so he was there alone.

The therapist explained, "As *you already know, I am invited to a planning meeting next week, and I think it is important to get your opinion about the school situation and how it affects your opportunities to participate in school activities. I would like to apply the SSI with you to identify school activities in which you may need support and accommodation to more easily participate.*" "*OK,*" Thomas said, "*I think it is strange that I am not invited to the meeting—they do not know anything about me.*" "*Well, I promise I will bring up the issues you emphasize in the SSI,*" the therapist answered. As the interview progressed, it was obvious that Thomas found being in the new school a negative experience. Things that he readily did in his former school were now difficult or impossible for him. He had tried hard to adapt to the new circumstances, and he had not wanted to complain because he was afraid of drawing too much attention to himself. During the SSI interview, Thomas identified unmet needs and problems with student–environment fit in several areas, as reflected in the Summary Form shown in Figure 17-7.

In his previous school, Thomas' homeroom teacher had taught the students in nearly all subjects. Therefore, she came to know his special needs and was able to integrate the accommodations he needed into her plans for the class. For example, in the area of writing, she always made a paper copy of any visual aids she used in class. She gave a copy of these to Thomas because he wrote slowly and needed additional time to take notes. Now, in secondary school, Thomas had different teachers in nearly all subjects. He had informed some of his teachers about his need for paper copies of slides and overheads. However, the information had not reached some teachers, or they had forgotten. Consequently, he rarely got paper copies of class audiovisuals. Thomas also needed access to a computer and more time for writing in exams, but no such arrangements had been made in the new school.

Thomas was used to being able to participate in activities like field trips or outdoor activities, because his previous teacher always tried to include his needs in her planning. He had a powered wheelchair he could use on outings, because his ambulation was too labored for such events. There had already been several occasions in the new school when plans for special events were made without consideration of his needs. This meant that he was excluded. On the other hand, Thomas was very happy that he did not have to participate in gym because he found it embarrassing that he could not dress himself.

Another big difference was that, in his former school, all of Thomas' classes were held in his home classroom. Now, in secondary school, he

SUMMARY SHEET

Date:
Student: Thomas

Summary of the initial assessment.

Item	Rating Scale			
	Perfect (4)	Good (3)	Partial (2)	Unfit (1)
1. Writing				✗
2. Reading		✗		
3. Speaking	✗			
4. Remembering things	✗			
5. Do mathematics		✗		
6. Do homework	✗			
7. Take exams				✗
8. Participate in sports activities				✗
9. Participate in practical subjects			✗	
10. Participate in the classroom			✗	
11. Participate in social activities during breaks				✗
12. Participate in practical activities during breaks			✗	
13. Go on field trips				✗
14. Get assistance		✗		
15. Access the school			✗	
16. Interact with staff				✗
Sum:	12	9	8	6

Total sum: 35

Summary of the re-assessment.

Item	Rating Scale			
	Perfect (4)	Good (3)	Partial (2)	Unfit (1)
1. Writing				
2. Reading				
3. Speaking				
4. Remembering things				
5. Do mathematics				
6. Do homework				
7. Take exams				
8. Participate in sports activities				
9. Participate in practical subjects				
10. Participate in the classroom				
11. Participate in social activities during breaks				
12. Participate in practical activities during breaks				
13. Go on field trips				
14. Get assistance				
15. Access the school				
16. Interact with staff				
Sum:				

Total sum:________

Rating scale:
4 = Perfect fit when the student perceives that the school environment fit is ideal and the student doesn't need any adjustments at all. The student has no need for adjustments.
3 = Good fit when the student perceives that the school environment has been adapted to meet his or her needs. Thus, the student has received needed adjustments and is satisfied with adjustments made. The student has the necessary adjustments.
2 = Partial fit when the student perceives that the school environment needs to be modified although he or she has already received some adjustments. The student already has some adjustments but additional adjustment is needed.
1 = Unfit when the student perceives that the school environment needs to be modified but he or she has not received any adjustments at all. The student needs new adjustments.

FIGURE 17-7 Thomas' Identified Needs for Accommodations on the SSI.

had to travel between classrooms. During the short breaks between classes, Thomas often had to go to a different floor or a different building. Ambulating made it difficult for him to carry books and other things that he needed in the next classroom. Neither his balance nor his strength was good enough to walk carrying a heavy bag. Of his own accord, Thomas had decided to start using his wheelchair at school, which made it possible for him to carry his things between classrooms. Using a wheelchair in school had also made lunchtime easier, because he had experienced difficulty standing in line in the lunchroom.

Using the wheelchair, however, created new problems. The organization of the school day required rather quick transfer between different classrooms. Using the elevator was time consuming, and he had difficulty opening the manual elevator door. Moreover, there was only one wheelchair-accessible toilet on the second floor of one building. Finally, there were only steps to the entrance of school, forcing him to take an otherwise unused side entrance that also increased the distance he had to travel when entering and exiting the building. Another problem related to frequent classroom changes was that Thomas and his personal equipment (e.g., assistive devices, special chair, special desk, and personal computer) were, unfortunately, seldom in the same classroom.

Finally, as part of the SSI interview, the therapist and Thomas collaboratively discussed ways in which the school might address his unmet needs in each content area. The therapist suggested that Thomas be given an assistant who would carry his bag and take notes when needed, or that he request a home classroom. However, Thomas did not want a personal assistant. He preferred to ask some classmates who were friends to assist him. He noted that they already helped him voluntarily sometimes, without him even asking. He also did not want to ask for a home classroom because he thought it would adversely affect his relationships with classmates who would find it childish. He was most satisfied with the idea that the school be asked to schedule as many of his courses as possible on the ground floor to minimize his need to use the elevator.

The therapist then brought up to Thomas the risk of immobilization. She explained that if he constantly used the wheelchair, he increased the risk of contractures in his hip flexors. She pointed out that, with his diagnosis, immobilization even for short periods may cause permanent loss of ambulation. She pointed out that his use of the wheelchair in school, in combination with avoiding gym, was a serious risk. It was obvious that Thomas did not want to think about this. However, the therapist got his permission to talk with the physical therapist and with the gym teacher about arranging an individual gym program for Thomas.

Finally, they discussed ways that the school could become more aware of and attentive to Thomas' special needs. Thomas and the therapist decided together that the therapist should share the information from the SSI with the other team members at the planning meeting. She would be responsible to report back to Thomas what happened.

Recommendations for Accommodation

At the staff meeting, the therapist presented the SSI results and discussed necessary accommodations for Thomas. The therapist recorded the results of this meeting on the SSI Intervention Planning Form that is shown in Figure 17-8 and discussed later. The therapist began by presenting Thomas' need for classroom scheduling to keep him mostly on one floor. Second, she emphasized that all of Thomas' teachers needed better information about his special needs. She recommended that there be a written document about Thomas' needs (i.e., copies of slides, a desk suitable for a wheelchair in all classrooms he was scheduled, extra time and access to a computer in examinations, and consideration of his physical limitations when planning outdoor activities and field trips). The therapist recommended that the principal give this document to any new teacher. In addition, Thomas would receive copies that he could give to teachers as a reminder. The therapist also requested the following accommodations on Thomas' behalf:

- Adapting one of the toilets on the ground floor
- A ramp at the entrance
- An automatic door opener to the elevator

Finally, the occupational therapist brought up the serious risk of immobilization from constant use of the wheelchair together with not attending gym lessons. Thomas' parents, teachers, and principal were surprised when the therapist described the results from the SSI. They had assumed that everything was fine, because Thomas had never complained. However, they appreciated the information and supported doing everything reasonable to adapt his learning environment. After discussion, the following decisions were made:

- The principal would investigate the logistics of reducing the number of classrooms and the number of teachers who taught in Thomas' classes. He was to consult with Thomas before he made any final decisions.

Content Area	Environmental Adjustments				Team Members	Steps for Implementation: whom, when, where, and how
	Space	Objects	Forms	Groups		
1. Writing			Thomas is given photocopies of visual aides.		• OT • Teacher • Thomas • Principal	• OT and Thomas write his special needs report. • Principal informs Thomas' teacher about helpful strategies decided in the planning meeting.
7. Taking exams			Thomas is given more time to take exams.		• OT • Teacher • Thomas • Principal	• Same as above • PT consults with P.E. instructor and parents.
8. Doing sport activities			Alternative P.E. activities at school and home.		• PT • Teacher • Thomas • Principal	• PT, parents, and P.E. instructor regularly remind Thomas of contracture risks. • Regular assessment of Thomas' mobility by P.T.
9. Doing practical subjects			More time needed to complete art projects.		• Art teacher	• Art teacher will prepare activities that students can complete at their own pace.
10. Participating in the classrooms		Desk adjusted to fit wheelchair in more than one classroom.	Minimize the use of different classrooms.		• OT • Teacher • Thomas • Principal	• Principal, Thomas, and teachers discuss how to minimize the use of different classrooms. • OT orders appropriate desks.
11. Participating in social activities during breaks				Provide assistance to and from social activities so more time is spent having fun and not getting around.		• Thomas will identify some friends that can provide assistance to lunchroom, between classrooms, etc.
12. Participating in practical activities at breaks		Raised toilet seat, in bathroom at ground floor.			• OT • Thomas	• Decide on type of toilet seat and OT to order.
13. Going on field trips			Select field trip sites that are accessible to powered wheelchair.	Thomas will be included in class field trips.	• OT • Thomas • Teacher • Parents	• OT consults on selections of field trip sites. • Prior information from school to Thomas and parents to provide powered wheelchair.
15. Accessing the school	Ramp to the main door entrance. Automatic door opener to elevator.		Reduce transfer between different classrooms.		• OT • Thomas • Principal	• OT to provide temporary ramp. • Principal arranges for permanent ramp.
16. Interacting with staff				The school nurse provides mentorship to Thomas.	• Thomas • School nurse • OT	• School nurse to advocate on behalf of Thomas when needed. • The school nurse to cooperate with OT when needed.

FIGURE 17-8 Thomas' Intervention Planning Form.

- **The team agreed that a written document about Thomas' special needs was a good idea. The therapist agreed to write the document in cooperation with Thomas. In addition, the principal should inform all relevant teachers that Thomas was allowed extra time and access to a computer in examinations. He should also emphasize teachers' obligation to consider wheelchair accessibility when planning outdoor activities and field trips.**
- **The principal agreed to install a ramp at the entrance. As a ramp was needed immediately, the therapist offered to obtain for the school a borrowed ramp from a rehabilitation center until the school installed something more stationary at the entrance. The principal believed that the elevator alterations were cost-prohibitive.**
- **The gym teacher indicated that because he had limited experience with students who had physical impairments, he would need support to meet Thomas' needs. The physiotherapist was identified as the best person to consult with him.**
- **The physiotherapist agreed to regularly assess Thomas' locomotion as well as consult with the school, Thomas, and his parents on how to avoid contractures.**
- **The school nurse was assigned the responsibility to serve as an advocate and coordinator to ensure that Thomas' needs were being met.**

Finally, they decided to invite Thomas to the next planning meeting.

As this case illustrates, the SSI can be particularly helpful in identifying unmet needs for accommodation in the school setting. The framework of the interview, which gives students the opportunity to talk about their experiences, preferences, and needs, is well suited to this end.

Work Environment Impact Scale

The Work Environment Impact Scale (WEIS) (Moore-Corner, Kielhofner, & Olson, 1998) focuses on the fit between a person and his or her work environment. The semistructured interview and the accompanying rating scale are designed to provide a comprehensive assessment of how qualities and characteristics of a given work environment affect a person's work performance, satisfaction, and well-being. After completing the interview, the therapist rates the 17 WEIS items on a four-point rating scale. The WEIS is often used in conjunction with the WRI, because the two interviews can be combined, saving time in administration. A detailed description of the assessment and a case study is provided in Chapter 24.

WORKER ROLE INTERVIEW

The Worker Role Interview (WRI) (Braveman et al., 2005) is designed to identify psychosocial and environmental factors that influence a client's ability to return to work, remain in work, or get employment in general, in other words, the client's psychosocial work potential. The WRI consists of a semistructured interview with an accompanying therapist-administered four-point rating scale. The 16-item scale is rated according to the implications of each item for the client's likelihood of work success. The WRI is designed for concurrent use with other assessments that provide work-related ability. The psychosocial factors identified by the WRI often reveal unique strengths and weaknesses and provide a solid foundation for planning client-centered interventions aimed at enabling the client achieve employment. A detailed description of the assessment and a case study are provided in Chapter 24.

Conclusion: Interviews in Perspective

This chapter presented and illustrated five interviews that have been developed for different clients and different contexts. The variety of interviews allows the therapist to select the one that will be most appropriate in a given setting or for a given client. These interviews are also designed to be flexible in use so that they can be adapted to each client.

Although interviews will not be feasible for use with all clients, many of the MOHO interviews are designed so that certain key questions may be administered without the need to administer the entire interview. It is important to keep in mind that eliciting a client's self-report through an interview does present opportunities to gather important information to achieve a client-centered focus. Hence, their use whenever possible is strongly encouraged. Interviews also actively engage clients in discussing and giving perspectives on their own situations, which helps them begin a collaborative role in their own therapy. Finally, they serve as important opportunities to build rapport. Although interviews take time, the time is well spent, given the kinds of information they yield and the opportunities they represent for beginning a true collaboration with the client.

Chapter 17 Review Questions

1. Describe the components of a semistructured interview.
2. Which of the MOHO interview assessments is a three-part assessment? What are the parts?
3. Which of the MOHO interview assessments provides a form for planning occupational therapy interventions?
4. Who may draw the narrative slope in the OPHI-II?
5. Which of the MOHO interview assessments is appropriate for use with school-aged children?
6. Why is the use of rating scales important?

HOMEWORK ASSIGNMENTS

1. Work in pairs, perform an OCAIRS interview with a person older than 35. One of you should perform the interview, and the other should act as an observer. After the interview, complete the rating form individually, compare the ratings, and discuss your rating choices.
2. Interview a school-aged child using the School Setting Interview, and reflect on differences and similarities in interviewing a child and an adult person.
3. Work in pairs, tell each other about your occupational performance history, make a slope for each of you, and discuss the results.
4. Read the three cases in this chapter and identify the occupational therapy intervention for each case. Group the type of interventions provided and give each group a label.

REFERENCES

Braveman, B., Robson, M., Velozo, C., Kielhofner, G., Fisher, G., Forsyth, K., et al. (2005). *Worker Role Interview (WRI)* [Version 10.0]. Chicago: Model of Human Occupation Clearinghouse, Department of Occupational Therapy, College of Applied Health Sciences, University of Illinois at Chicago.

Egilson, S., & Hemmingsson, H. (2009). School participation of pupils with physical and psychosocial limitations: A comparison. *British Journal of Occupational Therapy, 72*(4), 144–152.

Forsyth, K., Deshpande, S., Kielhofner, G., Henriksson, C., Haglund, L., Olson, L., et al. (2005). *The occupational circumstances assessment and interview rating scale, version 4.0.* Chicago, IL: Model of Human Occupation Clearinghouse, Department of Occupational Therapy, College of Applied Health Sciences, University of Illinois at Chicago.

Haglund, L., & Forsyth, K. (2013). The measurement properties of the Occupational Circumstances Interview and Rating Scale—Sweden (OCAIRS-S V2). *Scandinavian Journal of Occupational Therapy, 20*, 412–419.

Hemmingsson, H., Egilson, S., Lidström, H., & Kielhofner, G. (2014). *The School Setting Interview (SSI)* [Version 3.1]. Nacka, Sweden: Sveriges Arbetsterapeuter.

Kaplan, K. (1984). Short-term assessment: The need and a response. *Occupational Therapy in Mental Health, 4*(3), 29–45.

Kaplan, K., & Kielhofner, G. (1989). *The occupational case analysis interview and rating scale.* Thorofare, NJ: Slack.

Kielhofner, G., Dobria, L., Forsyth, K., & Basu, S. (2005). The construction of keyforms for obtaining instantaneous measures from the occupational performance history interview rating scales. *Occupational Therapy Journal of Research, 25*, 23–32.

Kielhofner, G., Mallinson, T., Crawford, C., Nowak, M., Rigby, M., Henry, A., et al. (2004). *Occupational Performance History Interview-II (OPHI-II)* [Version 2.1]. Chicago: Model of Human Occupation Clearinghouse, Department of Occupational Therapy, College of Applied Health Sciences, University of Illinois at Chicago.

Moore-Corner, R., Kielhofner, G., & Olson, L. (1998). *Work Environment Impact Scale (WEIS)* [Version 2.0]. Chicago: Model of Human Occupation Clearinghouse, Department of Occupational Therapy, College of Applied Health Sciences, University of Illinois at Chicago.

Assessments Combining Methods of Information Gathering

Sue Parkinson, John Cooper, Carmen-Gloria de las Heras de Pablo, Nichola Duffy, Patricia Bowyer, Gail Fisher, and Kirsty Forsyth

CHAPTER 18

EXPECTED LEARNING OUTCOMES

Upon completion of this chapter, the readers will be able to:

1. Recognize that information can be gathered from multiple sources and combined to inform a comprehensive occupational assessment.
2. Discriminate between MOHO assessments that combine methods of information gathering.
3. Identify when to use an assessment that combines methods of information gathering.
4. Understand how to administer these assessments.
5. Appreciate how these assessments can influence treatment.

This chapter discusses six assessments that combine various methods of information gathering (interview, observation, self-reporting, and liaison with key others). The first three are comprehensive assessments that summarize the occupational needs for different client groups:

- The Model of Human Occupation Screening Tool (MOHOST)
- The Short Child Occupational Profile (SCOPE)
- The Model of Human Occupation Exploratory Level Outcome Ratings (MOHO-ExpLOR)

The MOHOST and SCOPE are used when assessing the occupational needs of the general population, with the MOHOST being suitable for adolescents, adults, and older people, and the SCOPE being suitable for children and adolescents. Meanwhile, the MOHO-ExpLOR is suitable for adolescents, adults, and older adults whose occupational participation is severely impaired.

The remaining three assessments are either used in specific settings or have a more specific focus in terms of the MOHO concepts being analyzed:

- The Assessment of Occupational Functioning—Collaborative Version (AOF-CV)
- The Occupational Therapy Psychosocial Assessment of Learning (OT PAL)
- The Residential Environment Impact Scale (REIS)

Both the AOF-CV and the OT PAL have rating scales that focus primarily on volition and habituation. They differ in that the AOF-CV is administered as a self-report or an interview with adults, while the OT PAL gathers information on children in school settings through interviews and observation. The REIS, as its name suggests, can be used in residential settings to evaluate how well the environment meets the needs and interests of its residents.

Model of Human Occupation Screening Tool and the Short Child Occupational Profile

The Model of Human Occupation Screening Tool (MOHOST; Parkinson, Forsyth, & Kielhofner, 2006) and the Short Child Occupational Profile (SCOPE; Bowyer et al., 2008) gather information relevant to the majority of MOHO concepts, allowing the therapist to gain an overview of a person's occupational functioning. They are both therapist-rated tools, but whereas the MOHOST was designed for *adult* populations, the SCOPE was designed for *pediatric* populations. Both assessments may be used with adolescents, according to their needs, and can be used with a wide range of people with psychosocial and/or physical impairments. They are easy to administer and can be used flexibly and efficiently to record a person's occupational needs, identify areas for further assessment, and guide treatment planning, before being readministered and used as outcome measures.

The assessments aim to capture a person's relative strengths, highlighting the impact of volition, habituation, skills, and the environment on occupational participation. The MOHOST consists of 24 items divided equally between 6 sections, representing volition, habituation, communication and interaction, process skills, motor skills, and the environment. Volition has been renamed "motivation for occupation" and habituation has been renamed "pattern of occupation" to support the understanding of anyone who is not an occupational therapist reading the form.

The SCOPE is similar, but uses the original MOHO terms and has an additional item in the environment section. For both the MOHOST and SCOPE, each item is assessed using a 4-point rating scale. Figures 18-1A and B illustrate the rating scale and a selection of items from each of the assessments. As shown, the criteria for making the ratings are built into the forms, to make the rating process as straightforward as possible.

The MOHOST and the SCOPE can be ordered from the MOHO website at www.cade.uic.edu/moho

ADMINISTRATION

The data collection method for the MOHOST and SCOPE has been designed to be flexible to meet multiple needs in practice. Therapists may use any dependable source of information for completing the scales. This information is often gained through observation; however, it may be supplemented or achieved through talking to the person, workers, and/or relatives. Additionally, therapists may gather information from records, team meetings, or other available sources. The SCOPE also has parent and teacher reporting forms that can be used to obtain data.

Item	Rating	Criteria
Expectation of success Optimism & hope, self-efficacy, sense of control & self-identity	F	Anticipates success and seeks challenges, optimistic about overcoming obstacles
	A	Has some hope for success, adequate self-belief but has some doubts, may need encouraging
	I	Requires support to sustain optimism about overcoming obstacles, poor self-efficacy
	R	Pessimistic, feels hopeless, gives up in the face of obstacles, lacks sense of control
		Comments:
Routine Balance, organization of habits, structure, productivity	F	Able to arrange a balanced, organised and productive routine of daily activities
	A	Generally able to maintain or follow an organised and productive daily schedule
	I	Difficulty organising balanced, productive routines of daily activities without support
	R	Chaotic or empty routine, unable to support responsibilities and goals, erratic routine
		Comments:
Problem-solving Judgement, adaptation, decisionmaking, responsiveness	F	Shows good judgement, anticipates difficulties and generates workable solutions (rational)
	A	Generally able to make decisions based on difficulties that arise
	I	Difficulty anticipating and adapting to difficulties that arise, seeks reassurance
	R	Unable to anticipate and adapt to difficulties that arise and makes inappropriate decisions
		Comments:
Physical space Self-care, productivity and leisure facilities, privacy and accessibility, stimulation and comfort	F	Space affords a range of opportunities, supports & stimulates valued occupations
	A	Space is mostly adequate, allows daily occupations to be pursued
	I	Affords a limited range of opportunities and curtails performance of valued occupations
	R	Space restricts opportunities and prevents performance of valued occupations
		Comments:

A

Response to challenge The child engages in new activities and/or accepts the opportunity to achieve more, or perform under conditions of greater demand		
F	The child spontaneously seeks and persists in new or more challenging activities	*Comments:*
A	The child spontaneously attempts new or more challenging activities, but is easily frustrated and/or needs some support in order to persist	
I	The child usually requires significant support to engage in new and more demanding activities and to overcome frustration and persist during such activities	
R	The child avoids new or more challenging activities because they elicit a high level of frustration	

FIGURE 18-1 A. Sample Items from the MOHOST. **B.** Sample Items from the SCOPE.

Routine The child has an awareness of routines and is able to participate effectively in structured daily routines		
F	The child demonstrates an awareness of the sequence and structure of regular routines, and can anticipate, initiate, and/or cooperate with related activities	*Comments:*
A	The child requires occasional cueing and redirection in order to cooperate with the regular sequence and structure of routines in his/her life	
I	The child is often unable to participate in the sequence and structure of regular routines	
R	The child does not demonstrate an awareness of the sequence and structure of regular routines; does not participate, cooperate, and/or initiate routine activities	

Problem Solving The child demonstrates an appropriate ability to identify and respond to challenges		
F	The child consistently anticipates problems, generates workable solutions, and evaluates these solutions to determine the best course of action	*Comments:*
A	The child can identify difficulties but needs step-by-step cues to generate an effective response	
I	The child rarely anticipates and adapts to difficulties; needs ongoing reassurance when problems are encountered	
R	The child is unable to anticipate and adapt to difficulties; makes inappropriate decisions	

Physical space The layout and arrangement of physical space (at home, community, school, and/or hospital) supports the child's participation.		
F	Arrangement of physical environment is accessible and provides opportunities to engage in various activities; stimulates and supports occupational participation in child's valued roles.	*Comments:*
A	Arrangement of physical environment does not adequately support occupational engagement or is somewhat accessible; poses some limitations to the child's participation in valued roles.	
I	Arrangement of physical environment affords a limited range of opportunities with limited accessibility and support for occupational engagement and participation in child's valued roles.	
R	Arrangement of physical environment is not accessible, does not provide opportunities and prevents participation in the child's valued roles.	

B

FIGURE 18-1 (continued)

If necessary, therapists can build an understanding of a person's occupational participation over a period of time to complete the assessments. For this reason, the MOHOST and SCOPE include a Single Observation Form that therapists may use to record the observations made after a single intervention, for example, a kitchen assessment or a group attendance; a child in a classroom or community activity. (The MOHOST Single Observation Form is illustrated in Fig. 18-2A). Once the therapists have sufficient information, they may progress to completing the summary MOHOST or SCOPE form. All the MOHOST and SCOPE forms are easy to administer and rate and can therefore be used at regular intervals to document a person's progress.

MOHO Problem-Solver: Using the MOHOST in Community Mental Health

Bryony Robinson worked as an occupational therapist in a community mental health team in the UK and regularly completed the MOHOST to track the occupational needs of her clients. One of the strengths of using the MOHOST was that it allowed her to frame her feedback for the majority of her clients. Ultimately, however, she wanted to empower her clients to reflect on their own occupational participation, and she recognized that one of the limitations of using the MOHOST was that it is a therapist-rated tool.

When working with a group of men to facilitate their discharge from the service, she asked them, "How shall we evaluate this program?" Their response was that they should evaluate their own progress over the course of the intervention, using the MOHOST items that they had become familiar with. Rather than using the Occupational Self-Assessment to evaluate their sense of competence and identity across a broad range of occupational concerns, they wanted to use the MOHOST items that they had become familiar with to rate their participation in the group program.

Bryony worked with them to adapt the MOHOST Single Observation Form and create a non-standardized MOHOST Self-Assessment form (Fig. 18-2B). Although this process inevitably forfeited the reliability and validity of the assessment, it served to complement and reinforce the value of the original MOHOST.

Process skills	Chooses/uses equipment appropriately	N/S	F	A	I	R	*Comments:*
	Maintains focus throughout task/sequence	N/S	F	A	I	R	
	Works in an orderly fashion	N/S	F	A	I	R	
	Modifies actions to overcome problems	N/S	F	A	I	R	

Motor skills	Mobilizes independently	N/S	F	A	I	R	*Comments:*
	Manipulates tools and materials easily	N/S	F	A	I	R	
	Uses appropriate strength and effort	N/S	F	A	I	R	
	Maintains energy and appropriate pace	N/S	F	A	I	R	

Key: **N/S** = Not seen
A = Allows occupational participation
R = Restricts occupational participation
F = Facilitates occupational participation
I = Inhibits occupational participation

A

Process skills	I knew what needed to be done or asked as necessary	N/S	F	A	I	R	*Comments:*
	I followed the tasks and concentrated from beginning to end	N/S	F	A	I	R	
	I planned how to approach tasks, organised workspace & materials	N/S	F	A	I	R	
	I dealt with problems that arose and adapted if necessary	N/S	F	A	I	R	

Motor skills	I was able to stand and move (walk, bend and reach) easily	N/S	F	A	I	R	*Comments:*
	I handled any equipment, tools or objects securely and easily	N/S	F	A	I	R	
	I used appropriate strength and effort for the task	N/S	F	A	I	R	
	I maintained my energy levels throughout the session	N/S	F	A	I	R	

Key: **N/S** = Not seen
A = Allows occupational participation
R = Restricts occupational participation
F = Facilitates occupational participation
I = Inhibits occupational participation

B

FIGURE 18-2 A. Sample Sections from the MOHOST Single Observation Form. **B.** Sample Sections from the MOHOST Self-Assessment Form.

The resulting form can now be downloaded from the MOHO website at www.cade.uic.edu/moho

Andrew: Using the MOHOST to Evidence Progress

Andrew was diagnosed with schizophrenia in his late 20s, 10 years ago. He completed an art degree but never had a job or formed any major relationships, and he continued to receive substantial support from his parents. He had multiple psychiatric hospitalizations and was last admitted to an acute mental health hospital in a distressed and agitated state.

Why Was the MOHOST Chosen?

The occupational therapist was able to complete the Volitional Questionnaire (VQ) and the Assessment of Communication and Interaction Skill (ACIS), but Andrew's needs required more comprehensive assessment. He was unable to tolerate interviews, engage in a self-assessment procedure, or cooperate in a formal observational assessment process. When the occupational therapist attempted to interview Andrew on a previous admission, he answered most of the questions with "I don't know" or "I've never thought about it." The MOHOST allowed the therapist to gather a broad range of information with minimal intrusion.

How Was Information Gathered?

Initially, Andrew was observed on the ward, where he neglected both his hygiene and his diet, but would spend long periods writing furiously (and for the most part illegibly) or making seemingly random but energetic movements. The occupational therapist made contact with him and embarked on the Remotivation Process. She gathered information by reading his case notes and speaking with team members and Andrew's parents. In doing so, she was able to validate the opinion of others and was also able to educate them about the purpose of MOHOST and the focus of occupational therapy.

What Did the MOHOST Show?

The initial summary MOHOST reinforced the breadth of Andrew's needs, with most of the personal items *restricting* occupational participation other than the motor skills items and the volitional item: interest. Although the occupational therapist recognized some limitations in the institutional setting, Andrew clearly needed to be in safe surroundings and so the environmental items were rated as *allowing* occupational participation.

Could the MOHOST Record Progress?

Eventually, Andrew made some improvement and started to attend an art session on the ward for 10 minutes at a time. A single observation MOHOST indicated that his interest, choices, and communication might be improving, and he expressed an interest in attending further occupational therapy sessions. After much deliberation, the team agreed that he could be accompanied to activities in the main day therapy area. Andrew's initial program was based on his expressed interest in art, yoga stretches, and table tennis—activities where social interaction was not the primary focus. The occupational therapist used the summary MOHOST at this point to evaluate his progress, and the ratings are shown in Figure 18-3.

How Did the MOHOST Influence Treatment?

The nursing team had not identified much progress, and recommended transferring Andrew to a rehabilitation setting, but his parents were concerned as to whether Andrew would cope with the transition. They were unable to convince the nursing team that the small improvements they saw amounted to sustained progress. The MOHOST was pivotal in providing evidence of incremental changes, leading to an agreement that Andrew's admission to the acute hospital should continue and that the whole team would work to:

- Encourage Andrew's interests and values
- Provide Andrew with positive feedback
- Support Andrew to rebuild a satisfying routine

Was the MOHOST Discussed with Andrew?

In the initial stages of treatment, the occupational therapist provided verbal feedback to Andrew to reinforce his emerging strengths: his interest had improved; he made choices that supported occupational participation; he proved able to follow a routine with

ANALYSIS OF STRENGTHS & LIMITATIONS

Although Andrew does not verbalize his feelings, he has clear interests. He has proved able to tolerate new situations and to demonstrate a degree of responsibility. His interactions remain limited but improve when there is a practical focus, and he is able to plan and organize activities with support. He continues to be restless and has a marked hand tremor, but his movements show signs of improved coordination.

SUMMARY OF RATINGS

Motivation for Occupation				Pattern of Occupation				Communication & Interaction skills				Process skills				Motor skills				Environment: Inpatient ward			
Appraisal of ability	Expectation of success	Interest	Choices	Routine	Adaptability	Roles	Responsibility	Non-verbal skills	Conversation	Vocal expression	Relationships	Knowledge	Timing	Organization	Problem-solving	Posture & Mobility	Coordination	Strength & Effort	Energy	Physical space	Physical resources	Social groups	Occupational demands
F	F	F	F	F	F	F	F	F	F	F	F	F	F	F	F	F	F	(F)	F	F	(F)	F	F
A	A	(A)	A	A	(A)	A	A	A	A	A	A	(A)	A	A	A	(A)	A	A	A	(A)	A	(A)	(A)
I	I	I	(I)	(I)	I	I	(I)	I	(I)	(I)	(I)	I	(I)	(I)	I	I	(I)	I	I	I	I	I	I
(R)	(R)	R	R	R	R	(R)	R	(R)	R	R	R	R	R	R	(R)	R	R	R	(R)	R	R	R	R

Key: **F** = Facilitates occupational participation **A** = Allows occupational participation
I = Inhibits occupational participation **R** = Restricts occupational participation

FIGURE 18-3 Andrew's Analysis of Strengths and Limitations and MOHOST Ratings.

support, tolerated changes that occurred, communicated with others, and demonstrated improved processing skills. He also showed signs of increased responsibility and yet seemed unaware of his achievements and doubted that he would ever recover. At this point, the occupational therapist showed him evidence of his progress using the MOHOST ratings and was able to negotiate goals with Andrew to support continued improvement.

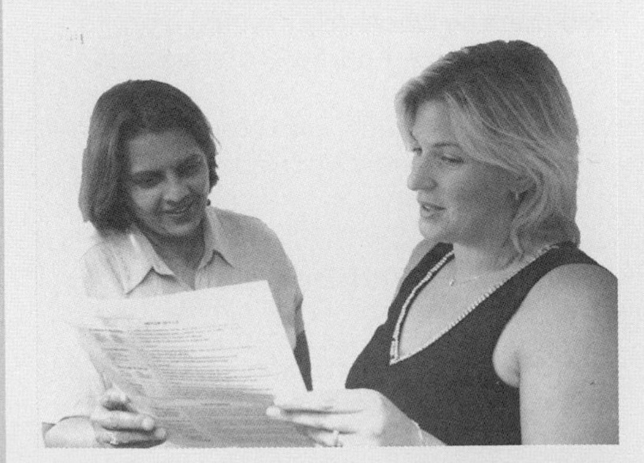

An occupational therapist, Katrina, reviews a MOHOST assessment with her manager, Lena

Ivan: Using the SCOPE to Guide Intervention

Ivan was 4 years old when he was admitted to the hospital due to a fever. He had been born at 32 weeks gestation and was diagnosed with gastroschisis at birth. This led to a small bowel transplant at age 1, but this transplant went into rejection and he required a second small bowel transplant at age 2 as well as a liver transplant. Consequently, he spent most of his first 2 years in the hospital, and had frequent hospital stays thereafter. When not hospitalized, he lived at home with his mother, father, and younger sister, where he receives 16-hour nursing care every day of the week.

Why Was the SCOPE Chosen?

Since his last hospitalization 2 months previously, Ivan appeared to have acquired many new skills. The occupational therapist working with Ivan chose to administer the SCOPE in order to evaluate his progress and to gain insight into new areas for intervention. The therapist specifically wanted to focus on interventions applicable to Ivan during his frequent hospitalizations, as well as to identify possible environmental modifications for his hospital room.

How Was Information Gathered?

The SCOPE was completed while observing Ivan in his hospital room as well as during play in the therapy room. Information was also gathered through informal discussions with the hospital staff that were familiar with Ivan from his current and previous hospitalizations and his parents filling out the parent forms.

What Did the SCOPE Show?

The results of the SCOPE (Fig. 18-4) indicated that Ivan's strengths were in the areas of volition (exploration, enjoyment, and response to challenge), habituation (daily activities, response to transitions, and routines), and process skills (understands and uses objects, orientation to the environment, and ability to make decisions). Ivan's limitations were noted to be in communication and interaction skills (verbal/vocal expression, conversation, and relationships), motor skills (posture and mobility, coordination, strength and energy/endurance), and environment (physical space, physical resources, social groups, occupational demands, and family routines).

How Did the SCOPE Influence Treatment Planning?

The SCOPE highlighted several of Ivan's strengths. These were his motivation to participate in play, his comfort level with daily activities and routines, and his ability to understand his environment. The SCOPE also helped Ivan's therapist to identify that many of Ivan's behaviors were due to the limited amount of control that he had in the hospital environment. Therefore, intervention strategies included modifying and adapting his physical and social environment in collaboration with the hospital staff to allow more active participation and opportunity to engage in play. Specific goals were introduced to:

- Increase effectiveness of nonverbal and verbal communication
- Improve muscle strength and gross motor coordination

How Did the SCOPE Shape Intervention?

The SCOPE helped Ivan's therapist to develop intervention strategies that utilized

SUMMARY OF RATINGS																								
Volition				Habituation				Communication & Interaction skills				Process skills				Motor skills				Environment				
Exploration	Expression of Enjoyment	Preferences & Choices	Response to Challenge	Daily Activities	Response to Transitions	Routines	Roles	Non-verbal Communication	Verbal/vocal Expression	Conversation	Relationships	Understands & Uses Objects	Orientation to Environment	Plans & Makes Decisions	Problem Solving	Posture & Mobility	Coordination	Strength	Energy/Endurance	Physical Space	Physical Resources	Social Groups	Occupational Demands	Family Routine
F	F	F	F	(F)	F	F	F	F	F	F	F	(F)	F	F	F	F	F	F	F	F	F	F	F	F
(A)	(A)	A	(A)	A	(A)	(A)	A	(A)	A	A	A	A	(A)	(A)	A	A	A	A	A	A	A	A	A	A
I	I	(I)	I	I	I	I	(I)	I	(I)	(I)	(I)	I	I	I	(I)	(I)	(I)	(I)	(I)	I	(I)	(I)	I	I
R	R	R	R	R	R	R	R	R	R	R	R	R	R	R	R	R	R	R	R	(R)	R	R	(R)	(R)

Key: **F** = Facilitates occupational participation **A** = Allows occupational participation
I = Inhibits occupational participation **R** = Restricts occupational participation

FIGURE 18-4 Profile of Ivan's Strengths and Limitations on the SCOPE Rating Form.

his strengths to address his communication and motor limitations.

- Hospital staff agreed to talk to Ivan during routine interventions by introducing themselves, describing what they were doing, naming things, offering him choices, and providing positive feedback when he communicated.
- Toys, including a small tricycle, were brought to Ivan's hospital room and placed in an area which was gated off, allowing him the freedom to move around and play without supervision. In addition, the therapist worked to involve Ivan's family, by setting up scheduled family play times and encouraging them to provide more stimulation in his hospital room.

How Did the SCOPE Aid Communication?

By providing a systematic framework for conceptualizing and documenting Ivan's occupational participation status, the SCOPE was able to highlight strengths on which therapeutic interventions could be built. It afforded a concrete means of documenting change and proved to be a useful communication tool between the therapist and other staff, caregivers, and family.

Model of Human Occupation Exploratory Level Outcome Ratings

The Model of Human Occupation Exploratory Level Outcome Ratings (MOHO-ExpLOR; Parkinson, Cooper, de las Heras de Pablo, & Forsyth, 2014) was designed to provide an alternative assessment to the MOHOST when a person's performance and participation are severely impaired. The person may have long-term disabilities that impact on all aspects of self-care, leisure and productivity, advanced cognitive deficits, or profound developmental conditions, such that future change is expected to remain at the exploratory level. They may be living in care facilities, or require substantial packages of care, or receive extensive family support, but they continue to be able to participate in the basic dimensions of doing. This may include experiencing their surroundings, contributing their skills in a shared activity, or performing one or two steps of an activity.

The MOHO-ExpLOR is similar to the MOHOST in that it is still a therapist-rated tool that gathers information relevant to the majority of MOHO concepts and allows the therapist to gain an overview of a person's occupational functioning. However, the items focus on more subtle indicators of volition, habituation, and performance, and the rating scale is a frequency scale that allows therapists to record whether items occur Reliably (R), Often (O), Sometimes (S), Infrequently (I), or Never/Not evident (N).

In addition, the authors of the MOHO-ExpLOR set out to link key environmental supports for volition, habituation, communication and interaction skills, process skills, and motor skills to the person's characteristics. The assessment therefore includes 10 personal factors relating to the person's participation in occupation and 10 items relating to contributory factors in the environment. Criterion statements are included on the form to guide the ratings according to the percentage of time that the item is observed. These are shown in Figure 18-5A, which illustrates the rating scale and a selection of items from the assessment.

At the time of writing, the MOHO-ExpLOR remains in development, but it is anticipated that it will be available to order via the MOHO website at www.cade.uic.edu/moho and directly from Firefly Research at www.fireflyresearch.ac.uk

ADMINISTRATION

In common with the MOHOST and the SCOPE, the data collection method for the MOHO-ExpLOR has been designed to be flexible to meet multiple needs in practice. Therapists may use any dependable source of information for completing the scales. This information is often gained through observation; however, it may be supplemented or achieved through talking to the person, workers, and/or relatives. Additionally, therapists may gather information from records, team meetings, or other available sources.

If necessary, therapists can build up an understanding of a person's occupational participation over a period of time to complete the assessments. For this reason, the MOHO-ExpLOR includes a *Single Observation Form* (Fig. 18-5B) that therapists may use to record the observations made after a single intervention (e.g., a dressing practice or a reminiscence session). Once the therapists have sufficient information, they may go on to complete the *Summary MOHO-ExpLOR* form. Both the MOHO-ExpLOR forms are easy to administer and rate and so they can be used at regular intervals to document a person's progress.

		Motivation for occupation	95%	75%	50%	25%	5%
Personal factors	**Exploring** inc., visual, tactile or oral exploration of objects, people and environment	The person notices/responds to changes in the environment (sound, lighting etc)	☐	☐	☐	☐	☐
		The person indicates curiosity by listening, looking, touching, smelling etc.	☐	☐	☐	☐	☐
		The person is attracted to certain objects, tasks or people	☐	☐	☐	☐	☐
	R O S I N	*Comments:*					
	Engaging inc., emotional investment in activity and accompanying intentional actions	The person responds to on-going action with enjoyment/satisfaction	☐	☐	☐	☐	☐
		The person shows an emotional connection by re-engaging over time	☐	☐	☐	☐	☐
		The person co-operates with tasks, readies self for assistance if required	☐	☐	☐	☐	☐
	R O S I N	*Comments:*					
Environmental factors	**Validation** inc., empathy, creating a sense of personal capacity/ significance and security	Personal uniqueness is recognised & subjective experience is appreciated	☐	☐	☐	☐	☐
		Personal strengths are identified, acknowledged and celebrated	☐	☐	☐	☐	☐
		The environment facilitates meaningful experiences / sensory preferences	☐	☐	☐	☐	☐
	R O S I N	*Comments:*					
	Encouragement inc., disposition of the environment to invite participation in new activities	The environment is attractive and invites exploration in novel contexts	☐	☐	☐	☐	☐
		Activities are adapted/selected to stimulate increased interest & engagement	☐	☐	☐	☐	☐
		Positive reinforcement is used effectively to convey hope and optimism	☐	☐	☐	☐	☐
	R O S I N	*Comments:*					

Key: **R** = Reliably **O** = Often **S** = Sometimes **I** = Infrequently **N** = Never or Not evident

Administration

In common with the MOHOST and the SCOPE, the data collection method for the MOHO-ExpLOR has been designed to be flexible to meet multiple needs in practice. Therapists may use any dependable source of information for completing the scales. This information is often gained through observation; however, it may be supplemented or achieved through talking to the person, workers, and/or relatives. Additionally therapists may gather information from records, team meetings or other available sources.

If necessary, therapists can build up an understanding of a person's occupational participation over a period of time to complete the assessments. For this reason, the MOHO-ExpLOR includes a Single Observation Form (shown in Fig. 18.5B) which therapists may use to record the observations made after a single intervention (e.g., a dressing practice or a reminiscence session). Once the therapists have sufficient information, they may go on to complete the Summary MOHO-ExpLOR form. Both the MOHO-ExpLOR forms are easy to administer and rate and so they can be used at regular intervals to document a person's progress.

A

Process skills	The person attended and responded to on-going action	R	O	S	I	N	*Comments:*
	The person used objects effectively	R	O	S	I	N	
	The environment provided optimum structure	R	O	S	I	N	
	The environment responded with appropriate flexibility	R	O	S	I	N	

Motor skills	The person endured throughout the session	R	O	S	I	N	*Comments:*
	The person moved objects safely and independently	R	O	S	I	N	
	The environment facilitated appropriate positioning	R	O	S	I	N	
	The environment aided mobility	R	O	S	I	N	

B **Key:** **R** = Reliably **O** = Often **S** = Sometimes **I** = Infrequently **N** = Never or Not evident

FIGURE 18-5 **A.** Sample Items from the MOHO-ExpLOR. **B.** Sample Sections from the MOHO-ExpLOR Single Observation Form.

MOHO Problem-Solver

Louise: Using the MOHO-ExpLOR to Advise Carers

Louise was diagnosed with Alzheimer's disease in her 80s and a decision was made for her to go into residential care. Prior to her referral to the occupational therapist, she had been moved three times due to her increasing needs. She often attempted to leave the care home and was described as "noncompliant" with personal care, becoming increasingly agitated and verbally aggressive with both staff and residents.

Why Was the MOHO-ExpLOR Chosen?

Given Louise's declining performance capacity and reduced engagement, the occupational therapist needed a flexible assessment that would allow information to be collected from family members and care staff and through observation. Louise retained various skills and could perform one or two steps of an activity but did not perform tasks independently or participate in any roles. Therefore, the assessment tool also needed to be sensitive enough to distinguish subtle changes and strengths/capabilities at the exploratory level, and include an analysis of the impact that the environment was having on Louise.

How Was Information Gathered?

The occupational therapist read case notes and documentation provided by the care home and conducted discussions with Louise, care staff, and family members to gain an initial understanding of Louise's occupational identity. In order to identify possible environmental triggers for Louise's behavior, she was also observed by a support worker when she was being supported to complete personal care tasks and being encouraged to participate in social activities. In addition, the therapist carried out a personal care assessment.

What Did the Therapist Discover?

The therapist realized that Louise valued having a sense of purpose and a meaningful role. She prided herself on having worked extremely hard to achieve her goals and had always been an assertive lady. Over her lifetime, she had taught a range of subjects including arts and textiles, mountaineering and music. She had always loved gardening and the outdoors and had spent many weekends wild camping and fell-walking.

Having engaged in a number of activities in her lifetime, Louise expressed that she was "not the type of person to have a hobby or do an activity for fun." Every activity had to have a purpose, such as completing textile projects for charity or for gifts. Staff within the home struggled to understand that Louise would not engage in activities such as quizzes or games as they held no value to her.

What Did the MOHO-ExpLOR Show?

Louise's responses were dependent upon her understanding of the environment and her role within it. She often believed that she was a staff member but she cooperated in personal care tasks around 50% of the time and was more likely to engage if staff gave her reasons for doing so, for example, "your visitors are coming," "it's time to go to bed." Unfortunately, staff interactions were inconsistent. In particular, many staff members did not take into account that Louise had held leadership positions in her life and misinterpreted her assertive nature as being hostile. They struggled to understand that Louise would not engage in activities such as quizzes or games as they held no value to her. Therefore, the environment did not facilitate meaningful experiences and the structure of the activities promoted disengagement. (Initial ratings are shown in Fig. 18-6A.)

How Did the MOHO-ExpLOR Influence Treatment?

The MOHO-ExpLOR highlighted the need for understanding Louise's life story, so that interventions could focus on meaningful activities and roles. This required adaptations to the physical and social environment. Personal objects were introduced into Louise's room, to reflect her unique identity, and staff began working with her to identify meaningful occupations. She was encouraged to assist in facilitating groups (including singing to the residents), cultivating the garden, and looking after the indoor plants. Louise began to participate in some activities related to these roles, to complete various tasks independently, and to express a sense of purpose.

Staff reported that she no longer fixated on the role of helping others in the home or trying to leave the property. Once the number of these incidents reduced, the care home agreed for Louise to become a permanent resident, which prevented another move.

Could the MOHO-ExpLOR Record Progress?

A second MOHO-ExpLOR (Fig. 18-6B) recorded

- increased validation and encouragement by introducing home-like features and offering activities that appealed to Louise's past interests, as well as increased engagement on Louise's behalf;
- increased continuity regarding how personal care routines were introduced and increased variety by offering opportunities for Louise to exercise choice;
- an increased emphasis on communicating with Louise in a way that enabled respect and increased opportunities to interact with others in valued roles;
- an unexpected decrease in Louise's energy levels and ability to focus on ongoing action. This was attributed to a change in medication that was subsequently reviewed.

Personal factors supporting occupational participation / Environmental factors supporting occupational participation (rating scale: R O S I N; circled rating shown)

Motivation for occupation				Pattern of occupation				Communication and interaction				Process function				Motor function			
exploring	engaging	validation	encouragement	maintaining	adapting	continuity	variety	indicating	relating	communication	variety	attending	using objects	structure	flexibility	enduring	moving	positioning	mobility
R	S	I	I	S	S	I	I	O	S	O	I	O	S	S	S	R	R	R	R

How did the MOHO-ExpLOR influence treatment?

The MOHO-ExplOR highlighted the need for understanding Louise's life story, so that interventions could focus on meaningful activities and roles. This required adaptions to the physical and social environment. Personal objects were introduced to Louise's room, to reflect her unique identity and staff began working with her to identify meaningful occupations. She was encouraged to assist in facilitating groups, (including singing to the residents), cultivating the garden and looking after the indoor plants. Louise began to participate in some activities related to these roles, to complete various tasks independently, and to express a sense of purpose. Staff reported that she no longer fixated on the role of helping others in the home or trying to leave the property. Once the number of these incidents reduced, the care home agreed for Louise to become a permanent resident, which prevented another move.

Could the MOHO-ExpLOR record progress?

A second MOHO-ExpLOR (see Fig. 18.6B) recorded

- increased validation and encouragement by introducing homelike features and offering activities that appealed to Louise's past interests, as well as increased engagement on Louise's behalf;
- increased continuity regarding how personal care routines were introduced and increased variety by offering opportunities for Louise to exercise choice;
- an increased emphasis on communicating with Louise in a way that enabled respect and increased opportunities to interact with others in valued roles;
- an unexpected decrease in Louise's energy levels and ability to focus on ongoing action. This was attributed to a change in medication which was subsequently reviewed.

A

FIGURE 18-6 A. Louise's MOHO-ExpLOR Ratings—Preintervention. **B.** Louise's MOHO-ExpLOR Ratings—Postintervention.

B

Domain	Personal factors supporting occupational participation	Rating (R O S I N)	Environmental factors supporting occupational participation	Rating (R O S I N)
Motivation for occupation	exploring	R	validation	O
	engaging	O	encouragement	O
Pattern of occupation	maintaining	O	continuity	S
	adapting	S	variety	O
Communication and interaction	indicating	O	communication	O
	relating	S	variety	O
Process function	attending	S	structure	O
	using objects	O	flexibility	O
Motor function	enduring	S	positioning	R
	moving	R	mobility	R

FIGURE 18-6 (continued)

Assessment of Occupational Functioning—Collaborative Version

The Assessment of Occupational Functioning—Collaborative Version (AOF-CV) is a semi-structured assessment that gives clients an opportunity to report on their occupational participation (Watts, Hinson, Madigan, McGuigan, & Newman, 1999). Although the assessment has been largely superseded by more recent assessments, its ability to be administered as either an interview or as a self-report with therapist follow-up means that it remains a flexible option. It yields a general overview of a person's occupational participation by collating qualitative information and providing a rating profile that reflects clients' views of their own strengths and limitations in personal causation, values, roles, habits, and skills.

The AOF-CV is a free resource that can be accessed via the MOHO website at www.cade.uic.edu/moho

ADMINISTRATION

The interview/questionnaire consists of 22 questions. When administered as a self-report, the client responds to the questions in writing. After reviewing the client's responses, the therapist briefly discusses them with the client to clarify and gather additional information necessary for completing the rating scale. When conducted as an interview, the therapist treats the questions as a semi-structured interview, probing and asking additional questions as necessary. The questions (whether used as an interview or self-report) are designed to elicit the client's perception of his or her occupational functioning.

After the interview or self-report with follow-up is finished, the therapist completes a rating scale, which is in the form of questions about the client's functioning (e.g., "Does this person demonstrate personal values through the selection of well-defined, meaningful activities?"). These are scored using a 5-point rating scale.

MOHO Problem-Solver

Phil: Using the AOF-CV to Develop Understanding

Phil was 36 years old and had been diagnosed with multiple sclerosis (MS) 4 years previously. He was previously employed full time as a roofer but had become progressively debilitated with no remission and was unable to work. He was divorced 2 years after his diagnosis was made and lived in a house with his two sons, aged 14 and 10. Having been hospitalized during an exacerbation of MS, he had subsequently been transferred to an intensive rehabilitation unit.

Why Was the AOF-CV Chosen?

The therapist administered the AOF-CV as an interview in order to gain insight into Phil's view of his situation and as a guide to make therapy more responsive to his needs. Phil's ratings on the AOF-CV rating scale are shown in Figure 18-7.

Volition

Values	5	4	3	2	1
Does this person demonstrate his/her values through the selection of well-defined, meaningful activities?				✗	
Does this person demonstrate his/her values through the selection of personal goals?				✗	
Does this person demonstrate socially appropriate values through the selection of personal standards for the conduct of daily activities?		✗			
Does this person demonstrate temporal orientation through expressed awareness of past, present, and future events and beliefs about how time should be used?	✗				
Personal Causation	**5**	**4**	**3**	**2**	**1**
Does this person demonstrate personal causation through an expressed belief in internal control?				✗	
Does this person demonstrate personal causation by expressing confidence that he/she has a range of skills?		✗			
Does this person demonstrate personal causation by expressing confidence in his/her skill competence at personally relevant tasks?					✗
Does this person demonstrate personal causation by expressing hopeful anticipation for success in the future endeavors?			✗		
Interests	**5**	**4**	**3**	**2**	**1**
Does this person clearly discriminate degrees of interests?		✗			
Does this person clearly identify a range of interests?			✗		
Does this person routinely pursue his/her interests?					✗

Habituation

Roles	5	4	3	2	1
Does this person demonstrate an adequate array of life roles (family member, student, worker, hobbyist, friend, etc.)?					✗
Does this person have a realistic concept of the demands and social obligations of his/her life roles?			✗		
Does this person express comfort or security in his/her major life roles?					✗
Habits	**5**	**4**	**3**	**2**	**1**
Does this person demonstrate habit patterns through well-organized use of time?			✗		
Does this person report that his/her habits are socially acceptable?				✗	
Does this person demonstrate adequate flexibility in his/her habits?			✗		
Occupational Performance Skills	**5**	**4**	**3**	**2**	**1**
Does this person have adequate motor skills necessary to move himself/herself or manipulate objects?					✗
Does this person have adequate skills for managing events, processes, and situations of various types?				✗	
Does this person have communications and interpersonal skills necessary for interfacing with people?				✗	

Key: **1** = Very little **2** = Little **3** = Highly **4** = Very highly

FIGURE 18-7 Phil's AOF-CV Ratings.

What Were the Key Issues Discussed?

Phil reported that his two most important sources of meaning were his family and his work. However, both had been disrupted in the past 4 years. Phil's future goals were to walk again and to participate in the things he did before the onset of MS. He avoided any suggestion that his illness was likely to progress and require accommodations. Consequently, he had no plans to adapt his home, which was not wheelchair accessible, and had not considered the possible impact on his children.

Prior to the onset of his illness, Phil had many roles including being a parent, husband, worker, friend, sports participant, church member, and club member. His remaining role was being a parent, and this was radically altered as he had become dependent on his sons for meeting his self-care needs and no longer had authority over them.

Up until 4 months before his hospitalization, he independently performed his morning self-care, and completed simple home management tasks such as cleaning and meal preparation. Since being admitted, he was using a powered wheelchair for mobility. He had very limited success with ambulation and stand pivot transfers even with maximal assistance. Yet despite obvious difficulties, he refused to discuss the future course of his illness. He had almost no knowledge about MS and rejected the idea of receiving education about the disease and its prognosis.

Phil's view of his skills was fraught with conflict. His mounting impairments and swift decline in performance conflicted with his need to believe his condition would markedly improve. He admitted that his anger and poor communication contributed to deteriorating relationships with friends and family.

What Were the Implications for Therapy?

The AOF-CV results made it clear that any successful rehabilitation had to begin with addressing Phil's view of his situation. Phil's unwillingness to address his physical limitations, combined with his poor prognosis, was his greatest liability.

How Did the AOF Influence Treatment?

- Volition—assisting Phil to identify his highest priorities for occupational participation and develop realistic goals
- Personal causation—increasing Phil's knowledge of MS
- Interests—introducing modifications to past interests and exploring new areas of interest
- Roles—working with Phil to plan a self-care management role and reestablish his parenting role despite his impairments
- Habits—educating Phil on energy conservation and adaptations to increase activity levels
- Skills—collaborating with Phil to adapt the environment and enhancing his ability to cope with his disability through better planning and communication

How Was the AOF-CV Received?

The whole team appreciated the insights gained by using the AOF-CV and worked to provide realistic information to Phil about his condition and prognosis. Phil returned to rehabilitation about 1 year later and the occupational therapist revisited some key questions from the AOF-CV with Phil. At this point, he had accepted the reality of his MS and expressed fears about what it would mean. He agreed to increased changes to his home environment, and the focus on how he could realize some of his values and interests in his everyday life gave him new hope. Although he died some months later, his sons were grateful for the improved final months with their father.

Occupational Therapy Psychosocial Assessment of Learning

The OT PAL (Townsend et al., 2001) is designed for use within a school-based setting with children aged 6 to 12 years who are experiencing difficulty fulfilling expectations and roles in the classroom. It captures information on 21 psychosocial factors that influence a child's learning, relating to a student's volition (ability to make choices) and habituation (roles and habits). In addition to the rating scale, the OT PAL also provides the structure to gather and report qualitative information on:

- The student's classroom
- The behavioral expectations in the classroom
- The teacher's style of teaching and managing the classroom
- The student's ability to meet these expectations
- The student's beliefs about his or her abilities as a learner within the school environment

It recognizes that the teacher, student, and parents offer different perspectives about the student's performance, behaviors, beliefs, and interests related to school, and it can be flexibly adapted to each child and school setting. Completing the OT PAL supports the occupational therapist to determine the quality of fit between the student and the classroom environment and how the latter affects the student's performance.

The OT PAL can be ordered from the MOHO website at www.cade.uic.edu/moho

ADMINISTRATION

The therapist collects information for completing the scale through observation supplemented with semi-structured interviews with the teacher, student, and parents. The following forms are then completed:

- A preobservation and environmental description worksheet that gathers information about basic characteristics of the student and the classroom
- The rating scale
- Brief summaries of the teacher, student, and parent interviews
- A summary of the student–environment fit, listing the students' strengths and weaknesses, and describing any intervention plan.

An observation of at least 40 minutes is generally necessary to gather sufficient information for completion of the rating scale. The teacher, student, and parent interviews are administered after the observation because part of their purpose is to gather information that supplements and confirms/corrects the observation. Each interview takes approximately 15 minutes. The parent interview may be conducted as a written questionnaire or via telephone. After the therapist finishes the information-gathering process, he or she completes the rating scale and forms. Other assessments may also need to be administered, because the OT PAL does not gather information on performance capacity or skills.

MOHO Problem-Solver

Gerald: Using the OT PAL to Evaluate Adjustment to First Grade

Gerald was 7 years old and was in first grade. He was diagnosed at age 5 with acute lymphocytic leukemia and received chemotherapy for 2 years. Although no longer receiving leukemia treatment, he still experienced fatigue and weakness, and had also been identified as having sensory integrative dysfunction. His symptoms affected his attention span, arousal levels, spatial orientation, postural control, visual motor skills, visual perceptual skills, and bilateral integration. He had several adaptations in his classroom environment to improve his organization and attention span, and had a classroom aide during half the school day to provide extra assistance.

Why Was the OT PAL Chosen?

Because Gerald faced numerous challenges in the classroom, the therapist decided to administer the OT PAL as a means of gathering information on his overall adjustment to first grade in anticipation of a school team review. This process leads naturally to development of intervention plans and recommendations to others in the school setting. Because of the comprehensive nature of the OT PAL, it is a useful assessment for giving input to the school team for planning how to best meet a child's educational needs.

What Issues Were Discovered?

The assessment illuminated both strengths and concerns for Gerald in the areas of making choices, habits/routines, and roles. Gerald displayed a positive sense of personal causation regarding his academic ability and took pride in his work, but relied heavily on his aide to help him organize his school materials and maintain the pace of his individual work. He struggled to participate in classroom duties requiring strength and endurance and his teacher reported that students often rejected him during recess because of his limited motor capacities.

Figure 18-8 illustrates the habituation portion of Gerald's OT PAL rating scale. Although he showed a good understanding of what to do throughout the day, his level of energy and difficulties with focusing, attending, and organizing hampered keeping up with routines. Another factor that contributed to his difficulty completing activities within the allotted time was his periodic removal from the classroom for occupational therapy, physical therapy, and social work. As a consequence of all these things, Gerald was often catching up on assignments during free time. This tended to mark Gerald as different from the other students, thus undermining his attempts to appear normal.

Gerald strongly identified with and attempted to meet the expectations of the student role in the classroom. He accepted the teacher's authority, asked for help appropriately, tried hard as a student, and participated in activities and class discussions. Opportunities for interaction with peers were more challenging for him, as he was sometimes teased and others did not defend him when this happened.

What Conclusions Were Drawn from the OT PAL?

Overall, Gerald's school environment supported his participation in school and learning. Gerald sat in the back of the room so he could move around at times, and he had been provided with a move-and-sit cushion that met his need for movement and improved his distractibility. Moreover, the desks in the classroom were arranged in groups of four, with assigned seating, facilitating positive interactions with students. Figure 18-8 summarizes Gerald's ratings.

What Were the Implications for Therapy?

Gerald's greatest strength was his volitional desire to be a good student and the sense of efficacy he had concerning some aspects of his classroom performance. Supporting Gerald's volition meant paying attention to the strong values he held about being a student and bolstering his sense of personal causation. His limited motor performance tended to make him stand out in certain situations, and these needed to be considered and minimized.

How Did the OT PAL Influence Treatment?

- Managing fatigue—for example, a cart was provided so that Gerald could assist with classroom duties
- Increasing organizational skills—for example, the aide and Gerald sought to find ways to increase his responsibility and autonomy
- Facilitating peer relationships—for example, therapy appointments were rescheduled so as not to interfere with free time

Section	Item	N/O	4	3	2	1
Volition Student chooses to:	Begin activity with direction	N/O	(4)	3	2	1
	Begin self-directed activity	N/O	4	3	2	(1)
	Stay engaged	N/O	4	(3)	2	1
	Continue/transition with direction	N/O	(4)	3	2	1
	Discontinue activity with direction	N/O	(4)	3	2	1
	Discontinue self-directed activity	N/O	4	3	(2)	1
	Engage with peers given direction	N/O	4	(3)	2	1
	Engage with peers self-directed	N/O	(4)	3	2	1
	Follow social rules	N/O	(4)	3	2	1
	Show preferences	N/O	(4)	3	2	1
Habits and Routines The student:	Demonstrates routines	N/O	4	3	(2)	1
	Adheres to routines	N/O	4	(3)	2	1
	Completes activities	N/O	4	3	(2)	1
	Maintains desk	N/O	4	3	(2)	1
	Maintains belongings	N/O	4	3	(2)	1
	Organizes projects and assignments	N/O	4	3	2	(1)
	Completes transitions	N/O	4	3	(2)	1
Roles The student:	Demonstrates student role	N/O	4	(3)	2	1
	Transitions smoothly between roles	N/O	(4)	3	2	1
	Responds to diverse roles	N/O	(4)	3	2	1
	Assumes school related roles	N/O	(4)	3	2	1

Key: **N/O** = Not Oserved **4** = Competent **3** = Questionable **2** = Ineffective **1** = Deficient

FIGURE 18-8 Gerald's OT PAL Ratings.

Residential Environment Impact Scale

The Residential Environment Impact Scale (Fisher et al., 2014) is a semi-structured assessment and consulting instrument designed to examine the impact of community residential facilities on residents. It supports the therapist to rate the facility in four different domains informed by the model of human occupation: everyday space, everyday objects, enabling relationships, and structure of activities. Each domain has five subareas that are rated on a 1 to 4 scale. A detailed rating guide is provided, allowing the therapist to indicate how well the home supports the residents' sense of identity and competence, in terms of opportunities, resources, demands, and constraints that promote engagement in meaningful and culturally appropriate activities.

Findings from the REIS can be used to guide recommendations aimed at improving the residents' sense of identity and competence. This is achieved through a focus on the opportunities, resources, demands, and constraints that promote engagement in meaningful and culturally appropriate activities. It includes short and long forms with global and probing interview questions for residents and caregivers, and an optional photo gallery to communicate with individuals who respond better to pictures.

The REIS can be ordered from the MOHO website at www.cade.uic.edu/moho

ADMINISTRATION

The REIS uses four data collection methods to gather the information needed to comprehensively evaluate how well the home provides the support and opportunities necessary to meet the needs and desires of its residents. The four strategies are:

- a walk-through of the home
- observation of three daily routines or activities
- an interview of the residents, and
- an interview of a caregiver, ideally both a manager and staff member if it is a group home situation

Several formats for data gathering are provided to support the data collection and rating by both novice and experienced therapists.

MOHO Problem-Solver

Acacia Avenue: Using the REIS to Assess a Group Home

Acacia Avenue used to provide long-term residential accommodation, but for the last 3 years it has operated as a house of multiple occupancy for six residents who have mild to moderate intellectual disabilities. It is staffed by two support workers throughout the day but is not staffed overnight. Although deemed to provide transitional living arrangements, some of the residents have lived there for 3 years.

Why Was the REIS Chosen?

One of the residents was referred to occupational therapy due to the perceived difficulties he experienced interacting with staff and fellow residents, to the extent that he tended to sleep during the day and get up at night. The therapist took the opportunity to evaluate the group home and demonstrate how changes to the whole environment could benefit all the individual residents. The REIS ratings are shown in Figure 18-9.

How Was the Information Gathered?

The therapist completed a walk-through of the home and an informal observation of the residents engaged in everyday routines (making breakfast, playing a game, and participating in a residents' meeting), as well as semi-structured interviews with the person who had been referred and two members of staff.

What Was the Everyday Space Like?

There was an abundance of space available, allowing for private and social space. However, the space had not been tailored to the needs of residents, for example, the layout of furniture in the sitting room did not promote social interaction and did not facilitate engagement in activities. Also, although the bedrooms were adequate in size, the location of the staff office beside a bedroom did not facilitate privacy. In addition, the space had an institutional feel due to the impersonal decoration of the walls (bland colors) and flooring (office-like carpet) that resulted in a lifeless quality to the space. Signage further conveyed an institutional feel, the garden had not been maintained, and paintwork was chipped and neglected.

Everyday Space					Everyday Objects					Enabling Relationships					Structure of Activities				
Accessibility of space	Adequacy of space	Homelike qualities	Sensory space	Visual supports	Availability of objects	Adequacy of objects	Homelike Qualities	Physical attributes of objects	Variety of objects	Availability of people	Enabling respect	Support and facilitation	Provision of information	Empowerment	Activity demands	Time demands	Appeal of activities	Routines	Decision making
4	4	4	4	4	4	4	4	4	4	4	4	4	4	4	4	4	4	4	4
(3)	(3)	3	3	3	3	3	3	3	3	3	(3)	3	3	(3)	3	3	3	3	3
2	2	2	(2)	(2)	(2)	(2)	(2)	(2)	(2)	(2)	2	(2)	(2)	2	2	(2)	(2)	(2)	(2)
1	1	(1)	1	1	1	1	1	1	1	1	1	1	1	1	(1)	1	1	1	1

Key:
4 = Environment strongly supports people's sense of identity & competence by providing exceptional opportunities, resources, and demands to engage in meaningful culturally appropriate activities.
3 = Environment supports people's sense of identity & competence by providing opportunities, resources and demands to engage in meaningful culturally appropriate activities.
2 = Environment interferes with people's sense of identity & competence by providing limited opportunities, resources, and demands to engage in meaningful culturally appropriate activities.
1 = Environment strongly interferes with people's sense of identity & competence by not providing opportunities, resources, and demands to engage in meaningful culturally appropriate activities.

FIGURE 18-9 Acacia Avenue's REIS Ratings.

. . . And the Everyday Objects?

While there was a good variety of equipment in the kitchen (e.g., a smoothie maker), which supported engagement in meal preparation, some items are inadequate (e.g., a rusty toaster). Meanwhile, there was a limited variety of objects in the communal sitting room and these were arranged in a mismatched manner (e.g., old catalogues, old computer keyboards), which did not support individuals to engage in activities. Furthermore, there was no emergency equipment in place that would make it difficult for residents to contact staff overnight.

What about the Enabling Relationships?

Staff members had established collaborative relationships based on mutual respect and understanding and were approachable and sensitive to individuals' needs and respectful of individuals' preferences. Formal tools were used to promote decision-making and goal setting and meetings took place twice a month to make household decisions. However, actions were not always implemented efficiently (e.g., the cleaning rostra was ineffective) and the notice board could be used in a clearer and more effective way. The residents spent the majority of their time in their rooms and peer interaction did not seem to be encouraged. The lack of overnight staff may also have impacted negatively on some of the residents.

. . . And the Structure of Activities?

Staff members were creating some opportunities for participation in community activities (e.g., swimming), but limited opportunities were being created to engage in meaningful activities within the home environment. Although the routine was flexible, a lack of structure resulted in unoccupied time. There was a potential for boredom due to a lack of interesting activities on offer, which matched personal needs and preferences.

How Could the Environment Be Improved?

Some of the issues raised required long-term solutions (e.g., nighttime staffing levels, redecoration, and acquiring new equipment). However, many of the changes could be implemented by reorganizing the communal spaces and notice boards, and refocusing the responsibility of the staff on engaging residents in everyday activities, including gardening and basic home maintenance as well as group meals and leisure activities.

What Was the Impact of the REIS?

Completing the REIS led to more open communication between the residents and the staff about how to rejuvenate the residential environment for the benefit of all and use daily opportunities to help residents plan their time. The staff showed enthusiasm about negotiating a shared vision for their work with the residents and had ideas for moving their office to a more central space. The residents requested a new television and interactive video game in the communal sitting room (the old one had not been replaced after a previous theft). In addition, residents agreed that using the equipment would be negotiated around shared interests, and that they would support each other by making and sharing refreshments and keeping the room tidy.

Conclusion

This chapter presents six diverse assessments that all use more than a single method of data collection. Each method of data collection has its strengths and limitations, and assessments that use a single method (interview, self-report, or observation) are designed to make the most of the methodology that they employ. These assessments, by combining or allowing alternative approaches to collecting information, are designed to maximize flexibility.

Chapter 18 Quiz Questions

1. Which assessment can be administered as a self-report or conducted as a semi-structured interview?
2. Which assessment comprises 24 items divided equally between 6 sections?
3. The SCOPE has one more item than the MOHOST in the environmental section. What is it?
4. Which assessment is used to help therapists determine the quality of fit between the student and the classroom environment?
5. The REIS is divided into four sections. What are they?
6. What is the rating scale for the MOHO-ExpLOR?

HOMEWORK ASSIGNMENTS

1. Describe the process of administering the MOHOST.
2. Explain how the environment impacts on occupational participation when a person has severe impairments.
3. Analyze your home environment using the REIS.

thePoint® For additional resources and exercises, visit http://thePoint.lww.com

Key Terms

AOF-CV: Assessment of Occupational Functioning—Collaborative Version.

MOHOST: Model of Human Occupation Screening Tool.

MOHO-ExpLOR: MOHO Exploratory Level Outcome Ratings.

OT PAL: Occupational Therapy Psychosocial Assessment of Learning.

REIS: Residential Environment Impact Scale.

SCOPE: Short Child Occupational Profile.

REFERENCES

Bowyer, P., Kramer, J., Ploszaj, A., Ross, M., Schwartz, O., Kielhofner, G., et al. (2008). *The Short Child Occupational Profile (SCOPE)* [Version 2.2]. Chicago: Model of Human Occupation Clearing House, Department of Occupational Therapy, College of Applied Health Sciences, University of Illinois at Chicago.

Fisher, G., Forsyth, K., Harrison, M., Angarola, R., Kayhan, E., Noga, P., et al. (2014). Chicago: Model of Human Occupation Clearing House, Department of Occupational Therapy, College of Applied Health Sciences, University of Illinois at Chicago.

Parkinson, S., Cooper, J., de las Heras de Pablo, C. G., & Forsyth, K. (2014). Measuring the effectiveness of interventions when occupational performance is severely impaired. *British Journal of Occupational Therapy, 77*(2), 78–81.

Parkinson, S., Forsyth, K., & Kielhofner, G. (2006). *The Model of Human Occupation Screening Tool (MOHOST)* [Version 2.0]. Chicago: Model of Human Occupation Clearing House, Department of Occupational Therapy, College of Applied Health Sciences, University of Illinois at Chicago.

Townsend, S. C., Carey, P. D., Hollins, N. L., Helfrich, C., Blondis, M., Hoffman, A., et al. (2001). *The Occupational Therapy Psychosocial Assessment of Learning (OT PAL)* [Version 1.0]. Chicago: Model of Human Occupation Clearing House, Department of Occupational Therapy, College of Applied Health Sciences, University of Illinois at Chicago.

Watts. J. H., Hinson, R., Madigan, M. J., McGuigan, P. M., & Newman, S. M. (1999). The Assessment of Occupational Functioning—Collaborative Version. In B. J. Hempill-Pearson (Ed.), *Assessments in occupational therapy in mental health.* Thorofare, NJ: SLACK.

PART IV

CASE ILLUSTRATIONS

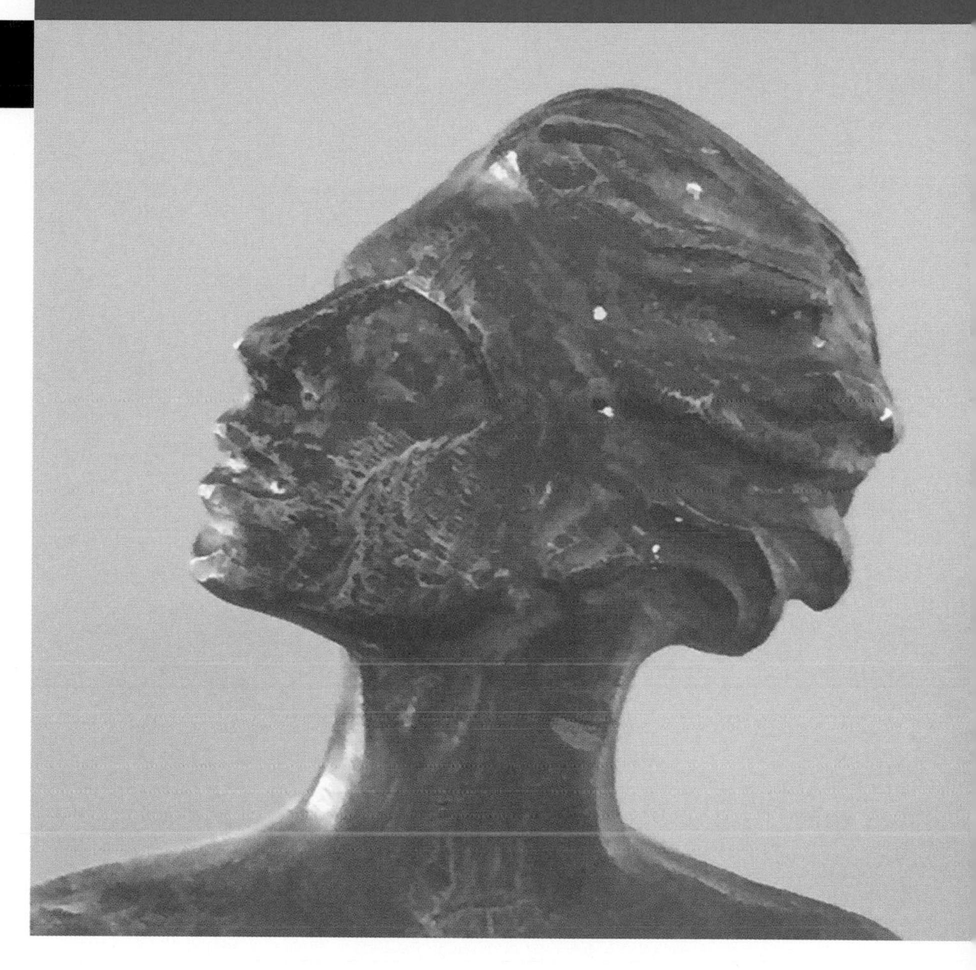

Rebuilding Occupational Narratives: Applying MOHO with Older Adults

Carmen-Gloria de las Heras de Pablo, Genevieve Pépin, and Gary Kielhofner (poshumous)

CHAPTER 19

EXPECTED LEARNING OUTCOMES

Upon completion of this chapter, the readers will be able to:

1. Understand the application of narrative thinking within the occupational therapy process.
2. Identify the most relevant interventions and therapeutic strategies for older adults.
3. Understand how the model of human occupation (MOHO) intervention process can be utilized in complex situations.
4. Identify the key competencies that therapists must develop when helping people to reconstruct their occupational narratives.

As explained in earlier chapters of this book, occupational history is dynamic, forming an occupational narrative over time. According to the Model of Human Occupation (MOHO; Kielhofner, 2008), an **occupational narrative** is a person's story of the ongoing interactions between his or her own volition, habituation, performance capacity, and environments over time. This story may be told and/or enacted and it is relayed through plots and metaphors that sum up and assign meaning to each person's volition, habituation, performance capacity, and environments (Kielhofner, 2008). A person's occupational identity and occupational competence are reflected and enacted in an occupational narrative (Kielhofner, 2008).

In the course of life people face many changes, some more difficult than others, but all requiring personal effort. The amount of effort people invest in changing will depend on the impact that these changes have on their unique personal occupational characteristics, cumulative experiences of change, and the supports or restrictions that the social and physical environment, cultural, economic, and political circumstances pose on them.

Some life events are extremely challenging for people, such as severe chronic illnesses, traumatic accidents, extreme natural events, wars, and personal losses. The changes provoked by these events have been identified as "catastrophic changes" because they represent a "destruction" of people's occupational narratives (Kielhofner, 2002). Events like these result in people losing a significant portion of all they have gained through their lives. As a consequence, these changes produce a large gap between a person's occupational identity and competence, and the uncertainty about what could be expected for the future. Under these circumstances people are challenged by having to *reinvent or rebuild their occupational lives*.

In the face of significant life challenges where people's occupational identity has been significantly eroded, occupational narratives must be rebuilt. This adaptation implies that the course of therapy must focus on helping people reconstruct their occupational narratives for themselves and find ways to put these narratives into action. Thus, *the evaluation and intervention process needs to be framed within a delicate and progressive facilitation of the volitional process* (de las Heras et al., 2002). In order to reconstruct narratives people need to go through a long process of recovery, in which *a new opportunity* to explore one's own strengths and limitations, as well as those of the environment, is presented. People also have the chance to slowly develop new roles and habit patterns, but must be provided with a physically and socially conducive environment.

The most effective occupational therapy *is timed according to the person's needs and readiness for change.* In these situations, therapists can realize that the course of therapy is not always linear. There are often times when a person will step back or have difficulty moving forward due to complex combinations of personal and environmental factors.

This chapter illustrates the reconstruction of the narrative process through three examples of work with older adults, highlighting key aspects that influenced occupational therapists' decision-making during the process of evaluation and intervention,

CASE EXAMPLE: AN OLDER ADULT WITH A CEREBRAL VASCULAR ACCIDENT

Haydée was the widowed mother of three grown children and a grandmother of seven. She led an active and independent life in Mar del Plata, Argentina, working as a school principal. Five days after her 50th birthday, she suffered a cerebral vascular accident, resulting in left hemiplegia. She received acute care services at a local hospital and was transferred to a rehabilitation institute where she made limited progress. The physician in charge of Haydée's rehabilitation wrote in her chart that she would be a wheelchair user for the rest of her life. Haydée was transferred to a nearby public geriatric residence. She was unable to get out of bed. Her impairments were significant. For example, she had lateral rotation and deviation of her neck due to contractures and she drooled uncontrollably. Haydée was severely depressed and withdrawn.

Because of her compromised volition, the only goal Haydée could see as possibly improving her life was to walk again. Although this goal was not realistic based on the severity of her stroke, her therapist decided not to negotiate a goal more in line with her current physical status. Rather, she met Haydée where she was and *validated* her one desire to walk again, agreeing to explore what might be done. The therapist attempted to refer her to physical therapy at the same institution, but Haydée *did not meet the criteria* because of her prognosis and because she lacked the economic resources to pay for private therapy. Therefore, the occupational therapist found an occupational therapy colleague who had the background to work with Haydée on ambulation and who agreed to see Haydée for a reduced fee that she could afford. As she began to experience the return of her motor function, her volition began to improve slightly. Unfortunately, during one of the regular exams to monitor her osteoporosis, a technician fell with Haydée while trying to assist her with a transfer. This accident provoked a fracture in Haydée's left arm, leaving her with more physical limitations than she had before. Realizing the effects of this fracture on her function, Haydée became despondent and was not able to identify a goal for herself. She "did not see how working toward something would really help her." She continued to report that she felt totally robbed of control over her life. She had no interest in anything around her. She felt all her life plans as well as the lifestyle she valued had been destroyed.

Working with Haydée

Under these circumstances, the therapist decided that she needed to begin Remotivation treatment within the exploratory stage (refer to Chapter 14). This would allow her to restore some sense of control, regenerate some feelings of satisfaction in doing things, and experience some sense of value. Because Haydée had such disrupted volition, it was clear that she would need a highly supportive environment that could scaffold her volition. The therapist also reasoned that a high level of environmental support could best be achieved in a group context.

At first Haydée was reluctant. However, with encouragement and statements of expectations from her therapist reminding her she should do this for herself, Haydée agreed to join a collective project called "The Puppet Workshop." With the leadership of an occupational therapist, a number of residents of the facility had planned to implement a musical puppet show for their grandchildren. For this project, they would make puppets and a stage, adapt the script of a musical for puppets, rehearse, and perform the show. Every resident collaborated in undertaking these activities according to the dimension of participation that they could achieve (refer to Chapter 8). *Becoming involved as an observer in this project provided the necessary momentum for Haydée.* After participating in the collective workshop twice she began to suggest some ideas to the rest of the participants when consulted. Thus, she became an essential part of the group so that the *group members began to expect that* Haydée would participate, an expectation that the therapist had previously stated. Over time, Haydée improved her sense of capacity and gained a feeling of satisfaction in doing this.

Because the therapist knew that Haydée was a strong writer, she was recruited to write the adaptation of the play's script. At first she hesitated to accept this responsibility, but with *constant encouragement* from the therapist, Haydée soon regained confidence in her writing skills. Bolstered by her success in this task, she also showed interest in performing with puppets. With some adjustments to the physical environment (providing adaptations to accommodate her left arm limitations and adjusting the stage for wheelchair access) and coaching, she was able to manipulate a puppet in the first show, which was presented to other residents and their families. Thus, *she became a puppeteer*. The puppet group was subsequently invited to perform seven more

shows hosted in different community settings. One of the settings was suggested by Haydée, a school where she had formerly been principal. Performing there meant that she had to face the emotionally difficult challenge of reencountering her former colleagues and students.

Going back to her old school was only one of many social and physical challenges Haydée faced. Overcoming a variety of architectural barriers made it difficult to get onto the stages. Involvement in working on the script and doing the performance promoted Haydée's feelings of efficacy and enjoyment in writing. She began writing poetry and other types of essays about her experiences in occupational therapy. Her excursions into the community provided her *with the opportunity to know that she could face and overcome many barriers, both physical and social.*

Because of Haydée's volitional progress, the therapist felt it was an ideal time to administer the Occupational Performance History Interview, Second Version (OPHI-II). The process of engaging in the interview was important for Haydée. It allowed her to put the experiences of her life into perspective and to be reminded of her own strengths. Furthermore, through the process of telling her life story, Haydée was able to identify goals she wanted to strive toward in the future, such as improving her walking, managing herself in a house, obtaining a disability pension, and working part-time as a writer. Haydée had faced adversity before and had used her determination to overcome obstacles in the past. It was clear that from this moment on, her narrative development could take a different path.

Haydée worked hard on her goals. She improved her performance of her self-care activities, and achieved independence in everything except bathing. She used her wheelchair to get around the facility and walked around her room with a tripod cane. Haydée took a 500-km trip on her own to complete the legal procedures to receive her pension. She completed a book of essays and prose, improving her motor skills for typing in occupational therapy. Haydée also began to go out alone to shop regularly, using a local taxi that accommodated her wheelchair. Finally, Haydée achieved one of her most important dreams. She traveled by bus with her three children back to her hometown. There, she reencountered relatives and old friends that she had not seen for years. She also visited the cemetery where her parents and husband were buried. Haydée returned very enthusiastically with the plan to move to her hometown within a short period of time.

After reviewing her achievements and reflecting on her future during occupational counseling with her occupational therapist, Haydée decided that she needed to focus on her main productive role as a writer and on her goal of living independently. She recognized that she had enjoyed writing and received positive feedback on her writing abilities. With her therapist's encouragement, she decided to take a university-sponsored writing course. She became the first student with a disability to attend a literary workshop called "Words Amidst Hands."

During this time she also continued in occupational therapy, *practicing her skills* in using the computer and in her self-care. After a couple of months she became totally independent in self-care, including bathing. She began to *practice* other activities of daily living such as sewing, washing, and ironing her clothes.

All of these efforts, which took place during a four-and-a-half-year period, not only moved Haydée closer to her goals, but also allowed her to realize her long-standing values of independence, vitality, and accomplishment in what she did. Haydée still had some highs and lows. Nonetheless, despite her occasional fears and uncertainties, Haydée continued to strive to live her occupational narrative.

and the turning point in the narratives of each of these unique individuals.

The case of Haydée illustrates how the most effective occupational therapy must be timed according to the client's needs and readiness for change. Haydée's therapist correctly reasoned that initial assessment was best done through informal means and only later chose to emotionally face and benefit from reviewing her life. Haydée also illustrates that the course of therapy is not always linear. There are often times when a client will regress or have difficulty moving forward as a result of complex combinations of personal and environmental factors. In particular, the process of rebuilding one's occupational narrative is extremely difficult when the onset of a disability has completely altered it.

CASE EXAMPLE: AN OLDER ADULT WITH MENTAL ILLNESS

Rebecca is 59 years old. She has been married for 34 years. Rebecca's husband, Lyle, runs the family plumbing business. The business has been in his family for three generations. Rebecca teaches English in secondary school. She loves her work

and is respected by her colleagues and appreciated by her students. Rebecca and Lyle have two sons, Lachlan, 25 and Patrick, 28. Both boys are very close, attend a local community college, and live at home. Patrick is very protective of his younger brother. The family participates in many activities together as often as they can, including eating dinner together. It is important for Rebecca to have this time with her family. For her it's an opportunity to spend quality time with everyone despite their busy schedules. At dinner, they talk about school, sports, friends, family, plans they have, and problems they face.

Rebecca worries about her children, especially Lachlan. He has a mild learning disability and she knows that he has a tough time in his classes at college. Lately, he has been hanging out with younger boys who left school but still spend their time around campus. Rebecca doesn't know any of them, but Lachlan tells her they are nice to him, treat him well, and make him feel smart. Her older son, Patrick, told her "these boys are not good—they drink and smoke, and party hard late into the evening." Rebecca feels she can't protect him and is failing him as a mother.

Work is also quite demanding on Rebecca. There have been budget cuts and it is hard for the teachers to provide varied and quality teaching and learning activities. There is talk that some subjects will be cut such as Indonesian and Arts. Extracurricular activities and trips will be dropped and there will need to be staff cuts too. Rebecca is the teachers' union representative. She is in the middle of several disputes and her colleagues come to her for advice and support. Although this is very stressful and demanding, it makes Rebecca feel useful and good about herself. She gets a rush of energy from being involved in and influencing decision-making.

When the budget cuts were implemented, Rebecca decided to take some money from the teachers' union petty cash fund to place a few bets in hopes of winning enough money to limit the impacts of the budget cuts. Rebecca spent the next month going to the casino to play black jack. She started with a few wins, which increased her excitement and made her feel she had definitely made the right decision. However, when she started losing money, she took more from the teachers' union bank account as well as from her and Lyle's joint bank account. Rebecca continued to gamble and, in the end, lost a total of $67,000. As her losses increased she felt increasingly anxious and trapped. She could not talk to anyone about what was going on because everyone looked up to her at work. She couldn't face her husband and tell him what she had done. She felt ashamed and could not see how she could fix this.

As Rebecca's distress and despair increased, she could not cope with what she had done. She considered ending her life, hoping her life insurance money would cover her debts. One morning, Rebecca left the house and pretended to go to work. She came back home when she was sure Lyle and the boys would be out for the day and took a large amount of over-the-counter medication and alcohol. Patrick came home from school early that day and found his mother unconscious with an empty bottle of alcohol and several empty bottles of different medications. He called an ambulance and Rebecca was rushed to the hospital. Following her suicide attempt, Rebecca was admitted to the psychiatric ward.

First Appreciations of Rebecca's Volition

Rebecca was diagnosed with bipolar disorder. After her admission to the ward, she became severely depressed. All she said to her psychiatrist was that she couldn't succeed at anything, "not even ending her life." She stayed in her room, in bed, and would not speak to anyone. It became clear that Rebecca's volition was severely compromised.

Michelle, the occupational therapist, decided to use the Volitional Questionnaire (VQ) with Rebecca to determine the severity of her volitional status. Rebecca did not meet with the most basic indicators of the volitional continuum even with encouragement and support from nurses and the rest of the staff.

Beginning the Intervention Process

Michelle's colleagues advised her to engage Rebecca in meaningful activities "by getting her out of bed and explaining to her that this would help her feel better." Michelle, knowing Rebecca's volitional conditions, decided to follow the first stage of the Remotivation Process's Exploratory Module: Validation.

Validation

Michelle focused on establishing a therapeutic relationship by respecting Rebecca's feelings and need for privacy. She began by spending brief periods of time sitting in a chair next to Rebecca's bed. She did this twice a day at the same time. She responded to Rebecca's requests, but remained silent. After a week, Rebecca became aware that Michelle was visiting her consistently and attending to her needs. She responded by changing her position in bed so she was facing Michelle with her eyes open. Michelle recognized this gesture as Rebecca accepting her company. This gave Michelle an opening to try to talk with her.

At first, conversations were very brief. Rebecca provided very short or vague responses to Michelle's comments and questions. These brief encounters provided Michelle with an opportunity to gather information about Rebecca's interests, values, and home and work environments. After a few days, Michelle went to see Rebecca in her bedroom (as usual), but Rebecca was not there. She had left her room and was having breakfast in the ward's dining room. Michelle brought her a cup of tea and asked Rebecca if she could sit with her. Rebecca and Michelle sat together and initiated a longer conversation. Every day after that, Michelle showed up to have breakfast and chat with Rebecca. During these conversations, Michelle learned about the importance of family dinners to Rebecca and how she and Lyle used to sit in their backyard with a cup of tea after a long day at work. She also shared that she enjoyed gardening and cooking with the produce from her veggie patch.

Michelle also talked to Rebecca's husband, Lyle, to find out more about Rebecca's interests and daily routine. Michelle was then able to comment and add information about Rebecca's family in their conversations. For example, when Rebecca was talking about her vegetable garden, Michelle would mention which vegetables Lyle or the boys preferred. At first, Rebecca was reluctant to engage in conversations about her family. She had not seen her sons in 2 weeks and only saw her husband on a couple of occasions and she was still feeling guilty and ashamed.

By the end of her third week in the ward, Rebecca and Michelle had established a trusting and respectful therapeutic relationship. Michelle thought it would be a good time to complete an occupational therapy evaluation and suggested the idea to Rebecca. Rebecca showed limited interest and wondered what the point was and what it would achieve. Michelle decided to complete the Occupational Performance History Interview, Second Version (OPHI-II). The interview format seemed suited to Rebecca and she seemed to find some comfort in not having to do anything specific. Because Rebecca's volition was still low, Michelle decided to administer the OPHI-II in sections, completing one scale at a time. There were some clear trends in Rebecca's results. She scored much higher when discussing her past roles and routines, interests and values, and occupational settings. Any question referring to the present or the future was met with low expectations, negation, or avoidance. The most interesting part of the OPHI-II contents for Rebecca was the section on critical life events and the resulting narrative slope. Rebecca was more engaged in this section of the assessment. She was more energetic when talking about important moments in her life like the birth of her children, a trip with her husband, and even losing money at the casino. The visual aspect of the narrative slope seemed to have more of an impact on Rebecca. This appeared to be the turning point in Rebecca's recovery.

After discussing her results on the occupational identity and the occupational competence scales with Michelle, Rebecca identified areas of her life that were important to her. Her roles as a mother and a wife were very important. She still felt she had failed her family. She didn't know where to start and how she could possibly face them, especially Patrick, her son who found her unconscious after her attempted suicide. Her role as a teacher was also something she was still passionate about, but she could not imagine going back to work after having gambled the teachers' union money away. Rebecca also expressed interest and found meaning in gardening.

Wanting to build on Rebecca's interests and self-confidence (personal causation), Michelle advised Rebecca to participate in gardening activities with other patients. The occupational therapy department had a small vegetable and herb garden as well as several plants. Rebecca agreed to have a look at the garden, but stated she wasn't ready to commit or engage in a group activity. Two days later, she left her room and came to the occupational therapy garden. Michelle was there with three other people. They were talking about a lemon tree and wondering why there were so few lemons. Rebecca made a few suggestions. One patient asked her opinion about pruning. There had been disagreement between the members of the group about how to do it, and considering her background in gardening, they sought her opinion. Later that day, Rebecca mentioned to a nurse that she enjoyed going to the garden.

Through participation in this meaningful collective project, Rebecca began to use her communication and interaction skills more and gradually identified and expressed different emotions related to her occupational performance. Eventually, Rebecca identified one clear and important goal: going home and having a cup of tea with Lyle in their garden.

Rebecca and Michelle made a plan for Rebecca to progressively take steps to help her go back home. She worked hard to build a positive occupational identity, find meaning and satisfaction in her life, and expect success when engaging in occupations. She sought to achieve the level of occupational competence she had envisioned for herself. There were moments when Rebecca doubted her ability to overcome the challenges she faced and she had a few setbacks. Nonetheless, with the help of her family and Michelle, Rebecca continued to strive to reconstruct her occupational narrative.

Rebecca's accomplishments would not have happened if the therapist had not recognized Rebecca's severe volitional conditions, and followed the necessary steps to validate her feelings before encouraging her to act. Michelle was flexible, focusing on Rebecca's subjective experiences and giving her a protagonist role in decision-making. Rebecca needed to rebuild her basic sense of being through others who appreciated her as she was. This approach made her feel able to try new things and consequently participate in something that was meaningful and part of her daily life.

CASE EXAMPLE: AN ADULT WITH SCHIZOPHRENIA

Alvaro, a Chilean man, was 33 years old when he began occupational therapy. This example summarizes his involvement in MOHO-based therapy until Alvaro reached the age of 55. Alvaro was the youngest of three children and lived with his mother, a homemaker, and his father, a pilot. As a child and adolescent, Alvaro was an outstanding student and showed musical talent from a young age. He was gregarious and had many friends.

When Alvaro was 18 years old, he had his first psychotic episode and was diagnosed with schizophrenia. He became paranoid and withdrawn. He experienced unpleasant side effects of prescribed medication and, consequently, was resistant to taking it. Alvaro's family did not understand his illness and his relationship with his father, who could not accept his illness, became particularly strained. Alvaro's mother was very supportive and stood by him through four suicide attempts. For 15 years Alvaro's psychosis continued unabated. He developed obsessive and delusional ideation. These symptoms, which he interpreted as blasphemous, were particularly unsetting to him due to his deep religious values. At this time he preferred death to having such thoughts and feelings. He felt overwhelming desperation, anxiety, and guilt.

When clozapine became available in Chile, Alvaro began to take it and for the first time his symptoms abated. Around this time Alvaro attended a participatory education–style conference *for* people with schizophrenia and their families. At the conference he met an occupational therapist and learned about the importance of people with mental illness and their families being active participants in their treatment and rehabilitation. Following the conference, Alvaro and a number of other young persons with mental illness asked the therapist to assist them in organizing a self-help group (refer to Chapter 14). Subsequently, the group began to meet regularly with the guidance of the occupational therapist who also provided MOHO-based occupational counseling (described in Chapter 14) to the members of the group who were ready for it. Alvaro was an active member of the group who took on the role of encouraging others in the group. Nonetheless, he still had difficulty concentrating and focusing.

Initial Assessment

Because Alvaro was not actively psychotic, had a long history of illness, was cognitively able to participate in an interview, and had developed trust with this therapist, she chose to begin his assessment with the Occupational Performance History Interview-Second Version (OPHI-II). Figure 19-1 shows his ratings on the OPHI-II scales.

Summary of the Results of the OPHI-II

After the onset of Alvaro's mental illness, he attempted to study at the University of Chile, School of Music. He began his studies four times. Each time, the demands of school work, exams, and relating to professors and classmates led to an exacerbation of his psychosis and subsequently led to him dropping out of the program. Despite these failed attempts, Alvaro still wanted to study music. He pursued, and with some difficulty finished a 1-year training to be a sound technician. During this time and when he was able, Alvaro also sang in the Chamber Chorus of Chile and volunteered in a nursing home, where he performed religious songs. Throughout this period Alvaro experienced a variety of psychotic symptoms including paranoid delusions (e.g., thinking that he was being followed). Despite his symptoms, Alvaro's faith, values, and intense passion for music carried him forward.

Occupational Identity

Alvaro's sense of efficacy was eroded by his repeated failures. Thus Alvaro's volition was characterized by a gap between his strong *values* ("living life and using [the] talents God gave me") *and interests* (a passion for music), and his *personal causation*,

Occupational Identity Scale	1	2	3	4
Has personal goals and projects				✗
Identifies a desired occupational lifestyle			✗	
Expects success	✗			
Accepts responsibility				✗
Appraises abilities and limitations		✗		
Has commitments and values				✗
Recognizes identity and obligations				✗
Has interests				✗
Felt effective (past)		✗		
Found meaning and satisfaction in lifestyle (past)			✗	
Made occupational choices (past)				✗
Occupational Competence Scale	**1**	**2**	**3**	**4**
Maintains satisfying lifestyle		✗		
Fulfills role expectations			✗	
Works toward goals				✗
Meets personal performance standards	✗			
Organizes time for responsibilities		✗		
Participates in interests		✗		
Fulfilled roles (past)		✗		
Maintained habits (past)		✗		
Achieved satisfaction (past)		✗		
Occupational Settings (Environment) Scale	**1**	**2**	**3**	**4**
Home life occupational forms			✗	
Major productive role occupational forms			✗	
Leisure occupational forms			✗	
Home life social group			✗	
Major productive role social group			✗	
Leisure social group			✗	
Home life spaces, objects, and resources				✗
Major productive role spaces, objects, and resources			✗	
Leisure spaces, objects, and resources				✗

Key: **1** = Extreme occupational functioning problems
2 = Some occupational functioning problems
3 = Appropriate satisfactory occupational functioning
4 = Exceptionally competent occupational functioning

FIGURE 19-1 Alvaro's Strengths and Weaknesses on the OPHI-II Occupational Identity, Competence, and Environmental Scales.

which was dominated by negative expectations for his future participation in valued occupations. He was particularly fearful that his schizophrenic symptoms would come back and ruin anything he attempted. Alvaro showed a high sense of obligation in what he perceived as his ongoing role responsibilities. These included being a good son and taking care of his mother, being an uncle to his nephews, volunteering, and being responsible for his own treatment and recovery. He was too fearful of the future to have goals or a vision for life that he really thought was possible. During the OPHI-II assessment interview, Alvaro stated that he still wanted to return to his studies at the University of Chile; however, he was extremely fearful that he would only fail again. His years of living with schizophrenia had led him to a compromised sense of his life story—one in which he struggled simply to enact his values as best he could.

Occupational Competence

Alvaro had difficulty reestablishing his occupational competency. He often felt that he could not meet these role obligations as he should. Moreover, his father continued to devalue him and Alvaro felt that he would never live up to his father's expectations. While he maintained a routine of self-care and family and volunteer involvement, he did not feel fulfilled with these occupations since they did not fit with his occupational identity. Overall, Alvaro was not living the life he had envisioned for himself due to his impairment. Instead he felt he was doing the best he could to live the best kind of life possible.

Environment

Alvaro's social environment consisted mainly of his mother, the singers of Chamber Chorus of Chile, and the group of elderly people he helped in his volunteer role. He identified them as being very supportive and giving. The major negative aspect of his social environment was his father's devaluing attitude toward him. The tasks he performed in each of these environments (groups) provided a level of satisfaction, but they did not meet alvaro's hopes for what he wanted. He was also aware that his strained relationship with his father made his mother very sad. Alvaro did have financial resources from his family that allowed him to have objects he needed and valued. He owned a classical guitar and had money to attend concerts.

Occupational Narrative

Alvaro's occupational narrative is dominated by a constant quest to realize his dreams, which were deeply rooted in his values. His narrative slope (Fig. 19-2) illustrates a downward trend followed by a period of steady struggle in which he fights against his symptoms, repeatedly fails at school, and yet maintains a level of participation. Given the significant impact of his impairment on his life course and all the failures Alvaro had accumulated since adolescence, his narrative is also dominated by a sense of fear about what the future will bring, even as he struggles on.

Additional Evaluation

Because informal observation had indicated that Alvaro was having difficulty with motor, process, and communication interaction skills, the occupational therapist decided to observe Alvaro using the formal Assessment of Motor and Process Skills (AMPS), and the Assessment of Communication and Interaction Skills (ACIS). She also decided to use the Volitional Questionnaire (VQ) in order to gather more details about his volition. Using these assessments together provided information about his personal causation and the impact of his occupational performance on volition and vice versa.

Information Gathered from the AMPS

The occupational therapist chose to modify the administration of the AMPS. She observed Alvaro outside the standardized AMPS tasks doing things he was highly motivated to do. She chose to approach the assessment in this way because she

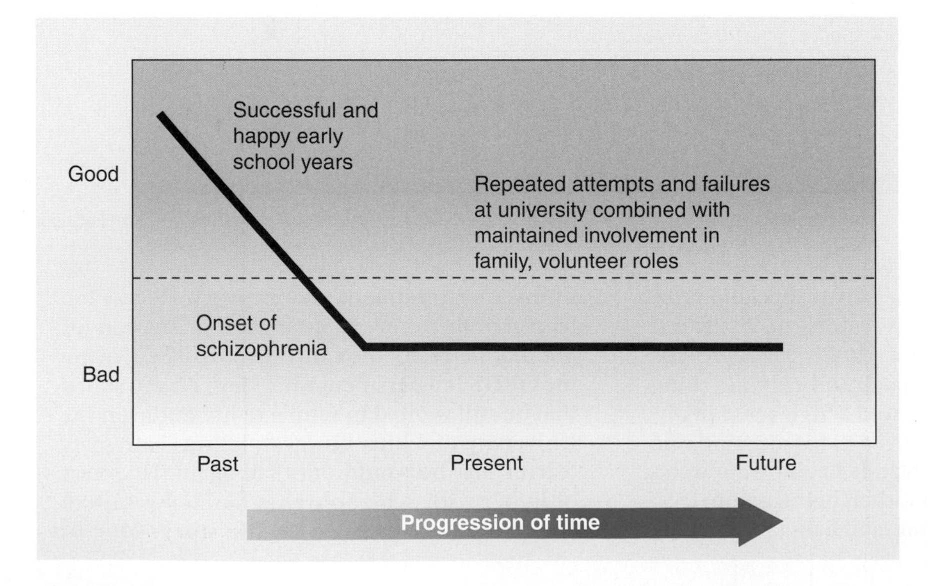

FIGURE 19-2 Alvaro's Narrative Slope.

had noted that Alvaro's performance was highly variable depending on his level of motivation to do the task. In addition to observing him making a sandwich (a standardized AMPS task) she also observed him serving tea for his mother and participating in a music rehearsal involving his peers.

During these observations Alvaro showed competence in seeking and using knowledge and organizing time. He had difficulty attending to the task at hand and could not effectively pace himself. He was generally competent at arranging his environment to support tasks. He was ineffective at adapting and often failed to notice circumstances in the environment that required him to modify his actions. He also had difficulty with motor skills. For example, he had trouble regulating the speed and force of his actions (calibration), and as a result he bumped into furniture, accidentally banged his guitar and dropped dishes. He did not appear to learn from his mistakes.

Information Gathered from the ACIS

Figure 19-3 shows the results of the ACIS observations of Alvaro. He was observed with his mother and father doing different activities and at a mental health conference. He was a charming person, very expressive and sensitive to others. He collaborated and related well. He demonstrated competence in the domains of physicality and relations. Alvaro's main problems were in the area of information exchange. He had difficulty being assertive, articulating, modulating, and speaking. Alvaro had problems voicing his opinions because he feared rejection and worried about offending other people. His problems with articulating (due to side effects of medications) meant that others often had to ask him to repeat what he said, but he still ended up confusing others. He vacillated between being too loud or almost silent when talking. Despite these areas of difficulty, he got along well with others because of his strengths in relating to people.

The one exception to these observations was when Alvaro interacted with his father. In this circumstance, his information exchange skills were inhibited in reaction to his father's attitudes. Alvaro was unable to finish a conversation with his father and retreated to his bedroom.

Skills	With his father				With his mother				With the group				Conference			
Physicality	1	2	3	4	1	2	3	4	1	2	3	4	1	2	3	4
Contacts				■				■			■					■
Gazes				■				■				■				■
Gestures				■				■				■				■
Maneuvers				■				■				■				■
Orients				■				■				■				■
Positions				■				■				■				■
Information Exchange	1	2	3	4	1	2	3	4	1	2	3	4	1	2	3	4
Articulates		■				■					■			■		
Asserts	■				■					■						■
Asks	■							■				■				■
Engages	■							■				■				■
Expresses	■							■				■				■
Modulates		■				■				■				■		
Shares				■				■				■				■
Speaks		■					■			■					■	
Sustains	■							■				■			■	
Relations	1	2	3	4	1	2	3	4	1	2	3	4	1	2	3	4
Collaborates				■				■				■				■
Conforms				■				■				■				■
Focuses				■				■				■				■
Relates				■				■				■				■
Respects				■				■				■				■

Key: **4** = Competent **3** = Questionable **2** = Ineffective **1** = Deficit

FIGURE 19-3 Alvaro's Rating from the First Administration of the ACIS in Four Observational Settings (Summary of All Ratings in Each Situation)

Information Gathered from the VQ

The occupational therapist conducted the VQ while observing Alvaro volunteering at a mental health conference, during a group activity with his peers, and doing activities with his mother and father. Figure 19-4 shows his VQ ratings.

When participating in known and supportive environments, Alvaro demonstrated spontaneous volition for most items, except for those most clearly related to personal causation (e.g., showing pride, trying to solve problems, and trying to correct his own mistakes). He received higher scores for items that ordinarily reflect high volition (e.g., staying involved and seeking additional responsibility) because the activities were so closely tied to his values. In this instance, he persisted despite worries about being ineffective. In contrast, his volition was very low when doing social activities with his father. The VQ observation confirmed the therapist's suspicions that Alvaro's motivation was largely bolstered by his strong values, despite lacking a sense of efficacy. The occupational therapist administered the VQ and tracked volitional changes twice more and across contexts (Figs. 19-5 & 19-8). Repeated administrations of the VQ revealed that after the first period of intervention Alvaro's volition still decreased when faced with situations that were unstructured and ambiguous, such as interacting with his father and waiting for a response from school to which he had applied. However, in his major roles, such as studying and working, he began to demonstrate spontaneity in volition.

Therapist's Conceptualization of Alvaro's Situation and Identification of Treatment Goals

The occupational therapist concluded that despite Alvaro's significant impairment, he had managed a level of occupational participation because of his volitional strength, in particular his values. As a consequence he had been able to participate in meaningful roles such as group member, coordinator, volunteer, family member, and amateur musician. Alvaro's challenges included his weak personal causation and difficulties with process and communication interaction skills. When the therapist shared this conceptualization with Alvaro and identified what she felt were his strengths and weaknesses, Alvaro agreed, and gained insight into his subjective experience. Together, they negotiated his goals:

- achieving a career as a musician at the University of Chile
- gaining the respect of his father,
- continuing with his volunteer role, and
- contributing to the development of *Reencuentros*, a Community Integration Center.

Working with Alvaro

Alvaro agreed with the therapist that he needed to develop his sense of efficacy in order to achieve

Indicators	Conference					Self-help group					Activities with mother					Activities with father				
Shows curiosity	P	H	I	**S**	N/A	P	H	I	**S**	N/A	P	H	I	**S**	N/A	**P**	H	I	S	N/A
Initiates actions/tasks	P	H	I	**S**	N/A	P	H	I	**S**	N/A	P	H	I	**S**	N/A	**P**	H	I	S	N/A
Tries new things	P	H	I	**S**	N/A	P	H	**I**	S	N/A	P	H	I	**S**	N/A	**P**	H	I	S	N/A
Shows preferences	P	H	I	**S**	N/A	P	H	I	**S**	N/A	P	H	I	**S**	N/A	**P**	H	I	S	N/A
Shows that an activity is special/significant	P	H	I	**S**	N/A	P	H	I	**S**	N/A	P	H	I	**S**	N/A	**P**	H	I	S	N/A
Stays engaged	P	H	I	**S**	N/A	P	H	I	**S**	N/A	P	H	I	**S**	N/A	**P**	H	I	S	N/A
Indicates goals	P	H	I	**S**	N/A	P	H	I	**S**	N/A	P	H	I	**S**	N/A	**P**	H	I	S	N/A
Shows pride	**P**	H	I	S	N/A	P	**H**	I	S	N/A	P	**H**	I	S	N/A	**P**	H	I	S	N/A
Tries to solve problems	P	H	I	S	**N/A**	P	H	**I**	S	N/A	P	H	I	**S**	N/A	**P**	H	I	S	N/A
Tries to correct mistakes	P	H	**I**	S	N/A	P	H	**I**	S	N/A	P	H	I	S	**N/A**	**P**	H	I	S	N/A
Pursues an activity to completion/accomplishment	P	H	I	**S**	N/A	P	H	I	**S**	N/A	P	H	I	**S**	N/A	**P**	H	I	S	N/A
Invests additional energy/emotion/attention	P	H	I	**S**	N/A	P	H	I	**S**	N/A	P	H	I	**S**	N/A	**P**	H	I	S	N/A
Seeks/accepts additional responsibilities	P	H	I	**S**	N/A	P	H	I	**S**	N/A	P	H	I	**S**	N/A	**P**	H	I	S	N/A
Seeks/accepts challenges	P	H	I	**S**	N/A	P	**H**	I	S	N/A	P	H	I	S	**N/A**	P	H	I	**S**	N/A

Key: **(1)** P = Passive **(2)** H = Hesitant **(3)** I = Involved **(4)** S = Spontaneous

FIGURE 19-4 Alvaro's Ratings from the First Administration of the Volitional Questionnaire.

his goals. His course of therapy followed the *remotivation process,* starting at the first stage of the Competence Module (de las Heras et al., 2002). This *meant* that Alvaro needed to begin with those goals that were closer to his volitional strengths and skills, in familiar environments, and doing tasks in which he felt satisfaction and efficacy. He progressively increased the level of challenge and took on new roles. It was important that his occupational therapist validate his fears and encourage him, demonstrating her belief that he could succeed.

Alvaro was very motivated by the idea of helping to develop the community-based center, Reencuentros. The occupational therapist was working at the center with eight members of a self-help group, including Alvaro, to create a collective occupational project. She invited each member to take on a different role according to their unique skills. Alvaro, who knew musicians and locations where music was performed, agreed to develop a strategy for holding concerts and other musical events to raise money. He even began to play his classical guitar during these events in front of many people. Alvaro was very anxious, anticipating problems and mistakes, but he faced these challenges and was always satisfied with and thankful for what he accomplished. After a few of these events, he told the therapist in an occupational counseling session, "I have never done so many things in my entire life." In response, the therapist gave Alvaro feedback, "Alvaro, you have done much in the past to continue functioning despite your illness! Have you realized that?" This helped Alvaro reexamine his tragic narrative of self-perceived failure (Fig. 19-5).

Over time, by participating in real-life tasks and activities that resonated with his values and interests, Alvaro showed an increased sense of efficacy. Alvaro's Volitional Questionnaire showed personal causation in progress so the therapist decided to continue with the Competence Module of the Remotivation Process. Alvaro was more spontaneous in trying new things and trying to solve problems. He was able to stick with increasingly challenging activities until they were completed. His therapist, through occupational counseling sessions, coached him and provided him feedback throughout the process in order to help him make choices to take on appropriate challenges and to recognize when he succeeded. Together, the occupational therapist and Alvaro decided that it was the right moment to begin with MOHO-based skill teaching. In his case, this needed to be done during occupational counseling and through direct coaching when Alvaro was performing tasks that were relevant to him. The therapist gave feedback to help Alvaro better understand the challenges he faced in motor, process, and communication interaction skills. They identified ways he could perform more effectively. At first the therapist had to coach Alvaro consistently

Indicators	Talking on the radio					Participation in fund-raising					Playing guitar at events					Learning skills				
Shows curiosity	P	H	I	**S**	N/A	P	H	I	**S**	N/A	P	H	I	**S**	N/A	P	H	I	**S**	N/A
Initiates actions/tasks	P	H	**I**	S	N/A	P	H	**I**	S	N/A	P	H	**I**	S	N/A	P	H	**I**	S	N/A
Tries new things	P	H	I	**S**	N/A	P	H	I	**S**	N/A	P	H	I	**S**	N/A	P	H	**I**	S	N/A
Shows preferences	P	H	I	**S**	N/A	P	H	I	**S**	N/A	P	H	I	**S**	N/A	P	H	I	**S**	N/A
Shows that an activity is special/significant	P	H	I	**S**	N/A	P	H	I	**S**	N/A	P	H	I	**S**	N/A	P	H	I	**S**	N/A
Stays engaged	P	H	I	**S**	N/A	P	H	I	**S**	N/A	P	H	I	**S**	N/A	P	H	I	**S**	N/A
Indicates goals	P	H	I	**S**	N/A	P	H	I	**S**	N/A	P	H	I	**S**	N/A	P	H	**I**	S	N/A
Shows pride	P	H	**I**	S	N/A	P	H	**I**	S	N/A	P	H	**I**	S	N/A	P	**H**	I	S	N/A
Tries to solve problems	P	H	I	**S**	N/A	P	H	**I**	S	N/A	P	H	I	**S**	N/A	P	H	**I**	S	N/A
Tries to correct mistakes	P	H	**I**	S	N/A	P	H	**I**	S	N/A	P	H	I	**S**	N/A	P	H	**I**	S	N/A
Pursues an activity to completion/accomplishment	P	H	I	**S**	N/A	P	H	I	**S**	N/A	P	H	I	**S**	N/A	P	H	I	S	N/A
Invests additional energy/emotion/attention	P	H	I	**S**	N/A	P	H	I	**S**	N/A	P	H	I	**S**	N/A	P	H	**I**	S	N/A
Seeks/accepts additional responsibilities	P	H	I	**S**	N/A	P	H	I	**S**	N/A	P	H	I	**S**	N/A	P	**H**	I	S	N/A
Seeks/accepts challenges	P	H	I	**S**	N/A	P	H	**I**	S	N/A	P	**H**	I	S	N/A	P	H	**I**	S	N/A

Key: (1) P = Passive **(2)** H = Hesitant **(3)** I = Involved **(4)** S = Spontaneous

FIGURE 19-5 Alvaro's Ratings from the Second Administration of the Volitional Questionnaire in More Challenging Situations.

and provide him feedback about environmental cues he had missed. Eventually he was able to perform, practice, and monitor himself and the environment. Together they identified that by writing down the steps and environmental demands of any new task, Alvaro became more aware and could better monitor himself and the environment while performing activities and tasks. Alvaro's improvements on his communication interaction skills, particularly in his communication exchange domain, are illustrated in Figures 19-6 and 19-7.

A New Challenge

Over time, Alvaro's improved occupational performance made his personal causation increase, allowing him to anticipate his future with hope. He internalized new habits of performance and committed to a new social role at Reencuentros: helping peers to initiate actions and try new things that were important but challenging to them.

After going through this process with his occupational therapist, he felt ready to tackle his goal of studying music at the University of Chile. Attending the university meant that he needed to prepare himself for a very demanding environment in which he would have to do such things as take exams in front of classmates and professors, learn classical guitar techniques that demand sophisticated motor and process skills, and interact and communicate in a new environment. Alvaro, conscious of all these challenges, decided he wanted to continue volunteering at Reencuentros while attending university on a part-time basis. Together Alvaro and his therapist inquired as to whether the School of Music at the university would allow part-time study. This was a very difficult process since the program was very selective and rigid. Over 2 months, Alvaro went to the school weekly, and called daily to remind administrative staff about his request. The therapist encouraged and sometimes accompanied him, especially at the beginning. During this time Alvaro continued helping Reencuentros to raise money and he engaged in helping his peers.

Skills	With his father				Forming center				Coordinating musical group				Applying to school			
Physicality	1	2	3	4	1	2	3	4	1	2	3	4	1	2	3	4
Contacts				■				■				■				■
Gazes				■				■				■				■
Gestures				■				■				■			■	
Maneuvers				■				■				■				■
Orients				■				■				■				■
Positions				■				■				■				■
Information Exchange	1	2	3	4	1	2	3	4	1	2	3	4	1	2	3	4
Articulates		■				■					■				■	
Asserts	■				■						■					■
Asks	■							■				■				■
Engages	■							■				■				■
Expresses	■							■				■				■
Modulates		■				■				■					■	
Shares				■				■				■				■
Speaks		■					■				■				■	
Sustains	■							■			■				■	
Relations	1	2	3	4	1	2	3	4	1	2	3	4	1	2	3	4
Collaborates				■				■				■				■
Conforms				■				■				■				■
Focuses				■				■				■				■
Relates				■				■				■				■
Respects				■				■				■				■

Key: 4 = Competent **3** = Questionable **2** = Ineffective **1** = Deficit

FIGURE 19-6 Alvaro's Rating from the Second Administration of the ACIS in Four Observational Settings (Summary of All Ratings in Each Situation).

Skills	With his father				Educational program				With professors				At work			
Physicality	1	2	3	4	1	2	3	4	1	2	3	4	1	2	3	4
Contacts				■				■				■				■
Gazes				■				■				■				■
Gestures				■				■				■			■	
Maneuvers				■				■				■				■
Orients				■				■				■				■
Positions				■				■				■				■
Information Exchange	1	2	3	4	1	2	3	4	1	2	3	4	1	2	3	4
Articulates			■				■				■				■	
Asserts	■						■				■					■
Asks	■							■				■				■
Engages	■							■				■				■
Expresses	■							■				■				■
Modulates			■			■				■					■	
Shares				■				■				■				■
Speaks		■					■				■				■	
Sustains		■						■				■				■
Relations	1	2	3	4	1	2	3	4	1	2	3	4	1	2	3	4
Collaborates				■				■				■				■
Conforms				■				■				■				■
Focuses				■				■				■				■
Relates				■				■				■				■
Respects				■				■				■				■

Key: **4** = Competent **3** = Questionable **2** = Ineffective **1** = Deficit

FIGURE 19-7 Alvaro's Rating from the Third Administration of the ACIS in Four Observational Settings (Summary of All Ratings in Each Situation).

He took on the role of coordinator of a musical group that performed in pediatric hospitals and nursing homes. This new role demanded higher level performance and personal causation.

Alvaro showed an increasing sense of efficacy in different environments; he needed less support and encouragement from his therapist to face challenges in new and much more demanding environments. He began taking initiative to apply strategies he had learned to improve his skills in these new occupational settings.

Despite this, the occupational therapist still observed that Alvaro's symptoms (objective performance capacity) interfered with his process skills. She met with and advised Alvaro, his family, and his psychiatrist that he was still having some difficulty with psychotic symptoms and suggested they consider a complementary medication. Alvaro and his mother agreed and the physician wrote him a new prescription. The change in medication helped Alvaro to better organize his thoughts and communication. Alvaro's sense of efficacy increased, even in demanding social situations such as interacting with his father.

At Reencuentros, Alvaro began to use the services of the Educational Integration Program, which helped members achieve their educational goals. In the program, every member was supported by an occupational therapist and the other participants to progressively enter a new role (refer to Chapter 14). They *examined* their volition, skills, habits, and environmental options and demands in relation to their desires. As Alvaro participated in this program, he continued applying to the university for part-time admission. He shared the process with his peers who encouraged him to continue.

Finally, the university accepted Alvaro into the program as a part-time student. Alvaro celebrated with his parents, who were both happy and a bit nervous about the news. Consequently, at one of the regular participatory education meetings with his parents, the therapist listened to their concerns and shared her assessment of how much Alvaro's volition and skills had improved, and the positive effect these improvements had on his occupational participation. She also explained that Alvaro would continue receiving support to help him succeed at school.

Alvaro's Occupational Life at School

Alvaro began to attend school on a regular basis, taking three courses each semester. As expected, the courses were difficult for him. However, Alvaro spoke with one of his professors who allowed the occupational therapist to observe some classes. The therapist informed the instructor of Alvaro's challenges in learning the music. The instructor agreed to modify his teaching style (refer to Chapter 14) and to provide individual classes for Alvaro. Together the instructor and Alvaro negotiated the pace and sequence of learning to accommodate his unique challenges.

This kind of flexibility was totally new to the music program at the university. However, when the director and professors met and got to know Alvaro and witness his strength and courage, they agreed to the necessary accommodations. Alvaro persisted at his studies and graduated 7 years later. During this time he continued to receive support at Reencuentros by participating once a week in his occupational counseling sessions with his therapist.

His psychiatrist, his therapist, his mother, and other people he met at Reencuentros attended Alvaro's final exam, which consisted of him giving a concert to a large audience at the University of Chile. He made a great effort playing four long pieces of classical music. While playing the last piece, the one he knew best, he began to make mistakes on pacing due to fatigue and anxiety. However, he continued playing the piece until it was done and received a warm and enthusiastic round of applause.

Alvaro's father died 2 years before he finished school. Although his father did not see his final achievement, Alvaro felt he would somehow know how much he had achieved. Alvaro took his father's death with pain but also with strength. He was the first to intone religious songs at his funeral. His memories of his father were realistic, emphasizing the best of him as a person.

Achieving the Integration of Work and Education

Following graduation, Alvaro committed to a new challenge, entering into the worker role. He was confident despite the lack of job opportunities that were available in Santiago. He applied for a job as sound technician and music coordinator of a youth center. The occupational therapist supported Alvaro to prepare a résumé and practice for the job interview. She helped him arrange for references and supported him by phone the day of the interview.

Alvaro got the job and began working part-time. He was responsible for arranging the sound for all musical plays and concerts given at the

Indicators	Talking in the radio					Participation in Fund-raising					Playing guitar at events					Learning skills				
Shows curiosity	P	H	I	**S**	N/A	P	H	I	**S**	N/A	P	H	I	**S**	N/A	**P**	H	I	S	N/A
Initiates actions/tasks	P	**H**	I	S	N/A	P	H	I	**S**	N/A	P	H	I	**S**	N/A	P	**H**	I	S	N/A
Tries new things	P	H	I	S	**N/A**	P	H	I	**S**	N/A	P	H	I	**S**	N/A	**P**	H	I	S	N/A
Shows preferences	P	H	**I**	S	N/A	P	H	I	**S**	N/A	P	H	I	**S**	N/A	**P**	H	I	S	N/A
Shows that an activity is special/significant	P	H	I	**S**	N/A	P	H	I	**S**	N/A	P	H	I	**S**	N/A	P	H	I	**S**	N/A
Stays engaged	P	H	I	**S**	N/A	P	H	I	**S**	N/A	P	H	I	**S**	N/A	P	**H**	I	S	N/A
Indicates goals	P	H	I	**S**	N/A	P	H	I	**S**	N/A	P	H	I	**S**	N/A	P	H	I	**S**	N/A
Shows pride	P	H	I	**S**	N/A	P	H	I	**S**	N/A	P	H	**I**	S	N/A	**P**	H	I	S	N/A
Tries to solve problems	P	H	**I**	S	N/A	P	H	I	**S**	N/A	P	H	I	**S**	N/A	**P**	H	I	S	N/A
Tries to correct mistakes	P	H	**I**	S	N/A	P	H	I	**S**	N/A	P	H	I	**S**	N/A	**P**	H	I	S	N/A
Pursues an activity to completion/accomplishment	P	H	I	**S**	N/A	P	H	I	**S**	N/A	P	H	I	**S**	N/A	P	H	**I**	S	N/A
Invests additional energy/emotion/attention	P	H	I	**S**	N/A	P	H	**I**	S	N/A	P	H	I	**S**	N/A	**P**	H	I	S	N/A
Seeks/accepts additional responsibilities	P	H	**I**	S	N/A	P	H	I	**S**	N/A	P	H	I	**S**	N/A	**P**	H	I	S	N/A
Seeks/accepts challenges	P	**H**	I	S	N/A	P	H	I	**S**	N/A	P	H	I	S	**N/A**	**P**	H	I	S	N/A

Key: **(1)** P = Passive **(2)** H = Hesitant **(3)** I = Involved **(4)** S = Spontaneous

FIGURE 19-8 Alvaro's Ratings from the Third Administration of the Volitional Questionnaire.

center. One night when working there, he did not notice a piece of furniture, tripped over it and fell, breaking his right leg. Although he had to be out of work for the month, the center waited for him to return. The staff and youth all valued Alvaro's personality and social attitudes. When the center closed because of financial problems, Alvaro went on to work as coordinator of music at different centers over the years (Fig. 19-8).

When Alvaro was 45 years old, 12 years after he helped to found Reencuentros, he remained involved. Any time his help was needed for different fund-raising events or to put on concerts, Alvaro was happy to volunteer. One day, his former therapist and director of Reencuentros shared with Alvaro that the center would have to close due to insufficient funding. As one of Reencuentros' founders, Alvaro tried desperately to find some means to prevent the closure. After it became clear that the center must close, Alvaro then helped with its closing. He prepared and ran the closing ceremony. It was a bittersweet ending for Alvaro, who had gained and given so much to the organization. Nonetheless, the story had come full circle and Alvaro was able to go on with confidence to do the things he valued, despite the acknowledged uncertainty about the future.

Alvaro's Occupational Life Today

When this case was written, Alvaro was 55 years old. His main productive occupational roles had changed due to his mother's advanced age and severe osteoarthritis. He became her caregiver, and also a home maintainer. He continued in his roles as a religious participant, and as a volunteer singing at his church choir and giving musical presentations in various nursing homes. He continued to encourage his friends to persist on working toward their goals. Alvaro periodically called his former therapist asking, "Do you need any help from me?" In fact, he was a guest in some occupational therapy classes and shared his lived experience and taught OT students how important occupational therapists are in helping people "feel alive again." He would finish his classes by playing a piece of classical music.

Conclusion

Each of the cases in this chapter illustrates the human potential that exists even in the face of extreme adversity and personal failure. Life stories can be retold and rebuilt. The extent of the devastation of life faced by each person in this chapter required substantial and long-term efforts collaborating with their occupational therapists. Although the process of rebuilding one's occupational narrative is difficult, the cases in this chapter show how occupational therapists, through therapeutic reasoning and advocacy, secure the best services and opportunities for their clients, despite facing environmental barriers.

Chapter 19 Review Questions

Describe an occupational narrative and how it may change over time as a result of major life events.

1. Identify at least three professional competencies necessary for a MOHO-oriented therapist that are reflected through the examples in this chapter.
2. What are attitudes that therapists need to display when facilitating the reconstruction of an occupational narrative?
3. Which MOHO principles do you think are crucial for the intervention process when reconstructing an occupational narrative?

HOMEWORK ASSIGNMENTS

1. In Haydée's story:
    - Why do you think the therapist recommended that Haydée participate in the collective project?
2. Reflect on Alvaro's case:
    - What was the turning point of his occupational narrative? Justify your response.

3. In Rebecca's story:
   - Identify the possible challenges Michelle had to face when she decided to apply the Remotivation process as an occupational therapist working in a traditional medical model context. Discuss the arguments that Michelle might use as a member of the treatment team to advocate for her intervention with Rebecca.

thePoint® For additional resources and exercises, visit http://thePoint.lww.com

Key Terms

Occupational narrative: A person's story of the ongoing interactions between his or her own volition, habituation, performance capacity, and environments over time.

REFERENCES

de las Heras, C. G., Llerena, V., & Kielhofner, G. (2002). *Remotivation process: Progressive intervention for individuals with severe volitional challenges* [Version 1.0]. Chicago: Model of Human Occupation Clearinghouse, Department of Occupational Therapy, College of Applied Health Sciences, University of Illinois at Chicago.

Kielhofner, G. (Ed.). (2002). *Model of Human Occupation: Theory and application*. Philadelphia, PA: Lippincott Williams & Wilkins.

Kielhofner, G. (Ed). (2008). *Model of Human Occupation: Theory and application*. Philadelphia, PA: Lippincott Williams & Wilkins.

Applying MOHO to Individuals with Dementia

Christine Raber, Takashi Yamada, and Sylwia Gorska

CHAPTER 20

EXPECTED LEARNING OUTCOMES

Upon completion of this chapter, readers will be able to:

1. Recognize the complexities of volition in older people living with dementia.
2. Identify how assumptions of others affect volition of PWD.
3. Describe at least three approaches to support volition of people living with dementia.
4. Value the importance of understanding life story and use of narrative when working with any older adult.
5. Apply an understanding of volition, habituation, and performance capacity to an older person and analyze how occupational participation is impacted by these areas.
6. Describe all elements of environment that impact occupational participation for older adults and discuss the importance of addressing the environment in all interventions for older adults.

> *I am fundamentally different from you. Different in ways I can't express and you can't fully perceive or understand. Our brains are different.*
>
> —Richard Taylor

> *Treat us as someone you love as we are, not who you wish we were or who you want and think we should be.*
>
> —Richard Taylor

Is it possible to understand the experience of dementia? Gaining a glimpse of the experience is a powerful path to developing greater empathy, and many excellent first-person accounts have been written that offer helpful insights into the lived experience of dementia (Bryden, 2005; Page & Keady, 2010; Taylor, 2007). These accounts challenge conventional, deficit-driven and diagnostic-based thinking, opening the window into everyday life of people living with dementia. Given all the complex impairments associated with dementia, it is widely believed that not only is a person with dementia unable to do things due to their cognitive impairment, but that the dementia also robs the person of their motivation and their identity (Menne, Kinney, & Morhardt, 2002). However, it is often lowered expectations from others combined with decreased opportunities for occupational participation that creates significant threats to occupational identity and occupational competence. Both of these threats can be addressed by promoting occupational adaptation, which requires a nuanced approach that emphasizes understanding the person and their narrative, as well as supporting and advocating for needs of the person experiencing dementia.

Supports and Threats to Occupational Identity

Mary

Mary, a 90-year-old widow with Alzheimer's disease and macular degeneration, had been living in an assisted living apartment in the Midwestern region of the United States for several years. She had Alzheimer's disease and needed the 24-hour supervision the apartment afforded, which included daily checks by staff members, having her meals prepared and sharing them with others in a community dining room, staff administration of her medications, housekeeping services for her apartment, assistance with her self-care as needed, and a schedule of activities she could attend on a daily basis. During her adult life, Mary and her husband had been prominent community members, and she was a watercolor artist and teacher, and quite involved in the arts. She was a mother of two children, a son and a daughter, and had adult grandchildren. Her son and his adult children lived near her, and her daughter lived over a thousand miles away. Her family was very close to her, with family members visiting her at the facility several times a week. Staff reported she was quite social, enjoyed participating in most activities, and had a keen sense of humor. She had always dressed meticulously and continued to do so while at the facility. Her appearance reflected her value of presenting herself with a positive appearance and gracious manners.

Mary met with an occupational therapist for the purpose of creating an educational training video for the Volitional Questionnaire (VQ), to which she and her family had consented. She was excited to be of help, and was happy to participate in the two activities selected by the therapist for the visit. The activity director shared that Mary enjoyed "flowers and painting," but that she needed help to initiate and stay engaged in most activities due to her cognitive impairments and macular degeneration. For the visit, the therapist chose a flower arranging activity that consisted of arranging

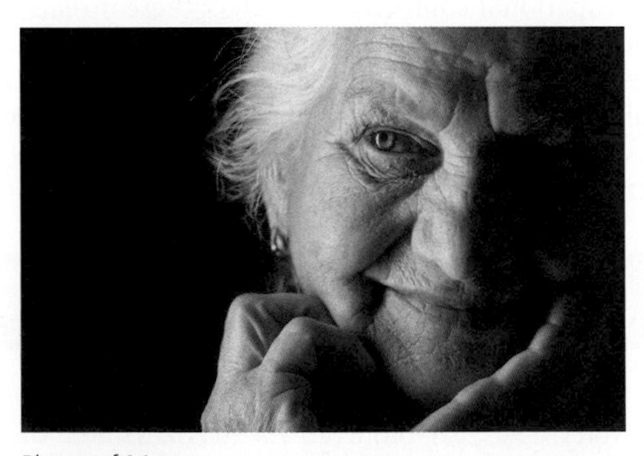

Photo of Mary

silk flowers into a small pail in which a block of florist foam had already been secured, and stenciling a greeting card using acrylic paints. The activity director set up the activities and worked with her on them, while the therapist observed, talked with Mary, and videotaped the session. Mary worked on the flower arranging activity for approximately 8 minutes, creating a pleasing arrangement and interacting positively with the activity director and the therapist, frequently making jokes and talking in an animated fashion about the "rules" of making floral arrangements, such as the number of blooms to use, how to position them, and where to place the tallest stem. While she had not previously handled silk flowers, whose stems were made of covered wire, she readily explored them, and fairly quickly she was bending and moving them to create the shapes and positioning she desired for the arrangement. Clearly enjoying the interactions, she talked in an animated fashion, joking and laughing, particularly when she noticed mistakes and felt challenged with handling the materials for the floral arrangement.

Transitioning into the unfamiliar task of stenciling a greeting card presented more challenges. Mary watched with interest as the activity director demonstrated the stenciling technique, and hesitantly began the card activity. While Mary was able to draw on well-established habits of handling her brush and mixing paints, she had never used a stiff stencil brush and her efforts with the new approach were disappointing to her, which she readily critiqued, making negative comments about her performance and the outcome of the card. Mary's VQ (Fig. 20-1) illustrates the subtle differences in her responses to the new activities, and how performance capacity issues (in her process skills for new learning, and in her low vision which impacted ability to see details in the stenciling activity) impacted her volition, particularly her sense of self-efficacy, as she was aware that she was not able to use past skills during the activity. This mismatch between previous sense of capacity in her painting abilities and her current lower self-efficacy created distress for Mary, as illustrated in the following exchange with the therapist, as she finished working on the card. She had been engaged in the stenciling activity for nearly 45 minutes, taking time to mix her paint colors and engage in her brush work on the card. Until the end of the activity, Mary had appeared to be enjoying the process of painting.

Mary finished applying paint to all parts of the stencil, and lifted the stencil off the card. She inspected it closely for about 30 seconds, held up the card in front of her face with the design facing out, and said loudly and emphatically "Blah!" Then Mary looked at the therapist, waiting. Therapist: "What don't you like about it, Mary?" Mary turned the card back to face her, and said "It's not my type of work (pause) . . . I like to do." Therapist: "um hmm," acknowledging Mary's disappointment. Mary quietly and intently looked at the finished

Client: **Mary**					Therapist:
Age: **90** Gender: **F**					Date:
Diagnosis: **Alzheimer's disease**					Facility:
Silk flower arranging and stenciling a card					**Comments**
Shows curiosity	P	H	I	**S**	*Readily explored, handled, and worked with flowers and brush/paint*
Initiates actions/tasks	P	H	I	**S**	*Arranged and adjusted flowers; used tapping motions with stencil brush*
Tries new things	P	H	**I**	S	*Stenciling activity was entirely new to her, and while she had experiencing arranging live flowers, working with the silk flowers was new to her. She engaged more readily with the flowers and some encouragement to try the stenciling activity*
Shows preferences	P	H	I	**S**	*Made clear statements about preferences for flower placement, type of brush, and type of painting she values (" this is not a creation", referring the stenciling, and "I don't copy")*
Shows that an activity is special or significant	P	H	**I**	S	*Smiling, pleasure with flower arranging; pleasure with brush use and paint (habitual ways of mixing paint, manipulating brush, creating strokes), but also required some support to verbalize the significance of both activities*
Indicates goals	P	**H**	I	S	*Needed encouragement to consider what to do with her flowers, and was reluctant to identify how she might use the card*
Stays engaged	P	H	**I**	S	*Emotional connection to familiar actions (positioning flowers, using brush/paint), but less connection to the end product (card)*
Shows pride	P	**H**	I	S	*With prompts and compliment from activity staff member, was accepting of flower arrangement ("It's okay...do you like it?"), but evaluated her performance on the stencil negatively, stating "Blah" when asked if she like the finished card*
Tries to solve problems	P	H	I	**S**	*Replaced flower that came out of arrangement; asked for help with brush when it began losing bristles*
Tries to correct mistakes	P	H	I	**S**	*Told activity staff member to reposition stencil repeatedly when it moved; stated frequently "what's wrong with this brush?" when brush needed more paint and pushed on brush with different pressure*
Pursues activity to completion/accomplishment	P	H	**I**	S	*While she demonstrated spontaneous rating for flowers, she required verbal supports and encouragement from activity staff member to finish the card*
Invests additional energy/emotion/attention	P	H	**I**	S	*Prompts and support from activity staff member to decide on colors to use for card and to place brush on stencil*
Seeks additional responsibilities	P	**H**	I	S	*Got up to wash brush and stencil when card finished*
Seeks challenges	P	H	**I**	S	*For doing video more than activities provided*

FIGURE 20-1 Mary's VQ.

card for a short time, and then said "I'd like to take a soft bristle brush . . . and, (pause) paint like . . . (pointing her brush at a watercolor landscape she had painted, which was hung on the wall near her) . . . those pictures." Therapist: "Um hum . . . like your paintings?" Mary continued looking at her painting on the wall, and said, with pride and a small smile "yeah." Therapist, approvingly: "Yeah. (pause). Have you been painting, recently?" Mary shifted in her seat, sighed audibly, shook her head, looked down at the card in her hands, and said with disappointment in her voice "No." Then she put her brush into the water, and swished it expertly, as the therapist asked gently "No? Why not? You certainly still have a lot of skills you could use for your painting." Mary left the brush in the water cup, sat back in her seat, looked down at the card, and drew a long breath: "Well, you couldn't tell from this." Therapist: "Oh, yes I can." *(pointing to a heart on the card which came out clearly).* Mary: "nah . . ." (pause, looking at the area therapist pointed out, then, with some pride) . . . *Well* . . . Mary gestured to the area above the heart and said ". . . but not up there." Mary turned the card around, held it out, and said "that stencil part . . . (indicating the heart) . . . I can show that off." Therapist: "Really, Mary, you did a wonderful job!" Mary smiled slightly, chuckled, laid the card down on the table, and said "That's for you. Now then, should we wash the stencil off? And these brushes?" Mary began gathering up the stencil and brushes, as the therapist replied "That's a good idea. Shall we go over to the sink?" Mary smiled, stood up, and said "Sure."

By responding to and validating her sense of capacity, Mary's initial negative appraisal of her performance was eased. While cleaning up, the therapist asked Mary to tell her about the watercolor landscape paintings hung in her room, which led to an animated discussion recalling creating her artwork, and her work giving private art lessons. The exchange reinforced Mary's prior capacity, helped support her interest in painting, and validated current efficacy by appreciating her willingness to try a new painting technique.

Mary's case has been used in training sessions about dementia and volition, and inspired the development of an international collaboration to share and build model of human occupation (MOHO) resources for occupational therapy practitioners working with people living with dementia (Forsyth, Melton, Raber, Burke, & Piersol, 2015). The Mary Collaborative was designed to assist practitioners and academics with the primary mission of supporting the provision of client-centered, occupation-focused, theory-driven, and evidence-based occupational therapy services for people living with dementia. The structure of the collaborative is an academic–practice partnership (Forsyth, Summerfield-Mann, & Kielhofner, 2005) based on principles of mentorship and collaboration and, at this writing, includes three academic organizations and three provider organizations. To date, participating organizations in the Mary Collaborative have presented the ideas of the collaborative at international venues, and supported research efforts of several dementia-focused projects (Górska et al., 2013; Raber, Quinlan, Neff, & Stephenson, 2016). These projects are grounded in MOHO, focus on the needs of people living with dementia, and have inspired clinicians to deepen their understanding and applications of MOHO in daily practice. Alice's case illustrates the importance of understanding volition using multiple perspectives.

Why MOHO?

Worldwide the number of people living with dementia is growing exponentially (Batsch & Mittelman, 2012), and this growth means that occupational therapists who work with older adults will almost certainly be faced with navigating the complexities of addressing their needs while advocating for their fullest engagement and occupational participation. The MOHO is particularly well suited to understanding people living with dementia, despite challenges they may have with communicating their wants, preferences, and desires. In addition to the impact of dementia, the aging process and common health conditions present their own challenges to daily life. In all instances, the physical, social, and cultural environment affect a person as they age. Unfortunately environmental impacts often detract from the person's ability to use their volition, habituation, and performance capacity in ways that are satisfying and effective. This chapter presents four cases that illustrate the use of MOHO to understand and effectively address the needs of older adults, particularly those living with dementia.

VOLITION AND OLDER ADULTS WITH DEMENTIA

While much of the research on Alzheimer's disease and related dementias (ADRD) is currently focused on finding a cure, the fact remains that people with dementia have pressing needs that are complex and present challenges to their care partners, whether they live in their home and have family and friends helping them, or live in some form of care home, such as nursing homes, assisted living, domiciliary care, and so forth. Optimal care approaches for people living with dementia resonate with the philosophical position of MOHO, making occupational therapy practitioners essential health care providers for this group of older adults. For example, understanding a person's life story is advocated for dementia care providers (McKeown, Clark, Ingleton, Ryan, & Repper, 2010), to help mitigate the communication challenges and effectively respond to confusing and problematic behaviors that are universal in the experience of dementia. By knowing the person's key relationships, past life roles, and valued occupations, along with preferences about habits and routines that support their daily engagement in life and with a chronology of life experiences, care partners are able to decipher the meaning and relevance of current behaviors, support their identity, and preserve dignity (Fraker, Kales, Blazek, Kavanagh, & Gitlin, 2014). Each of these approaches is embedded within MOHO, and the therapeutic reasoning process elicits the key connections between these elements, offering care partners a connection into the world of the person with dementia. Therapists using MOHO have a responsibility not only to make and communicate these connections, but also to develop and provide effective interventions for people living with dementia and their care partners.

Research exploring the experience of volition in people with dementia (Raber, Teitelman, Watts, & Kielhofner, 2010) indicates that the hierarchical view of volition is actually much more nuanced and bears additional scrutiny when working to understand the volitional narrative of a person with dementia. One essential aspect of therapeutic reasoning involves marrying knowledge about conditions and diagnoses with the person and their life experiences and situations. Examining and understanding volition contains many layers that are dynamic, ever-changing, and quite sensitive to the micro- and macro-realities of the person and their current life situation (de las Heras, Llerena, & Kielhofner, 2003). For example, a person living with dementia has developed and possessed

MOHO Problem-Solver Case: Redefining Volitional Hierarchy–Acknowledging Competence

Alice, an 80-year-old widow with dementia and delusions, resided in a memory care facility in the Midwestern United States. Alice had a large, supportive family (10 children and 14 grandchildren), half of whom lived near the facility and visited regularly. For 2 years after her initial dementia diagnosis, she had lived alone, but experienced growing distress from her deep suspicions that people were following her, trying to harm her, and take her money. She received occupational therapy as part of a day treatment program in which she was enrolled. The therapy included her eldest daughter acting as a caregiver and focused on organizational skills and memory aides to help her compensate for her cognitive dysfunction. However, despite the usefulness of the therapy in these aspects, Alice was reluctant to share her suspicions with her therapist. As her paranoid delusions increased, Alice began to mistrust her therapist and, when her daughter was not with her, repeatedly called her daughter and her other adult children, asking them to help her with the people who were "after her." Medication was prescribed, but Alice refused to take it.

Over time, her paranoia increased to the point that she became very unsafe in her home, often wandering from home and walking into the path of oncoming traffic, failing to eat, and experiencing persistent and high levels of anxiety from her paranoid delusions. Her family sought emergency guardianship and placement in the facility after a major incident involving Alice indiscriminately giving away large amounts of money.

The MOHO-based therapist within the facility began learning about Alice's life and about the people most important to her within her environment. Alice's husband had been a successful dentist in their hometown. The worker role was highly valued by Alice, as evidenced by multiple careers during her life. In addition to raising her children, Alice managed her husband's dental office. When her youngest child was in middle school, Alice earned an associate's degree in business along with a real estate license, becoming a successful real estate agent in the area for nearly 20 years. She intermittently continued to help her husband in his office, and her last paid position was for a state tax collection agency. Alice clearly valued productivity and being active, and both she and her family stated how important it was for her to "keep busy."

During her retirement, Alice was an active volunteer at a local Catholic monastery, where she ran the gift shop. This capitalized on skills she had developed in her other careers, and she took great pleasure in her responsibilities, making sales as well as ordering, stocking, and organizing the merchandise. Her faith and religious participation was very important to her. Alice attended Mass daily and belonged to several church groups. Alice's room was decorated with many religious icons, and she regularly carried several prayer books and rosaries with her. Part of being busy for Alice included caring for several friends and church members when they were ill, completing their cooking and cleaning and driving them to medical appointments. Most of Alice's interests involved others, and she preferred leisure activities that were social in nature.

While an immediate benefit of her admission to the facility was a significant reduction in her paranoia in response to medication, her early adjustment was slow. Initially, Alice spent a fair amount of time either in her room or trying to leave the facility, and she wore her coat and carried her purse constantly. Within a month, she was spending most of the time out of her room, socializing with other residents and joining in all the groups led by the activity therapist. She particularly enjoyed the morning exercise group. As she became comfortable in her new environment, Alice began going into other residents' rooms, collecting their belongings, carrying them around with her, and then hiding them in her room and other small spaces on the unit. These items included loose papers, magazines, newspapers, personal items (such as glasses), toiletries, blankets, and clothing. Most staff members interceded when Alice went into other residents' rooms by telling her to leave, then taking away the items she had collected. However, her occupational therapist noticed that the use of verbal redirection and taking of the items often upset alice, resulting in bewilderment and agitation. She responded more positively to being transitioned into an activity, such as folding laundry or helping set tables in the dining room. Alice's collecting behaviors typically occurred when she was not engaged in structured activities.

Alice still experienced paranoid delusions, albeit less intensely than upon admission, which caused periods of increased anxiety. Whenever she felt anxious, Alice frantically asked others (staff, residents, and visitors) to help her since an elusive "they" were following her, or had stolen her money. At these times, her preoccupation with a desire to leave or fix a perceived problem was not easily abated. Although many staff viewed Alice as having a mostly pleasant, easy-going disposition, they expressed frustration with the inconsistent effectiveness of their attempts to redirect Alice away from her "hoarding" or attempting to leave the facility. Most staff labeled her collecting behavior as hoarding, and did not perceive Alice's collecting activity as an expression of her desire to be active, but as a problem to be managed. Alice's response to redirection varied from being cooperative to becoming argumentative and resistant to leaving other residents' rooms or relinquishing their belongings. When Alice felt she was being genuinely listened to and that her concerns were being heard, she was more likely to cooperate. However, redirection that ignored her emotions, or pushed her too quickly into another activity often created more distress and resistance.

Occupational therapy was initiated to determine options for behavior management. Evaluation began with interviewing Alice, family, and staff, and completion of the VQ during unstructured time in Alice's day. The following exchange illustrates how the therapist acknowledged Alice's beliefs about productivity. Beliefs and values are a key aspect of volition that require careful assessment in people experiencing dementia. Therapist: *I understand you worked in your husband's office*? Alice: *Oh yes, I did a lot there*. Therapist: *And you were a realtor*? Alice: *What?* Therapist: *You sold houses? Helped people buy a new house?* Alice (very animatedly): "That, yes, that was fun. I was good." (pause, as she watched therapist smile in response to the comment). "Oh yes, I loved to work . . . you have to." Then Alice spontaneously added "I like being busy . . . they called me, what you call, a busy body." Therapist: "What happens when you're not busy?" Alice replied very clearly, without skipping a beat in the conversation "When I'm not busy, I get nervous." She placed strong emphasis on the word "nervous," and turned and looked directly at the therapist, with strong eye contact, to punctuate her remark. Alice then repeated several times how important it was to be busy.

During a treatment session, the therapist focused on uncovering strategies that caregivers could use to support Alice's desire to be engaged and feel productive while respecting other residents' space and belongings. Alice and the therapist were walking to Alice's room, to find her purse, when Alice stopped, looked into the open doorway of her neighbor's room, and said "I'm going to check over here." Alice walked into the neighbor's room and approached the dresser, which was covered with a stack of folded clothing. Alice reached out and began to riffle through the clothes, picking up a nightgown and stating authoritatively, "I'd better take these or they'll be taken by them." The therapist slowly approached her, and said calmly "The gown is fine there," pointing to the nightgown. Alice reluctantly put the gown back down on the dresser and looked worriedly at the therapist, who replied "let's go next door. . . . I know where your purse is." Alice followed the therapist out of the room and into her room, where the therapist walked over to the sofa, and retrieved her purse and handed it to her, saying "here it is." Alice took the purse, walked over to her bed, and began rummaging through a small pile of linens on the bed, saying seriously "Well, we've got to get these out of here, or they'll take them for sure . . . you don't know how they are around here." Alice rummaged in the linens for several minutes, while the therapist stood quietly at the end of the bed, and then asked "Can I help?" The therapist picked up a pillowcase and began folding it, then handed Alice a blanket, which she took and folded. The therapist then quietly began to straighten the sheets on the bed, and Alice joined in, helping to finish making the bed and stacking the folded linens on the end of the bed. After the task was done, the therapist said "that looks good" and Alice nodded, and sat down in her chair, looking relieved.

The therapist shared with staff what was learned from this interaction, highlighting the strategy of working along with Alice whenever she began collecting, rather than only redirecting her away from the occupation she was creating. One key aspect that the therapist observed about Alice's volition was that she seemed to generally perceive herself as effective, even when feeling distressed. Her sense of ill-being typically related to her experience that "they" (persons of her delusions) were the main barrier to being able to engage in preferred activities and maintain a sense of peace. This feeling would extend to others when Alice did not feel her distress was acknowledged and understood. Because of her belief that she was effective in solving problems, Alice was not often perturbed for long about staff's insistence that she relinquish other residents' belongings or leave their rooms. Her persistent initiation of collecting objects was an outward demonstration of how she created occupation that aligned with her sense of personal causation, values, and interests. Through collecting, Alice was acting on a desire to accomplish what she felt needed to be done, regardless of how others viewed this activity. Her collecting occupation also reflected her values of being busy and productive, related to her past interests of cleaning up and organizing, and reinforced her view of herself as being a competent, efficient person. As the therapist worked with staff to understand the strength of Alice's sense of capacity and self-efficacy, they were able to adjust their approaches to acknowledge and validate her need "to be busy."

different capacities than an individual with an intellectual disability, and the symptoms of dementia impact performance capacities at varying levels and degrees, resulting in threats to the volitional cycle. One phenomenological study explored the experience of volition in eight people with moderate dementia, who were all residing in an assisted living facility in the United States (Raber et al., 2010). Three major themes (Fig. 20-2) were revealed, including: variation in the demonstration of volition in the participants; the importance of modifying occupations; and the potency of the social environment impacting all aspects of volition. One key finding about volitional expression was that it is often subtle, usually behavioral (rather than verbal), and frequently contradictory. Additionally, modifying the task demands of occupations is essential and needs to be carefully tailored and matched to the abilities of the person with dementia. Finally, both of these elements are dependent upon the social environment, namely, people who both recognize and respond to demonstrations of volition in the person with dementia.

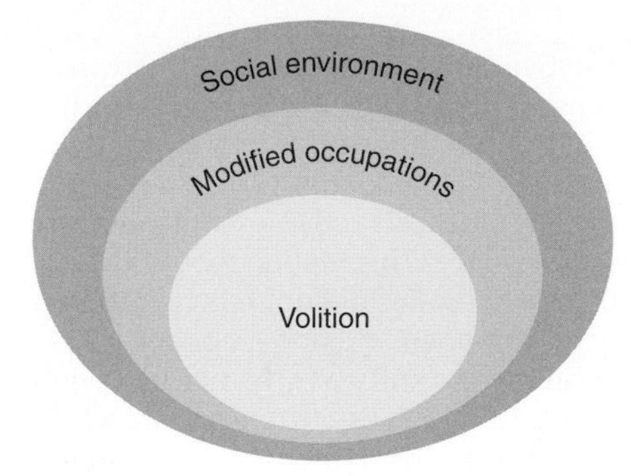

FIGURE 20-2 Themes of the Experience of Volition in Dementia.

For example, a person may shake their head side to side and reply "not today" when invited to participate in washing their face, but may at the same time reach for, and handle, the washcloth being held by the care partner, making rubbing motions with their hands and so forth. At this instant, a care partner who focuses only on the verbal reply assumes the person is "not motivated" to complete their morning grooming routine and may either stop the activity or wash the person's face without their active participation, effectively "doing for" rather than "doing with" the person. However, if the care partner *recognizes* the nonverbal behaviors as an indication of preference (exploring and handling the wash cloth, moving their hands in a familiar habitual way associated with face washing), *responds* to these actions by replying "let's give it a try," and *modifies the occupation* using hand-over-hand assistance to guide the person to bring the washcloth under the faucet that had been turned on and then to their face, the person may begin the familiar task of washing their face.

Recognizing and **responding to volition** are skills embedded in the therapeutic use of self and are an essential aspect of a supportive social environment. As dementia erodes the ability to plan, initiate, and sustain engagement in valued occupations, a person becomes increasingly dependent upon caregivers to support their innate desire to engage in their world, and this dynamic underscores the potency of the social environment (Teitelman, Raber, & Watts, 2010). However, despite significant impacts to multiple aspects of performance capacity, a person's volition and habituation remain present and can be tapped into and supported, in order to elicit engagement, support occupational identity, and reinforce competence. Identifying the key elements of the person can be facilitated through use of the Remotivation Process intervention (de las Heras, Geist, Kielhofner, & Li, 2007). The Remotivation Process outlines specific strategies to address volitional challenges and incorporates understanding of the volitional cycle to guide intervention. Since the Remotivation Process targets volitional change, it is essential that volition be assessed to gain a baseline and develop goals for improving volition. Assessment of volition is best accomplished by using the VQ, which uses a 4-point scale to rate 14 behaviors indicative of volition. An Environmental Characteristics Form is completed in addition to the item ratings, which offers more detailed information about the qualities of the environment and tasks that were present during the observed situation. VQ results allow a therapist to create a volitional profile and to identify the complex interplay between the person and the environment. Occupational therapy practitioners can become better advocates for people with dementia when equipped with a deeper, clearer understanding of volition and its relationship to engagement in occupation. Assessing volition, habituation, performance capacity, and environment also has potential to be accomplished using the MOHO-ExpLOR, which is in development (Parkinson, Cooper, de las Heras de Pablo, & Forsyth, 2014). Mary's case, from the beginning of this chapter, and Alice's case, which follows, illustrate a continuum of exploring volition for people with dementia.

Alice's case raises questions about volition as a hierarchical construct for this population, as do the experiences of others with dementia (Raber et al., 2010). Alice's collecting occupation demonstrated that a contradiction exists when a person's motivation to act on their environment conflicts with the social expectations generated by others regarding definitions of appropriate and acceptable behavior, even in the face of cognitive disability. In Alice's case, her motivation to act on her world and create occupation in the face of occupational deprivation, despite the negative feedback from the social environment, illustrates the complexity of volition, and the significance of how it is named and framed by others. Volition has been conceptualized using a developmental continuum consisting of three phases: *exploration*, *competency*, and *achievement*, where lower levels of volition are exhibited in the exploration phase, and the highest levels are seen in the achievement phase (de las Heras et al., 2003). Although a developmental continuum is acknowledged, understanding micro- and macro-realities is emphasized for people with dementia. **Micro-realities** refer to the "client's perception of past and present involvement in occupations; his/her experience of physical and cognitive capacities and environmental opportunities and conditions; his/her experience of social and physical aspects of the environment; his/her sense of capability for future involvement" (de las Heras et al., 2003, p. 39). *Macro-realities* involve factors external to the person, including contextual aspects of the physical and social environment (de las Heras et al., 2003).

Since people with dementia have usually attained the highest developmental phases of the volitional process prior to experiencing the cognitive impairments associated with dementia, a clear identification and recognition of prior volitional strengths can help acknowledge behaviors that are indicative of higher levels of current volition. Therefore, it is recommended that in addition to using VQ ratings, a careful consideration of the Environmental Characteristics Form along with a strong assessment of the physical and social environment be completed. One assessment tool that may prove useful to understand the environment is the Residential Environmental Impact Scale (REIS) 4.0 (Fisher et al., 2014). This assessment systematically evaluates the multidimensional layers of the environment and its impact on opportunities for engagement in occupation and, by extension, the quality of life. The REIS 4.0 is designed to be used in care homes and facilities of various sizes and is appropriate for use in an individual's home. Since the REIS 4.0 is not diagnosis specific, it may be used in a range of environments to better understand the impact of environment on the well-being of older adults.

In many instances, care partners, both family and paid caregivers in facilities, assume that people with dementia have little to no motivation, or volition, to engage in their environments. These beliefs are often reinforced, inaccurately, by intrinsic symptoms of the condition, namely, difficulty initiating actions and apathy. When caregivers believe that motivation is low or nonexistent, fewer opportunities are offered, and failed attempts to engage the person with dementia can perpetuate beliefs in poor volition. Once begun, this negative cycle is difficult to break, as it requires changing the attitudes and beliefs of caregivers, the social environment. The complexities of volition and its inherent reliance on the dynamics of the social environment were highlighted in a qualitative study (Raber & Stone, 2015) that explored caregivers' perceptions of volition relative to observed volition, as rated using the VQ. Eight formal caregivers, which included nurses, care assistants, and activity assistants, were interviewed about their perceptions about the volition of three residents in the memory care facility. Two major themes emerged from the analysis of the interviews and residents' VQ scores. These were: (1) staff possesses varying insights about volition of residents, and (2) staff uses scripts to share information about residents (Raber & Stone, 2015). The themes underscored the potency of the social environment, noting that caregivers' beliefs play an important role in both the ongoing volition of people with dementia and in the types of supports that caregivers may, or may not, use to support engagement in everyday occupations.

Family caregivers' perceptions and skills contribute to the well-being of people living with dementia, and occupational therapy services that target caregivers' needs have demonstrated efficacy (Gitlin et al., 2008; Graff et al., 2007). The case of Judi and John illustrates applying MOHO to an exploration of the needs of people with dementia who live in the community.

MOHO Problem-Solver Case: The Need for Access to Family-Centered Dementia Interventions to Support Habituation

Judi is an 81-year-old woman with dementia, who was described by her husband John as an extremely intelligent and highly sociable and amenable person. She lives with John and their pet dog, Jazz, in a semidetached town house in Scotland, UK. She has a son and a daughter who live locally. For years Judi enjoyed her demanding job as a civil servant, from which she retired about 20 years ago. Between her job and family life she successfully and with ease managed multiple responsibilities. Music has always been a source of great pleasure to Judi and for many years she was an active member of a choir through which she was involved in various charitable activities.

John shared: "She used to sing quite a bit. She was into operetta; she had her own group for about 30, nearly 40 years. They used to tour the old folks' homes, even been to Germany with her group."

She was also a talented artist and painted for pleasure, but some of her work also found keen buyers. Judi is very proud of her paintings, especially the portrait of her husband, which is displayed with pride of place in her living room. Doing jigsaw puzzles also used to be one of her favorite pastimes. About 3 years ago John noticed his wife's problems attending to and retaining information. At first he thought she was simply not paying attention. But with time he noticed Judi's increasing confusion, and marked deterioration in the volume and the content of the information she could recall. John shared his concerns with the local GP who referred Judi to a consultant psychiatrist for specialist assessment. John explained: "About three years ago [I noticed] she wasn't retaining what you were saying to her, you know, I just put it down she's not listening to me. But it gradually got worse and I mentioned it to the doctors." As a result, shortly after, Judi was given a diagnosis of dementia. Soon after the diagnosis Judi was assigned a community psychiatric nurse (CPN) from the Care of the Elderly Team who has since been involved in Judi's care and assists the couple in organizing the necessary support. At present the CPN is the only source of professional support as, according to Judi and John, there is no need for further assistance. Despite this claim, Judi gives a conflicting account of her experience related to dementia. On the one hand she states that she is well and dementia does not have an impact on her life: ". . . things are more or less the same way they have ever been." She describes her ability to attend to household-related tasks and satisfaction with her current routine: "I do my ironing . . . I always do the washing up." On the other hand, however, both Judi and John speak about Judi's loss of interest in her past activities of singing, painting, and doing jigsaw puzzles. Judi shared: "I used to do a lot of painting. I can't be bothered with it now," and John confirms this change: "Before [dementia] she's done jigsaws, puzzles, paint, you know, and that all stopped."

Judi describes her dissatisfaction with her limited social involvement and inability to engage in previously enjoyed activities: "I am not happy because I can't do what I used to do . . . I used to be able to go out myself and things like that. I can't do that now. And it used to be quite the thing to just go out along the road, get the [shopping] and come back." Judi described how she gradually stopped going to her local church. She believes a recent knee injury and her damaged hip are contributing factors: "with getting this leg in a mess I can't go out the same now." Additionally, she spoke about missing her close friend who passed away recently and with whom she used to meet weekly for coffee and a chat. John also noted his wife's withdrawal from engagement in activities and from social interactions. He associates it with Judi's physical deterioration and with her desire to remain in their familiar and safe home environment. John related a recent outing: "[We went for a drive], we stopped in [a local village] and I had fish and chips, she had macaroni and she enjoyed it, you know, but she's always dying to get back to her bed. We'll go out maybe at eleven [o'clock], we're back [at home] at two o'clock and she goes straight upstairs [to bed]." He also described changes in Judi's daily routine which, previously filled with various social and household-related activities, was now limited to watching TV and doing a few housekeeping chores. John's account of her daily routine is: "She'll get up [in the morning], have her breakfast, go back to bed. She'll get up at lunchtime, have her lunch, maybe sit around for an hour or so, then she'll go back to bed. She'll get up, sit around, maybe watch television with me, you know. I'll go and make the dinner, she'll do the washing up, come back, sit down there until nine o'clock and that's when we go to bed. That's our normal day."

Changes in Judi's health and related changes in her routine also had impact on John's daily activities. Both Judi and John acknowledged that he rarely goes out with his friends since the diagnosis, something that he did regularly for years. Judi shared: "[John] used to go out with some chaps on a Monday; they used to go out at night. But he has given that up. He just feels he can't cope with it anymore." John spoke about his reluctance to leave his wife at home without supervision for any extended period of time. He admitted that these factors, in combination with his deteriorating physical health (cardiac problems), result in his gradual withdrawal from previously enjoyed social commitments, leaving him isolated and feeling resigned to the situation. John explained: "I used to go fishing . . . a chap and me used to go fishing away in the morning until about four at night. [. . .] I think I'm getting now to the stage I don't like leaving her too long on her own. [. . .] I'm just resigning myself. This is going to be me for the rest of my life the way we're going on and it will get worse." Additionally, over the last 2 years John has gradually taken over responsibility for the majority of household tasks, such as cooking and shopping, which previously were strictly Judi's domain. John shared that he does "Cooking and shopping. I've got to make sure there's money in her account, things like that, you know. I'm doing things now I'd never done in my life before." Although John perceives these new responsibilities as part of his commitment in marriage, he admits that the additional pressures, at times, take a toll on both his relationship with Judi and his own health.

Judi's CPN shared these changes during a team conference, and the occupational therapist felt that a referral for occupational therapy services should be considered to assist them with developing more satisfying routines that address the performance capacity changes each has been experiencing due to multiple age-related conditions. The occupational therapist presented this perspective to Judi's CPN, to make the case for an OT referral: "Based on the information you're sharing, occupational therapy could be of benefit to both Judi and John. By assessing Judi's current abilities and motivation, as well as looking at Judi and John's daily routines, I could make some recommendations and develop interventions that would support Judi in re-activating her interests, which may help her energy level. I can also help John look at ways he could involve Judi more effectively in household chores and outings in the community, which may help each of them." Through careful assessment of Judi's performance capacity, and both Judi and John's habituation using interview, observation, and the Role Checklist, the occupational therapist would be able to develop adaptations and interventions to support occupational competence of both John and Judi, before a precipitating event creates a crisis that may threaten their ability to maintain their lifestyle in their own community. Judi and John's story illustrates how thinking with MOHO can promote referrals for community-based interventions and the potential to develop community-based programs.

Preventive Occupational Therapy Using MOHO

The MOHO can effectively be applied to older adults in order to promote wellness and prevent disability. One example that highlights this application is a MOHO-based preventive health promotion program developed in Japan and tested in a randomized clinical trial (Yamada et al., 2010). The foundation of the MOHO program was teaching participants the basic components of the model through lecture and discussion, followed by seminar experiences that facilitated personal application of the concepts. The program was designed for healthy older adults living in the community. Using 10 basic components of MOHO (personal causation, value, interest, habit, role, motor skill, process skill, communication and interaction skill, physical environment, and social environment), 15 sessions were developed and provided using a group (lecture/discussion) and an individual format (seminar). The 15 sessions of this moderate-intensity program were offered every other week over 8 months. For example, to address the MOHO component "interest," the lecture focused on defining "what are interests?" and "relationships between interests and aging," and during the seminar, participants completed assessments of interest, including an interest checklist.

Thirty older adults received the experimental MOHO-based preventive health promotion program, and 33 older adults in the control group participated in health promotion activities consisting of completing traditional crafts in a social group situation. The use of crafts in this manner is culturally relevant and typical of health promotion programs in Japan. Outcomes of the study were quality of life and psychological well-being, which were measured using the Japanese versions of the Life Satisfaction Index, Z (LSI-Z; Nakazato, 1992) and the World Health Organization Quality of Life-26 (QOL26; Tazaki & Nakane, 1997), respectively. Yamada and colleagues demonstrated that the MOHO-based health promotion program created positive changes in the outcome measures supporting the conclusion that MOHO-based occupational therapy interventions can promote wellness effectively in Asian older people by having an impact on quality of life and sense of well-being (Yamada et al., 2010).

MOHO Problem-Solver Case: Promoting Positive Aging Using MOHO

Fumi is an 82-year-old woman with primary aging. Fumi participated in the MOHO preventive health promotion program that was implemented at a university setting in greater Tokyo. She participated actively in 14 of the 15 sessions and always arrived properly dressed and made up for going out in the community. Her home was near the university and she had the balance and vitality to come to the sessions by bicycle. During the program, Fumi completed these assessments during different session seminars to help her understand more about herself using the MOHO perspective: NPI Interest Checklist, Role Checklist, the Occupational Questionnaire, the Occupational Self-Assessment (OSA), worksheets assessing her Belief in Skills, Values, and Environment, and development of a life narrative.

Fumi's strongest interests on the NPI Interest Checklist were identified as gardening, sewing, embroidery, knitting, crafts, foods, puzzles, mahjong, reading, and classic music, and she regularly engaged in all of these occupations (Fig. 20-3). Using the Role Checklist (Fig. 20-4), she identified five roles (student, caregiver, home maintainer, family member, and hobbyist/amateur) that she has done in the past and present, and in which she sees herself participating in the future. Fumi also rated each of these

Name: **Fumi / Female** Age: **82** Occupation: **None** Date: **Sept. 12, 2008**

	Activity	Strong	Casual	No		Activity	Strong	Casual	No
1	Gardening	✔			41	Exercise			✔
2	Sewing	✔			42	Volley ball			✔
3	Trump game		✔		43	Woodworking			✔
4	Foreign languages			✔	44	Billiards			✔
5	Social clubs			✔	45	Driving		✔	
6	Radio			✔	46	Dusting		✔	
7	Japanese chess			✔	47	Jewelry making			✔
8	Car repair			✔	48	Tennis			✔
9	Writing			✔	49	Cooking	✔		
10	Dancing			✔	50	Basketball			✔
11	Needlework	✔			51	History			✔
12	Golf			✔	52	Guitar			✔
13	Football			✔	53	Science			✔
14	Popular music			✔	54	Collection			✔
15	Puzzles	✔			55	Ping Pong			✔
16	Holiday			✔	56	Leather work			✔
17	Solitaire			✔	57	Shopping		✔	
18	Movies		✔		58	Photography			✔
19	Lectures		✔		59	Painting		✔	
20	Swimming			✔	60	Television		✔	
21	Bowling			✔	61	Concerts		✔	
22	Visiting		✔		62	Ceramics			✔
23	Mending			✔	63	Camping			✔
24	Go (Japanese chess)			✔	64	Laundry		✔	
25	Barbecues		✔		65	Dating			✔
26	Reading	✔			66	Mosaics			✔
27	Traveling			✔	67	Politics			✔
28	Manual arts	✔			68	Scrabble			✔
29	Parties			✔	69	Decorating		✔	
30	Dramatics			✔	70	Math			✔
31	Shuffleboard			✔	71	Service groups			✔
32	Ironing		✔		72	Piano			✔
33	Social studies			✔	73	Scouting			✔
34	Classical music	✔			74	Play			✔
35	Floor mopping			✔	75	Clothes		✔	
36	Model building			✔	76	Knitting	✔		
37	Baseball			✔	77	Hair styling		✔	
38	Mah-Jongg	✔			78	Religious			✔
39	Singing		✔		79	Drums			✔
40	Home repairs			✔	80	Conversation		✔	

FIGURE 20-3 Fumi's Results of NPI Interest Checklist.

Role Checklist Summary Sheet

Name: Fumi Age: 82 Date: Oct. 20, 2008

Gender: Male (Female) Are you retired? (Yes) No

Role	Role identity			Value you put on roles		
	Past	Present	Future	Not at all valuable	Somewhat valuable	Very valuable
Student	✔	✔	✔			✔
Worker	✔			✔		
Volunteer				✔		
Caregiver	✔	✔	✔			✔
Home maintainer	✔	✔	✔			✔
Friend					✔	
Family member	✔	✔	✔			✔
Religious participation				✔		
Hobbyist/Amateur	✔	✔	✔			✔
Participant in organizations				✔		
Other						

FIGURE 20-4 Fumi's Role Checklist.

roles as "very valuable" to her, in the past, present, and future. Being a friend was rated as somewhat valuable, but she did not identify participating in this role in the past, present, or future. Her Occupational Questionnaire (Fig. 20-5) indicated that she primarily engaged in productive activities by herself, and that her daily routine was interspersed with mostly solitary daily activities, recreation, and rest. She rated the majority of activities in her daily routine as pleasurable. With regard to her volition, Fumi believed in her skills and discovered that while her communication and interaction skills rated the highest (Fig. 20-6), she was not regularly engaging in leisure activities that used these abilities. Reflecting on her values, Fumi was asked to think of five activities very important to her during the program, which she stated were working on knitting eagerly, having enjoyed gardening, having learned new cooking, replacing clothes, and adjusting the new electric rice cooker. Her value ratings for these activities revealed she experienced personal satisfaction that aligned with her values.

Her environment was assessed using a comprehensive environmental questionnaire, and Fumi viewed environment as largely good to excellent, with the exception of the ease of going out. While she uses her bicycle easily, she shared that "walking for a long time is difficult, so for me, I cannot go out freely. But I think that is ordinary in terms of age." Fumi participated actively in preparing her life narrative, and told the following story; her narrative slope is shown in Figure 20-7.

Fumi's Narrative

"On January 1, 1926, I was born in Osaki, Shinagawa-ku. In the kindergarten, I studied English by an English leader. As a fourth grader, my father died after a two month hospitalization. Then, my family moved in Kamakura and I entered the normal elementary school. Then I entered the girls' junior

Date: Oct. 24, 2008 Name: Fumi Date of Birth: January 1, 1926

Typical Activities Time	Question 1 I consider this activity to be: W: Work D: Daily Living task R: Recreation RT: Rest	Question 2 I think that I do this: VW: Very well W: Well AA: About average P: Poorly VP: Very poorly	Question 3 For me this activity is: EI: Extremely important I: Important TL: Take it or leave it RN: Rather not do it TW: Total waste of time	Question 4 How much do you enjoy this activity? LVM: Like it very much L: Like NLD: Neither like nor dislike D: Dislike SD: Strongly dislike
5:00	W D R RT	VW W AA P VP	EI I TL RN TW	LVM L NLD D SD
5:30	W D R RT	VW W AA P VP	EI I TL RN TW	LVM L NLD D SD
6:00 Waking up and brushing teeth	W **D** R RT	VW W **AA** P VP	**EI** I TL RN TW	LVM L **NLD** D SD
6:30 Preparing meal	**W** D R RT	VW W **AA** P VP	**EI** I TL RN TW	LVM **L** NLD D SD
7:00 Cleaning entrance	**W** D R RT	VW W AA P VP	EI **I** TL RN TW	LVM **L** NLD D SD
7:30 Breakfast	**W** D R RT	VW W **AA** P VP	EI **I** TL RN TW	LVM **L** NLD D SD
8:00 Reading newspaper	W D R **RT**	VW W **AA** P VP	EI **I** TL RN TW	LVM **L** NLD D SD
8:30 Laundry	**W** D R RT	VW W **AA** P VP	**EI** I TL RN TW	LVM **L** NLD D SD
9:00 Watching TV	W D R **RT**	VW W **AA** P VP	EI **I** TL RN TW	**LVM** L NLD D SD
9:30 Taking a walk with dog	**W** D R RT	VW **W** AA P VP	**EI** I TL RN TW	**LVM** L NLD D SD
10:00 Taking a walk with dog, cont'd	**W** D R RT	VW **W** AA P VP	**EI** I TL RN TW	**LVM** L NLD D SD
10:30 Visiting doctor's office	W **D** R RT	VW W **AA** P VP	**EI** I TL RN TW	LVM **L** NLD D SD
11:00 Shopping	**W** D R RT	VW **W** AA P VP	**EI** I TL RN TW	LVM **L** NLD D SD
11:30 Resting	W D R **RT**	VW W **AA** P VP	EI **I** TL RN TW	LVM **L** NLD D SD
12:00 Resting, cont'd	W D R **RT**	VW W **AA** P VP	EI **I** TL RN TW	LVM **L** NLD D SD
12:30 Lunch	W **D** R RT	VW W **AA** P VP	EI **I** TL RN TW	LVM **L** NLD D SD
1:00 Needlework	W D **R** RT	VW W **AA** P VP	EI **I** TL RN TW	LVM **L** NLD D SD
1:30 Needlework, cont'd	W D **R** RT	VW W **AA** P VP	EI **I** TL RN TW	LVM **L** NLD D SD
2:00 Needlework, cont'd	W D **R** RT	VW W **AA** P VP	EI **I** TL RN TW	LVM **L** NLD D SD
2:30 Ironing	**W** D R RT	VW **W** AA P VP	**EI** I TL RN TW	LVM L **NLD** D SD
3:00 Putting laundry away	**W** D R RT	VW W **AA** P VP	EI **I** TL RN TW	LVM L **NLD** D SD
3:30 Taking a walk with dog	**W** D R RT	VW **W** AA P VP	**EI** I TL RN TW	**LVM** L NLD D SD
4:00 Taking a walk with dog, cont'd	**W** D R RT	VW **W** AA P VP	**EI** I TL RN TW	**LVM** L NLD D SD
4:30 Resting, watching TV	W D R **RT**	VW W **AA** P VP	EI **I** TL RN TW	LVM **L** NLD D SD
5:00 Resting, watching TV, cont'd	W D R **RT**	VW W **AA** P VP	EI **I** TL RN TW	LVM **L** NLD D SD
5:30 Resting	W D R **RT**	VW W **AA** P VP	EI **I** TL RN TW	LVM **L** NLD D SD
6:00 Preparing dinner	**W** D R RT	VW **W** AA P VP	**EI** I TL RN TW	LVM **L** NLD D SD
6:30 Preparing dinner, cont'd	**W** D R RT	VW **W** AA P VP	**EI** I TL RN TW	LVM **L** NLD D SD
7:00 Preparing dinner, cont'd	**W** D R RT	VW **W** AA P VP	**EI** I TL RN TW	LVM **L** NLD D SD
7:30 Preparing dinner, cont'd	**W** D R RT	VW **W** AA P VP	**EI** I TL RN TW	LVM **L** NLD D SD
8:00 Resting, watching TV	W D R **RT**	VW W **AA** P VP	EI **I** TL RN TW	**LVM** L NLD D SD
8:30 Dinner	W **D** R RT	VW **W** AA P VP	**EI** I TL RN TW	LVM **L** NLD D SD
9:00 Cleaning up	**W** D R RT	VW **W** AA P VP	**EI** I TL RN TW	LVM L **NLD** D SD
9:30 Resting, watching TV	**W** D R RT	VW **W** AA P VP	**EI** I TL RN TW	LVM L **NLD** D SD
10:00 Resting	W D R **RT**	VW W **AA** P VP	EI **I** TL RN TW	LVM **L** NLD D SD
10:30 Taking a bath	W **D** R RT	VW W **AA** P VP	EI **I** TL RN TW	LVM L NLD D SD
11:00 Sleeping	W D R RT	VW W AA P VP	EI I TL RN TW	LVM L NLD D SD
11:30	W D R RT	VW W AA P VP	EI I TL RN TW	LVM L NLD D SD

FIGURE 20-5 Occupational Questionnaire.

OBJECTIVE
To examine a component of personal causation – belief in skill – and its relationship to the pattern of occupation in your daily life.

STEP ONE: Beside each activity below enter the code that best describes how well you think you do. If you have never done the activity, rate how well you think you would do it after having some experience with it. Don't consider whether you'd like to do it or not; just indicate what you think your abilities would be. Use the following codes:

G = I am (would be) good at this
O = I am (would be) okay at this
P = I am (would be) poor at this

Item no.	Activity	Code
1	Archery	P
2	Ask someone for help	G
3	Lead a discussion group	O
4	Plan a party	O
5	Exercise	O
6	Balance a checkbook	P
7	Run in a race	P
8	Give helpful criticism to others	O
9	Find resources in a new city	O
10	Participate in a job interview	G
11	Thread a needle	G
12	Decide between two job interviews	G
13	Roller skate	G
14	Budget money for the year	P
15	Introduce myself to strangers	G

STEP TWO: Now, using the following key, enter scores for each activity by the appropriate number:

G = 3
O = 2
P = 1

Item no.	Score	Item no.	Score	Item no.	Score
1	1	2	2	4	2
5	2	3	2	6	1
7	1	8	2	9	2
11	3	10	3	12	3
13	3	15	3	14	1
Total	10	**Total**	12	**Total**	9

STEP THREE: Add up the scores in each column to find a total. Your first score represents your belief in your perceptual-motor skills; the second, your belief in your interpersonal/communication skills; and the third, your belief in your process (planning and problem-solving) skills. In looking over these scores, consider the following questions.

Question	Yes/No
Are your three scores equal or very similar?	Yes
Do your current leisure interests overlap with the category(s) in which you have your highest score?	No
Do the scores reflect your own ideas about your abilities?	Yes

FIGURE 20-6 Volition: Fumi's Personal Causation.

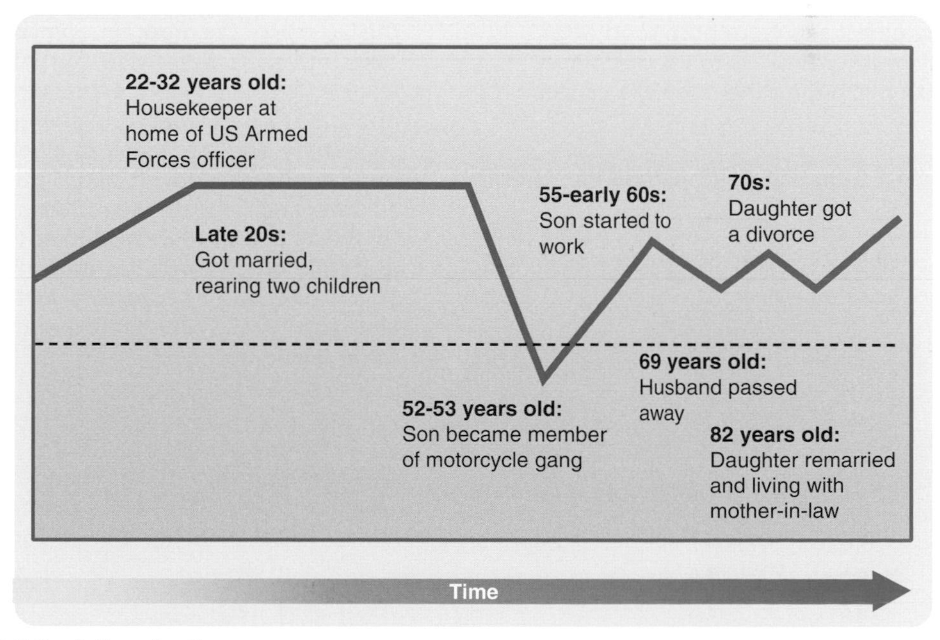

FIGURE 20-7 Fumi's Narrative Slope.

school at Kamakura and studied as a military and government affairs girl. From 18 years old to the end of the Second World War, I worked for the aviation fuel Research Institute in Ofuna. I was attacked by the airplane of the United States Armed Forces, and was scared. A lot of officers who worked there were from the faculty of science and engineering at the university. At the end of the war, I remember that I was in high spirits about when we can live freely in the future. I began to work as a housekeeper in the house of an officer of the US Armed Forces. I studied English again, during the days with the children, and commanded five maids. The officer's wife liked foods, and taught me the way of foods, so I studied to make foods. The abundant supplies were available since the employer was an officer of the United States Armed Forces. We continued the life that forgot Japanese for ten years. When the officer returned to the U.S., he said that I could go to the U.S. with them, and I was determined to go, but did not go because mother objected to it. Then, I got married at the age of 32 years old. Our first child was born dead. The eldest daughter and the eldest son were born soon after. My mother took us to various places with her, but mother died of a cancer after a 3-month hospitalization. The eldest daughter entered St. Paul (Rikkyo) University in Tokyo and advanced to the graduate school. She married a classmate in graduate school. The eldest son became part of the motorcycle gangs when I was the age of 52 years old. I lost it . . . how should we receive it as a parent? I thought that I brought you up well. We said to a neighboring person, 'Please call out to me with hello if you saw a son.' Then later my son started to work, got married, and the children were born, too. At my age of 69 years old, my husband suffered from a cancer, and I was hospitalized. He left [died] six months later. My daughter went to Indonesia and enjoyed Java printed cotton. My son folded the shop which did business and moved out toward another city in Tokyo. My daughter got a divorce soon. The daughter married again, living with [his] mother."

The occupational therapists leading the program observed that through reflection and learning about herself using the lens of MOHO, Fumi was changing. During the last sessions, the posttests were completed and she had improvements in several areas (Tables 20-1 to 20-3). Most importantly, on the last day of the program, Fumi brought a cake with a letter attached, to the program leaders: "I would like to express that it was good that I participated in the activity of your study, and thank you so much for this opportunity to study. It was significant at all times and I was able to reflect on myself, for me. Thank you very much and I was very grateful. This is a small present from me. This is one's way of life, life as the work learned, all which I had not thought about so far including."

Table 20-1 Fumi's SF-36 (Japanese Version)

	PF	BP	GH	VT	SF	RE	MH
Pretest	30.5	29	44.6	56.4	43.9	31.1	62.4
Posttest	34	29	49	57	50.2	31.1	65.1

BP, bodily pain; GH, general health; MH, mental health; PF, physical functioning; RE, emotional role functioning; SF, social role functioning; VT, vitality.

Table 20-2 Fumi's WHO-QOL26 (Japanese Version)

	Total	Physical Domain	Psychological Domain	Social Domain	Environment Domain
Pretest	4.5	3.4	3.7	4	4.4
Posttest	4.5	3.6	3.7	2.8	4.1

Table 20-3 Fumi's Activity Competence Scale (TMIG), Geriatric Depression Scale (GDS), Life Satisfaction Index (LSI-Z) (Japanese Versions)

	TMIG	GDS	LSI-Z	Mean	Social Activity
Pretest	5	4	3	1[a]	25
Posttest	5	4	4	1[a]	26

[a]Indicates no depression.

Conclusion

For older adults, the experience of aging brings changes and potential problems to occupational adaptation. Understanding the richness of an older adult's life using the lens and tools of MOHO can help the older adult navigate challenges within themselves, and outside of themselves. By embracing and comprehending the volitional complexities of clients with dementia, occupational therapists can support meaningful engagement and positive occupational participation, as Alice and Mary's cases illustrate. Occupational therapists must also be prepared to thoroughly assess the environments in which older adults are situated because environmental change, particularly in social contexts, requires therapists to work collaboratively with all types of care partners to create the person-centered care that clients need and deserve. Judi's and Fumi's cases highlight the need for therapists to advocate for community-based programs that support clients to successfully age in place. Understanding and honoring life story narratives, using multiple means, is the essential foundation for effective occupational therapy services with older adult clients.

Final Case Study for Contemplation

Frank is 85 years old and lives with his wife in a retirement community in rural southern Ohio. They have been married over 60 years, and have no children. They do have a close relationship with one niece and her family, and an extensive network of friends. Frank was diagnosed with dementia 2 years ago, and has been living with Parkinson's disease for 12 years. His wife, Jean, has high blood pressure and a history of recurrent depression, for which she takes maintenance antidepressant medication. Jean and Frank have lived in the retirement community for 1 year, where they moved when Jean decided that their small farm was too much for her to manage as Frank's physical ability declined and he experienced decreasing judgment about his skills. Frank retired from his work as an electrician at age 65, shortly before purchasing their farm. Having the farm was a dream fulfilled for both Frank and Jean, and Frank developed three major occupations during his retirement: beekeeping, gardening, and writing humorous short stories. In spring, summer, and fall seasons, Frank spent the majority of his time engaged in taking care of 30 hives of bees, growing pumpkins and tomatoes in his 1 acre garden, and mowing and caring for their remaining 5 acres of land and home. Frank was very mechanically inclined, and Jean reported: "He can fix anything, he's so good with his hands. Always has been." During the winter, Frank repaired his hives and wrote short stories. His writing was an unexpected occupation, which he began after attending a writing weekend with Jean, who was a poet and novelist. She encouraged him to write down some of his jokes and funny stories, because she felt others would enjoy them as much as she did. Before their move, Frank had published a book of his short stories, and Jean was working on organizing his manuscripts for a second book. Six months after moving into their apartment in the retirement community, Frank began to sleep poorly, and he regularly left their apartment in the middle of night, thinking it was time to go to the dining room for dinner. On several occasions, he wandered on the outside grounds, and security staff brought him back to the apartment. To keep him from leaving during the night, Jean installed a slide lock at the top of their external door, but Frank was able to operate the lock and he continued to get out, and became more belligerent when staff tried to redirect him back to the apartment. After an incident in which he hit Jean when she tried to keep him from leaving one night, a referral for occupational therapy services was ordered to assess his ability to safely remain in the independent apartment with Jean. Frank's doctor and the admission team wanted to keep him with Jean, but they were concerned that safety issues may require a transfer to the secure memory unit in the community.

Questions About This Case

1. Generate a list of questions you would ask Frank, Jean, and the team. Label the question(s) that would assist you with understanding Frank's volition, habituation, performance capacity, and environment.

2. Describe Frank's volition. What strategies would you use to learn more about his volition, and assess its role in his current functioning?
3. Discuss a plan for occupational therapy evaluation, including selection of assessment tools, and potential interventions for Frank and Jean. Explain your rationale for these choices.
4. Compare and contrast Frank's past and current environments. Discuss the role of physical and social environment and ways it could be adapted to support Frank at this time.

Chapter 20 Review Questions

1. All of the following statements are common assumptions that others often make about the volition of people with dementia, *except:*
   a. Levels of motivation for occupation increase
   b. Lack of interests occurs due to decreased ability
   c. Verbal statements are always an accurate reflection of preferences
   d. Low motivation is a normal consequence of the condition
2. The micro-reality underlying Alice's collecting occupation would best described as:
   a. Lack of opportunities to engage in meaningful activity
   b. Staff's use of redirection to keep her out of other residents' rooms
   c. Valuing productivity, such as needing to be busy and solve problems
   d. Paranoid thoughts
3. Which of the following is NOT a phase of volition?
   a. Achievement
   b. Mastery
   c. Competence
   d. Exploration
4. In Mary's case, the therapist talked with Mary about her watercolor landscape paintings. This was an example of which type of volitional support?
   a. Reinforcing prior capacity
   b. Validating change in ability
   c. Acknowledging change of interests
   d. Honoring preferences
5. Impairments caused by dementia result in declines in volition to exploration level in all people with the condition.
   a. TRUE
   b. FALSE

HOMEWORK ASSIGNMENTS

1. Observe a person with dementia in their home situation for 30 minutes. Take notes about what they are doing, how they go about it, objects used, and the environment. Note what you understand, and don't understand, about what they are doing. Based on your observation, label their volition, habituation, and performance capacity. What parts of the environment supported their doing, and what parts limited their engagement?
2. Active learning assignment: Working with one to two colleagues/students, obtain the VQ. After each team member has read the manual thoroughly, identify an older adult volunteer who has at least one chronic condition that is impacting their volition. Together select two

situations to observe your volunteer, and complete the VQ for situation one using Form B (including the Summary), the Environmental Characteristics Form, and Form D. Each group member should independently rate and complete the VQ forms. After completing the ratings and forms for situation one, compare your ratings and discuss the following:

1. For all items rated the same, have each team member explain their rationale for assigning the rating and discuss notes and observations made for these items.
2. For all items rated differently, have each team member explain their rationale for assigning the rating and discuss notes and observations made for these items.
3. What aspects of completing the VQ were challenging? What aspects were easier? What would you change about your approach to completing the VQ the next time you use it?

3. After comparing completed VQ for situation one, as a group observe situation two, and complete ratings and compare again, answering questions 1–3, and this additional question:
   1. Did agreement on item ratings change between situation one and situation two? Discuss your ideas about the changes. How useful do you feel the VQ was to help you understand your volunteer's volition?
   2. As a group, use your VQ findings to write a short narrative describing your volunteer's volition. How does this volitional narrative help you understand your volunteer's current occupational participation?

thePoint® For additional resources and exercises, visit http://thePoint.lww.com

Key Terms

Recognizing volition: Ability of others in the environment of a person with dementia to observe subtle behavioral expressions (body language, nonverbal expression and actions) of choices, likes, and dislikes. Acknowledging contradictory expressions between verbal and nonverbal behaviors.

Responding to volition: Ability of others in the environment of a person with dementia to discern preferences in the face of contradictory information and select and offer responses that support interests, values, and personal causation of the person.

REFERENCES

Batsch, N. L., & Mittelman, M. S. (2012). *World Alzheimer report 2012: Executive summary: Overcoming the stigma of dementia.* London, United Kingdom: Alzheimer's Disease International.

Bryden, C. (2005). *Dancing with dementia.* London, United Kingdom: Jessica Kingsley.

de las Heras, C. G., Geist, R., Kielhofner, G., & Li, Y. (2007). *A user's manual for the Volitional Questionnaire.* Chicago: The Model of Human Occupation Clearinghouse, Department of Occupational Therapy, College of Applied Health Sciences, University of Illinois at Chicago.

de las Heras, C. G., Llerena, V., & Kielhofner, G. (2003). *A user's manual for remotivation process: Progressive intervention for individuals with severe volitional challenges.* Chicago: The Model of Human Occupation Clearinghouse, Department of Occupational Therapy, College of Applied Health Sciences, University of Illinois at Chicago.

Fisher, G., Forsyth, K., Harrison, M., Angarola, R., Kayhan, E., Noga, P. L., et al. (2014). *Residential Environment Impact Scale* [Version 4.0]. Chicago: The Model of Human Occupation Clearinghouse, Department of Occupational Therapy, College of Applied Health Sciences, University of Illinois at Chicago.

Forsyth, K., Melton, J., Raber, C., Burke, J., & Piersol, C. (2015). Scholarship of practice in the care of people with dementia: Creating the future through collaborative efforts. *Occupational Therapy in Health Care, 29*(4), 429–441.

Forsyth, K., Summerfield-Mann, L., & Kielhofner, G. (2005). Scholarship of practice: Making occupation-focused, theory-driven, evidence-based practice a reality. *British Journal of Occupational Therapy, 68*, 261–268.

Fraker, J., Kales, H. C., Blazek, M., Kavanagh, J., & Gitlin, L. N. (2014). The role of occupational therapist in the management of neuropsychiatric symptoms of dementia in clinical settings. *Occupational Therapy in Health Care, 28*(1), 4–20.

Gitlin, L., Winter, L., Burke, J., Chernett, N., Dennis, M., & Hauck, W. (2008). Tailored activities to manage neuropsychiatric behaviors in persons with dementia and reduce caregiver burden: A randomized pilot study. *The American Journal of Geriatric Psychiatry, 16*, 229–239.

Górska, S., Forsyth, K., Irvine, L., Maciver, D., Prior, S., Whitehead, J., et al. (2013). Service-related needs of older people with dementia: Perspectives of service users and their unpaid careers. *International Psychogeriatrics, 25*(7), 1107–1114.

Graff, M. J. L., Vernooij-Dassen, M. J. M., Thijssen, M., Dekker, J., Hoefnagels, W. H. L., & Rikkert, M. G. M. (2007). Effects of community occupational therapy on quality of life, mood, and health status in dementia patients and their caregivers: A randomized controlled trial. *Journal of Gerontology, 62*(9), 1002–1009.

Kawamata, H., Yamada, T., & Kobayashi, N. (2012). Effectiveness of an occupational therapy program for health promotion among healthy elderly: A randomized controlled trial. *Japanese Journal of Public Health, 59*(2), 73–81.

McKeown, J., Clarke, A., Ingleton, C., Ryan, T., & Repper, J. (2010). The use of life story work with people with dementia to enhance person-centred care. *International Journal of Older People Nursing, 5*, 148–158. doi:10.1111/j.1748-3743.2010.00219.x

Menne, H., Kinney, J., & Morhardt, D. (2002). "Trying to continue to do as much as they can": Theoretical insights regarding continuity and meaning making in the face of dementia. *Dementia: The International Journal of Social Research and Practice, 1*, 367–382.

Nakazato, K. (1992). An approach to quality of life from the point of view of psychology [in Japanese]. *Nursing Study, 25*, 193–202.

Page, S., & Keady, J. (2010). Sharing stories: A meta-ethnographic analysis of twelve autobiographies written by people with dementia between 1989 and 2007. *Ageing and Society, 30*, 511–526.

Parkinson, S., Cooper, J. R., de las Heras de Pablo, C. G., & Forsyth, K. (2014). Measuring the effectiveness of interventions when occupational performance is severely impaired. *British Journal of Occupational Therapy, 77*(2), 78–81.

Raber, C., Quinlan, S., Neff, A., & Stephenson, B. (2016). A phenomenological study of occupational therapy practitioners using the remotivation process with clients experiencing dementia. *British Journal of Occupational Therapy, 79*(2), 92–101.

Raber, C., & Stone, M. (2015). An exploration of volition: Caregiver perceptions of persons with dementia. *Open Journal of Occupational Therapy, 3*(1), Article 3. doi:10.15453/2168-6408.1075

Raber, C., Teitelman, J., Watts, J., & Kielhofner, G. (2010). A phenomenological study of volition in everyday occupations of older people with dementia. *British Journal of Occupational Therapy, 73*(11), 498–506. doi:10.4276/030802210X12892992239116

Taylor, R. (2007). *Alzheimer's from the inside out.* Baltimore, MD: Health Professions Press.

Tazaki, M., & Nakane, M. (1997). *Manual of World Health Organization QOL26* [in Japanese]. Tokyo, Japan: Kaneko-Shobou.

Teitelman, J., Raber, C., & Watts, J. (2010). The power of the social environment in motivating persons with dementia to engage in occupation: Qualitative findings. *Physical & Occupational Therapy in Geriatrics, 28*(4), 321–333.

Yamada, T., Kawamata, H., Kobayashi, N., Kielhofner, G., & Taylor, R. R. (2010). A randomized clinical trial of a wellness program for healthy older people. *British Journal of Occupational Therapy, 73*(11), 540–548.

Applying MOHO to Individuals with Mental Illness

Jane Melton, Kirsty Forsyth, Susan Prior, Donald Maciver, Michele Harrison, Christine Raber, Laura Quick, Renée R. Taylor, and Gary Kielhofner (posthumous)

CHAPTER 21

EXPECTED LEARNING OUTCOMES

Upon completion of this chapter, readers will be able to:

1. Gain an understanding of the application of the model of human occupation (MOHO) with and for individuals experiencing mental illness.
2. Acknowledge the importance of therapists' adopting an empathically grounded and empowering approach in MOHO-based therapy.
3. Explain the dynamic and interconnected nature of the key components of MOHO.
4. Describe the importance of the impact of the social and physical environment to support an individual to make occupational choices, to gain a sense of occupational identity, and to achieve occupational participation.
5. Explain how MOHO assessments and interventions can be used to support recovery and occupational participation of persons with mental illness.

This chapter considers how occupational therapy practitioners, working with individuals experiencing mental illness, facilitate engagement and participation in occupation. A common theme throughout the chapter is how therapy-enabled persons with mental illness to envision and live their lives differently. Although the nature of the clients' impairments varied, they shared a common challenge. Each had to reorganize volition, reconstruct habit patterns, revise or reengage in life roles, and find new ways to effectively perform and participate in occupational life—in other words, to occupationally adapt in order to participate in meaningful pursuits. The concept of recovering occupation through understanding occupational identity and competence is built upon in this chapter. The importance of the therapist's considered approach as part of the individual's therapeutic environment is also referenced through case study narrative. In this chapter, exemplars of model of human occupation (MOHO) assessments that assist therapists to gain a rich understanding of the needs and aspirations of persons with mental illness are provided. Examples of MOHO-based intervention structures for this client group are also woven into the chapter narrative.

The purpose of this chapter is to:

- Introduce how MOHO is applied to individuals experiencing mental illness;
- Reinforce the dynamic and interconnected nature of the key components of MOHO;
- Emphasize the need to understand the social and physical environment to support occupational choice, participation, and adaptation;
- Consider the importance of remotivation for occupation in therapy practice; and
- Acknowledge the importance of an empathically grounded approach by therapists in MOHO-based therapy.

Chapter 9 introduced the concept of occupational narrative or, in other words, how a client's volition, habituation, performance capacity, and environment dynamically interact over time to influence what a client does with his or her occupational life. The focus of this chapter is to explain how the MOHO practice concepts, assessments, and interventions support positive therapy outcomes with persons experiencing mental illness. Therapists explain the progress of enabling occupational adaptation through MOHO-based therapy in situations where complexity is evident. Through MOHO-based therapy, clients and their caregivers can incrementally move toward new ways of seeing and experiencing occupations, recognize painful realities, and make hard decisions and compromises. Occupational therapists (OTs) featured in this chapter were able to help their clients to change through careful understanding of their situation made possible through the concepts and tools provided by MOHO. The problem-solver that follows illustrates the impact of illness and disability on the occupational adaptation of two people. The couple featured struggled to undertake the things that were important to them and preserve their sense of identity, competence, participation, and, ultimately, well-being. The therapist describes her approach to understanding their shared situation and the intervention that supported their occupational participation within their environment.

CASE EXAMPLE: AN OLDER ADULT WITH DEMENTIA

Libby and Sam, both 81 years, lived in a studio apartment within a retirement community. They were familiar with their physical environment, which was designed to assist with the strengths and limitations of their motor and process skill ability. Married for 63 years, they had two adult sons, one of whom lived nearby. Libby, diagnosed with unspecified dementia, did not acknowledge any difficulties. Family members suspected that she also had an undiagnosed personality disorder, as her interpersonal style has always been experienced as "difficult." Her ongoing dependence on her husband, Sam, had been noted. Libby's cognitive challenges included significant short-term memory loss, decreased decision-making ability, and inhibition. Any changes in her daily routine would lead to an expression of frustration and agitation. Apart from Sam, Libby had no friendships with peers, and this was historically consistent for her. Sam was Libby's long-time caregiver but had maintained a wealth of social connection.

Changes in the couple's circumstances had an impact on their ability to manage their individual occupational identity.

- A long-standing routine of sharing mealtimes with another couple at the retirement community came to an end when discomfort was expressed with Libby's reduced ability to be appropriate in her communication and interaction skills.
- Sam experienced a fall that resulted in a significant wrist fracture of his nondominant hand. This resulted in a limit to his own competency in occupational performance because of significant pain and a limited ability to use his arm and hand temporarily.
- The change in circumstances and Sam's ability to participate in usual leisure occupations led Sam to express how stressful his caregiving *role* had become. The circumstances had a negative effect on his emotional resilience in addition to his belief in his ability (personal causation) to continue his caring role.

An occupational therapy evaluation was sought. An interview was undertaken with the couple followed by a standardized, observational assessment using Residential Environment Impact Scale 4.0 assessment (Fisher et al., 2014). This provided further understanding of the impact of the physical and social environment on Libby and Sam's occupational participation. During the evaluation, Sam shared information about their daily routines:

> I usually wake up an hour or so before Libby. I get dressed and prepare breakfast for us. Now that I'm wearing this plaster I find dressing myself very difficult. I'm proud that I managed to figure out how to get my socks on with one hand . . . that was tricky! This change has affected us.
>
> Libby is less settled because we have to do things differently. It's made us both a bit fearful.
>
> I used to go to the exercise room and work out using the machines for half an hour or so, usually with friends. After exercising, I would stay with friends and watch game shows before lunch. I miss doing that now.
>
> We have lunch in the assisted dining room now. Libby can't go far; her walking is really unsteady. After lunch, Libby likes to be alone to watch her favorite television shows. I need to rest in the afternoon, but I miss going for a drive and my contact with my friends.

Libby's connection with Sam was clearly very strong. The only comments Libby made without prompting or waiting for Sam's input during the occupational therapy consultation were:

> "Sam helps me with everything. Everybody should have a Sam."

As the therapist was leaving, Sam shared:

> It's really hard to help her now . . . she does not understand, no matter how many times I tell her, the things I can't do now. She keeps getting angry that we are going to the other dining room, but I can't carry the trays. She doesn't see her memory problems.

The therapist replied:

> "Yes, it can be very hard when she can't remember things. It sounds like Libby's memory problems are hard for you to manage right now. Would you like some ideas about how to help her, and yourself, more?"

Sam gratefully replied, "That would be good, thank you."

After the evaluation, the therapist's consultation consisted of providing Sam and his daughter-in-law with caregiver education booklets for information and tips about facilitating communication and interaction opportunities as well as involvement in and daily activities for people with dementia. The therapist encouraged Sam to develop a different routine to visit his son in the afternoon for a break while Libby watched her shows before the evening meal. This supported the occupations and created the environments and occupational forms (i.e., specific instances of performance) that both individuals valued and the roles that were familiar to them. The therapist also provided Sam with suggestions for adapting the morning routine for less effort (for example, using paper bowls for oatmeal to eliminate dishwashing), and discussed adaptive equipment options, such as reachers, elastic shoelaces, a button hook, and a shower bench.

The therapist was able to provide clear information to Sam and his family to help them recognize the physical and social environmental challenges impacting Libby and Sam. The therapist used the findings to support the family to develop a plan to respond to the aspects of the environment that were interfering with Libby and Sam's opportunities to engage in meaningful activities. Immediate priorities focused on safety to reduce the risk of falls for Libby and Sam, and longer range strategies focused on helping Sam access information and staff supports within the retirement community to help maintain their current living situation and prepare for transition to assisted living when necessary. This example highlights the importance of considering the physical and social environment when working with persons with mental illness alongside other strategies of occupational participation.

Working with Persons with Mental Illness

Occupational therapy makes a difference in the lives of persons with mental illness (College of Occupational Therapists, 2007). One in four individuals will encounter mental illness in any given year (World Health Organization, 2001). Common experiences include mild anxiety and depression, whereas other, less prevalent illnesses include severe and enduring conditions involving psychosis or cognitive decline. It is not unusual for such illness to have a detrimental impact on the person's occupational pursuits of self-care, leisure, and work (Creek, 2003; Prior et al., 2013).

Mental illness is frequently associated with other illness experience. The literature notes that individuals with serious mental illness are more likely to have significant issues with, for example, cardiovascular disease and related risk factors compared with members of the general population (Ward, White, & Druss, 2015). This point reinforces the importance of conceptualizing the occupation-focused assessment of and intervention with persons defined as having "mental illness" with mind–body unity. Essentially, persons' needs should be considered in relation to their total lived experience. In addition, there is evidence that environmental factors have an impact on the recovery from mental illness (Milan, 2010; Prior et al., 2013). Scholars agree that attending to the limitations within the environment for persons with mental illness is also a key consideration so that living, working, and leisure environments are of optimal support of engagement in meaningful daily activities (Harrison, Angarola, Forsyth, & Irvine, 2015).

THE LIVED EXPERIENCE

People with a diagnosis of mental illness describe their lived experience in a variety of individual ways. Feelings of hopelessness, loss of control, disempowerment, and disconnection are common themes (Tew et al., 2012).

Milan (2010) provides an example through personal commentary about her experiences and perspectives of psychiatric intensive care in a hospital environment:

> When I went to bed at night I was so medicated that as soon as my head hit the pillow I was in a deep sleep. There was no time for reflection on the day's events, no processing of thoughts or emotions, no dreams and then a new day began all over again. It felt like a terrible nightmare existence. Part of what makes me who I am and human is my ability to reflect upon my experiences and interactions and I felt robbed of this ability to get in touch with what was going on in life. Milan (2010)

Such experiences, where all sense of normality is removed through changes to routines, roles, the social and built environment, and the lived body experience can combine to induce a sense of volitional vacuum. Persons with mental illness have described their illness as forming a barrier to occupational identity, occupational participation, and recovery. For example, in a qualitative study (Kelly, Lamont, & Brunero, 2010) to establish occupational perspectives of people experiencing mental illness, a participant shared:

> You've no one to talk to, no one to explain anything to, and I really stopped partaking in everything. (Kelly et al., 2010)

In another commentary, persons who experience mental illness have explained how involvement in occupational pursuits in an environment where the MOHO guides practice created a sense of hope, recovery, and social inclusion (Hitchman, 2010).

> It helped me to rebuild the confidence and belief in myself that had diminished while I was unwell. Slowly, I began to understand the journey of recovery and the obstacles that one has to jump, to move onto the next place. I knew I felt safe if I did make mistakes, and this was vital to my ongoing recovery programme. Hitchman (2010)

Persons involved in educational approaches to develop ability to live with their mental illness have reported positive impact. They speak of benefit to their sense of well-being, hope, inclusion, and involvement in occupations (Burhouse et al., 2015). An enhanced sense of personal causation and occupational identity has been the result. For example:

> I found a sense of fun during the college, of optimism and mutual support and respect that helped me feel safe and able to contribute to the discussions. I found a place and a group of people that I could trust and be trusted in reverse. A feeling of belonging sums it up really, another gift. I do miss the recovery college, it formed such an important part of my week, but it's definitely a case of gone but not forgotten! As I begin to look and move forwards in my life, I take with me that precious sprinkling of hope. With that on my side I'm in a much stronger position to deal with whatever life throws at me. I'm on a journey, one of recovery, of living, and of believing that life holds something more for me than just surviving. (Graduate of the 2013 Gloucester Recovery College)

THE USE OF MOHO IN PRACTICE WITH PERSONS WITH MENTAL ILLNESS

The MOHO is a well-known conceptual model in occupational therapy practice (Duncan, 2006). Lee, Forsyth, Menton, Kielhofner, and Taylor (2011) established that the vast majority of the respondents to their survey of an English sample of OTs reportedly use MOHO to guide their practice. It has also been reported that OTs who used MOHO acknowledge its utility and value for themselves and their clients (Lee, Taylor, Kielhofner, & Fisher, 2008). These strengths included the perceived support for a client-centered approach, provision of a strong base for planning and monitoring treatment and client outcomes, and also noting it as a framework for professional identity in practice. Other research suggests that therapists who have implemented the MOHO acquire a deep understanding of the complexities of enabling occupational participation with persons with mental illness (Melton, Forsyth, & Freeth, 2010; Pépin, Guérette, Lefebvre, & Jacques, 2008). Described as an empathic understanding of the client, Kielhofner (2008) emphasized the need to approach the understanding of each element of MOHO as it unfolds within a client's experience from the client's perspective. Establishing a relationship that is grounded in an empathic understanding is particularly important with clients with mental illness. Exceptional and considered judgment and care needs to be taken when supporting people with highly challenging circumstances. Therapists need to understand their own influence as part of an individual's social environment.

The MOHO has been applied with reported success to many areas to guide and develop mental health practice (Kielfhofner, 2008). Examples include practice for people with eating disorders (Abeydeera, Willis, & Forsyth, 2007; Barris, 1986); people with dementia (Borell, Gustavsson, Sandman, & Kielhofner, 1994; Raber, Teitelman, Watts, & Kielhofner, 2010); people living with HIV/AIDS (Anandan, Braveman, Kielhofner, & Forsyth, 2006; Braveman, Kielhofner, Albrecht, & Helfrich, 2006); and people with severe mental illness (Aubin, Hachey, & Mercier, 1999; Heasman & Atwal, 2004; Kavanagh & Fares, 1995). The MOHO is also of value when used with persons of varying ages and has been reported to be of relevance in services for children (Basu, Jacobson, & Keller, 2004; Harrison & Forsyth, 2005), adolescents (Baron, 1987), adults (Braveman, 1999), and older adults (Burton, 1989a, 1989b). Furthermore, the MOHO has been successfully utilized to guide change from a "supervisory" style to an "occupation-focused" style culture within institutions for people experiencing mental illness (Melton et al., 2008) and to tackle mental health stigma in communities (Melton & Clee, 2009).

ASSESSMENT AND INTERVENTION TO ENABLE OCCUPATIONAL PARTICIPATION

OTs working with people experiencing mental illness have concluded that MOHO-based assessment and intervention support clients to feel more secure and hopeful about therapy and to appreciate how engagement in occupational therapy can help (Melton et al., 2010; Pépin et al., 2008). By being actively involved in setting a plan of occupational therapy intervention, clients can make choices about their use of time and build upon their motivation for occupation. In some services, occupational therapy is defined through a pathway of care (Melton et al., 2008). MOHO-based assessments in mental health practice are selected initially to gain baseline information about the person's overall occupational performance or participation. Where more detailed information is indicated, further assessments are selected and introduced (Melton et al., 2008). Many of the MOHO-based assessments have an evaluative element that enables a measure of outcome to be outlined following a program of intervention. In relation to intervention, OTs introduce one or more occupation-focused interventions to reflect the individual circumstances, interest, values, roles, routines, and environmental influences of the individual. For example, the Volitional Questionnaire (de las Heras, Geist, Kielhofner, & Li, 2003a) assessment and the associated intervention manual of the Remotivation Process (de las Heras, Llerena, & Kielhofner, 2003b) may be selected where the therapist needs a deep understanding of the impact of volition and environment on an individual's performance followed by a structured approach to remotivation to occupation.

Illustrative Exemplars—MOHO Problem-Solvers

A series of problem-solvers follows that outline the application of MOHO for persons with mental illness. The first represents a MOHO approach in school-based Occupational Therapy. The second describes MOHO-based intervention with a young man with mental illness living in a residential facility.

The final problem-solver describes a young woman seeking to reengage with employment following an experience of mental illness.

MOHO Problem-Solver: A Boy with Attention-Deficit Hyperactivity Disorder

Robbie is an 8-year-old boy. His parents describe him as a "whirlwind" with a great deal of energy but very little focus. Robbie enjoys watching TV, swimming, and playing sports with his friends. He lives with his parents and his two older brothers. His parents had been concerned about him from an early age. He appeared to have a very short attention span, did not enjoy quiet or complex activities, and needed constant supervision. Robbie was always "on the go," and he enjoyed rolling around on the floor, running, and jumping. He seemed to stop only when he was tired out. Robbie's teachers reported that he had serious problems with school work and social interaction and that these issues were interfering with his ability to learn.

As a result of these concerns, Robbie was seen by a family doctor, pediatrician, and children's mental health agency who diagnosed attention-deficit hyperactivity disorder (ADHD). Robbie's doctor referred the family to the Occupational Therapy service. The OT met with Robbie and his parents, who indicated their greatest concern was with Robbie's school work. They were afraid that Robbie was missing out on important parts of his education. The therapist knew that for ADHD treatment to be most effective, consistency and communication with Robbie's school was very important. She was working to a consultative approach, knowing that the teacher was the best placed person to implement supports and strategies. The OT then began working with Robbie's teacher.

During their meetings, the therapist and teacher discussed Robbie. The teacher had noticed poor reading skills, such as phonological awareness, vocabulary, and letter recognition. Robbie could not sit still and found it hard to give focused attention to the teacher. He often became frustrated and upset during the school day. Robbie's teacher said he had particular difficulty concentrating and would struggle to remember routines and sequences for tasks and activities.

> Robbie just cannot sit still! He seems able and has good general knowledge, but he is all over the place. If the task is something active, interactive, or something he enjoys, then he can focus quite well. He seems to learn by doing rather than listening. But sometimes listening work is inevitable and at these times he has real difficulty concentrating. (Robbie's teacher)

The teacher said that multistep or complex instructions were difficult for Robbie to follow and that Robbie was easily distracted by other children. The teacher said that Robbie's behavior improved on days with a very clear routine, and when Robbie knew the structure of the day (e.g., on Tuesdays, go to Gym class). Robbie had strengths in terms of his motivation. He was particularly motivated when completing activities including movement.

The therapist, experienced in using MOHO, knew there could be a tendency to focus on how discrete physical, sensory, or behavioral challenges were impacting on Robbie. She also knew that this was usually only a small part of the picture. Drawing on MOHO, she knew that Robbie's participation in school was influenced by a combination of factors including the physical environment, attitudes, expectations, opportunities, and motivation. The therapist used a resource—*Occupational Therapists Manual* (Forsyth, 2010)—to support her clinical reasoning in making intervention decisions. This manual provided the therapist with a set of intervention techniques for young people in schools based on MOHO. The therapist also wanted to work collaboratively, and the manual provided a guide to collaborating with the teacher, and supports and strategies for the teacher to use in class.

The therapist, in collaboration with the teacher, identified four techniques (CIRCLE Collaboration, 2009) to use with Robbie:

1. **Modifying school environment:** Changing Robbie's physical, social, or sensory school environment (including equipment and/or a consistent change in adult behavior) to support his occupational participation.
2. **Role scripting:** Providing opportunities for Robbie to extend, change, alter, or develop his school role repertoire, and supporting him to understand and meet a range of responsibilities.
3. **Reconstructing habits:** Providing opportunities for Robbie to extend, change, alter, or develop effective school habit patterns.
4. **Sensory support:** Sensory and motor supports, strategies, and occupations provided throughout the school day, specifically selected for Robbie.
5. **Recreating volition:** Changing Robbie's appraisal of his values, his perceptions of what is enjoyable, and the accuracy of his perception of his abilities and limitations.

The therapist and the teacher worked collaboratively to develop an intervention plan for Robbie.

- Starting with the *environment*, they agreed that the teacher would always use Robbie's name to make sure she had his attention. They also agreed that the teacher would use short, simple instructions and support them with demonstration when necessary. The teacher and therapist agreed that Robbie's seating should be carefully considered, and where possible, he should be close to the teacher's desk, away from the window, and with learners who are not easily distracted. They planned to set up a "quiet" workstation for Robbie when he needed to focus on his work.
- In terms of *role*, the therapist and the teacher both identified that Robbie needed to physically move between tasks. They asked Robbie what he would like to do that involved moving around the class. He responded that he wanted to collect the jotters, so he was given that role for the school term.
- For *habits*, the therapist and the teacher identified that Robbie was supported by having a clear routine. A detailed visual timetable was developed that Robbie could keep on his desk. This would allow a habit pattern to form, ensuring more consistent success in completion of his routine.
- For sensory support, the therapist recommended a sit-and-move cushion and also a fidget toy to squeeze when Robbie needed to concentrate.
- For *volition*, it was agreed that Robbie could choose (when appropriate) when to use his quiet space and his sensory supports. The teacher suggested use of an incentive chart, which Robbie would complete, based on good behavior.

Finally, the therapist and the teacher agreed to make sure that Robbie's parents were fully informed of the work in school. A review meeting was set for 3 months, at which they would again discuss Robbie's progress.

SUMMARY

The theoretical assumptions of MOHO stress the interrelationships between people, environments, and outcomes, focusing on practice that requires actions at multiple levels. Working with the *Occupational Therapists Manual*, the therapist considered that the child's underlying skill set or difficulties were only part of the picture and that issues also arose from surroundings (the physical and social environment), routines, and motivation. Working together, the teacher and the therapist supported Robbie's participation by putting in place supports and strategies to overcome challenges at multiple levels.

CASE EXAMPLE: A YOUNG ADULT WITH SCHIZOPHRENIA

Ross is a 28-year-old man who has a diagnosis of schizophrenia. He hears voices that can cause him to be preoccupied and become distracted when engaging in activity or speaking with people. Ross currently lives in a residential facility with five other people who also have a mental illness. Ross has his own room, which includes a sleeping area and a bathroom en suite. The house has a communal kitchen where he and the other residents can prepare meals, and a lounge area where the residents have arranged that they can watch TV, play computer games, or listen to music together. Ross gets on well with one of the other residents, Jimmy, who is similar in age to him, and will spend time in the lounge watching TV or playing computer games with him or sit outside in the garden smoking cigarettes and talking with his friend.

All the residents receive 4 hours' support on a daily basis from staff with routine activities of daily living and to access leisure interests. Ross attends a community football group and visits his family once a week to spend a day with them and catch up with his brother and sister who are younger than him.

Ross has been talking with his keyworker about living in his own flat. He is keen to follow an interest in gardening, think about opportunities for volunteering, and reduce the amount of support he receives with daily living activities. His keyworker has some concerns about how Ross will cope living on his own with less support. He knows that Ross can sometimes be poorly motivated to look after his room, not eat on a regular basis, and stop attending the community football group. His keyworker refers him to the Community Occupational Therapist based in the local mental health service to assess what intervention may support Ross's transition to move to less supported living.

The OT wants to understand what Ross's motivation, performance, and organization of occupation are and whether Ross's environment is impacting on his ability to engage in occupations. The OT talks with Ross, his keyworker, and the staff who support him at the residential facility and uses the Wayfinder Intervention (Wayfinder Collaboration, 2014) to understand whether Ross's current living environment is supporting his sense of identity and competence by providing exceptional opportunities, resources, and demands to engage in meaningful and culturally appropriate activities. To identify this, the OT completes the Model of Human Occupation Screening Tool (MOHOST) (Parkinson, Forsyth, & Kielhofner, 2004) and the Residential Environment Impact Survey (REIS) (Fisher et al., 2014).

The MOHOST identifies that Ross is able to manage most daily living activities with some encouragement, and that Ross lacks confidence to complete some activities when staff are not present. He recognizes that he has some limitations with managing his money and using the bus to visit his family and attend his football group. He is keen to pursue other leisure interests and begin to think about options for work. He wants to think about his role as a brother, organizing social activities that he could do together with his brother and sister.

The REIS identifies that there are several pieces of broken kitchen equipment that make it difficult for Ross to increase the range of meals he could prepare. It also identifies that Ross does not have anywhere he could store personal items securely, and often toiletries and other items go missing. The structure of Ross's daytime activities is inhibited by the availability and flexibility of support staff time at the residential facility. This particularly impacts their availability to support daily meal preparation with Ross, support him to attend his football group, and accompany him to pursue new interests. Ross identifies that this often leaves him with long periods of time that he fills by playing computer games, sleeping, or talking with his friend. He does not find these activities provide him with enough challenge.

Ross and the OT identify that it would be helpful to create a more organized and productive routine, taking on more responsibility within current activities and increasing opportunities for him to engage in new interests. They discuss this with the support staff as it will involve changes in how support to Ross is organized and used.

PLAN

- Changes within the environment including the structure of Ross's activities; negotiating regular support times with staff, creating a weekly plan, staff organizing new kitchen equipment to support meal preparation; and Ross having a lock on the drawers in his room to store personal items.

- **Ross taking increasing responsibility for daily living activities including meal preparation and cleaning his living space.**
- **Ross identifying and organizing a social activity he and his brother and sister can do together.**
- **Ross pursuing a new interest.**

Ross describes how the plan is working.

I found it hard to get into the plan at first. It's great that the support workers have been encouraging me to do things like cooking my meals on my own. Now that we have more pans and a microwave that works in the kitchen, I can make four different hot meals. I sometimes cook with my pal Jimmy who lives here, and I have taught him some of my recipes. I have started going to the community gardening project. I really enjoy it there and get on well with Mike who runs the garden. I've decided to go there three times a week as well as my football group. I really enjoy digging the plots, and I have planted vegetables.

Because I go to groups, I have to be more organized about things like cleaning my room and making sure I get up on time. I have started setting the alarm on my phone to get me up in the morning. It's a lot better now that I can lock up my things in my drawer, 'cos I don't have to worry about whether my stuff will still be there when I get back from my groups. I don't sleep as much in the day anymore because I have a lot more things to do. I am getting better at using the bus to get to my groups. The staff helped me get a transport pass so that I don't need to worry about having the right money with me, which I find a lot easier.

I organized to meet my brother and sister at the cinema a few weeks ago. We saw a horror film because we all like those. We also met up at the pub last week, and it was good to be out with them.

My keyworker and the OT have been talking to me about planning to move to my own place where I would still get some support every day. Me and the OT have talked about if I could volunteer at the garden project, which I am really happy about.

SUMMARY

The theoretical assumptions of MOHO inform the Wayfinder Intervention. The intervention aims to ensure that there is an exceptional fit between the person and their environment to support their engagement in a pattern of meaningful daily routines that provide them with a sense of identity and competence. The OT identified that Ross's environment was having an impact on his engagement in routine daily living activities and pursuing his interests. The inflexibility of support time impacted on Ross's satisfaction with activities, such that he found activities were underdemanding and that he had a lot of unoccupied time. Further, there were not enough objects in the kitchen to support Ross with meal preparation, and he was unable to secure personal items to ensure they were available to him when he required them.

The plan supported Ross taking on increasing role responsibility, organizing social outings with his brother and sister, and establishing a new role at the community garden and sharing his cooking skills with his friend.

A review meeting was agreed for 3 months, and the OT agreed to complete the MOHOST and REIS with Ross, the support staff, and his keyworker to identify Ross's progress. The outcome of the assessments will assist in identifying the level of supported living environment that would facilitate Ross to maintain community living skills, routines, and meaningful activities.

CASE EXAMPLE: A YOUNG ADULT WITH BIPOLAR DISORDER

Sally referred herself to the occupational therapy vocational rehabilitation program, seeking support when she initially felt she was ready to return to employment. Sally is 24 years old and lives independently in a rented flat with weekly support from her community psychiatric nurse (CPN). Sally has a bipolar disorder, which she first experienced while in university in her late teens; she has been admitted to hospital on several occasions, but at the time of referral felt she had the best strategies in place to manage her condition and was ready to return to employment on a part-time basis. Sally's CPN and mother were both concerned that Sally's recently stable mental health may be adversely affected by the additional stress of employment and tried to discourage her from contacting the occupational therapy team.

The occupational therapy service adopted the ActiVate Collaboration Intervention (ActiVate Collaboration, 2014) based on the MOHO, integrating the principles of evidence-based supported employment (Dartmouth IPS Supported Employment Centre, 2010). At initial appointment, the occupational therapy service routinely uses the Worker Role Interview (Braveman et al., 2005) to gain an understanding and baseline assessment of psychosocial and environmental factors influencing a person's ability to return to or sustain work. When interviewing Sally, the OT explored Sally's

views of previous work experiences and how current circumstances were influencing her motivation to return to employment, her current roles and routines, and her ability to perform a work role.

Following the worker role interview, the OT completed the scoring form and a case formulation. This case formulation was shared with Sally to ensure that the OT had a good understanding of Sally's strengths supporting returning to employment and problem areas that may interfere with Sally accomplishing her goals.

Case Formulation

Sally had a strong work ethic and was keen to return to employment, which she felt would

- increase her independence, reducing her reliance on state benefits,
- widen her social network,
- give an improved structure and purpose to her routine, and
- provide an opportunity to develop new skills and abilities.

Sally felt confident that her mental health had improved to a point where she was ready to take on a new challenge and that she would be successful. However, this confidence was undermined by the concerns of her family and CPN, who did not support her goal.

Sally filled her days with home maintenance chores and spending time with family members. She had lost contact with many friends and was keen to widen her social network. Sally struggled to find enough to do to keep her routine active; she recognized that a purposeful routine is helpful for maintaining her mental health.

Sally was undertaking veterinary training at university when she initially became unwell; she had a strong interest in animal care, recognized she had knowledge and skills in the field, and was keen to return to a related area of employment.

Intervention Planning

Sally and the OT spoke about the importance of emotional and practical support that Sally perceived as important to maintaining her motivation for employment. The OT provided a range of information and materials demonstrating the positive effect of employment on health and encouraged Sally to share this information with her family. The occupational therapy team worked closely with the community mental health services, and therefore the OT decided to plan a repeat of the regular employability training to update the whole team on the importance of supporting the vocational aspirations of individuals with mental health problems.

Recognizing that seeking employment would require a regular routine of time and effort, Sally committed to a regular routine of reviewing job opportunities, completing an up-to-date CV, and completing applications. The OT linked Sally up with a member of support staff in the team who could offer practical help and advice in these activities. In addition, Sally attended an appointment with a financial advisor who was able to provide advice about moving from state benefits to a wage.

Sally was also keen to improve her CV with some current experience; she had not been in employment since a part-time job at school and at university. The OT suggested volunteering at a local animal shelter, pointing out that this would also allow Sally to widen her social network with people with shared interests. Sally and the OT visited the animal shelter and arranged 3 half-days per week unpaid role at the shelter. The OT had previously linked other individuals with the shelter and knew that the manager and team had previously offered successful opportunities to people with mental health problems.

Sally also consented to the OT contacting local employers on her behalf to seek work opportunities. The OT set up appointments with local kennels and veterinary surgeries.

After 6 Months

Sally thrived in the volunteering role, and her confidence in her abilities to return to employment increased; her mother and CPN also recognized how much happier Sally was with her new regular routine. She developed a CV, which the OT shared with several employers. A local doggy day care service had trouble recruiting reliable staff willing to work early mornings, and the OT felt this might be a good fit for Sally, so she arranged an introductory meeting.

In preparation for the meeting, the OT and Sally discussed the work environment in the animal shelter. The OT wanted to help Sally identify the environmental characteristics that had facilitated such a positive experience. To structure this discussion and provide a measurement, the OT used the Work Environment Impact Scale (Moore-Corner, Kielhofner, & Olson, 1998). During the interview, they discussed the social and physical environment, support available, task and time demands, objects used, and daily job functions. Key aspects that Sally noted, which the OT was confident would be replicated, were the appeal of work tasks, the task demands, and the physical and sensory

qualities of the environment. Sally was keen that she had the opportunity to discuss the social environment, she was aware that she responded well to constructive and regular feedback, and although she enjoyed working autonomously, she preferred working alongside colleagues. Sally felt her work schedule volunteering had offered some flexibility, allowing her to attend health appointments, and she needed to know this would be possible in a new role.

Sally and the employer got on well and felt that the center could offer similar work environment to the rescue shelter. After an initial trial, Sally commenced work on a part-time basis. Sally continued to volunteer one session a week, and she recognized the value of the role and the positive relationships she had made with other volunteers. Sally spoke about doing veterinary nursing training in the future, but was continuing to consolidate her current roles and was appreciating the greater independence, social life, and time with animals.

Conclusion

Throughout this chapter, we demonstrated the unique and synergistic application of MOHO concepts to individuals with mental illness. We emphasized the role of volition and how to understand it within the remotivation process. In addition, we provided examples of how habituation may be used to enable a person to establish more productive habits and routines in order to create more structure within one's life. We discussed the roles of providing opportunities for the further development of communication and interaction skills within the social and physical environment. We identified additional environmental barriers that need to be addressed in order to ensure the most comprehensive and successful treatment outcomes.

The case examples described represent complex challenges faced by individuals with mental illness. Because of the multifactorial issues faced by each client, success in therapy required very considered understanding of the individual and their environment. The successes that occurred in each case reflect the fact that the therapist took the time and used the necessary tools to fully understand clients and how best to approach them. Thus, the cases represent valuable examples of how to actively use MOHO to make sense of clients' circumstances and to devise a thoughtful approach to the therapy process.

BOX 21-1: Client characteristics addressed in this chapter

- Older man (age 81 years) and older woman (age 81 years)—with fracture and dementia, respectively
- Boy (8 years old)—attention-deficit hyperactivity disorder (ADHD)
- Young man (28 years)—schizophrenia
- Young woman (24)—bipolar disorder
- Older man (83)—depression

CASE EXAMPLE: TO TEST YOUR KNOWLEDGE: AN OLDER ADULT WITH DEPRESSION

Lawrence described his reflections about his occupational circumstances and his involvement in occupational therapy:

I'm 83 years old, you know, that's getting on a bit now. Back then I was thinking, 'It's no fun when you can't do what you're used to. I can't be bothered really, what am I good for now?'

It's true, I used to be well regarded for being one of the lads at the farm, I had lots of friends from my military services too.

I was always a cheerful and sociable personality, well known and respected in my local community. When I retired from my job on the farm I thought that me and the wife would have a ball. I was so sad that I lost her. I was thinking for a long time that there was just not a lot of point anymore. My children had grown up, they didn't need me.

I can see now that the depression was getting hold of me. It changed everything, changed my life. I was a strong man before. In fact, I was a military veteran too and very proud of what I did as service for my nation. But all of that didn't seem to matter at the time of the depression.

My daughter came and helped me to get some tablets from the doctor. That helped to sort my mood out but I'd lost my confidence. When the occupational therapist came to see me, she asked me all about what was important to me, past, now and going forward. She really listened to me. I got the idea that she was interested to help me live my life again. She did some tests to look at my skills, the AMPS I think she said it was , and we went from there!

The occupational therapist helped to get me motivated again. It took a bit of time, but I'm joining in with life again now. I'm doing little jobs in my garden every day and growing some lovely beans at the minute. I'm walking into town to get my paper every day, and I've even made some new chums at the Old Age lunch that I look forward to going to every Tuesday. I feel a lot more confident now. I've got some enjoyment again and a plan for my week. My daughter says that she'd be glad to have her dad back, and my neighbor says I'm the 'chirpy-chappy' again! (Fisher & Bray Jones, 2010)

Questions to Encourage Critical Thinking and Discussion

- **Articulate Lawrence's narrative plot using the key concepts of the MOHO before his experience of depression.**
- **Provide a statement, articulated through MOHO, describing Lawrence's experience of occupational performance during his depression.**
- **Explain, in as much depth as possible, Lawrence's regressive narrative plot, paying attention to his volition, habituation, performance capacity, and the interface with his physical and social environment.**
- **Comment on the dynamic nature of the interface of MOHO concepts in Lawrence's circumstances.**
- **Describe the changes that Lawrence has made with his therapist to achieve a more positive experience of valued occupation.**
- **Speculate on the MOHO-based assessments and interventions that could have been of use in Lawrence's Occupational Therapy experience.**

Chapter 21 Quiz Questions

1. Consider how the experience of mental illness impacts occupational performance and occupational narrative.
2. Describe how volition is inextricably linked with the experience of mental health. How can this be explained using MOHO theory and concepts?
3. How might you characterize the connection between physical well-being and mental health?
4. How important are techniques of validation and remotivation in therapy with persons with mental illness?
5. What are your observations about the therapists in the case examples using themselves as part of the social environment to facilitate understanding of circumstances and ultimately occupational participation?

HOMEWORK ASSIGNMENTS

1. Review literature that provides insight into the occupational narrative of persons with mental illness. Note the similarities and differences in experience and how the environment supports or hinders occupational engagement. Note the importance of hope and the environmental impact of the stigma of mental illness.
2. Review cases where persons' primary "condition" is framed as "physical." Use MOHO concepts to consider the potential for emotional impact of such illness/disability and/or environmental circumstances on the individual(s) concerned. Reflect on the dynamic nature of physical and mental illness experience.
3. Reflect on the way that you have used your own skills and characteristics when interacting with persons with mental illness. What was the key to building a therapeutic relationship to support their occupational performance?

thePoint® For additional resources and exercises, visit http://thePoint.lww.com

Key Terms

Modifying school environment: Changing Robbie's physical, social, or sensory school environment (including equipment and/or a consistent change in adult behavior) to support his occupational participation.

Role scripting: Providing opportunities for Robbie to extend, change, alter, or develop his school role repertoire, and supporting him to understand and meet a range of responsibilities.

Reconstructing habits: Providing opportunities for Robbie to extend, change, alter, or develop effective school habit patterns.

Recreating volition: Changing Robbie's appraisal of his values, his perceptions of what is enjoyable, and the accuracy of his perception of his abilities and limitations.

Sensory support: Sensory and motor supports, strategies, and occupations provided throughout the school day, specifically selected for Robbie.

REFERENCES

Abeydeera, K., Willis, S., & Forsyth, K. (2007). Occupation focused assessment and intervention for clients with anorexia. *International Journal of Therapy and Rehabilitation, 13*(7), 22–24.

ActiVate Collaboration. (2014). *Vocational rehabilitation intervention manual.* Edinburgh, Scotland: Queen Margaret University.

Anandan, N., Braveman, B., Kielhofner, G., & Forsyth, K. (2006). Impairments and perceived competence in persons living with HIV/AIDS. *Work: A Journal of Prevention, Assessment, and Rehabilitation, 27,* 255–266.

Aubin, G., Hachey, R., & Mercier, C. (1999). Meaning of daily activities and subjective quality of life in people with severe mental illness. *Scandinavian Journal of Occupational Therapy, 6*(2), 53–62.

Baron, K. (1987). The model of human occupation: A newspaper treatment group for adolescents with a diagnosis of conduct disorder. *Occupational Therapy in Mental Health, 7*(2), 89–104.

Barris, R. (1986). Occupational dysfunction and eating disorders: Theory and approach to treatment. *Occupational Therapy in Mental Health, 6*(1), 27–45.

Basu, S., Jacobson, L., & Keller, J. (2004, June). Child-centered tools: Using the model of human occupation framework. *School System Special Interest Section Quarterly, 11*(2), 1–3.

Borell, L., Gustavsson, A., Sandman, P., & Kielhofner, G. (1994). Occupational programming in a day hospital for patients with dementia. *Occupational Therapy Journal of Research, 14,* 4.

Braveman, B. (1999). The model of human occupation and prediction of return to work: A review of related empirical research. *Work: A Journal of Prevention, Assessment, and Rehabilitation, 12*(1), 13–23.

Braveman, B., Kielhofner, G., Albrecht, G., & Helfrich, C. (2006). Occupational identity, occupational competence and occupational settings (environment): Influences on return to work in men living with HIV/AIDS. *Work: A Journal of Prevention, Assessment, and Rehabilitation, 27,* 267–276.

Braveman, B., Robson., M., Velozo, C., Kielhofner G., Fisher, G., Forsyth K., et al. (2005). *A user's manual for Worker Role Interview (WRI)* [Version 10.0]. Chicago: Model of Human Occupation Clearinghouse, Department of Occupational Therapy, University of Illinois at Chicago.

Burhouse, A., Rowland, M., Niman, H. M., Abraham, D., Collins E., Matthews H., et al. (2015). Coaching for recovery: A quality improvement project in mental health care. *British Medical Journal, 4*(1), 1–11.

Burton, J. E. (1989a). The model of human occupation and occupational therapy practice with elderly patients, Part 1: Characteristics of aging. *British Journal of Occupational Therapy, 52,* 215–218.

Burton, J. E. (1989b). The model of human occupation and occupational therapy practice with elderly patients, Part 2: Application. *British Journal of Occupational Therapy,* 52, 219–221.

Circle Collaboration. (2009). Queen Margaret University, Scotland, United Kingdom.

College of Occupational Therapists. (2007). Recovering ordinary lives: The strategy for occupational therapy in mental health services 2007 to 2017. London, United Kingdom: Author.

Creek, J. (2003). *Occupational therapy defined as a complex intervention.* London, United Kingdom: College of Occupational Therapists.

Dartmouth IPS Supported Employment Centre. (2010). *IPS overview, characteristics and practice principles.* Retrieved from http://www.dartmouth.edu/~ips2/styled/styled-2/page70.html

de las Heras, C.G., Geist, R., Kielhofner, G., & Li, Y. (2003a). *The Volitional Questionnaire (VQ)* [Version 4.0]. Chicago: Model of Human Occupation Clearinghouse, Department of Occupational Therapy, University of Illinois at Chicago.

de las Heras, C.G., Llerena, V., & Kielhofner, G. (2003b). *Remotivation process: Progressive intervention for individuals with severe volitional challenges* [Version 1.0]. Chicago: Model of Human Occupation Clearinghouse, Department of Occupational Therapy, University of Illinois at Chicago.

Duncan, E. A. S. (2006). An introduction to conceptual models of practice and frames of reference. In Duncan, E. A. S. (Ed), *Foundations for practice in occupational therapy.* London, United Kingdom: Elsevier.

Fisher, G., Forsyth, K., Harrison, M., Angarola, R., Kayhan, E., Noga, P. L., et al. (2014). *Residential Environment Impact Scale* [Version 4.0]. Chicago: University of Illinois at Chicago.

Forsyth. (2010). *CIRCLE therapy manual: Occupational therapy.* Edinburgh, Scotland: Queen Margaret University, City of Edinburgh.

Harrison, M., & Forsyth, K. (2005). Developing a vision for therapists working within child and adolescent mental health services: Poised of paused for action? *British Journal of Occupational Therapy, 68*(4), 181–185.

Harrison, M., Angarola, R., Forsyth, K., & Irvine, L. (2015). Defining the environment to support occupational therapy intervention in mental health practice. *British Journal of Occupational Therapy,* 1–5. Retrieved from http://bjo.sagepub.com/content/early/2015/04/17/0308022614562787.full.pdf+html

Heasman, D., & Atwal, A. (2004). The active advice pilot project: Leisure enhancement and social inclusion for people with severe mental health problems. *British Journal of Occupational Therapy, 67*(4), 511–514.

Hitchman, M. (2010). Volunteering within an acute care setting—Its role in promoting hope, recovery and social inclusion. *Mental Health and Social Inclusion, 14*(2), 24–27.

Kavanagh, J., & Fares, J. (1995). Using the Model of Human Occupation with homeless mentally ill clients. *British Journal of Occupational Therapists, 58*(10), 419–422.

Kielhofner, G. (2008). *Conceptual foundations of occupational therapy practice* (4th ed.). Philadelphia, PA: F. A. Davis.

Kelly, M., Lamont, S., & Brunero, S. (2010). An occupational perspective of the recovery journey in mental health. *British Journal of Occupational Therapy, 73*(3), 129–135.

Lee, S. W., Forsyth, K., Menton, J., Kielhofner, G., & Taylor, R. (2011). Practice development efforts impact on mental health rehabilitation: Results-based health care implications. *International Journal of Therapy and Rehabilitation, 18*(11), 602–609.

Lee, S. W., Taylor, R. R., Kielhofner, G., & Fisher, G. (2008). Theory use in practice: A national survey of therapists who use the Model of Human Occupation. *American Journal of Occupational Therapy, 62*, 106–117.

Melton, J., & Clee, S. (2009). Mechanisms to engage communities I fostering social inclusion: a provider perspective. *The International Journal of Leadership in Public Services, 5*, 29–37.

Melton, J, Forsyth, K., & Freeth, D. (2010). A study of practitioners' use of the Model of Human Occupation: Levels of theory use and influencing factors. *British Journal of Occupational Therapy, 73*(11), 549–558.

Melton, J., Forsyth, K., Metherall, A., Robinson, J., Hill, J., & Quick, L., (2008). Program redesign based on the Model of Human Occupation: Inpatient services for people experiencing acute mental illness in the UK. *Occupational Therapy in Healthcare*, 22(2/3), 37–50.

Milan, S. (2010). Personal experience and perspectives of psychiatric intensive care and recovery. *Journal of Psychiatric Intensive Care*, 1–5.

Moore-Corner, R. A., Kielhofner, G., & Olson, L. (1998). *A user's manual for Work Environment Impact Scale (WEIS)* [Version 2.0]. Chicago: Model of Human Occupation Clearinghouse, Department of Occupational Therapy, University of Illinois at Chicago.

Parkinson, S., Forsyth, K., & Kielhofner, G. (2004). *Model of Human Occupation screening tool* [Version 2.0]. Chicago: University of Illinois at Chicago.

Pépin, G., Guérette, F., Lefebvre, B., & Jacques, P. (2008). Canadian therapists' experience while implementing the Model of Human Occupation remotivation process. *Occupational Therapy in Health Care, 22*(2-3), 115–124.

Prior, S., Maciver, D., Forsyth, K., Walsj, M., Meiklejohn, A., & Irvine, L. (2013). Readiness for employment: Perceptions of mental health service users. *Community Mental Health, 49*, 658–667.

Raber, C., Teitelman, J., Watts, J., & Kielhofner, G. (2010). Phenomenological study of volition in everyday occupations of older people with dementia. *British Journal of Occupational Therapy, 73*(11), 498–506.

Tew, J., Ramon, S., Slade, M., Bird, V., Melton, J., & LeBoutillier, C. (2012). Social factors and recovery from mental health difficulties: A review of the evidence. *British Journal of Social Work, 42*(3), 443–460.

Ward, M. C., White, D. T., & Druss, B. G. (2015). A meta-review of lifestyle interventions for cardiovascular risk factors in the general medical population: Lessons for individuals with serious mental illness. *The Journal of Clinical Psychiatry, 76*(4),477–486.

Wayfinder Collaboration. (2014). *Rehabilitation for people with complex needs: A user's guide for occupational therapists*. Edinburgh, Scotland: Queen Margaret University.

World Health Organization. (2001). The World Health Report. Retrieved from http://www.who.int/whr/2001/media_centre/press_release/en/

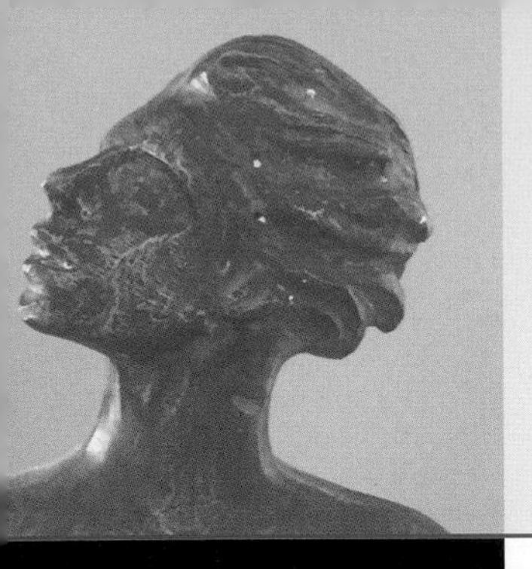

Applying MOHO in Pediatric Practice: Working with Children with Sensory Processing, Motor, Medical, and Developmental Issues

Susan M. Cahill, Patricia Bowyer, Jane C. O'Brien, Lauro Munoz, and Gary Kielhofner (posthumous)

CHAPTER 22

EXPECTED LEARNING OUTCOMES

Upon completion of this chapter, readers will be able to:

1. Describe how the four components of model of human occupation (MOHO) apply to children with a variety of issues.
2. Describe how MOHO components guide the occupational therapy process during screening, evaluation, intervention, and discharge planning in pediatric practice.
3. Identify appropriate methods for collecting data for different pediatric MOHO assessment tools.
4. Discuss how MOHO can be used to enable children's participation in meaningful life roles and occupations.

MOHO Problem-Solver: Lisa

Lisa is a 13-year-old girl who receives school-based occupational therapy services to address concerns related to her performance in the student role. Lisa's special education team believes that Lisa's lack of organization, poor history of homework completion, and difficulty with emotional self-regulation contribute to her performance difficulties. The occupational therapist uses the model of human occupation (MOHO) to better understand Lisa's occupational performance difficulties, as well as her strengths and to prioritize her needs. In using MOHO, the occupational therapist is able to move beyond simply focusing on organizational skills, homework completion, and emotional self-regulation and begin to focus on Lisa's occupational identity, occupational competence, performance skills, volition, and habituation. In addition, the occupational therapist is able to take into consideration factors in Lisa's environment that facilitated or restricted her participation at school. Lisa and the occupational therapist often have discussions during treatment sessions. During the discussions, the occupational therapist tries to ask probing questions that help her to understand Lisa's sense of identity and competence. The occupational therapist also probes to better understand how the environment influences Lisa's performance skills, as well as her volition, and habituation. The following dialogue includes some questions that Lisa's occupational therapist asked her, as well as Lisa's responses.

Occupational therapist: Lisa, how do you think your teacher would describe you?

Lisa: My teachers think I'm lazy and that I don't try hard enough at school.

Occupational therapist: Do you think you're lazy and that you don't try hard enough?

Lisa: No. I try really hard, but I just don't get some things. I get so tired of trying hard sometimes and that's when I think about giving up. But my mom says that I have to keep working hard so that I'm ready for high school. I don't know why she thinks high school is going to be different for me. I think it is still going to be hard.

Occupational therapist: What sorts of school things are hard for you now?

Lisa: Homework is hard. I try to pay attention in class and sometimes I feel like I understand what the teacher wants. Then when I get home and start to work on my homework, I just forget what I'm supposed to do. I do what I remember, but sometimes when I turn assignments in my teachers give me incompletes. Sometimes I don't even bring home the right textbooks. When I don't have my books, I can't do my homework at all.

Occupational therapist: How long has this been going on?

Lisa: I've always had trouble with homework. It seems like we get more homework in middle school than we used to in elementary school. I think it's been worse since I've been in middle school. I'm worried it will be even worse in high school.

Occupational therapist: Can you tell me about a time when you got an incomplete on an assignment?

Lisa: Last week we were supposed to find five sources for our research paper. I found five sources and wrote them down on my reference list. I didn't know or I forgot that we were supposed to summarize the information from each source and turn that in too. I didn't summarize the sources and I failed the assignment.

Occupational therapist: Do you think you know how to summarize the sources?

Lisa: My teacher gave me a worksheet to follow after I turned in the incomplete assignment. She actually gave me five copies of the worksheet. She said I can just fill out the worksheets because there are headings for all of the details that I need to include in my summary.

Occupational therapist: Was that helpful?

Lisa: Well, I guess it was helpful after I calmed down. I got so mad that she had these worksheets and didn't give them to me in the first place that I tore up my reference list right in front of her. Then, I got sent to the Dean's office and had to sit for detention.

Occupational therapist: Besides worksheets, do you think anything else would help you to be able to complete homework assignments?

Lisa: In elementary school, we used to have assignment notebooks and the teacher used to tell us to take out our assignment notebooks and write down our homework. My teachers now don't do that. I don't even have an assignment notebook. We also used to gather all of our books and things to take home together as a class. Now, I try to grab what I need from my locker before I have to run to catch the bus.

Occupational therapist: What are your habits around keeping track of your homework assignments and bringing home the right books and materials for your assignments now?

Lisa: I just try to remember what I need to do and what books I need to bring. That's what I see everyone else doing. Sometimes I've written down assignment due dates on a scrap piece of paper, but I usually lose the paper.

Occupational therapist: How effective do you feel like those habits are?

Lisa: They aren't effective. I think I need help coming up with a new system. I want to be a good student and I want to be able to turn in complete assignments on time when I start high school.

Occupational therapist: I think we could work together to come up with a new system and I think I could support you in a few of your different classes so that you can try it out. Then, we can work together to fine-tune your system and keep practicing it until it becomes more automatic for you. I think we could also work together to come up with ways that you can use with your time in between classes to get yourself organized for what you need to bring home. Do you think that if we worked together, you might be able to turn in some complete assignments?

Lisa: I think I might be able to turn in some complete assignments if I get a little help with keeping track of my assignments and my books. I'm willing to try it out anyway.

This scenario provides an example of how an occupational therapist used the Model of Human Occupation (Kielhofner, 2008) to move beyond typical reasons for referral in the school systems and address the child's occupational identity and occupational competence.

Pediatric occupational therapy practice has historically focused on the attainment of developmental milestones (Humphry, 2002). Consequently, many pediatric occupational therapy practitioners have developed an overreliance on remedial or developmental approaches (Ashburner, Rodger, Ziviani, & Jones, 2014; Humphry, 2002; Spencer, Turkett, Vaughan, & Koenig, 2006). The concentration of interventions focused on developmental outcomes has caused some occupational therapy practitioners to move away from occupation-focused and occupation-based interventions in favor of more impairment-focused interventions (Fisher, 2013; Miller Kuhaneck, Tanta, Coombs, & Pannone, 2013). While the remediation of deficits remains a valid pursuit in pediatric practice, there is a growing impetus for occupational therapy practitioners to address the occupational performance and engagement of children and youth with and at risk for disabilities (Cahill & Lopez-Reyna, 2013; Kiraly-Alvarez, 2015; Kramer, Bowyer, O'Brien, Kielhofner, & Maziero-Barbosa, 2009).

Children's engagement in occupation is determined by many factors. The Model of Human Occupation (Kielhofner, 2008) can provide a basis for addressing the factors that inhibit occupational performance and engagement in children and youth experiencing sensory processing, motor, medical, and developmental issues. Further, MOHO can help practitioners understand how their pediatric clients view their own impairments (O'Brien et al., 2010). Pediatric occupational therapy practitioners can use MOHO to guide every aspect of the occupational therapy process (i.e., screening, evaluation, intervention, progress monitoring, and discharge planning; American Occupational Therapy Association [AOTA], 2014). Embracing theory-driven therapeutic reasoning aligns pediatric occupational therapy with evidence-based practice (Lee, 2010; Lee, Taylor, Kielhofner, & Fisher, 2008) and allows practitioners to fully address the complex factors associated with a child's restricted or inhibited occupational performance and engagement.

Applying MOHO

The application of MOHO with pediatric clients begins with the therapeutic reasoning process. When using MOHO to guide therapeutic reasoning, the therapist focuses on understanding the child's unique sense of occupational identity and competence and how these factors are influenced by the child's volition, habituation, and performance capacity. In addition, the therapist also attends to how the environment influences the child's perspectives.

Forsyth and Kielhofner (2008) outline six steps that can be used to guide the therapeutic reasoning process:

- Getting to know the client through the process of asking MOHO-based questions
- Collecting data about the client
- Developing a clinical hypothesis to explain the client's occupational performance difficulties
- Developing intervention goals and strategies to be used in occupational therapy
- Monitoring the client's progress in therapy
- Evaluating the outcomes of therapy

Although the above steps are presented sequentially, many therapists find **therapeutic reasoning** to be an iterative and dynamic process (Forsyth & Kielhofner, 2008). Such a process challenges the therapist to constantly reassess his or her clinical hypotheses and subsequent interventions based on new and emerging information.

GETTING TO KNOW THE CLIENT

Pediatric occupational therapists often rely on parents, teachers, and other caregivers to construct their view of a child's strengths and needs. While this information is important, relying solely on these perspectives prevents the therapist from developing a sophisticated understanding of the child as an occupational being. The major concepts in MOHO can be used to construct questions to orient the therapist to concerns that stem beyond the typical reasons for pediatric referrals. The clinical questions that the therapist uses to guide clinical reasoning should be specific to the situation, the client, and the treatment.

CASE EXAMPLE: A YOUNG CHILD WITH CANCER

Jon is a 5-year-old boy who was recently diagnosed with acute lymphoblastic leukemia and is being treated with chemotherapy. He was referred to outpatient occupational therapy for decreased engagement in self-care activities at home. The intake coordinator interviewed Jon's mom and reported her concerns to the therapy department's intake coordinator. She indicated that Jon quit dressing himself after two chemotherapy treatments because he was tired. Jon also stopped participating in play with his sister and asked to stay home from school, which he previously enjoyed.

Prior to meeting Jon and his mother for the first time, the occupational therapist developed a list of clinical questions to frame an understanding of Jon's occupational needs based on the major MOHO concepts (Table 22-1).

The therapist may refine the clinical questions as more information is learned about the child. For example, a therapist may have difficulty conceptualizing a child's volition until the child is presented with a challenging task in therapy. Once the therapist sees how the child responds to a challenge, additional questions may emerge, such as:

- What other occupations or skills might produce a similar reaction from this child?
- What other occupations or skills might produce an opposite reaction from this child?
- How does the child's demonstration of volition during occupational engagement change if features of the environment are altered?

Table 22-1 Clinical Questions Guiding the Therapist's Understanding of Jon's Occupational Needs

MOHO Concept	Clinical Question
Occupational identity	• What is Jon's sense of who he is and what's happening with his leukemia diagnosis? • Who does Jon wish to be as a son, a student, and a friend? • Does Jon have any hobbies or interests that he associates with current or future roles?
Occupational competence	• Was Jon previously able to sustain a pattern of satisfying occupational participation? • Does Jon feel that he can do all of the things that he needs and wants to do at home, at school, and in the community? • Given Jon's age, how much has Jon been taught or allowed to do for himself and how much is done for him?
Participation	• Does Jon currently engage in play, self-care, and educational or other productive pursuits? • Does Jon engage in social participation?
Performance	• Does Jon perform self-care, play, and school occupations in a similar way to his peers? • Does Jon perform certain activities in keeping with the expectations established by the adults (i.e., parents and teachers) in his life?
Skill	• Does Jon have the necessary motor, process, and communication/interaction skills necessary to do what he needs and wants to do?
Environment	• What expectations do the adults in Jon's life hold for his participation and performance related to self-care, play, and education? • How do the adults in Jon's life support or restrict his development of motor, process, and communication/interaction skills? • How do the adults in Jon's life support or restrict the development of his volition and habituation? • What other people or social groups does Jon encounter? How do these people or groups support or restrict his occupational performance and participation? • How do the supports or constraints in the environment influence Jon's sense of his abilities and his potential? • What spaces and objects support or restrict Jon's occupational performance or participation?
Volition	• What does Jon think he's good at? • What does Jon think he's not good at? • How does Jon respond when he encounters a challenge? • What values or interests does Jon have? • What obligations does he perceive? • What does Jon think is important?
Habituation	• What are Jon's typical routines? • Who initiates Jon's routines? • What causes disruptions in these routines? • How does Jon respond to disruptions in routines? • What habits does Jon have that supports his occupational performance and participation? • What habits does Jon have that do not support his occupational performance and participation? • With what roles does Jon identify? • How do Jon's roles influence how he spends his time?

Based on the table originally presented in Forsyth and Kielhofner (2008).

COLLECTING DATA ABOUT THE CLIENT

The second step to clinical reasoning is gathering data about the client. Therapists use the clinical questions they developed to guide their collection of this information from a variety of sources in order to obtain a holistic view of the child. Pediatric clients will generally use an array of strategies and assessment tools in order to identify the child's strengths and needs. When using MOHO, the therapist should adopt a top-down approach (Coster, 1998) and consider first how to assess the child's occupational participation before moving on to assessing skill deficits. The Short Child Occupational Profile Evaluation (SCOPE) (Bowyer, Kramer, Kielhofner, Maziero-Barbosa, & Girolami, 2007; Bowyer, Ross, Schwartz, Kielhofner, & Kramer, 2005) is often used by therapists to start their process of data collection. Data for the SCOPE can be obtained from multiple sources and provide the therapist with an understanding of how the child's volition, habituation, skills, and environment support or inhibit participation. Using this tool may help the therapist understand which areas may warrant further evaluation.

Standardized assessment tools are very common in pediatric practice (Bagatell, Hartmann, & Meriano, 2013; Kramer et al., 2009). Depending on the practice setting, such tools may be required to establish eligibility for services (Bazyk & Cahill, 2015). However, a great deal of information can be ascertained from viewing the child in his or her natural environment. Certain practice settings, like the school systems and home-based early intervention, afford therapists such an opportunity. Therapists working in medical settings and clinics may not be able to observe the child in his or her natural circumstances. Regardless of practice setting, a comprehensive occupational therapy evaluation always includes the therapist viewing the child while he or she is engaging in occupation. The therapist might also interview the child's caregiver, ask the caregiver to complete a checklist, or review the child's records.

In addition to these methods, a therapist using MOHO to guide clinical reasoning should always consider how to gather information directly from the child. Depending on the child's age and condition, he or she may be able to provide a traditional self-report. Examples of MOHO assessment tools that provide an opportunity to collect a self-report include the Child Occupational Self-Assessment (COSA; Keller, Kafkes, Basu, Federico, & Kielhofner, 2005; Keller, Kafkes, & Kielhofner, 2005; Keller & Kielhofner, 2005) and the School Setting Interview (SSI; Hemmingsson, Egilson, Hoffman, & Kielhofner, 2005; Hemmingsson, Kottorp, & Bernspang, 2004). Other children, due to their communication and interaction skills, may not be able to provide a self-report. When that is the case, the occupational therapist may rely on systematic observations of the child during occupations. The Pediatric Volitional Questionnaire (PVQ; Anderson, Kielfhofner, & Lai, 2005; Basu, Kafkes, Schatz, Kiraly, & Kielhofner, 2008) is one example of an observation-based assessment tool that can be used with children with a wide range of abilities and conditions. Table 22-2 includes a list of pediatric MOHO assessment tools, the type of information that can be collected by using them, and the manner in which data are collected.

Table 22-2 Pediatric MOHO Assessment Tools

MOHO Assessment Tool	Type of Information Collected	Manner in Which Information Is Collected
Assessment of communication and interaction skills	Performance skills	Observation
Assessment of motor and process skills	Performance skills	Observation
Child occupational self-assessment	Values and competence	Self-report
Occupational therapy psychosocial assessment of learning	Students' adaption to the student role and associated demands	Observation
Pediatric interest profiles	Interests, perceived competence, participation	Self-report
Pediatric volitional questionnaire	Volition	Observation
Short child occupational profile evaluation	Volition, habituation, performance skills, influence of the environment	Observation, caregiver interviews, client interviews, review of records
School setting interview	Student–environment fit	Interviews with client

Based on the table originally presented in Forsyth and Kielhofner (2008).

DEVELOPING A CLINICAL HYPOTHESIS

The therapist should be able to construct a **clinical hypothesis** related to the child's occupational needs and their causes based on the answers they have formulated related to their guiding clinical questions. This clinical hypothesis should be framed around the major concepts related to MOHO and cover the major areas of occupation (i.e., play, education, work/volunteer, and self-care). As this is just a hypothesis, the therapist should review the hypothesis with the child's caregivers and, when possible, with the child. During this review more information may be gathered and this could lead to a refined hypothesis. In some cases, the therapist and the caregiver, or the child, might have a different view of why the child is experiencing occupational performance difficulties. The therapist needs to balance his or her perspectives with those of the client's and the caregiver's.

DEVELOPING INTERVENTION GOALS AND STRATEGIES

The therapist's clinical hypothesis will serve as a basis for the client's intervention goals, as well as the strategies the therapist will employ to help the client achieve these goals. As with the clinical questions and the selection of methods to gather data, the client's therapy goals should be directly related to the therapist's clinical hypothesis. For example, consider that a therapist asks clinical questions about a child's habituation and, through the process of assessment and hypothesis generation, determines that the child's afterschool routine inhibits his ability to get a restful night's sleep. The therapist would then establish a goal that is related to the cause of the identified problem, which is the child's unsupportive afterschool routine. The therapist's intervention would then be targeted at working with the child and the family to establish a supportive afterschool routine. The therapist would use the other information that is known about the child as a result of the clinical questions and the data gathering process to craft unique and responsive intervention strategies that would support the development of a positive routine.

MOHO Problem-Solver: Adam

Adam is a 19-year-old male who lives in a small town in the country. He has spastic quadriplegia. He attends high school and receives special education services, including assistive technology. He is able to operate his own wheelchair, but does not drive a car. He lives at home with his mother and twin brother. His other brother graduated from high school last year and is working at a mechanics shop in town and living with friends.

The school-based occupational therapist received a request for consultation to assist the special education team with developing a transition plan for Adam from high school. This transition was to take place in 2 years. The therapist was also charged with determining how assistive technology might be useful to Adam. The occupational therapist conducted a comprehensive occupational therapy evaluation guided by MOHO.

First, the therapist developed specific questions to find out about Adam's occupational desires and identity. Overall, the therapist wanted to gain an understanding of Adam's occupational identity by inquiring about the child's and family's sense of who he has been, is, and wishes to become in relation to family life, school, friendships, hobbies, and interests. The therapist used the SCOPE to collect the following information about Adam:

Volition

Adam enjoys people, always smiling when a friend walks by. He is difficult to understand but waves, says hello, and attempts to communicate. Adam likes cars, watching police shows, and being the center of attention. He enjoys going to school and especially his history and music classes. Adam stated he did not like math class and struggled with reading and writing. However, he enjoys books on tape. When asked what he wanted to be when he grew up, Adam stated "a policeman." Adam is fascinated with cars. He likes going to dances and hanging out with friends. He states he is "close with his brother."

Habituation

Adam is able to transfer from his bed to a wheelchair using a stand-pivot transfer; he gets himself dressed in the morning, with some assistance with fasteners. He eats independently with adapted feeding utensils after set up. He handles toileting independently. At school, Adam attends the special education classroom for the majority of his classes. He spends time after school with friends playing computer games, watching television, and socializing. He likes competitive sports.

Adam enjoys school events such as dances, and hopes to attend the prom.

Performance Capacity

Adam has spastic quadriplegia. He uses an electric wheelchair for mobility. He is able to stand and walk a few steps with difficulty. He is involved in the Special Olympics and enjoys the competition. He communicates verbally although he exhibits some articulation difficulties. Adam is able to hold objects in both hands using a gross grasp. His coordination and timing are imprecise. He uses an adapted keyboard to type responses for academics. Cognitively, Adam struggles with academics. He has difficulty paying attention to details. Socially, Adam shows a good sense of humor and has a core group of friends who enjoy his company.

Environment

Adam's home is wheelchair accessible and the school provides transportation to and from school and to school events as needed. His mother and brother are available to transport him to events as well. The town does not have accessible sidewalks and snow limits his mobility outside in the winter. The school offers a police training class through the sheriff's office.

The therapist used the above information to create an understanding of Adam's situation and as a basis for an intervention plan. The therapist described Adam's situation in terms of the interactions between volition, habituation, performance capacity, and environment. Adam's increased muscle tone in all four extremities and poor postural stability interfere with his engagement in physical activity. His poor coordination, timing, and strength interfere with work abilities for certain jobs (such as police work). Adam shows a desire to work as a policeman upon graduation; however, he shows physical difficulties interfering with this choice. Adam's strong volitional desires, social nature, cognitive abilities, and desire to give back to his community in addition to vocational resources at the school will allow him to learn work skills for the future. Adam would benefit from one-on-one mentoring to develop work habits.

The therapist determines that Adam's love for people and being the "center of attention" can be met in an office situation. Adam needs to learn some basic work habits and skills to work in an office setting but this could provide him with employment upon graduation. Adam may require assistive technology to perform in the workplace. He will benefit from a setting where he is supervised, provided with clear feedback, and allowed to socialize throughout the day. Furthermore, the school offers a police training program which appeals directly to his career aspiration. The program can be adapted to meet Adam's cognitive, physical, and social needs. The following therapy goals were created with Adam (and input from his family) after several sessions.

- Demonstrate effective work habits and routines to prepare for worker roles
- Participate in training program at sheriff's department to develop experience and establish self-efficacy and awareness of strengths
- Adapt work duties to match client's performance capacity (skills and abilities)
- Develop verbal communication skills for office work
- Use assistive technology to complete work routines as necessary
- Complete the requirements to graduate with a high school degree
- Receive positive evaluations from mentors at the vocational placement (Deputy Assistant)
- Become involved with community social group

Intervention

Adam will participate in the police training program to meet his educational needs and develop skills for future employment. He will work with a mentor and answer the phones, file, and assist with office duties. Assistive technology will be provided to allow Adam to successfully complete tasks. For example, Adam will use a built-up handled stapler; headset for phone; and adapted keyboard. Adam will receive specific and direct feedback regarding his performance on a regular basis. The occupational therapist will provide Adam with practice on social rules for the workplace through role playing. The therapist will consult with the police program to adjust the challenges or adapt tasks to encourage success. Each week, the therapist will review Adam's work performance with him to allow him to reflect and develop essential work skills. Adam will work with the speech therapist to more clearly articulate speech for work. The occupational therapist will reinforce articulation during all sessions. Overall, developing performance skills and a belief in one's skills will allow Adam to develop an occupational identity that will help him transition to worker roles of adulthood. Secondly, the occupational therapist will role play social situations to facilitate social relationships. Together, they will establish situations that allow Adam to engage in social interactions with an emphasis on groups or clubs in the community (for older teens).

MONITORING THE CLIENT'S PROGRESS IN THERAPY

Monitoring the client's progress in therapy happens on a regular basis and is used for various reasons. First, monitoring progress can help the therapist understand whether or not the clinical hypothesis can be accepted. Monitoring progress can also help to provide insights related to the child's engagement in the therapy process, as well as the influence of the child's caregivers on the therapy process. Finally, reviewing the client's progress can be used to refine the therapy strategies being used, refine the client's goals, or establish a basis for discharge from therapy services.

It is important that the therapist reviews the client's progress with the client, as well as with the client's caregivers. It is not uncommon for the therapist and the caregiver to have differing perspectives regarding the rate of the child's progress, the success of different intervention strategies, or the need for continued therapy. Engaging in an ongoing dialogue about progress may help the therapist to understand the child's and the caregiver's commitment to the therapy process. This dialogue also often serves as a foundational element to a strong therapeutic relationship. Providing accurate feedback is essential and doing so will help the child to develop a sense of his or her personal capacity. Actively talking about the gains made in therapy and celebrating them may help support a child's volitional development. Conversely, informing clients and their caregivers of slow progress and instances of regressions is also important. However, when possible, the therapist should consider the framing of this information so as not to disrupt the therapeutic relationship or inadvertently compromise the child's volition.

EVALUATING THERAPY OUTCOMES

Therapy outcomes are typically evaluated after a course of therapy has been completed. Generally, therapists will assess whether or not a client has achieved the stated therapy goals. In addition, the therapist may also readminister all or some of the assessment tools that were used during the initial data gathering phase. Some pediatric settings may require specific methods for reporting therapy outcomes. For example, a therapist working in an outpatient clinic setting might be asked to generate a discharge report and a therapist working in early intervention might be asked to develop a transition plan for when the child enters the school system. Regardless of setting, therapists using MOHO may frame their outcome documentation based on the major MOHO concepts and the clinical questions that they generated at the start of the occupational therapy process.

MOHO Problem-Solver: Mary

Mary is a friendly and social 17-year-old who attends high school. Mary was diagnosed with a moderate intellectual disability and a speech and language impairment when she was 8 years old. Mary has been receiving the majority of her education in self-contained special education classrooms since her diagnosis. As part of her transition plan, Mary's occupational therapist recently recommended that she begin taking an elective consumer science class with general education students. The occupational therapist believes that this experience will help prepare Mary for eventually attending community college classes. The rest of Mary's special education team agreed with this recommendation.

Mary's transition to the consumer science class did not go smoothly. For the first week of consumer science, Mary entered the classroom with her head down and walked to a far corner of the classroom. Mary sat alone and did not respond when the teacher called her name. Twice during class, Mary became tearful and began saying "go," indicating that she wanted to leave the room. A paraprofessional followed Mary to consumer science and attempted to sit with her to provide assistance. Mary refused the paraprofessional's assistance by turning her body away from her and shaking her head "no." After observing Mary in the consumer science class and again in her special education classroom, the occupational therapist determined that her occupational performance was supported when she had the opportunity to engage in peer interactions. Because Mary did not know anyone in the consumer science class and none of the students knew her, she did not have the opportunity to initiate or reciprocate any social interactions.

The occupational therapist recognized Mary's desire to interact with her peers, as well as her strengths associated with being friendly and social. The occupational therapist devised goals and strategies for the special education team to implement based on Mary's desire for social interaction. The focus of these goals was to introduce Mary to another student who would serve as a consumer science mentor. The mentor would serve as an ambassador to the other students in consumer science and help Mary make more connections. In addition, the mentor would serve as a model for when and how to follow the teacher's instructions. The occupational therapist believed that the addition of a peer mentor would help Mary to demonstrate her volition in consumer science class and help her to develop the habits and routines needed to support her eventual transition to community college.

The special education team worked to identify a peer that was strong in consumer science, friendly, and willing to support Mary. Sophia was selected to serve as Mary's mentor. The occupational therapist introduced Sophia and Mary and began to work with them on developing a routine for entering the consumer science classroom and getting settled into a workspace. The occupational therapist also coached Sophia on how best to provide short and simple verbal cues to Mary.

After several weeks, the occupational therapist spoke with Mary about her experience being in consumer science class. Mary was clearly pleased with being in the class.

Occupational therapist: How is consumer science going?

Mary: Good. I like Sophia. She helps me.

Occupational therapist: How does Sophia help you?

Mary: She tells me to open my book and smiles.

Occupational therapist: Sophia is friendly. Did you make any other friends in consumer science?

Mary: Sophia's friends are my friends. I'm friends with Christine and Megan too.

Occupational therapist: What did you learn in consumer science?

Mary: Me and Sophia made an omelet.

Occupational therapist: Did you like making the omelet?

Mary: I liked cracking the eggs. Sophia let me crack the eggs.

The special education team was pleased with Mary's success in consumer science class and Sophia enjoyed serving as Mary's peer mentor. After two more weeks of class, Sophia approached the occupational therapist and asked if she, rather than the paraprofessional, might be able to walk Mary to her next class. The occupational therapist brought this suggestion to the special education team and the team agreed that Sophia could walk Mary to the class that followed consumer science. The occupational therapist was pleased that Mary had the opportunity to interact with Sophia in the hallway during a passing period.

Conclusion

MOHO can be used by pediatric occupational therapy practitioners to guide every aspect of the occupational therapy process (i.e., screening, evaluation, intervention, progress monitoring, and discharge planning; AOTA, 2014). Using MOHO allows occupational therapy practitioners to construct a theory-driven therapeutic reasoning approach that is aligned with best practice. Using MOHO allows pediatric therapists to fully address the complex factors associated with a child's restricted or inhibited occupational performance and engagement.

MOHO Problem-Solver: Jack

Jack was referred to outpatient occupational therapy due to sensory processing concerns and difficulty with written expression. Jack's mother provided the occupational therapist with Jack's school records, including his recently completely multidisciplinary evaluation. His multidisciplinary evaluation included a report from the occupational therapist. In the report, Jack's school therapist indicated that he had average visual motor and visual perceptual skills and that he was frequently off task. The report also stated that Jack continued to struggle with written communication at school despite being instructed with an evidence-based handwriting curriculum. Recently, Jack had undergone extensive testing to determine his academic needs. Prior to the first occupational therapy session, the therapist interviewed Jack and Jack's mom separately.

Interview with Jack's Mom

Prior to the first occupational therapy session, the therapist interviewed Jack's mom.

Occupational therapist: What are you and Jack hoping to get out of outpatient occupational therapy?

Jack's Mom: Jack hates handwriting. He's beginning to feel bad about himself because of the quality of his written work. He used to love school and now I have to drag him out of bed to get him to go. His teacher thinks he has an attention problem and his school OT thinks he has a sensory problem. I think he just feels like quitting. He's stopped turning in homework and I know that he understands the material. I just want him to like school again.

Interview with Jack

Occupational therapist: Jack, why do you think your mom brought you to see me?

Jack: I hate handwriting. I'm bad at it. My teacher makes me redo my work all the time and I hate it. It's so boring. I do have a little trouble with cursive, but everyone's handwriting is sloppy. I guess I thought I was like everybody else, but my teacher thinks I'm not good at it at all. They think I don't pay attention, but I'm just bored.

Occupational therapist: What has your OT at school tried with you so far?

Jack: Practice. We just practice and practice all the time. I hate that too. I could be at recess and instead I'm writing. Then, when I get back to class, I want to run around and I can't. I always get in trouble on the days that I miss recess.

Applying MOHO to Jack's Case

Given the information that was collected from Jack and his mom, the occupational therapist developed an assessment plan guided by the Model of Human Occupation. MOHO was used to discover Jack's strengths and prioritize his needs. In using MOHO, the focus of Jack's occupational therapy intervention expanded from being one strictly focused on increasing legible written communication to one that focused on Jack as an occupational being.

The occupational therapist devised a list of clinical questions to collect more data about Jack from him and his mom. The occupational therapist also used the Pediatric Volitional Questionnaire to guide observations.

Table 22-3 presents a list of findings from the occupational therapist's evaluation of Jack.

Follow-up Questions: Use the Preceding Case Example to Answer the Following Questions

1. What other pediatric MOHO assessment tools might the occupational therapist use to gather more information about Jack? What information would the additional tool or tools provide to the therapist? How might this information inform intervention planning?
2. What other information about the environment would a MOHO-based occupational therapist want to know in order to plan intervention?
3. Describe three recommendations that the occupational therapist could make to support Jack with handwriting at school. Align the recommendations to MOHO concepts.
4. What other intervention approaches could be used in conjunction with MOHO to support Jack?

Table 22-3 Jack's Evaluation Findings

MOHO Concept	Data about Jack
Occupational identity	Jack has a strong occupational identity. He identifies with being part of a loving family in which he is both a son and a brother. Jack also identifies with the role of friend, baseball player, day camper, and student. Jack expressed pride in being part of a "smart family" and shared that he knows that he is smart too. Jack indicated that he wanted to be a chemical scientist or an engineer.
Occupational competence	In general, Jack experiences occupational competence in many of his roles. Jack feels that he can do the things that he needs and wants to do to be a good big brother (like play with and look after his little sister) and a good son (listen to mom and dad). Jack also expressed feelings of competence related to playing sports (e.g., baseball) and swimming. Jack makes fewer positive statements related to his occupational competence when he talks about his school performance. Jack regularly states that he has to "try harder" and "try to work better."
Performance skills	**Motor** Jack is able to grip objects without finger slips. He is able to coordinate two or more body parts together to stabilize and manipulate objects. Jack has some difficulty with regulating and grading force on his writing utensils. He may benefit from writing on top of a notebook and practicing with mechanical pencils. Jack may also benefit from hand stretch breaks when being asked to produce long writing assignments as his hand may ache after several minutes of writing. Jack has some difficulty with regulating speed while writing. Jack tends to write quickly and needs cues to slow down. When writing quickly, Jack often skips letters and needs reminders to go back and fill them in. **Process** Jack requires some encouragement to continue handwriting tasks. Jack logically sequences his stories when he writes. He is also able to complete graphic organizers in a logical fashion. Jack needs some assistance to spatially arrange information on a page. He sometimes tries to squeeze letters or words into spaces that cannot accommodate them. Jack responds better to proactive cuing (e.g., "The end of your page is coming up, maybe you want to go down to the next line") versus reactive corrections (e.g., "You squeezed your word in and now I can't tell what it says. Would you please erase it and move down to the next line?"). Jack sometimes requires cues to notice/respond to feedback regarding task progression (e.g., alignment of words on a page). However, when his attention is drawn to the situation, he is able to correct it independently. Jack is able to change his work environment in anticipation of or in response to problems that arise. Jack is beginning to anticipate problems that arise related to his written communication.
Volition	The Pediatric Volitional Questionnaire was used to examine Jack's volition during early OT sessions. Jack demonstrates hesitancy with staying engaged, demonstrating task directedness, expressing mastery pleasure, and practicing skills.
Habituation	Jack's habits around written communication are not well established. Jack sometimes begins a worksheet in the middle of the page because he [in his words] "likes that question." Jack was also observed to form letters inconsistently, which reduces automaticity with writing.
Environment	Jack is in his last quarter of 1st grade. Jack is in the advanced reading and math groups. There are 24 other children in Jack's class. Jack uses a green folder to take papers to and from school. The teacher sets aside time on a weekly basis for the students to clean out their desks. Jack's desk is somewhat unkempt at times, but this is in keeping with the rest of his peers. Jack has identified several friends in his class. He sometimes gets into trouble for talking to his friends during quiet work time. At home, Jack does his homework at the kitchen table and usually when his mother is preparing dinner.

Chapter 22 Quiz Questions

1. Describe the therapeutic reasoning process that MOHO-based therapists use when working with children.
2. Write a list of MOHO-based clinical questions that could be used to gather more information about Lisa from the first MOHO Problem-Solver case in this chapter.
3. Name three pediatric MOHO assessment tools and describe how they can be used by pediatric therapists in practice.

HOMEWORK ASSIGNMENT

Use MOHO concepts to develop a clinical question interview guide for a child you know. Conduct the interview with the child. Document the child's answers. Then, write a reflection on how you might reframe your questions. Also consider other MOHO-based pediatric assessment tools that you could use to gain more information about the child.

thePoint® For additional resources and exercises, visit http://thePoint.lww.com

Key Terms

Clinical hypothesis: The clinical hypothesis is the occupational therapist's explanation of why the child is having occupational performance difficulties.

Therapeutic reasoning: The process the occupational therapist goes through to understand the child in terms of his or her own sense of occupational identity, occupational competence, volition, and habituation. In addition, the therapist considers the child's perspectives related to occupational performance in the context of his or her own typically occurring environments.

REFERENCES

American Occupational Therapy Association. (2014). Occupational therapy practice framework: Domain and process (3rd ed.). *The American Journal of Occupational Therapy, 68*(Suppl. 1), S1–S48. doi:10.5014/ajot.2014.682006

Anderson, S., Kielhofner, G., & Lai, J. (2005). An examination of the measurement properties of the Pediatric Volitional Questionnaire. *Physical & Occupational Therapy in Pediatrics, 25*(1), 39–57. doi:10.1080/j006v25n01_04

Ashburner, J., Rodger, S., Ziviani, J., & Jones, J. (2014). Occupational therapy services for people with autism spectrum disorders: current state of play, use of evidence and future learning priorities. *Australian Occupational Therapy Journal, 61*(2), 110–120. doi:10.1111/1440-1630.12083

Bagatell, N., Hartmann, K., & Meriano, C. (2013). The evaluation process and assessment choice of pediatric practitioners in the Northeast United States. *Journal of Occupational Therapy, Schools, and Early Intervention, 6*(2), 143–157. doi:10.1080/19411243.2012.750546

Basu, S., Kafkes, A., Schatz, R., Kiraly, A., & Kielhofner, G. (2008). *A user's manual for the Pediatric Volitional Questionnaire* [Version 2.1]. Chicago: MOHO Clearinghouse, Department of Occupational Therapy, College of Applied Health Sciences, University of Illinois at Chicago.

Bazyk, S., & Cahill, S. (2015). School-based occupational therapy. In J. Case-Smith & J. O'Brien (Eds.), *Occupational therapy for children* (7th ed., pp. 664–703). St. Louis, MO: Elsevier.

Bowyer, P., Kramer, J., Kielhofner, G., Maziero-Barbosa, V., & Girolami, G. (2007). The measurement properties of the Sort Child Occupational Profile (SCOPE). *Physical & Occupational Therapy in Pediatrics, 27*(4), 67–85. doi:10.1080/J006v27n04_05

Bowyer, P., Ross, M., Schwartz, O., Kielhofner, G., & Kramer, J. (2005). *The Short Child Occupational Profile (SCOPE)* [Version 2.1]. Chicago: Model of Human Occupation Clearinghouse, Department of Occupational Therapy, College of Applied Health Sciences, University of Illinois at Chicago.

Cahill, S., & Lopez-Reyna, N. (2013). Expanding school-based problem-solving teams to include occupational therapists. *Journal of Occupational Therapy, Schools, and Early Intervention, 6*(4), 314–325. doi:10.1080/19411243.2013.860763

Coster, W. (1998). Occupation-centered assessment of children. *The American Journal of Occupational Therapy, 52*(5), 337–344. doi:10.5014/ajot.52.5.337

Fisher, A. (2013). Occupation-centered, occupation-based, occupation-focused: Same, same, or different? *Scandinavian Journal of Occupational Therapy, 20*(3), 162–173. doi:10.3109/11038128.2012.754492

Forsyth, K., & Kielhofner, G. (2008). Therapeutic reasoning: Planning, implementing, and evaluating the outcomes of therapy. In G. Kielhofner (Ed.), *Model of Human Occupation: Theory and application* (pp. 143–154). Baltimore, MD: Lippincott Williams & Wilkins.

Hemmingsson, H., Egilson, S., Hoffman, O., & Kielhofner, G., (2005). *School Setting Interview (SSI)* [Version 3.0]. Nacka, Sweden: Swedish Association of Occupational Therapists.

Hemmingsson, H., Kottorp, A., & Bernspang, B. (2004). Validity of the School Setting Interview: An assessment of the student-environment fit. *Scandinavian Journal of Occupational Therapy, 11*(4), 171–178. doi:10.1080/11038120410020683

Humphry, R. (2002). Young children's occupations: Explicating the dynamics of developmental processes. *The American Journal of Occupational Therapy, 56*(2), 171–179. doi:10.5014/ajot.56.2.171

Keller, J., Kafkes, A., Basu, S., Federico, J., & Kielhofner, G. (2005). The Child Occupational Self-Assessment (COSA) [Version 2.1]. Chicago: Model of Human Occupation Clearinghouse,

Department of Occupational Therapy, College of Applied Health Sciences, University of Illinois at Chicago.
Keller, J., Kafkes, A., & Kielhofner, G. (2005). Psychometric characteristics of the Child Occupational Self-Assessment (COSA), Part 1: An initial examination of psychometric properties. Scandinavian Journal of Occupational Therapy, *12*(3), 118–127. doi:10.1080/11038120510031752
Keller, J., & Kielhofner, G. (2005). Psychometric characteristics of the Child Occupational Self-Assessment (COSA), Part 2: Refining the psychometric properties. *Scandinavian Journal of Occupational Therapy, 12*(4), 147–158. doi:10.1080/11038120510031761
Kielhofner, G. (2008). *Model of Human Occupation: Theory and application* (4th ed.). Baltimore, MD: Lippincott Williams & Wilkins.
Kiraly-Alvarez, A. (2015). Assessing volition in pediatrics: Using the Volitional Questionnaire and the Pediatric Volitional Questionnaire. *Open Journal of Occupational Therapy, 3*(3), Article 7. doi:10.15453/2168-6408.1176
Kramer, J., Bowyer, P., O'Brien, J., Kielhofner, G., & Maziero-Barbosa, V. (2009). How interdisciplinary pediatric practitioners choose assessments. *Canadian Journal of Occupational Therapy, 76*(1), 56–64. doi:10.1177/000841740907600114
Lee, J. (2010). Achieving best practice: A review of evidence linked to occupation-focused practice models. *Occupational Therapy in Health Care, 24*(3), 206–222. doi:10.3109/07380577.2010.483270
Lee, S., Taylor, R., Kielhofner, G., & Fisher, G. (2008). Theory use in practice: A national survey of therapists who use the Model of Human Occupation. *The American Journal of Occupational Therapy, 62*(1), 106–117.
Miller Kuhaneck, H., Tanta, K., Coombs, A., & Pannone, H. (2013). A survey of pediatric occupational therapists' use of play. *Journal of Occupational Therapy, Schools, & Early Intervention, 6*(3), 213–227. doi:10.1080/19411243.2013.850940
O'Brien, J., Asselin, E., Fortier, K., Janzegers, R., Lagueux, B., & Silcox, C. (2010). Using therapeutic reasoning to apply the Model of Human Occupation in pediatric occupational therapy practice. *Journal of Occupational Therapy, Schools & Early Intervention, 3*, 348–365. doi:10.1080/19411243.2010.544966
Spencer, K., Turkett, A., Vaughan, R., & Koenig, S. (2006). School-based practice patterns: A survey of occupational therapists in Colorado. *The American Journal of Occupational Therapy, 60*(1), 81–91. doi:10.5014/ajot.60.1.81

PRACTICING WITH THE MODEL OF HUMAN OCCUPATION

PART V

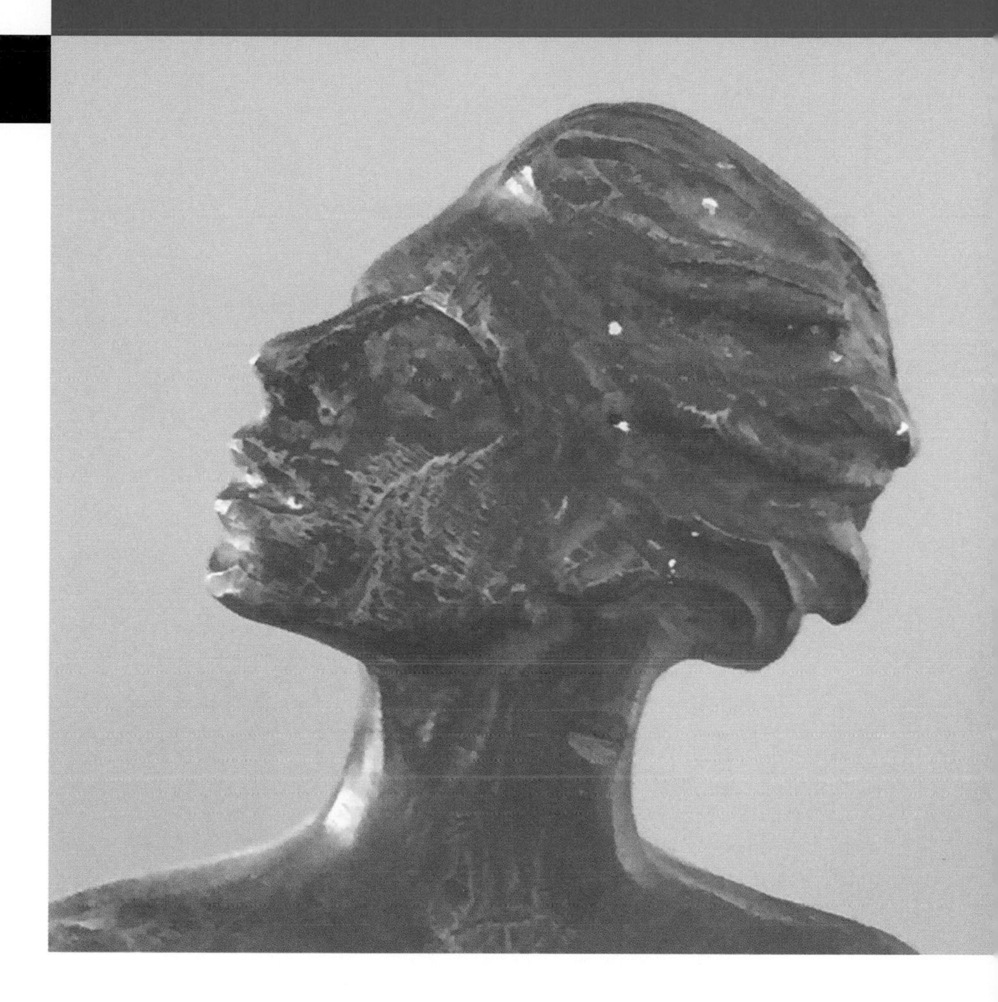

Applying the Model of Human Occupation to Vocational Rehabilitation

Jan Sandqvist and Elin Ekbladh

CHAPTER 23

EXPECTED LEARNING OUTCOMES

Upon completion of this chapter, readers will be able to:

1. The assessment of work ability/functioning is a complex task for the occupational therapist (OT), requiring the use of several assessments, each with a different focus.
2. The assessor should focus on the individual as well as the environment when assessing work ability and when planning interventions.
3. Model of human occupation (MOHO)-based instruments are an important aid in the process of intervention planning.
4. MOHO offers a unique theoretical foundation for interpretation of assessment results and helps the user integrate different work-related variables in an informed approach to therapeutic reasoning.

Occupational Therapy and Vocational Rehabilitation

Daily life consists of engaging in performance of activities required by various occupations (Harvey & Pentland, 2004). The concept of occupation has a central place within occupational therapy practice, theory development, and research. Occupation relates to doing, but there is no confirmed definition of the concept in the field. In other disciplines, occupation often refers to paid work (Persson, 2001), while occupation in occupational therapy concerns all occupations in the domain of play, self-care, and **work** (paid and unpaid). The doing of occupations can be subdivided into the following three levels: occupational participation, occupational performance, and skills. "Occupational participation" refers to overall engagement in play, self-care, and work and is part of the individual's sociocultural context and is desired and/or necessary to one's well-being. "Occupational performance" refers to the doing of tasks that are part of the specific occupation, and 'skills' are the observable purposeful actions that are carried out within the occupational performance (Kielhofner, 2008). The actual occupational performance depends upon the interaction between the characteristics of the individual, the occupations the individual engages in, and the environment (Law & Baum, 2005).

A person's ability to perform different kinds of activities in life is central in occupational therapy (Law, 1995, Smith, 1992), and one of these activities is work (Brintnell, Harvey-Krefting, Rosenfeld, & Friesen, 1998). Then, what is "work?" The term "work" is usually used to mean paid employment. The opposite is then play, rest, free time, and recreation (Wilcock, 1998). However, to have only one definition of work is not necessary or desirable. Various definitions of work can be used for different purposes and situations (Karlsson, 1986). A broader definition of work is presented by Karlsson (Karlsson, 1986, p. 119): "Work is the doing in the sphere of necessity." Thus, this broader definition includes the work done outside a paid employment such as household duties. A person's paid employment can be largely affected by the housework situation. A person may have major expectations from the family, for example, with respect to specific housework duties. Therefore, it is always important to consider the total amount of workload for a person—both paid employment as well as other obligations in life such as housework – when assessing a client's work functioning.

Work fulfils a central and valued role in people's everyday lives (Brown et al., 2001), and besides sleep, it is the activity that consumes most time per day in adult life (Harvey & Pentland, 2004). To be working has practical purposes in the form of economic possibilities and symbolic functions since it implies the ability to participate in society in a socially accepted manner. In the early 40s, Marie Jahoda (1942) conducted research on incentives to work. She found that work had other important meanings besides economic compensation, such as providing a structure for how to handle time, providing daily social contacts with others outside the family, giving social status and identity, and offering the possibility of taking part in common strivings (Jahoda, 1942). Her findings that work has other meanings than solely economic ones is still relevant at the beginning of the 21st century (Brown et al., 2001; Ekbladh et al., 2010; Lindin, Roos, & Björklund, 2007; Polanyi & Tompa, 2004; Svensson, Müssener, & Alexanderson, 2006). Work can have positive health implications for the individual as a result of well-functioning social interactions in the workplace (Lindin et al., 2007; Polanyi & Tompa, 2004), and the worker role contributes significantly to an individual's identity, sense of meaning, and satisfaction in life (Brown et al., 2001; Ekbladh et al., 2010; Svensson et al., 2006).

The concept of work has been fundamental to occupational therapy theory and practice ever since the birth of the profession in the beginning of the 20th century (Brintnell, 1998; Harvey-Krefting, 1985; Holmes, 1985; Jacobs, 1991; Lohman & Peyton, 1997; McCracken, 1991; McCuaig & Iwama, 1989; Schmidt & Walker, 1992). Furthermore, the term occupational therapy indicates that the profession works with the rehabilitation of disabled workers (Brintnell, 1998). For example, Karen Jacobs (Jacobs, 1991) states that:

> Work is at the heart of the philosophy and practice of occupational therapy. In its broadest sense, work, as productive activity, is the concern in almost all therapy. (p. 11)

The last decades have shown a great need for vocational rehabilitation when persons' **work functioning**[1] has been reduced by injury or illness, resulting in high levels of sickness absence and disability pension (Hansen, Edlund, & Bränholm, 2005; Hansen, Edlund, & Henningsson 2006; Marnetoft, Selander, Bergroth, & Ekholm, 2001; Selander & Marnetoft, 2005; Stubbs & Deaner, 2005; WHO, 2000). When an individual's ability to work is reduced, there are social and economic consequences for both the individual and the society. Therefore, reduced work functioning is not only a medical problem but also a socioeconomic one (Hansen et al., 2006, Kielhofner, 1993; Lechner, Roth, & Straaton, 1991; Marnetoft et al., 2001; McCracken, 1991).

Vocational rehabilitation provides medical, psychological, social, and/or vocational interventions for people with functional impairment to help them recover the best possible functional capacity and to sustain it. This type of rehabilitation also creates circumstances so a person can find, obtain, and/or retain a job. The aim of "obtaining and retaining a job" must be viewed in relation to the job market situation. Because functional impairment varies according to the capabilities of the individual, services and competencies need to be tailored to the varying needs of the clients (Höök & Grimby, 2001; Vahlne, Bergroth, & Ekholm, 2006). Vocational rehabilitation is a complex process and often involves, apart from the client, various professionals and rehabilitation actors. For the employed, the rehabilitation actors who usually participate in the vocational rehabilitation process include the employer, medical professionals, and officers from a social insurance office. For unemployed persons, the previously named actors, as well as representatives from the public employment services office, and sometimes social workers from the social services, participate in the vocational rehabilitation process (Jakobsson, Bergroth, Shüldt, & Ekholm, 2005).

OTs can play a major role in the vocational rehabilitation process through the assessment and rehabilitation of persons with reduced work functioning (Deen, Gibson, & Strong, 2002; Gibson & Strong, 2003; Holmes, 1985; Jundt & King, 1999; Keough & Fisher, 2001; Lysaght, 2004). To facilitate return to work or prevent loss of work, the use of multidisciplinary interventions is a prerequisite. In this area, OTs represent a professional group (Gobelet, Luthi, Al-Khodairy, & Chamberlain, 2007) that can make a valuable contribution to the rehabilitation process (Jackson, Harkess, & Ellis, 2004; Keough & Fisher, 2001; Thurgood & Frank, 2007).

ASSESSMENT OF WORK FUNCTIONING

To sufficiently understand an individual's work functioning, it is not enough to assess the efficiency and appropriateness of an individual's work performance. It is also necessary to find out *why* the person functions in a certain way. To find the answers to these questions, there are several factors that must be considered. These factors could be *personal*, *environmental*, or *temporal* (Sandqvist & Henriksson, 2004).

Personal factors can be both physical and psychological. Research has identified the impact of a number of personal factors. In addition, a number of *environmental factors* affect an individual's work functioning (Corner, Kielhofner, & Lin, 1997). They can be divided into two groups: environmental factors related to working life and environmental factors related to private life (Table 23-1). By assessing personal and environmental factors, an assessor may gain a better understanding of the individual's present work situation. However, an individual's ability to work may also be affected by *temporal factors* (Table 23-1). The

[1] In this chapter, *work functioning* is an umbrella term for all forms of work-related functioning and includes functioning in different dimensions and on different levels—body, individual, and society levels.

Table 23-1 Work Functioning in Comparison with the ICF

Work Functioning	ICF
Work participation[a]: The person's ability and possibility to fulfill a worker role and acquire or maintain/retain a work position in society.	Participation (society level)
Work performance[a] (including working skills): The ability to satisfactorily handle and carry out different work activities and tasks.	Activities (individual level)
Individual capacity[a]: Different physical and psychological attributes that enable the person to perform work tasks and activities, e.g., muscle strength, joint motion, sensibility, memory, and cardiopulmonary functions.	Body functions and structures (body level)

[a]Work functioning.
From Sandqvist and Henriksson, 2004.

client's past experiences and expectations about the future could also influence the client's current work conditions. His or her earlier work experience, work history, education, and other life experiences could greatly affect his or her present ability to work (Kaplan & Kielhofner, 1989; Söderback & Jacobs, 2000). When assessing personnel, it is important for an assessor to consider the individual's hopes and expectations for his or her future work situation and his or her larger life goals and beliefs about his or her own work functioning in the future. The constant changing demands of some work places or the general condition of the labor market (Kielhofner et al., 1999; Westmorland, Zeytinoglu, Pringle, Denton, & Chouinard, 1998) also influence an individual's future work prospects.

An assessment of work functioning can affect an individual on many levels and his or her whole life situation. (Kielhofner, 1993; Lechner et al., 1991). Gary Kielhofner (1993) explained why a reliable assessment of work functioning is important:

> . . .functional assessment is often used to determine what freedoms a person will and will not have, what roles he or she may take on, what activities he or she may do, and what benefits or resources he or she will receive. (p. 248)

There are several reasons why gaining an understanding of work functioning may be problematic as it is a multidimensional concept that concerns a relationship between several elements. Sandqvist and Henriksson (2004) identify various elements of work functioning. One of these elements is the different dimensions of work functioning: (1) **work participation** that pertains to society, (2) **work performance** that pertains to the individual, and (3) **individual capacity** that pertains to physical and psychological functioning. The dimensions of functioning were also related to the International Classification of Functioning, Disability, and Health (ICF) (WHO, 2001; Table 23-1). The ICF provides a unified language and framework for the description of human functioning and disability as an important component of health. It classifies functioning and disability according to an individual's life circumstances. The ICF organizes information into two dimensions: body functions and structures, and activities and participation. The body functions and structures dimension refers to the physiological or psychological functions of body systems and the anatomical parts of the body such as organs, limbs, and their components. The activity and participation dimension refers to the performance of tasks or actions by an individual and to the individual's ability to function in various life areas (WHO, 2001).

Furthermore, it is possible to outline and relate different dimensions of functioning presented in various conceptual frameworks: (a) work-related assessments (Innes & Straker, 1998a), (b) Lohman and Peyton's conceptual models of practice (i.e., the medical model, the prevocational model, and the biopsychosocial model) (Lohman & Peyton, 1997), (c) WHO's ICF (WHO, 2001), (d) a model of human occupation, and (e) specified rehabilitation areas (Table 23-2).

Because work assessments are complex, there is confusion over work assessment concepts. One of the concepts causing confusion is *work ability* (Franche & Krause, 2002; Innes & Straker, 1998a, 1998b). In an analysis of the concept of work ability, mainly from a health perspective, Tengland (2006) suggests that work ability could be divided into *general work ability* and *specific work ability*. The *general work ability* refers to a person's ability to perform any kind of work, work that any person at the same age and of the same sex could manage in an acceptable work environment. The *specific work ability* refers to a person's ability to manage the demands of a specific work in an acceptable work environment.

Table 23-2 Comparison of Concepts in Different Conceptual Frameworks

"Work Related Assessments—Individual Factors"	"Conceptual Models of Practice"	ICF	Model of Human Occupation	Rehabilitation Areas
Role	The biopsychosocial model	Participation (society level)	Participation	Vocational rehabilitation
Activity, task, skill	The prevocational model	Activities (individual level)	Performance (including skills)	Prevocational rehabilitation
Body system	The medical model	Body functions and structures (body level)	Performance capacity	Medical rehabilitation

Furthermore, Tengland points out that work ability could be seen as connected to the individual in relation to an acceptable environment. According to Tengland (2006), it is reasonable to understand work ability as something placed within the individual, as the work ability determines whether a person is entitled to compensation from the sickness insurance system. The work environment is considered to be something outside the individual and creates a platform for work-related actions.

Another concept worth considering when assessing work functioning is *employability*. Employability is conceptualized as a form of work-specific active adaptability that enables a person to identify and realize career opportunities (Fugate, Kinicki, & Ashfort, 2004). Having employability does not assure actual employment for the individual, but the concept focuses on the individual's likelihood of gaining employment. An individual is employable to the extent that he or she can effectively handle personal factors and manage environmental demands. The authors Fugate et al. (2004) attach great importance to the influence of individual characteristics in the person's adaptation to a work situation. According to Fugate et al. (2004), three component dimensions constitute employability: *career identity*, *personal adaptability*, and *social and human capital*.

Career identity represents a person's career experiences and aspirations and may include the following aspects: goals, hopes, and fears; values, beliefs, and norms; and interaction styles. Career identity refers to how people define themselves in a particular work context.

Personal adaptability refers to the individual's ability to adapt to changing demands in a work situation.

Social and human capital refers to the goodwill inherent in social networks (e.g., at a workplace) and employees' ability to make use of their unique resources to realize opportunities in the workplace. Human capital factors include age and education, work experience and training, and cognitive ability.

Similar to Tengland (2006), Fugate et al. (2004) claim that the concept of employability is closely connected to individual characteristics. However, it is reasonable to argue that an individual's work ability as well as employability, to a great extent, are affected by the contextual circumstances that exist at the time of an assessment.

Is it possible to arrange the concepts general work ability, specific work ability, and employability in relation to each other and in relation to other conceptual frameworks and concepts? In an attempt to do so, Table 23-3 was constructed to serve as a foundation for further discussion about the concepts and their relation to assessment of work functioning (Sandqvist & Henriksson, 2004).

ASSESSMENT IN OCCUPATIONAL THERAPY PRACTICE

Occupational therapy aims to maximize the client's ability to engage in valued occupations. An ideal way in which OTs can conceptualize client's difficulties and shape and evaluate intervention in a structured and theoretical manner is by using conceptual models of practice (Duncan, 2006). Conceptual practice models in occupational therapy focus on explaining clients' occupational problems such as how people choose, experience, and engage in occupations. To be able to explain occupational problems and guide practice, the models need to be built on an interdisciplinary base, have a technology which supports applying the model into practice, and must have been tested through research. Assessments in the form of gathering and analyzing data about the phenomenon addressed by the model are an important way to apply models into practice (Kielhofner, 2004). Assessment instruments in occupational therapy are used to improve clinical decisions. Information gathered through assessment instruments helps OTs to design interventions and evaluate outcomes, and it enables the OT to include the client in the reasoning about selecting the most compatible and effective intervention for the unique individual. Thus, a valid assessment process is essential in providing effective occupational therapy (Dunn, 2005).

Table 23-3 The Concepts *General Work Ability, Specific Work Ability*, and *Employability* in Relation to Some Conceptual Frameworks

Dimensions of Work Functioning	Concepts Describing Levels of Client Performance	Environment	Financial Compensation from Society Due to Loss of Earnings	ICF
Work participation[a]: The person's ability and possibility to fulfill a worker role and acquire or maintain/retain a work position in society.	Employability	Regular labor market	Unemployment compensation	Participation (society level)
Work performance[a] (including Working skills): The ability to satisfactorily handle and carry out different work activities and tasks.	Specific work ability General work ability	Actual/realistic workplace Artificial work context	Sickness compensation	Activities (individual level)
Individual capacity[a]: Different physical and psychological attributes that enable the person to perform work tasks and activities, e.g., muscle strength, joint motion, sensibility, memory, and cardiopulmonary functions.	Work capacity	Clinic (medical rehabilitation)	Sickness compensation	Body functions and structures (body level)

[a]Work functioning.

ASSESSMENT IN VOCATIONAL REHABILITATION

Assessment is everywhere in vocational rehabilitation and plays an important role in the return-to-work process (Gobelet et al., 2007; Matheson, Kaskutas, McCowan, & Webb, 2001). It aims to help people with disabilities to find, return to, or remain in work (Jackson et al., 2004). In fact, many interventions for clients are based on information yielded by some kind of assessment instrument (Matheson, 2001; Pransky & Dempsey, 2004; Strong et al., 2004). Assessment involves the collection, appraisal, and classification of gathered information, usually in an organized manner using an assessment instrument (formal assessment). Such methods or tools for collecting information include observation, interview, and self-report (Law & Baum, 2005). Objective assessments assess work ability from an outside perspective and are often gathered by professionals by observation. Subjective assessments assess work ability from an inside perspective, and information is often gathered by self-reports or interviews. Optimally, a combination of objective as well as subjective assessments should be used for assessment in vocational rehabilitation (Sandqvist & Henriksson, 2004; Shaw, Segal, Polatajko, & Harburn, et al., 2002).

Then, what is an assessment instrument? In this application, one can define an instrument as the device that an assessor uses to collect data and interpret information (Law & Baum, 2005; Polit & Beck, 2004). Assessment instruments are developed and tested to ensure that they can be applied consistently and gather valid and reliable information (Law & Baum, 2005).

Assessment instruments in vocational rehabilitation inform us about a wide range of things – from a person's beliefs and expectations about work and how an individual performs a work task to the demands of a work setting on a client (Corner et al., 1997; Ekbladh, Haglund, & Thorell, 2004; Kielhofner et al., 1999; Linddahl, Norrby, & Bellner, 2003; Sandqvist, Törnquist, & Henriksson, 2006; Velozo et al., 1999). Often this information is expressed as numbers, giving it an air of objectivity and trustworthiness. Converting concepts to numbers also generates a need for expert interpretation, giving the information a certain authority. These qualities have led assessors to rely on assessment instruments for credible and useful information.

Although vocational rehabilitation professionals use assessment instruments to develop a course of intervention for clients (Matheson, Isernhagen, & Hart, 1998; Pransky & Dempsey, 2004), evidence suggests that inconsistent assessment practice can arise from problems associated with the design, administration, and interpretation of work-related assessments (Travis, 2002). Accurate assessment helps disabled workers return to suitable employment or receive other adequate interventions. Unreliable and inadequate assessment instruments may complicate the rehabilitation process and result in immediate and latent health issues and socioeconomic consequences for workers, their employers, and society (Lechner et al., 1991; Matheson, 2001; Travis, 2002). To improve consistency in the assessment process and accuracy in assessment outcomes, rehabilitation professionals should use valid, reliable, and useful assessment instruments (Innes & Straker, 1999a, 1999b; Pransky & Dempsey, 2004; Schult, Söderback, & Jacobs, 2000; Travis, 2002).

PSYCHOMETRIC PROPERTIES OF RELEVANCE FOR WORK-RELATED ASSESSMENTS

Essential psychometric properties in work-related assessment instruments are *validity*, *reliability*, and *utility* (Innes & Straker, 2003). To be able to claim with acceptable certainty that an instrument is valid or reliable, it is necessary to examine several different forms of validity and reliability (Innes & Straker, 1999a; 1999b).

Validity is the degree to which an instrument measures what it is intended to measure (Dimitrov, Rumrill, Fitzgerald, & Hennessey, 2001; Gross, 2004, Innes & Straker, 1999a; McDowell & Newell, 1996; Polit & Beck, 2004). In general terms, it refers to the extent to which assessments lead to correct and meaningful interpretations (Dimitrov et al., 2001). Validity refers to the results of an assessment and how they are interpreted, not to the instrument itself (Innes & Straker, 1999a; Sim & Arnell, 1993). Successfully determining a disabled worker's ability to return to work performing suitable tasks is based on a valid interpretation of assessment results (Innes & Straker, 1999a). Validity is considered the most important characteristic of an assessment instrument (Benson & Schell, 1997; Clark & Watson, 1995; Dimitrov et al., 2001). Furthermore, a single study is not sufficient to determine an assessment's validity. This implies that multiple studies of various forms of validity are required (Benson & Schell, 1997; Innes & Straker, 1999a; McDowell & Newell, 1996). Validation is considered a continual process. Thus, for an instrument to remain valid over time, its validity must be reestablished periodically (Benson & Schell, 1997).

All forms of validity are appropriate for work-related assessments (Innes & Straker, 1999a). However, of the various forms of validity, *face*, *content*, *construct*, and *criterion-related* (*predictive* and *concurrent*) have been judged most relevant (Gross, 2004; Innes & Straker, 1999a; Velozo, 1993).

Face validity is evident when an assessment appears to measure what it intends to measure (Innes & Straker, 1999a; Polit & Beck, 2004; Portney & Watkins, 1993). It can be seen as the general relevance of an instrument to the overall purpose of an assessment (Innes & Straker, 1999a). Face validity can be established by a panel or group of experts who examine the assessment and reach a consensus that it does or does not represent a particular assessment domain (Dane, 1990). In addition, face validity can also be established by clients, therapists, and consumers of test results, such as an employer (Innes & Straker, 1999a). Face validity is considered the most basic and least rigorous form of validity, and there are no statistical measures or standards for determining whether an instrument has sufficient face validity (Dunn, 1989; Portney & Watkins, 1993). However, some qualitative interpretation can be made indicating whether good, moderate, or poor face validity exists (Innes & Straker, 1999a). Therefore, it is not sufficient to only have evidence of an instrument's face validity. Other forms of validity must also be established to determine the validity of an instrument. However, it is important to establish face validity for an assessment instrument. If not, users of the instrument may consider the instrument irrelevant and inadequate (Innes & Straker, 1999a; Portney & Watkins, 1993).

Content validity is the degree to which assessment items represent the assessment domain the instrument is intended to measure. Content validity is usually established by a panel of experts who examine the relationship between the purpose of the instrument and its content—the assessment items (Johnston et al., 1992; Thorn & Deitz, 1989). Content validity is not usually indicated by a statistical measure; rather it is inferred from judgments of experts (Dunn, 1989). It considers whether the test incorporates a sample of assessment items representing the assessment domain in question (Innes & Straker, 1999a). The level of content validity can be considered in the same way as face validity, with good, moderate, and poor levels of face validity according to agreement by content experts reviewing the specific items in relation to the instrument's assessment domain. Content validity is considered a prerequisite for construct and criterion-related validity and should generally be established before either of these (Thorn & Deitz, 1989).

Construct validity refers to the extent that the items of an instrument accurately measure a theoretical construct (Innes & Straker, 1999a; McDowell & Newell, 1996; Polit & Beck, 2004). There is no single method to determine construct validity, and often numerous studies are needed to provide an accumulation of evidence (Innes & Straker, 1999a; McDowell & Newell, 1996). Several methods are used to collect evidence for construct validity: *factor analysis* (FA) (Clark & Watson, 1995; Innes & Straker, 1999a; McDowell & Newell, 1996, Polit & Beck, 2004), *principal component analysis* (PCA) (Henningsson, Sundbom, Armelius, & Erdberg, 2001), and the *Rasch measurement model* (Benson & Schell, 1997; Fischer, 1993; Velozo et al., 1999). Demonstrating good construct validity enables greater generalization over various populations and situations (Innes & Straker, 1999a).

Criterion-related validity comprises *concurrent* and *predictive validity*. It is the extent to which assessment results from a new assessment instrument is related to (1) assessment results yielded by some other valued instrument ("gold standard") (i.e., *concurrent validity*) or (2) an external criterion such as return to work (i.e., *predictive validity*). Results from the new assessment instrument being evaluated are compared and correlated with those from the selected criterion. It is considered to be the most practical approach to validity testing and the most objective (Innes & Straker, 1999a).

Although validity is considered the most important characteristic of an assessment instrument that allows correct and meaningful interpretations, the instrument must also be accurate and consistent (i.e., reliable; Dimitrov et al., 2001). Reliability is the degree of consistency or dependability with which an instrument measures the attribute it is designed to measure (Gross, 2004; Innes & Straker, 1999b, McDowell & Newell, 1996; Polit & Beck, 2004; Streiner & Norman, 2003; Thorndike, 1987). The reliability of an assessment instrument is crucial to clinicians when assessing clients, evaluating the efficacy of an intervention, and planning future intervention. If an assessment is reliable, then changes noted in a client's performance over time are likely to be due to real improvement or deterioration, and not just due to measurement error (Innes & Straker, 1999b).

There are several forms of reliability, and the most common forms associated with work-related assessments are *test–retest reliability* and *interrater reliability* (Innes & Straker, 1999b). *Test–retest reliability* determines the consistency of an assessment instrument from one assessment occasion to another. It assumes that the characteristic being assessed does not change over the time between the assessment occasions. *Interrater reliability* examines the variation between several raters assessing the same phenomenon, for example, a client (Gross, 2004; Innes & Straker, 1999b).

Furthermore, in the assessment of performance a very important characteristic of an instrument is its *utility* (usefulness; Matheson, Gaudino, Mael, & Hesse, 2000). *Utility* represents the overall value of the instrument for the users in terms of its relevance, usefulness, efficiency, practicality, ease of administration, and flexibility (Innes & Straker, 2003; Matheson et al., 2000).

MOHO-Based Work-Related Assessment Instruments

Adequate and reliable methods for evaluation of clients with work disabilities are crucial for both the individuals who are assessed and for society as a whole. Sound and precise work assessments are needed to guide clients to suitable interventions using a minimum of rehabilitation resources (Innes & Straker, 1998b; Lechner et al., 1991; Matheson et al., 1998; Timpka, Hensing, & Alexanderson, 1995).

Because each work assessment instrument normally has a specific focus, a single instrument generally does not address all the multiple factors involved in a client's work functioning. Therefore, assessors should use several instruments in combination. This means that assessors must understand both what each specific instrument offers and what its limits are. In the vast majority of circumstances, a single instrument will not address all the work-related problems faced by a client, requiring the assessor to use other instruments along with it. Due to the specific purpose and delimitation of specific instruments, they should be incorporated into a methodology that considers the client's work functioning from a wider perspective to get a more complete and correct understanding of the client's strengths and weaknesses (Sandqvist & Henriksson, 2004; Shaw et al., 2002).

An adequate assessment of a client's work functioning is characterized by the following:

- a use of multiple data sources (e.g., client, employer, coworker, other health professionals, or assessing personnel);

- a use of multiple data collection methods (e.g., interview, observation, or measurement using different assessment instruments for data collection); and
- triangulation of the data collected.

The use of multiple data collection methods across multiple data sources provides deep and useful information, which combines an objective with a subjective assessment of performance (Innes & Straker, 2002; Travis, 2002). Using single methods, such as a structured interview, with single sources, such as an injured worker, does not always ensure that the data collected are adequate and reliable. Triangulation is essential in the assessment process involving the systematic analysis of the interrelationships of collected data in order to interpret and, finally, make judgments regarding the client's work functioning (Travis, 2002).

Vocational rehabilitation professionals often use assessment instruments to develop a course of intervention for clients (Matheson, 2001; Pransky & Dempsey, 2004). However, there may be a risk that assessors ascribe assessment instruments too much significance and importance. There may be a risk that assessors have a "blind faith" in assessment instruments, where just the fact that an instrument is used is believed to be enough to guarantee the quality of an assessment. The assessor must always keep in mind what the purpose of an instrument is and what information it can contribute. An assessment instrument is not "the solution for everything," but merely a tool in the hands of a professional—the assessor. A sound and precise instrument helps the assessor collect information in a valid, reliable, and structured way, but it is the assessor who must evaluate the information yielded by the used instruments, interpret its meaning, and evaluate in what way it contributes to the total understanding of a client's work functioning.

Assessment instruments are only as good as the manner in which they are applied in practice, but through application and use of tools that are usable, reliable, and valid, practitioners can feel more assured that the assessment also has some degree of credibility. The possibilities of assisting clients to achieve a safe, early, and durable return to work are dependent upon being able to identify the complex interrelationships of multiple factors that comprise and influence work functioning. When assessing a complex phenomenon such as work functioning, a single assessment instrument is not enough to capture all aspects of a client's work ability. It is the professional assessor's responsibility to bear in mind what the assessment instrument can contribute (i.e., to consider which aspects of work functioning it does and does not address). Without sound clinical reasoning and critical thinking, assessment results will lack relevance to individual workers and their futures.

McMillan (2006) states that, in order to understand clients' occupational problems, clients need to be viewed as occupational beings and conceptual practice models that focus on occupation should be used (McMillan, 2006). Furthermore, to articulate the theoretical thinking behind the doing and the decisions in daily work is also a prerequisite if scientifically sound occupational therapy is to be offered to the clients (Duncan, 2006). The use of theory in practice provides necessary understanding in occupational therapy (Kielhofner, 2004) and also helps the OT to explain actual intervention alternatives and strategies to the client (Law & Baum, 2005). The MOHO offers a comprehensive explanation of how occupation is motivated, patterned and performed in interaction with the surrounding physical and social environment. There are a number of work-related MOHO-based assessment instruments that can be used to assess various aspects of work functioning in vocational rehabilitation. Assessors who combine instruments based on MOHO in their practice will probably use the model to put together all the information yielded by the different instruments, a strategy that can make it easier for the assessor to create a more complete picture of the client's work functioning, as well as a foundation for the design and implementation of client-centered rehabilitation interventions.

ASSESSMENT OF WORK PERFORMANCE

The Assessment of Work Performance (AWP) (Sandqvist et al., 2006; Sandqvist, Lee, & Kielhofner, 2010) is an assessment instrument originally developed in Sweden. The purpose of the AWP is to assess an individual's observable (working) skills during work performance (i.e., how efficient and appropriate the client performs a work task). The data collection method is observation, and it is the assessor who interprets assessment results and the client's work performance (i.e., an assessment from an objective perspective).

The AWP can be used to assess the working skills of clients with different kinds of work-related problems. The instrument is not designed for any particular diagnosis or deficits. The AWP does not target any special tasks or contexts, and assessment can be made of any work tasks performed in realistic or real-life work situations, or in more constructed or artificial environments.

The AWP assesses the client's observable **working skills** in three domains: motor skills, process skills, and communication and interaction skills. These three domains contain 14 different skills in total: 5 in the domain of motor skills, 5 in the domain of process skills, and 4 in the domain of communication and interaction skills. The motor skills domain contains skills such as mobility, coordination, and strength. The process skills domain includes skills such as organization of time, planning of the work situation, and adaptation. Finally, the communication and interaction skills domain consists of skills such as social contacts and information exchange. The skills are numerically and individually assessed on a Likert-type four-point ordinal rating scale (1 = deficient performance, 4 = competent performance).

Various psychometric properties such as validity, reliability, and utility have been tested for the AWP (Fan, Taylor, Ekbladh, Hemmingsson, & Sandqvist, 2013; Sandqvist, et al., 2006; Sandqvist, Henriksson, Gullberg, & Gerdle, 2008; Sandqvist, Björk, Gullberg, Henriksson, & Gerdle, 2009). The instrument was developed in Sweden, but has so far been translated to English, Dutch, and Icelandic, and translations to other languages are planned or in progress (for example Chinese, Danish, German, and Finnish).

The AWP may also be combined with the instrument Assessment of Work Characteristics (AWC) (Sandqvist, 2007). The AWC describes the extent to which a client has to use different working skills to perform a work task in an efficient and appropriate way. The AWC is based on the AWP as the 14 assessment items in both instruments are mutual. However, there are major differences between the instruments:

- the instruments have different purposes, as the AWP focuses on the person and assessment of the client's work performance, whereas the AWC focuses on environmental attributes and assessment of the demands on a client when performing a work task;
- the instruments have different rating scales; and
- the procedure for assessment is not the same.

The AWC is only available in Swedish at present, and initial evaluations of content validity and utility of the AWC have been executed.

WORKER ROLE INTERVIEW

The Worker Role Interview (WRI) (Braveman et al., 2005) is designed to identify psychosocial and environmental factors that influence a client's ability to return to work, remain in work, or become employed in general. In other words, it assesses the client's psychosocial work potential. The WRI consists of a semistructured interview with an accompanying therapist-administered Likert-type four-point rating scale. The 16-item scale is rated according to the implications of each item for the client's likelihood of work success. The WRI is designed to collect data on sixteen items, included in the following six content areas, personal causation, values, interests, roles, habits, and the environment. "Personal causation" refers to the feeling of competence and effectiveness in relation to doing work tasks and facing challenges at work. "Values" refer to the feeling of importance and meaningfulness obtained from one's job and from being a worker, and "interests" refer to the enjoyment and stimuli one finds inside and outside work. The influence of lifestyle patterns on work behavior is conceptualized by the two theoretical constructs: roles and habits. "Roles" refer to attitudes and ways of behaving in a manner that is socially relevant. An internalized role is a support for understanding which behavior is appropriate in a specific situation. "Habits" refer to ways of doing things, which are internalized through repeated performance and which become semiautonomous and efficient when they are performed in familiar environments. The environment includes the physical and social features inside and outside work that provide opportunities and/or resources on one hand, but that constrain and/or make demands on the person on the other. This environmental impact results from the interaction between features of the environment and the characteristics of the person and thus affects what one does and how it is done. The WRI is designed to be relevant to use with any person with a disability. In the WRI manual, detailed instructions for administration are provided. The WRI has two interview guides for collection of information, one that can be used when the client has a specific job to relate to, and the other when the client has limited, or no work history. The interviews are semistructured, and the recommended questions in the interview guides are designed to help the interviewer keep track of the content of the interview, but they need to be adapted in relation to the unique situation of the clients who are interviewed, and so the questions are not standardized. After the interview, each item is rated and comments can be written as explanations of the reason for the actual rating. The WRI is designed for concurrent use with other assessments that provide data on work-related ability. The psychosocial factors identified by the WRI often reveal unique strengths and weakness and provide a solid foundation for planning client-centered interventions aimed at enabling the client achieve employment.

The first version of the WRI was developed in 1991 and has subsequently been translated and adapted to other languages and cultures (Chinese, Danish, Dutch, Finnish, French, German, Icelandic, Japanese, Korean, Norwegian, Persian, Portuguese, Slovenian, Spanish, Swedish). Since the early 1990s the WRI's reliability, validity, and utility have been investigated and developed through research (Biernacki, 1993; Haglund, Karlsson, Kielhofner, & Lai, 1997; Velozo et al., 1999; Ekbladh et al., 2004; Fenger & Kramer,

2007; Forsyth et al., 2006; Ekbladh et al., 2010; Köller, Niedermann, Klipstein, & Haugboelle, 2011; Lohss, Forsyth, & Kottorp, 2012, Yngve & Ekbladh, 2015).

WORK ENVIRONMENT IMPACT SCALE

The Work Environment Impact Scale (WEIS) (Moore-Corner, Kielhofner, & Olson, 1998) focuses on the fit between a person and his or her work environment. The semistructured interview and the accompanying Likert-type rating scale is designed to provide a comprehensive assessment of how qualities and characteristics of a given work environment affect a person's work performance, satisfaction, and well-being. Typical candidates for this assessment are persons who are experiencing difficulties on their job and those whose work is interrupted by an injury or illness. The WEIS interview focuses on the unique individual's perception of opportunities and constraints in the work environment related to physical spaces, social groups, objects, and tasks. How the client perceives the environmental impact at work is dependent upon the social and physical characteristics of the work environment and on each person's values, interests, personal causation, habits, roles, and performance capacities. Thus, the same environment has different impacts on different individuals. The WEIS yields the client's subjective perception of a specific work environment and is not an objective assessment of the work environment. After completing the interview, the 17 WEIS items are rated on a four-point rating scale by the therapist. In addition to the rating, qualitative information on each item can be added to the rating form by the interviewer in the form of a note explaining the participant's perception of the actual item and the reason why the actual rating has been chosen. The notes could consist of illuminating citations that the client had given during the WEIS interview or could be a summary of the interviewee's perceptions of the actual item. This information yields important information in planning for further client-centered intervention strategies since it describes the client's subjective perception of his or her work environment. The WEIS is designed for concurrent use with other assessments that measure work-related ability. WEIS is often used in conjunction with the WRI, since the two interviews can be combined, saving time in administration.

The first version of the WEIS was developed in 1998 and has subsequently been translated and adapted to other languages and cultures (Chinese, Danish, Dutch, Finnish, French, German, Icelandic, Japanese, Korean, Norwegian, Portuguese, Slovenian, Spanish, Swedish). Psychometric properties of the WEIS have been investigated (Corner et al., 1997; Kielhofner et al., 1999; Ekbladh et al., 2014).

Example of MOHO-Based Work-Related Interventions

Guidelines for vocational rehabilitation have been developed based on the MOHO. One example is the ActiVate Collaboration manual of vocational rehabilitation (ActiVate Collaboration, 2014). One vocational rehabilitation service using the ActiVate Collaboration manual and integrating the principles of evidence-based supported employment is the Dartmouth IPS Supported Employment Centre (Dartmouth, 2010). The service promotes the principal that being in employment is good for everyone's physical and mental health. Strong working relationships with local health and social care agencies ensure that all mental health service users are encouraged to consider employment goals and to approach the occupational therapy service if additional support is required to achieve goals.

MOHO Problem Solver: An Adult with Unexplained Fatigue and Pain

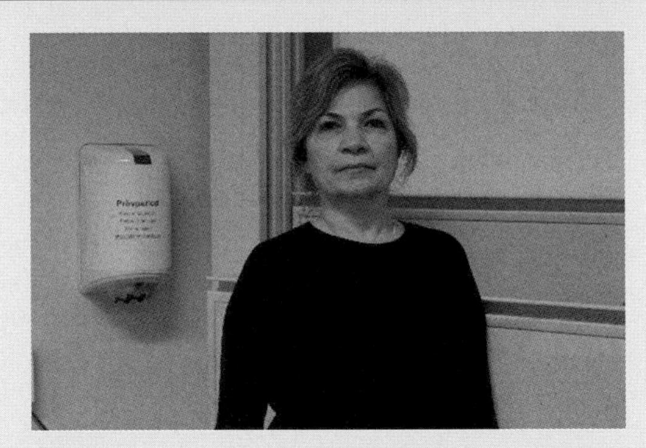

Maria

Maria (49 years) came to Sweden from Syria when she was 16 years old. Her whole family was then still remaining in their homeland, and many times she felt alone. She got married and had children at age 21. She has three children aged 28, 26, and 23, and none of them are living at home anymore. Maria lives with her husband in a house in a medium sized city in Sweden. Several of her seven siblings and her parents now live in Sweden or Germany. She says she has a good marriage, good relationships with her family, and a social network.

When the children were small, Maria worked as a nursing assistant in elderly care, where she spent most of the time working night shifts at full-time. When she was 31 years, she began to read courses to obtain the necessary level of education to be able to seek university studies, and then she started education to become a secondary school teacher of mathematics, physics, and chemistry. She completed her studies when she was 37 years old and immediately got employed as teacher at a local high school in their hometown, where she has worked for the last twelve years. The last couple of years she's had increasing symptoms of pain and tension in her right arm, neck, shoulders, and head. Maria's problems worsened successively with dizziness and severe headache, and she also experienced emotional stress. She also had trouble sleeping and felt "burned-out." She underwent a thorough medical examination, but no physical causes to her problems were found. Finally the situation became untenable, and her physician referred her to a physical therapist to work on building her endurance and to administer various modalities to address the pain. The physical therapy regime only resulted in Maria experiencing multiple crashes, resulting in increased fatigue and pain, and in feelings of invalidation. Two months ago, she had to go on full-time sick leave due to her problems.

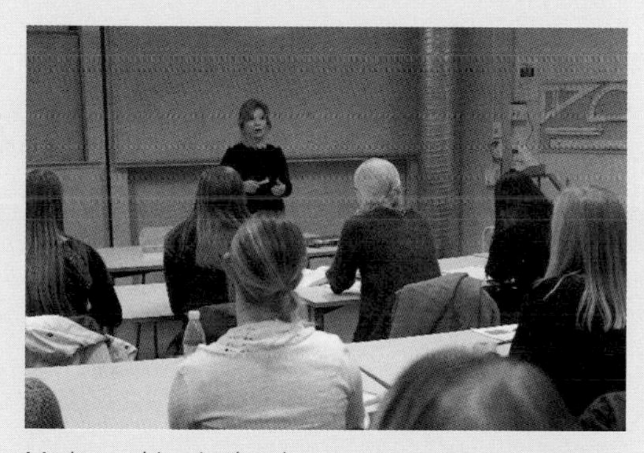

Maria teaching in the classroom

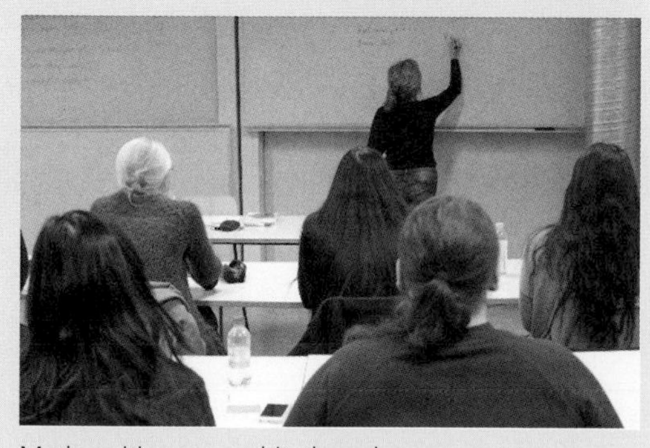

Maria writing on a white board

Assessment and Interventions for Maria

When Maria had been on sick leave for three months, she was referred to an OT working at a vocational rehabilitation setting.

The first step in the rehabilitation process was to assess Maria's work functioning from different perspectives. The OT used several MOHO-based instruments in combination for the assessment, including interviews and observations. The OT started by doing an interview with WRI and WEIS in order to identify psychosocial and environmental factors that influenced Maria's work potential. The following information was gathered.

To work is important and significant for her and she likes her work tasks, especially teaching and interacting with the students. She understands what is expected of her in the role as a teacher and how her difficulties affect her performance of the work tasks, which is one reason why she has begun to doubt her capacity in her job. She likes her colleagues, and they try to help each other and show that they understand her situation. Maria feels that the workload is constantly too high. It has been hard for her to concentrate and get her job done at school since it's never calm at the teachers' office, which she shares with three other colleagues. She has often had to bring unfinished jobs home with her after the work day. Now Maria has the feeling that the headmaster is thinking more and more about the fact that they are lacking personnel than about how they can adjust to help Maria manage her job with the problems she has. She is also in some way disappointed in her husband and family since they do not really understand why she can't do the things she has done before, such as taking care of almost all of the domestic duties.

Maria feels that she has chosen the right profession, but has experienced her work situation as very demanding and stressful in the past 5 years. Her responsibilities have increased over the years, and she has taken on tasks from former colleagues, tasks that she often feels are outside her field of competence. She has also been given an increased responsibility for administrative tasks at the school, while she constantly had to cover for colleagues who quit their work or have been sick or had other engagements. She really wanted to perform well and do a good job, and pressed herself hard.

Maria was observed when teaching as well as when working with administrative tasks at her workplace using the AWP as assessment instrument (Tables 23-4 and 23-5). Several strengths and limitations were identified in her work performance. When it came to her motor skills, Maria showed problems with reaching, lifting, and carrying objects, and she sometimes had problems with manipulation and with using her right arm when, for example, writing on her computer. However, the most evident problem was her lack of endurance (physical energy), and that she became so tired during her working days. She also had significant problems with her mental energy (process skills), which severely affected her ability to concentrate and focus on her work tasks. Furthermore, Maria sometimes had problems with performing actions in a logical order and she maintained a high tempo even when she did not have to. Stress made her pressured approach to work worse, and she

Table 23-4 AWP Ratings

1 Incompetent Performance	2 Limited Performance	3 Questionable Performance	4 Competent Performance
The performance of the work task a. is inefficient, b. is inappropriate, and c. gives an unacceptable result. The problems are major and all parameters (a–c) are clearly affected.	The performance of the work task a. is inefficient, b. is inappropriate, *and/or* c. gives an unacceptable result. One/several (1 or 2) of the parameters (a–c) are clearly affected.	The performance of the work task is not fully competent with respect to the parameters a–c, but none of them are clearly affected. Normally, the assessor has a vague feeling that the performance is reduced.	The performance of the work task a. is efficient, b. is appropriate, and c. gives an acceptable result.

Key: LI = Lack of information; NR = Not relevant.

Table 23-5 AWP Ratings for Maria

Motor Skills

Item	LI	NR	1	2	3	4
1. Posture (stabilize, position)	LI	NR	1	2	3	(4)
Comments: Maria has no problems placing herself in relation to the environment and maintaining balance and trunk control in the work situation.						
2. Mobility (walk, reach, bend)	LI	NR	1	(2)	3	4
Comments: Maria has obvious problems to reach and lift her arm to be able to write on the whiteboard in the classroom.						
3. Coordination (coordinate, manipulate, flow)	LI	NR	1	2	(3)	4
Comments: Some days, when she has more pain, Maria has problems with manipulation and using fine motor control (right hand) to handle objects such as pencils or the computer keyboard.						
4. Strength (grip, push, pull, lift, transport, calibrate)	LI	NR	1	(2)	3	4
Comments: Maria has problems with lifting and carrying objects, such as paper packages, when she has to load the copying machine with papers.						
5. Physical energy (endure, pace)	LI	NR	(1)	2	3	4
Comments: It is not possible for Maria to manage her teaching as she gets so tired, and the problems become worse as time goes on during her working days. Furthermore, she can't manage to sit and work at her computer and operate the computer mouse without getting very tired.						

Table 23-5 AWP Ratings for Maria (*continued*)

Item						
Process Skills						
6. Mental energy (endure, pace, attend)	LI	NR	(1)	2	3	4
Comments: *It gets harder and harder for Maria to concentrate and to maintain adequate attention throughout the performance of her work tasks, in both her teaching as well as administrative tasks. She gets extremely tired and can't maintain pace, for example in the administrative tasks.*						
7. Knowledge (choose, use, inquire, heed)	LI	NR	1	2	(3)	4
Comments: *Sometimes, Maria lacks necessary knowledge for work tasks, especially when she has to take over work tasks from her colleagues that are outside her field of competence.*						
8. Temporal organization (initiate, continue, sequence, terminate)	LI	NR	1	(2)	3	4
Comments: *When Maria gets stressed, she sometimes can't perform actions in a logical order or interruption for efficient use of time and energy, for example in her administrative work tasks.*						
9. Organization of space and objects (plan, restore)	LI	NR	1	2	3	(4)
Comments: *Maria has no problems with the ability to organize space and objects in the workplace.*						
10. Adaptation (notice/respond, adjust behavior, adjust environment)	LI	NR	1	(2)	3	4
Comments: *Maria notices when the progression of her work task is not optimal, but sometimes lacks the ability to appropriately change her actions to avoid undesirable outcomes.*						
11. Physicality (gesture, gaze, approximate, posture, contact)	LILI	NR	1	2	3	(4)
Communication and Interaction Skills						
12. Language (adjust language, adjust speech, focus)	LII	NR	1	(2)	3	4
Comments: *Maria has a good ability to use language in communication with others. However, sometimes she loses her focus on the conversation in her teaching sessions, leading to misunderstandings and a loss of interest from her students.*						
13. Relations (engage, relate, respects, collaborate)	LI	NR	1	2	3	(4)
Comments: *No problems with interaction or collaboration with others at her workplace.*						
14. Information exchange (ask, inform)	LI	NR	1	2	(3)	4
Comments: *Maria has no problems with the physical expression or interaction with others.*						

lacked the ability to change her actions according to the demands of her work situation.

Additionally, Maria sometimes lacked the necessary knowledge for her work tasks, especially when the work tasks were unfamiliar to her. Regarding Maria's communication and interaction skills, she had distinguished social skills when it came to interaction and collaboration with others, for example with her coworkers. However, Maria sometimes showed a tendency to try to solve everything herself and avoided asking for help from her colleagues, which made her work situation more difficult than necessary. Maria had a good ability to use language in communication with others. However, sometimes she lost her focus on the conversation in her teaching sessions, leading to misunderstandings and a loss of interest from her students.

After the assessments, the OT discussed the findings and situation with Maria. This was an opportunity for Maria to validate and reflect on the assessment results and also to facilitate her engagement and participation in the rehabilitation process. Together, they identified and formulated long- and short-term goals. Her long-term goal was to achieve a satisfactory balance between activities in her working and private life, and she aimed to work full-time again.

Maria and her therapist had a meeting with Maria's employer to inform about the rehabilitation plan and to involve the employer in the process. In relation to this visit to Maria's workplace, the OT observed and analyzed the work environment in relation to findings from previous assessments, followed by a discussion with Maria. Based on this, they formed a number of interventions related to personal as well as environmental factors.

The main interventions were as follows:

- The employer was able to offer Maria an office of her own to make it easier for her to focus on her work tasks. It was now possible for her to shut the door and put a "Do Not Disturb" sign on the door when she wanted to work without distractions.
- The new room was not furnished as an office. Therefore it was possible to purchase an ergonomic height-adjustable desk and chair and a forearm support in order to reduce strain and relieve her shoulders.
- In discussion with the employer, it was planned that Maria should focus on her primary work tasks to plan for her lessons and to teach. As much as possible, Maria should avoid covering for colleagues and replacing them in tasks that she's not so familiar with.
- She was encouraged to take short breaks regularly as a natural part of her working day.
- The employer approved Maria to have flexible working hours for the administrative tasks, depending on how Maria was feeling.
- An activity diary was used to help Maria reflect on her priorities for activities in her life, and how she experiences the balance between work, play, and activities of daily living.
- In collaboration with the employer, Maria and the OT agreed on a plan for a gradual return to work for Maria, where she started to work only a few hours a day in the beginning followed by a phased increase of her working hours over a period of time.
- During the return-to-work process, the OT had regular contact with Maria to follow and evaluate progress, in order to offer support and coaching in the return-to-work process.

WRI and WEIS ratings for Maria are shown in Tables 23-6 and 23-7, respectively.

Table 23-6 WRI Ratings for Maria

Rating						Brief Comments that Support Ratings
Personal Causation						
1. Assesses abilities and limitations	SS	**S**	I	SI	N/A	*Maria is mostly aware of her strengths and weaknesses. Can describe the tasks she can handle and not handle.*
2. Expectation of job success	SS	S	**I**	SI	N/A	*She hopes that she will be healthy and able to work again, but is not so sure she will manage. Doesn't think she will cope in the long run at her present job.*
3. Takes responsibility	SS	**S**	I	SI	N/A	*She has recently talked to her boss about the possibilities for change in her service and duties. "Must come to a change at work, but first of all I need to be healthy again."*
Values						
4. Commitment to work	**SS**	S	I	SI	N/A	*The work is very important "first and foremost for the supply, but also for the satisfaction of having accomplished something." She feels ashamed of being on sick leave.*
5. Work-related goals	SS	**S**	I	SI	N/A	*Want to do a good job, want to be a person that the employer can rely on.*
Interests						
6. Enjoys work	SS	S	**I**	SI	N/A	*"After all that has been" (illness, high demands from her boss, financial cutbacks at the workplace) has her job satisfaction decreased.*

Table 23-6 WRI Ratings for Maria (*continued*)

Rating						Brief Comments that Support Ratings
7. Pursues interests	SS	S	**I**	SI	N/A	*She has no energy and desire anymore. She previously had many interests and has been engaged. "Now I mostly lie on the couch". She can't cope with more than socializing with her family. Has lost her interests because of the pain and tiredness.*
Roles						
8. Appraises work expectations	**SS**	S	I	SI	N/A	*Can describe in detail the expectations of her in the work role such as being clear and calm, accessible, helpful.*
9. Influence of other roles	SS	S	I	**SI**	N/A	*Combining her work role with other roles has worked out badly for a long time. "I have given everything on the job, and thus have been completely exhausted when I come home." She is the one who always has taken care of all the practical home duties, but she has no energy for it anymore.*
Habits						
10. Work habits	**SS**	S	I	SI	N/A	*High degree of organization of the habits and routines of work. Can describe in detail what she does.*
11. Daily routines	SS	S	I	**SI**	N/A	*Loses her routines because she no longer does the tasks she previously has done. She finds it difficult to deal with the housework.*
12. Adapts routine to minimize difficulties	SS	S	I	**SI**	N/A	*Maria is aware of that the workload has been unreasonably high, but does not know how she shall resolve it. She has not been able to adapt routines to her current problems.*
Environment						
13. Perception of work setting	SS	S	I	**SI**	N/A	*For her to be able to return to work changes in responsibilities and duties are required but she does not believe that it will be possible to arrange.*
14. Perception of family and peers	SS	S	**I**	SI	N/A	*She has some support from family and friends and they say that they want her to go back to work. But she feels that they do not always understand and her husband finds it strange that she can't manage things she has done before.*
15. Perception of boss	SS	S	I	**SI**	N/A	*Her boss has phoned her a few times, but she perceived that the main point from the boss is that she put others in trouble by being on sick leave.*
16. Perception of co-workers	SS	**S**	I	SI	N/A	*She finds support and understanding from her colleagues. "They are in similar situations and know how it can be like."*

Key: SS = Strongly supports client returning to job; S = Supports client returning to job; I = Interferes with returning to job; SI = Strongly interferes with returning to job; N/A = Not applicable or not enough information to rate.

Table 23-7 WEIS Ratings for Maria

Rating						Brief Comments that Support Ratings
1. **Time demands:** Time allotted for available/expected amount of work	4	3	2	**1**	N/A	Maria has constantly high workload and it is stressful, the time assigned is never enough.
2. **Task demands:** The physical, cognitive, and/or emotional demands/opportunities of work tasks	4	3	2	**1**	N/A	The work tasks cause pain and fatigue in the back that increases during the afternoon. She is experiencing emotional stress of not being sufficient for the students.
3. **Appeal of work tasks:** The appeal/enjoyableness or status/value of work tasks	4	**3**	2	1	N/A	Stimulating and rewarding work. She finds it valuable and enjoyable to work with adolescents.

(*continued*)

Table 23-7 WEIS Ratings for Maria (*continued*)

Rating						Brief Comments that Support Ratings
4. **Work schedule:** The influence of work hours upon other valued roles, activities, transportation, and basic self-care needs	4	3	<u>2</u>	1	N/A	Expected to work unpaid beyond working hours. She is available for students and colleagues all the time even during breaks and evenings.
5. **Co-worker interaction:** Interaction/collaboration with co-workers required for job responsibilities	4	<u>3</u>	2	1	N/A	They try to help each other in the team, all have a high work load.
6. **Work group membership:** Social involvement with coworkers at work/outside of work	<u>4</u>	3	2	1	N/A	Get on well with her colleagues.
7. **Supervisor interaction:** Feedback, guidance and/or other communication/interaction with supervisor(s)	4	3	2	<u>1</u>	N/A	She feels that she is not treated in a respectful and fair way of her boss.
8. **Work role standards:** Overall climate of work setting expressed in expectations for quality, excellence commitment, achievement, and/or efficiency	4	3	2	<u>1</u>	N/A	Maria experience an unreasonable work demands.
9. **Work role style:** Opportunity/expectations for autonomy/compliance when organizing, making requests, negotiating, and choosing how and what work tasks will be done daily	4	<u>3</u>	2	1	N/A	She has the freedom to control the arrangement of her lessons within reasonable limits.
10. **Interaction with others:** Interaction/communication with subordinates, customers, clients, audiences, students or others, excluding supervisor or co-workers	<u>4</u>	3	2	1	N/A	The contact with students is the best part of the job.
11. **Rewards:** Opportunities for job security, recognition/advancement in position, and/or compensation in salary or benefits	4	3	2	<u>1</u>	N/A	She never gets a "thank you" for a great job from her boss and does really miss it. She cannot point out any direct benefits.
12. **Sensory qualities:** Properties of the work place such as noise, smell, visual, or tactile properties, temperature/climate, or air quality and ventilation	4	3	<u>2</u>	1	N/A	It is sometimes high noise level in the classroom and it is poor ventilation in the teacher' office, which leads to headaches.
13. **Physical arrangement:** Architecture or physical arrangement of and between work spaces and environments	4	3	2	<u>1</u>	N/A	She shares the teachers' office with three colleagues and it's far too small and crowded which makes it hard for her to concentrate.
14. **Social atmosphere:** The feeling/mood associated with the degree of privacy, friendliness, morale, excitement, anxiety, frustration at the workplace	4	<u>3</u>	2	1	N/A	The atmosphere between her colleagues is good but all have too much to do.
15. **Properties of objects:** The physical, cognitive or emotional demands/opportunities of tools, equipment, materials, and supplies	4	3	2	<u>1</u>	N/A	Static load and locked sitting postures during computer work. Her computer mouse do not work properly which all causing increased pain in her neck and shoulders.
16. **Physical amenities:** Non-work specific facilities necessary to meet personal needs at work such as restrooms, lunchrooms, or break room	4	3	2	<u>1</u>	N/A	Lacking a relaxation room where she can "take a breather" when needed.
17. **Meaning of work:** What work signify to a person	4	<u>3</u>	2	1	N/A	Maria perceives her work as very important.

Key: 4 = Strongly supports work performance, satisfaction, and well-being; S = Supports work performance, satisfaction, and well-being; I = Interferes with work performance, satisfaction, and well-being; SI = Strongly interferes with work performance, satisfaction, and well-being; N/A = Not applicable or not enough information to rate the actual item.

Acknowledgments

We thank professor Kirsty Forsyth for providing information about the ActiVate Collaboration manual of vocational rehabilitation.

The assessment instruments presented in this chapter, that is, AWP, WEIS ,and WRI, can all be found at MOHO website: http://www.cade.uic.edu/moho/

thePoint® For additional resources and exercises, visit http://thePoint.lww.com

Key Terms

Individual capacity: Different physical and psychological attributes that enable the person to perform work tasks and activities, for example, muscle strength, joint motion, sensibility, memory, and cardiopulmonary functions.

Work: Activities (both paid and unpaid) that provide services or commodities to others such as ideas, knowledge, help, information-sharing, entertainment, utilitarian or artistic objects, and protection.

Work functioning: Work functioning is an umbrella term for all forms of work-related functioning and includes functioning in different dimensions and on different levels—body, individual, and society levels.

Work participation: The person's ability and possibility to fulfil a worker role and acquire or maintain/retain a work position in society.

Work performance: The ability to satisfactorily handle and carry out different work activities and tasks.

Working skills: Discrete elements of action with implicit functional purposes that can be observed during work performance. Three types of skills can be observed during work performance: motor skills, process skills, and communication and interaction skills.

REFERENCES

ACTIVATE Collaboration. (2014). *Vocational rehabilitation intervention manual.* Edinburgh, Scotland: Queen Margaret University.

Benson, J. B., & Schell, B. A. (1997). Measurement theory: Application to occupational therapy and physical therapy. In J. Van Deusen & D. Brunt (Eds.), *Assessment in occupational therapy and physical therapy*. Philadelphia, PA: WB Saunders.

Biernacki, S. D. (1993). Reliability of the Worker Role Interview. *The American Journal of Occupational Therapy, 47*, 797–803.

Braveman, B., Robson, M., Velozo, C., Kielhofner, G., Fisher, G., Forsyth, K., et al. (2005). *Worker Role Interview (WRI)* [Version 10.0]. Chicago: Model of Human Occupation Clearinghouse, Department of Occupational Therapy, College of Applied Health Sciences, University of Illinois at Chicago.

Brintnell, E., Harvey-Krefting, L., Rosenfeld, M., & Friesen, M. (1998). Position paper on occupational therapist's role in work related therapy. *The Canadian Journal of Occupational Therapy, 55*, 2–4.

Brown, A., Kitchell, M., O'Neill, T., Lockliear, J., Vosler, A., Kubek, D., et al. (2001). Identifying meaning and perceived level of satisfaction within the context of work. *Work: A Journal of Prevention, Assessment, and Rehabilitation, 16*, 219–226.

Clark, L. A., & Watson, D. (1995). Constructing validity: Basic issues in objective scale development. *Psychological Assessment, 3*, 309–319.

Corner, R., Kielhofner, G., & Lin, F. L. (1997). Construct validity of work environment impact scale. *Work: A Journal of Prevention, Assessment, and Rehabilitation, 9*, 21–34.

Dane, F. C. (1990). *Research methods*. Pacific Grove, CA: Brooks/Cole Publishing.

Dartmouth IPS Supported Employment Center. (2010). *IPS overview, characteristics & practice principles*. Retrieved from www.dartmouth.edu/~ips2/styled/styled-2/page70.html

Deen, M., Gibson, L., & Strong, J. (2002). A survey of occupational therapy in Australian work practice. *Work: A Journal of Prevention, Assessment, and Rehabilitation, 19*, 219–230.

Dimitrov, D., Rumrill, P., Fitzgerald, S., & Hennessey, M. (2001). Reliability in rehabilitation measurement. *Work: A Journal of Prevention, Assessment, and Rehabilitation, 16*, 159–164.

Duncan, E. (2006). *Foundations for practice in occupational therapy* (4th ed.). Edinburgh, Scotland: Elsevier.

Dunn, W. (1989). Reliability and validity. In L. J. Miller (Ed.), *Developing norm-referenced standardised tests*. New York, NY: Haworth Press.

Dunn, W. (2005). Measurement issues and practice. In M. Law, C. Baum, & W. Dunn, (Eds.), *Measuring occupational performance: Supporting best practice in occupational therapy*. Thorofare, NJ: SLACK.

Ekbladh, E., Fan, C. W., Sandqvist, J., Hemmingsson, H., & Taylor, R. (2014). Work environment impact scale: Testing the psychometric properties of the Swedish version. *Work: A Journal of Prevention, Assessment, and Rehabilitation, 47*, 213–219.

Ekbladh, E., Haglund, L., & Thorell, L. H. (2004). The Worker Role Interview—Preliminary data on the predictive validity of return to work of clients after an insurance medicine investigation. *Journal of Occupational Rehabilitation, 14*, 131–141.

Ekbladh, E., Thorell, L.-H., & Haglund, L. (2010a). Return to work—The predictive value of the Worker Role Interview (WRI) over two years. *Work: A Journal of Prevention, Assessment, and Rehabilitation, 35*, 163–172.

Ekbladh, E., Thorell, L.-H., & Haglund, L. (2010b). Perceptions of the work environment among people with experience of long term sick leave. *Work: A Journal of Prevention, Assessment, and Rehabilitation, 35*, 125–136.

Fan, C. W., Taylor, R., Ekbladh, E., Hemmingsson, H., & Sandqvist, J. (2013). Evaluating the psychometric properties of a clinical vocational rehabilitation outcome measurement—The Assessment of Work Performance (AWP). *Occupational Therapy Journal of Research, 3*, 125–133.

Fenger, K., & Kramer, J. M. (2007). Worker Role Interview: Testing the psychometric properties of the Icelandic version. *Scandinavian Journal of Occupational Therapy, 14*, 160–172.

Fischer, A. (1993). The assessment of IADL motor skills: An application of many faceted Rasch analysis. *The American Journal of Occupational Therapy, 47*, 319–329.

Forsyth, K., Braveman, B., Ekbladh, E., Kielhofner, G., Haglund, L., Fenger, K., et al. (2006). Psychometric properties of the Worker Role Interview. *Work: A Journal of Prevention, Assessment, and Rehabilitation, 27*; 313–318.

Franche, R. L., & Krause, N. (2002). Readiness for return to work following injury or illness: Conceptualizing the interpersonal impact of health care, workplace, and insurance factors. *Journal of Occupational Rehabilitation, 12*, 233–256.

Fugate, M., Kinicki, A., & Ashfort, B. (2004). Employability: A psycho-social construct, its dimensions, and applications. *Journal of Vocational Behavior, 65*, 14–38.

Gibson, L., & Strong, J. (2003). A conceptual framework of functional capacity evaluation for occupational therapy in work rehabilitation. *Australian Occupational Therapy Journal, 50*, 64–71.

Gobelet, C., Luthi, F., Al-Khodairy, A. T., & Chamberlain, M. A. (2007). Vocational rehabilitation: A multidisciplinary intervention. *Disability and Rehabilitation, 29*, 1405–1410.

Gross D. P. (2004). Measurement properties of performance-based assessment of functional capacity. *Journal of Occupational Rehabilitation, 14*, 165–174.

Haglund, L., Karlsson, G., Kielhofner, G., & Lai, J. S. (1997). Validity of the Swedish version of the Worker Role Interview. *Scandinavian Journal of Occupational Therapy, 4*, 23–29.

Hansen, A., Edlund, C., & Bränholm, I. B. (2005). Significant resources needed for return to work after sick leave. *Work: A Journal of Prevention, Assessment, and Rehabilitation, 25*, 231–240.

Hansen, A., Edlund, C., & Henningsson, M. (2006). Factors relevant to a return to work: A multivariate approach. *Work: A Journal of Prevention, Assessment, and Rehabilitation, 26*, 179–190.

Harvey, A. S., & Pentland, W. (2004). What do people do? In C. H. Christiansen & E. A. Townsend (Eds.), *Introduction to occupation—The art and science of living*. Upper Saddle River, NJ: Prentice Hall.

Harvey-Krefting, L. (1985). The concept of work in occupational therapy: A historical review. *The American Journal of Occupational Therapy, 39*, 301–307.

Henningsson, M., Sundbom, E., Armelius, B. Å., & Erdberg, P. (2001). PLS model building: A multivariate approach to personality data. *Scandinavian Journal of Psychology, 42*, 399–409.

Holmes, D. (1985). The role of the occupational therapist—Work evaluator. *The American Journal of Occupational Therapy, 39*, 308-313.

Höök, O., & Grimby, G. (2001). Rehabiliteringsmedicin—Målsättning och organisation. In O. Höök (Ed.), *Rehabiliteringsmedicin* [in Swedish]. Stockholm, Sweden: Liber AB.

Innes, E., & Straker, L. (1998a). A clinician's guide to work-related assessments, Part 2: Design problems. *Work: A Journal of Prevention, Assessment, and Rehabilitation, 11*, 191–206.

Innes, E., & Straker, L. (1998b). A clinician's guide to work-related assessments, Part 3: Administration and interpretation problems. *Work: A Journal of Prevention, Assessment, and Rehabilitation, 11*, 207–219.

Innes, E., & Straker, L. (1999a). Validity of work-related assessments. *Work: A Journal of Prevention, Assessment, and Rehabilitation, 13*, 125–152.

Innes, E., & Straker, L. (1999b). Reliability of work-related assessments. *Work: A Journal of Prevention, Assessment, and Rehabilitation, 13*, 107–124.

Innes, E., & Straker, L. (2002). Strategies used when conducting work-related assessments. *Work: A Journal of Prevention, Assessment, and Rehabilitation, 19*, 149–165.

Innes, E., & Straker, L. (2003). Attributes of excellence in work-related assessments. *Work: A Journal of Prevention, Assessment, and Rehabilitation, 20*, 63–76.

Jackson, M., Harkess, J., & Ellis, J. (2004). Reporting patients' work abilities: How the use of standardised work assessment improved clinical practice in Fife. *British Journal of Occupational Therapy, 67*, 129–132.

Jacobs, K. (1991). *Occupational therapy: Work-related programs and assessments* (2nd ed.). Boston, MA: Little, Brown and Company.

Jahoda, M. (1942). Incentives to work: A study of unemployed adults in a special situation. *Occupational Psychology, 16*, 20–30.

Jakobsson, B., Bergroth, A., Shüldt, K., & Ekholm, J. (2005). Do systematic multiprofessional rehabilitation group meetings improve efficiency in vocational rehabilitation? *Work: A Journal of Prevention, Assessment, and Rehabilitation, 24*, 279–290.

Johnston, M. V., Keith, R. A., & Hinderer, S. R. (1992). Measurement standards for interdisciplinary medical rehabilitation. *Archives of Physical Medicine and Rehabilitation, 73*, 3–23.

Jundt, J., & King, P. M. (1999). Work rehabilitation programs: A 1997 survey. *Work: A Journal of Prevention, Assessment, and Rehabilitation, 12*, 139–144.

Kaplan, K. L., & Kielhofner, G. (1989). *Occupational case analysis and rating scale*. Thorofare, NJ: SLACK.

Karlsson, J. (1986). *Begreppet arbete: Definitioner, ideologier och sociala former* [in Swedish]. Lund, Sweden: Studentlitteratur.

Keough, J. L., & Fisher, T. F. (2001). Occupational-psychosocial perceptions influencing return to work and functional performance of injured workers. *Work: A Journal of Prevention, Assessment, and Rehabilitation, 16*, 101–110.

Kielhofner, G. (2004). *Conceptual foundations of occupational therapy* (3rd ed.). Philadelphia, PA: F. A. Davis.

Kielhofner, G. (2008). *A model of human occupation: Theory and application* (4th ed.). Philadelphia, PA: Lippincott Williams & Wilkins.

Kielhofner, G., Braveman, B., Baron, K., Fisher, G., Hammel, J., & Littleton, M. (1999). The model of human occupation: understanding the worker who is injured or disabled. *Work: A Journal of Prevention, Assessment, and Rehabilitation, 12*, 3–11.

Kielhofner, G., Lai, J. S., Olson, L., Haglund, L., Ekbladh, E., & Hedlund, M. (1999). Psychometric properties of the work environment impact scale: A cross-cultural study. *Work: A Journal of Prevention, Assessment, and Rehabilitation, 12*, 71–77.

Kielhofner, K. (1993). Functional assessment: Toward a dialectical view of person environment relations. *The American Journal of Occupational Therapy, 47*, 248–251.

Köller, B., Niedermann, K., Klipstein, A., & Haugboelle, J. (2011). The psychometric properties of the German version of the new Worker Role Interview (WRI-G 10.0) in people with musculoskeletal disorders. *Work: A Journal of Prevention, Assessment, and Rehabilitation, 40*(4), 401–410.

Law, M. (1995). Evaluation of occupational performance. In C. A. Trombly, *Occupational therapy for physical dysfunction* (4th ed.). Baltimore, MD: Williams & Wilkins.

Law, M., & Baum, C. (2005). Measurement in occupational therapy. In: M. Law, C. Baum, & W. Dunn (Eds.), *Measuring occupational performance: Supporting best practice in occupational therapy*. Thorofare, NJ: SLACK.

Lechner, D., Roth, D., & Straaton, K. (1991). Functional capacity evaluation in work disability. *Work: A Journal of Prevention, Assessment, and Rehabilitation, 1*, 37–47.

Linddahl, I., Norrby, E., & Bellner, A. L. (2003). Construct validity of the instrument DOA: A dialogue about ability related to work. *Work: A Journal of Prevention, Assessment, and Rehabilitation, 20*, 215–224.

Lindin, A. I., Roos, S., & Björklund, A. (2007). Constituents of healthy workplaces. *Work: A Journal of Prevention, Assessment, and Rehabilitation, 28*, 3–11.

Lohman, H., & Peyton, C. (1997). The influence of conceptual models on work in occupational therapy history. *Work: A Journal of Prevention, Assessment, and Rehabilitation, 9*, 209–219.

Lohss, I., Forsyth, K., & Kottorp, A. (2012). Psychometric properties of the Worker Role Interview in mental health [Version 10.0]. *British Journal of Occupational Therapy, 75*(4), 171–179.

Lysaght, R. M. (2004). Approaches to worker rehabilitation by occupational and physical therapists in the United States: Factors impacting practice. *Work: A Journal of Prevention, Assessment, and Rehabilitation, 23*, 139–146.

Marnetoft, S. U., Selander, J., Bergroth, A., & Ekholm, J. (2001). Factors associated with successful vocational rehabilitation in a Swedish rural area. *Journal of Rehabilitation Medicine, 33*, 71–78.

Matheson, L. N. (2001). Disability methodology redesign: considerations for a new approach to disability determination. *Journal of Occupational Rehabilitation, 11*, 135–142.

Matheson, L. N., Gaudino, E. A., Mael, F., & Hesse, B. W. (2000). Improving the validity of the impairment evaluation process: A proposed theoretical framework. *Journal of Occupational Rehabilitation, 4*, 311–320.

Matheson, L. N., Isernhagen, S. J., & Hart, D. L. (1998). Functional capacity evaluation as a facilitator of social security disability program reform. *Work: A Journal of Prevention, Assessment, and Rehabilitation, 10*, 77–84.

Matheson, L., Kaskutas, V., McCowan, S. H., & Webb, C. (2001). Development of a database of functional assessment measures related to work disability. *Journal of Occupational Rehabilitation, 11*, 177–199.

McCracken, N. (1991). Conceptualizing occupational therapy's role within vocational assessment. *Work: A Journal of Prevention, Assessment, and Rehabilitation, 1*, 77–83.

McCuaig, M., & Iwama, M. (1989). When daily living becomes a challenge in the work place: Occupational therapy: The profession that connects. *The Canadian Journal of Occupational Therapy, 56*, 161–162.

McDowell, I., & Newell, C. (1996). *Measuring health—A guide to rating scales and questionnaires* (2nd ed.). New York, NY: Oxford University Press.

McMillan, I. R. (2006). Assumptions underpinning a biomechanical frame of reference in occupational therapy. In E. Duncan (Ed.), *Foundations for practice in occupational therapy* (4th ed.). Edinburgh, Scotland: Elsevier.

Moore-Corner, R., Kielhofner, G., & Olson, L. (1998). *Work Environment Impact Scale (WEIS)* [Version 2.0]. Chicago, IL: Model of Human Occupation Clearinghouse, Department of Occupational Therapy, College of Applied Health Sciences, University of Illinois at Chicago.

Persson, D. (2001). *Aspects of meaning in everyday occupations and its relationships to health-related factors* (Doctoral dissertation). Lund, Sweden: Department of Clinical Neuroscience Division of Occupational Therapy, Lund University.

Polanyi, M., & Tompa, E. (2004). Rethinking work-health models for the new global economy: A qualitative analysis of emerging dimensions of work. *Work: A Journal of Prevention, Assessment, and Rehabilitation, 23*, 3–18.

Polit, D. F., & Beck, C. T. (2004). *Nursing research—Principles and methods*. Philadelphia, PA: J. B. Lippincott.

Portney, L. G., & Watkins, M. P. (1993). *Foundations of clinical research: Applications to practice*. Norwalk, CT: Appleton & Lange.

Pransky, G., & Dempsey, P. (2004). Practical aspects of functional capacity evaluations. *Journal of Occupational Rehabilitation, 14*, 217–229.

Sandqvist, J. (2007). *Development and evaluation of validity and utility of the instrument Assessment of Work Performance (AWP)*. Linköping, Sweden: Department of Social and Welfare Studies, Division of Health, Education and Welfare Institutions, Linköping University.

Sandqvist, J., Björk, M., Gullberg, M., Henriksson, C., & Gerdle, B. (2009). Construct validity of the Assessment of Work Performance (AWP). *Work: A Journal of Prevention, Assessment, and Rehabilitation, 2*, 211–218.

Sandqvist, J., & Henriksson, C. (2004). Work functioning—A conceptual framework. *Work: A Journal of Prevention, Assessment, and Rehabilitation, 2*, 147–157.

Sandqvist, J., Henriksson, C., Gullberg, M., & Gerdle, B. (2008). Content validity and utility of the Assessment of Work Performance (AWP). *Work: A Journal of Prevention, Assessment, and Rehabilitation, 4*, 441–450.

Sandqvist, J., Lee, J., & Kielhofner, G. (2010). *The assessment of work performance*. Chicago, IL: Model of Human Occupation Clearinghouse, Department of Occupational Therapy, College of Applied Health Sciences, University of Illinois at Chicago.

Sandqvist, J., Törnquist, K., & Henriksson, C. (2006). Assessment of Work Performance (AWP)—Development of an instrument. *Work: A Journal of Prevention, Assessment, and Rehabilitation, 4*, 379–387.

Schmidt, H. C., & Walker, K. F. (1992). The history of work in physical dysfunction. *The American Journal of Occupational Therapy, 46*, 56–62.

Schult, M. L., Söderback, I., & Jacobs, K. (2000). Multidimensional aspects of work capability. *Work: A Journal of Prevention, Assessment, and Rehabilitation, 15*, 41–53.

Selander, J., & Marnetoft, S.-U. (2005). Case management in vocational rehabilitation: A case study with promising results. *Work: A Journal of Prevention, Assessment, and Rehabilitation, 24*, 297–304.

Shaw, L., Segal, R., Polatajko, H., & Harburn, K. (2002). Understanding return to work behaviours: Promoting the importance of individual perceptions in the study of return to work. *Disability and Rehabilitation, 24*, 185–195.

Sim, J., & Arnell, P. (1993). Measurement validity in physical therapy research. *Physical Therapy, 73*, 102–115.

Smith, R. O. (1992). The science of Occupational Therapy Assessment. *The Occupational Therapy Journal of Research, 12*, 3–15.

Söderback, I., & Jacobs, K. (2000). A study of well-being among a population of Swedish workers using a job-related criterion-referenced multidimensional vocational assessment. *Work: A Journal of Prevention, Assessment, and Rehabilitation, 14*, 83–107.

Streiner, D. L., & Norman, G. R. (2003). *Health measurement scales: A practical guide to their development and use* (3rd ed.). Oxford, United Kingdom: Oxford University Press.

Strong, S., Baptiste, S., Cole, D., Clarke, J., Costa, M., Shannon, H., et al. (2004). Functional assessment of injured workers: A profile of assessor practices. *The Canadian Journal of Occupational Therapy, 71*, 13–23.

Stubbs, J., & Deaner, G. (2005). When considering vocational rehabilitation: Describing and comparing the Swedish and American systems and professions. *Work: A Journal of Prevention, Assessment, and Rehabilitation, 24*, 239–249.

Svensson, T., Müssener, U., & Alexanderson, K. (2006). Pride, empowerment, and return to work: On the significance of promoting positive social emotions among sickness absentees. *Work: A Journal of Prevention, Assessment, and Rehabilitation, 27*, 55–65.

Tengland, P. A. (2006). *Begreppet arbetsförmåga, IHS Rapport 2006:1* [in Swedish]. Linköping, Sweden: Institutionen för hälsa och samhälle, Linköpings universitet.

Thorndike, R. M. (1987). Reliability. In B. Bolton (Ed.), *Handbook of measurement and evaluation in rehabilitation* (2nd ed.). London, United Kingdom: Paul H. Brookes Publishing.

Thorn, D. W., & Deitz, J. C. (1989). Examining content validity through the use of content experts. *Occupational Therapy Journal of Research, 9*, 334–346.

Thurgood, J., & Frank, A. O. (2007). Work is beneficial for health and wellbeing: Can occupational therapists now return to their roots? *British Journal of Occupational Therapy, 70*, 49.

Timpka, T., Hensing, G., & Alexanderson, K. (1995). Dilemmas in sickness certification among Swedish physicians. *European Journal of Public Health, 5*, 215–219.

Travis, J. (2002). Cross-disciplinary competency standards for work-related assessments: Communicating the requirements for effective professional practice. *Work: A Journal of Prevention, Assessment, and Rehabilitation, 19,* 269–280.

Vahlne, W. L., Bergroth, A., & Ekholm, J. (2006). *Rehabiliterings-vetenskap—Rehabilitering till arbetslivet i ett flerdisciplinärt perspektiv* [in Swedish]. Lund, Sweden: Studentlitteratur.

Velozo, C. A. (1993). Work evaluations: Critique of the state of the art of functional assessment of work. *The American Journal of Occupational Therapy, 47,* 203–208.

Velozo, C. A., Kielhofner, G., Fisher, G., Gern, A., Lin, F. L., Ahzar, F., et al. (1999). Worker Role Interview: Toward validation of a psychosocial work related measure. *Journal of Occupational Rehabilitation, 9,* 153–168.

Westmorland, M. G., Zeytinoglu, I., Pringle, P., Denton, M., & Chouinard, V. (1998). The elements of a positive workplace environment: Implications for persons with disabilities. *Work: A Journal of Prevention, Assessment, and Rehabilitation, 10,* 109–117.

Wilcock, A. A. (1998). *An occupational perspective of health.* Thorofare, NJ: SLACK.

World Health Organization. (2000). *Occupational medicine in Europe: Scope and competencies.* Copenhagen, Denmark: WHO Regional Office for Europe.

World Health Organization. (2001). *International classification of functioning, disability and health (ICF).* Geneva, Switzerland: Author.

Yngve, M., & Ekbladh, E. (2015). Clinical utility of the Worker Role Interview—A survey study among Swedish users. *Scandinavian Journal of Occupational Therapy, 22,* 416–423.

MOHO-Based Program Development

Carmen-Gloria de las Heras de Pablo, Judith Abelenda, and Sue Parkinson

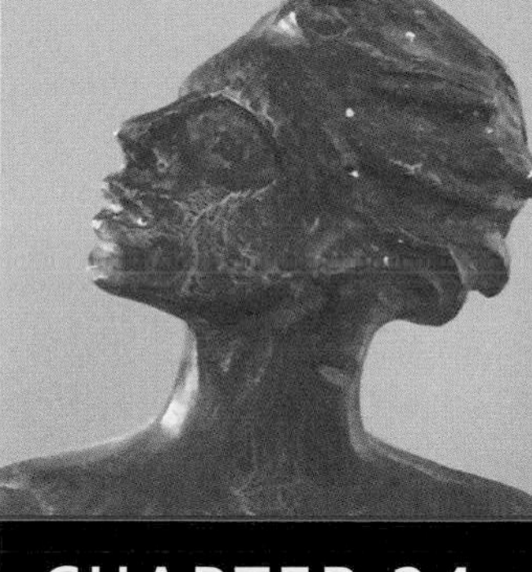

CHAPTER 24

EXPECTED LEARNING OUTCOMES

Upon completion of this chapter, readers will be able to:

1. Recognize the implications that model of human occupation (MOHO)-based program development has on occupational therapy practice.
2. Learn about the continuum of stages that influence MOHO-based program development.
3. Appreciate the role of assessment, planning, implementation, and evaluation when implementing a MOHO-based program.
4. Reflect on the contents of the chapter and translate them into one's own work or practice contexts.

During the past 15 to 20 years, international program development with model of human occupation (MOHO) has continued to grow and expand, to promote occupational participation, and to facilitate the natural flow of people's occupational narratives into their daily lives. Just as people's lives are diverse and complex, so are the contexts in which occupational therapists use MOHO programs multiple and dynamic, and the programs have been designed to enhance persons' satisfaction and well-being in a range of settings. These include: the community (de las Heras, 2015; Echeverría, 2014; Kielhofner, de las Heras, & Suarez Balcazar, 2011), hospitals (Borell, Gustavsson, Sandman, & Kielhofner, 1994; de las Heras, Dion, & Wash, 1993; Melton et al., 2008), and other closed institutions (Catalán & Cavieres, 2014). They focus on working with mothers (Avrech Bar & Jarus, 2015; Avrech Bar, Labock-Gal, & Jarus, 2011), with families (Abelenda & Helfrich, 2003), with children who are at risk (D'Angello, 1998; de las Heras, Manghi, Acevedo, & Prieto, 2013; Kielhofner et al., 2011), with children on wellness promotion with adolescents living with occupational deprivation (Girardi, 2010); and with older people (Yamada, Kawamata, Kobayashi, Kielhofner, & Taylor, 2010; Ziv & Roitman, 2008). They target the needs of people who have AIDS (Kielhofner et al., 2004), schizophrenia (Briand et al., 2005), and anorexia (Abeydeera, Willis, & Forsyth, 2006); who are blind (Du Toit, 2008); who have borderline personality disorder (Lee & Harris, 2010); who have experienced stroke (Shinohara, Yamada, Kobayashi, & Forsyth, 2012); who have long-standing physical illnesses (Olson & Kielhofner, 1998); who experience combat reactions (Gindi, Galili, Adir, Magen, & Volovic-Shusham, 2015); or who are victims of family violence through life span and sexual abuse (Helfrich, 2001).

MOHO-based programs are defined as created social spaces that offer a dignifying and meaningful opportunity for a collective or group of people to enhance, continue, change, or reinvent the course of their occupational life in progress.

When developing a program based on MOHO, occupational therapists engage in a series of tasks. These tasks are guided by a theoretical context for framing occupational strengths and challenges of collectives and environments. The theoretical context of MOHO also allows for conceptualizing the services and their intended impact. This involves seeking empirical evidence to support claims regarding the relevance and likely impact of services, identifying relevant assessments for use in their evaluation process and for determining the outcomes of the program, and creating protocols of interventions to deliver the best services possible. Evaluators must undertake to propose, create, implement, and evaluate service programs that are efficient, effective, and cost-effective, responding to the pressures and needs of consumers, employers, third-party payers, and accrediting bodies (Kielhofner, 2008).

The main goal of this chapter is to provide new information about MOHO-based program development that is based on a systematic analysis of the growing body of experience emerging from diverse areas of practice. Additionally, guidance is provided about developing, implementing, and assessing MOHO-based programs, as well as the integration of theory and practice in private and public settings around the world (de las Heras, 2011, 2015).

MOHO-Based Program Development: Implications for Occupational Therapists

Program development based on MOHO follows the same therapeutic reasoning process as when working with individuals. MOHO principles and theory guide the occupational therapist to coherently think, feel, and do with groups in the joint needs assessment and planning, implementation, and evaluation of these programs. These principles infuse problem-solving and decision-making processes regarding a wide range of issues in order to create meaningful contexts that facilitate optimal participation of a group and its members in occupations. When considering whether to implement a MOHO-based program, practitioners may query whether such a complex and subtle model can be translated into practice. A number of practical questions need answering, regarding the capacity of the occupational therapy service to deliver the program. Examples of such questions include:

"How many therapists are needed?"
"What physical resources are required?"
"Who might benefit from the program?"
"Will the program be client centered?"
"Can a program work succeed in the setting I work in?"

Let's begin by addressing these basic issues in order to understand what MOHO-based program development means.

NUMBER OF THERAPISTS REQUIRED

The principles and faithful application of this model require that occupational therapists give some serious thought to the number of professionals, therapeutic companions, aides, and others necessary to support people to reach their therapy goals. But if we think about creating social spaces, we really need to reflect on who makes the program come alive. Is it the staff or the participants? To focus on the MOHO perspective, consider the elements of the model (volition, habituation, performance capacity, and environment). In the same way that MOHO follows the best client-centered procedures in individual interventions, the process of program development is guided by the people who are participating in the program.

Thus, when deciding on a program, we must make an effort to consider the strengths of each participating individual in relation to the group's occupational needs. If we do this, a program based on MOHO will use as few professionals and aides as possible, because the program participants should be considered the key facilitators of change. The role of peer support and self-help in which the participants take on the roles of monitors, guides, and leaders is essential to the success of MOHO-based programs. It is through the participants' own doing and their exchanges with other members of the group that a dynamic force is created in the process of change. Therefore, therapists and their teams' best action is to avoid the risk of "overdoing" by offering more support than is necessary. This might restrict the participants' process of exploration and, as a consequence, their self-knowledge and sense of competence. As we know, these aspects of a person (i.e., person variables) are crucial to the development of occupational identity and competence (de las Heras, 2011, 2015; Parkinson, Cooper, de las Heras de Pablo, & Forsyth, 2014).

The development of a program based on MOHO requires generating vibrant and natural social spaces. "Doing with" implies trusting and working as a team with the program participants, to build upon their real-life experiences, which, in turn, helps them consider those spaces as contributing to the continuity of their occupational narratives (de las Heras, 2015).

NECESSARY PHYSICAL RESOURCES

MOHO-based programs have been developed in all kinds of urban and rural settings, and have come to life with and without funding. On the one hand, having enough funding, a proper space, and plenty of objects supports the prolonged continuity of a program and the peace of mind of the occupational therapist. On the other hand, having everything freely available may hinder creativity, skills development, a sense of working toward personal and common goals, and a sense of belonging to a program. As stated in Chapter 14, more is not always better, and when promoting occupational participation it is often more important to focus on the cultural relevance and versatility of the physical resources than on their quantity.

When health policies or insurance restrictions limit the availability of physical resources, occupational therapists and participants using MOHO have still been able to prove the value of their programs, and encourage policy makers to fund them. Fund-raising and efforts to gather resources have been ongoing, even while the process of change occurs in these social groups. Fund-raising has enabled these projects to come to life and thrive with the full collaboration of program participants in a variety of practice settings (Kielhofner et al., 2011; de las Heras, 2006; de las Heras et al., 1993; Du Toit, 2008). Active participation of participants in these projects allows clients to develop a deeper appreciation of the nuances and efforts involved in accomplishing life goal. It leads to the discovery of creative problem-solving skills that, in turn, strengthen the group's cohesion (de las Heras & Cantero Garlito, 2009).

With MOHO's conceptualization of the dimensions of the environment and environmental impact, it offers occupational therapists the opportunity to gain a deep understanding of what might represent an optimal balance between physical and human resources to ensure the progressive occupational participation and the consistent development of occupational identity and competency.

INCLUSION CRITERIA

Occupational therapy programs have often been geared to persons with specific medical diagnoses and narrow age ranges, or have been limited to those who can attend by the adoption of various admission requirements such as compliance with certain "norms" of personal hygiene or the demonstration of specific skills. Arguments to support such practices are often lacking and we should question the convictions and theories that guide these decisions. Do we, as occupational therapists, have a poor tolerance for diversity? MOHO helps us to be critical of ourselves and be careful not to cause segregation or denial of occupational opportunities without first reflecting on the consequences (de las Heras, 2015).

Although institutions such as hospitals and community centers vary regarding how inclusive they are, the role of occupational therapists using MOHO has been pivotal to changing these very systems, helping them become more inclusive for people with a diverse range of conditions and ages when their common concern has been their occupational needs (D'Angello, 1998; de las Heras, 2006, 2011, 2015; de las Heras et al., 1993; Dion, Skerry, & Lovely, 1996; Kielhofner et al., 2011; Poletti, 2015).

The inclusion criteria for MOHO-based programs propose some basic requirements so that a program is effective and efficient for all participants. This will depend on the results of a rigorous occupational needs assessment. For example, *Reencuentros*, a community integration program in Chile (de las Heras, 2006; Braveman, Kielhofner, Bélanger, de las Heras, & Llerena, 2002), was opened to individuals with a wide range of personal circumstances linked to their abilities, education, place of residency, culture, and age (from young adolescents up). What they had in common was, in fact, their occupational needs. Together with *Rumbos*, another community center that followed the roots of *Reencuentros* in Argentina, the two centers worked to ensure that their programs were beneficial to everyone. Both programs determined that exclusion criteria would be related to difficulties in developing a sense of belonging and difficulties relating to one another, or simply not liking the program. These occupational issues underpinned restrictions related to having unstable psychotic symptoms or having cognitive abilities that would make it more appropriate for the person in question to attend a different type of program. One requisite agreed upon by the whole group of initial members, and that applied to each person who wanted to be admitted and to remain in the program, was that of mutual respect. Working as a collective with the participants, the therapists developed a document describing rules of coexistence in a clear and detailed fashion (de las Heras, 2015, 2006).

Of course, some MOHO-based programs have been developed very specifically for people who have the same illness, disability, or age range, when they have needed specialized interventions that would otherwise have been impossible to achieve. Even so, these programs have often accepted diverse conditions, cultures, and social origins, and it is acknowledged that these aspects have enriched the interventions and their focus on occupational identity and competence (Abeydeera et al., 2006; Braveman et al., 2002, 2008; Briand et al., 2005; Kielhofner, 2009; Lee & Harris, 2010; Quick, Melton, Critchley, 2012).

INTERACTION WITH PARTICIPANTS

One of MOHO's basic beliefs is that an empathic and open relationship between the therapist and the person is essential for client-centered therapy and for the therapist to develop the confidence necessary to facilitate participants' active participation in their process of change. A program's social climate (environment) can be "breathed," and "felt," inviting the person to explore it or to reject it. Therefore, a MOHO-based program must fulfill this condition: every person must be respected and validated as a unique human being who holds his or her own beliefs about the meaning of life, and who belongs to a collective that is valuable, in itself, for what the individuals have in common, for their strengths, and for what they are seeking in life. Just as when working with a single person, the interaction between the occupational therapist, participants, and their meaningful social groups must generate feelings of worth, control, and hope. Thus, the occupational therapist and other facilitators are required to be part of this collective. This is the attitude that enables a natural and equal relationship where each party agrees upon respect, rights, and responsibilities, offering their strengths for the attainment of individual and collective goals (de las Heras, 2015; de las Heras, Sanz, & Robio, 2012; Kielhofner, 2002, 2008, 1983).

THE DOMINANT CULTURE

MOHO fully acknowledges the importance of culture, its impact on volition and, consequently, on occupational participation. Social groups develop a culture of their own that enables cohesion among the members. MOHO principles underlying the promotion of occupational participation in social groups and how they may facilitate or hinder occupational participation of all their members were reviewed in Chapter 14. The occupational therapist using MOHO needs to be a cultural expert, with an obligation to know, investigate, and discover the historical trajectory and development of the values, customs, and rituals that permeate each participant's worldviews, as well as their social environments.

The fact that occupational therapists work with a diversity of people and groups of people in different settings makes it worth taking some time to understand the concept of immersion. Immersion is a procedure used in ethnographic qualitative research in various fields of study. The core goal of immersion is to gain access and to be an active part of a social group through an attitude of genuine collaboration and respect, and the actions associated with them. This provides the opportunity to get to know in depth some aspects of the human group, its culture, its subjective perception of its needs, and its visions.

Stages of MOHO-Based Program Development

The process of program development based on MOHO includes an ongoing sequence of stages to ensure the program's meaningfulness and appropriateness to the different occupational conditions and needs of the collectives and their relevant environments.

ASSESSMENT OF A GROUP'S OCCUPATIONAL NEEDS: PERSONAL AND ENVIRONMENTAL FACTORS

As with the first stages of the assessment of a person, a thoroughly performed assessment of the occupational needs of a group or collective affords the occupational therapist the opportunity to focus on the group's unique real-life interactions with its environments. The development of different types of programs, integrating MOHO-based interventions alongside other occupational therapy models and other disciplines' knowledge, as needed, is based on these real-life experiences.

When completing a needs assessment, occupational therapists must use the immersion process (mentioned above), be it with the group of people or collective, with the directors, with persons in charge of existing programs, with the professional team, or with social community groups. In so doing, the therapist would be able to link realities and visions of the groups with concepts and principles of MOHO, while establishing relationships and taking into account any element that has supported a positive process of change within the previous programs or intended practices. The immersion process could turn out to be a fertile ground for meaningful participatory education with social groups (refer to Chapter 14). In addition, the process of immersion, which is fully in agreement with the principles of MOHO, allows for the integration of the assessment of personal occupational factors (volition, habituation, performance capacities) that are representative of the group or collective, the assessment of the global and specific environmental factors, and their interaction process. Occupational needs assessment brings an understanding of the emergence of occupational participation and stages of change, as well as of the occupational adaptation of a unique group of persons.

In addition, when assessing environmental factors, the therapist must consider all characteristics of the specific environmental dimensions specified in Chapter 7 of this book, to understand their impact on facilitating or restricting groups' occupational participation. Following a detailed analysis, occupational therapists learn to integrate those aspects of the environment that support occupational participation, thereby sustaining the progress of the participants and the life of the program itself.

Needs Assessment Methods for Groups

The needs assessment methods utilized during the immersion period could be structured, nonstructured, or mixed, and are selected according to the group's needs and the environmental context.

- Nonstructured methods include conversations with individual persons and with groups of potential participants, participant observation, informal interviews with local social groups and with key persons from the group and social groups (selected informants), revision of relevant documents, and gathering knowledge about strategic places of the community network.
- Mixed methods include participatory action research and focus groups (Braveman et al., 2008; de las Heras, 2015),
- Structured methods include the administration of MOHO-based assessment tools. In this regard,

the self-assessment tools most commonly used in the context of focus groups are the Occupational Self-Assessment (OSA), the Role Checklist, and the Interest Checklist. These have proven to be of great utility to collect information about groups' occupational needs and have been joined more recently by the Residential Environmental Impact Scale (REIS). This instrument has been implemented in a variety of residential facilities for older adults, with inmates in jails, in hospitals, in residencies for orphan adolescents at risk, and in private homes as the main tool to evaluate the needs for intervention (Catalán & Cavieres, 2014; Chateau, Etchebarne & Rubilar, 2013; Echeverría, 2014; Quintanilla, 2014; Seguell, Arriagada, & Donoso, 2013). The Work Environment Impact Scale (WEIS; refer to Chapter 23) has also been useful in the process of assessing the occupational needs of groups of workers in a variety of work contexts (de las Heras, 2015). The Occupational Performance History Interview (OPHI-II; refer to Chapter 17) has guided therapists' understanding of the ongoing occupational history of potential participants and any social groups that may be involved (de las Heras, 2015). Discussing the scoring criteria of the OPHI-II has helped to foster openness and trust and to arrive at a shared conceptualization of the information collected regarding the overall occupational identity and competence of the group, and the impact of the environment (de las Heras, 2015).

How Can I Record Information Gathered through Nonstructured Methods?

When nonstructured methods are used to gather information, occupational therapists may organize the gathered information using the content and scoring forms of selected MOHO assessments. This procedure supports therapeutic reasoning and the process of conceptualizing the information together with participants. For example, the rating scales of the Model of Human Occupation Screening Tool (MOHOST) and the Short Children Occupational Profile (SCOPE) provide relevant information about occupational participation, and could be supplemented by the observational indicators of the Volitional Questionnaire (VQ). Indeed, when the group members do not have sufficient cognitive or verbal abilities, the use of the VQ and the Pediatric Volitional Questionnaire (PVQ) is central to giving them voice and creating a meaningful program design consistent with the observed volition of the group and the environmental impact on it (de las Heras, 2010, 2015).

The assessments above have all been used with the goal of establishing a global visual occupational profile of the group in order to support conclusions reached in a qualitative fashion. For example, in Argentina and Chile, occupational therapists who work with children have been able to use the SCOPE for this purpose and, by showing the analysis to school teams, have been able to explain MOHO expand their role in these occupational settings (Margaría & Weidmann, 2008; Vera, 2014).

PROGRAM PLANNING

Before planning a program, it is necessary to reach a conceptualization of the occupational needs of the group or collective and of the environment. Conceptualization should be done in collaboration with the group whenever participants' capacities and timing conditions of the program settings allow. Shared conceptualization might be accomplished within the context of a focus group to discuss the gathered and recorded information. The occupational therapist must facilitate active participation of everyone involved, sharing the process of identification and organization of available information, and highlighting the analysis of strengths and weaknesses of both the collective and the environment.

After reaching a conceptualization of occupational needs, the program's goals and objectives can be established through the facilitation of shared problem solving and decision making based on the previous needs assessment. This process requires prioritization of goals according to the assessed reality, which makes the use of mutual negotiation indispensable. When therapists carry out this MOHO strategy skillfully and facilitate its use by the participants, they enrich the therapeutic relationship and the spirit of teamwork that is so necessary for the success of a program.

An important task in the planning stage is the establishment of a timeline for goal accomplishment, including program the initiatives and the interventions selected to attain them. Because MOHO is a model that works in parallel to and in an integrated fashion with people and their relevant social groups, it is necessary to establish two or more timelines. This allows for a realistic perspective regarding the program goals of facilitating occupational change, and a realistic view of the goals established to facilitate participants naturally moving in and out of their relevant social groups. Creating a Gantt chart with this information may help the occupational therapist to implement and assess the program alongside the participants (Abelenda et al., 2005; Braveman et al., 2002; Kielhofner et al., 2011).

MOHO Problem-Solver Case: A Program for School-Aged Children with Sensory, Motor, and Communication Difficulties

In Caracas, Venezuela, an occupational therapist created an open program (Therapeutic Space) for children and their families to support their occupational participation and performance as family members, students, and friends. After evaluating the children's needs, it was noted that the educational policies on which school programming was based were not inclusive. Moreover, they discriminated against disabled children, including those with temporal or permanent disorders that affected their learning processes and their communication and interaction skills. This open program was a therapeutic space where children and their families were supported on an individual and group basis using Sensory Integration and Motor Control Models, and other rehabilitation and developmental approaches. Her intervention at the school was focused on applying these models, always in a playful context and coordinating with teachers for planning. Although evaluating the existing program, families had expressed their wish that occupational therapists might be more actively involved in the schools.

The therapist asked the important question, "Why?" and received the following answers: "The school doesn't listen to our needs as parents"; "I don't see my child being happy"; "My child is afraid to attend school"; "You have tried so hard to support our children by being loving and helping them with their mobility and writing, but they don't seem to feel good at school"; "My child is isolated at school and does not want to play." Listening to them, the occupational therapist realized that the existing educational programming lacked a theoretical foundation that could offer a wide vision of occupational participation. Such a program could explain and guide her to solve the needs of these families and their children. The therapist was very clear about her role as a professional, and always intended to follow occupational therapy principles in each and every intervention with both the children and their families. However, the main problem was a collective one and the needs of the whole group needed to be addressed.

She looked for training on MOHO and read the books and materials that were, at that time, translated into her language. Then, in 2008, she developed a program called "Terapeuta Amigo" (Friendly Therapist) with seven other colleagues. This program integrated MOHO with the other models and established a parallel timeline for a program with teachers and directors of schools. The occupational therapists changed their approach to the school into one that was more integrative. They started to share MOHO with the teachers by using the SCOPE with children so they could feel more confident and foster this group of children's occupational participation at school. At the same time, at "Terapeuta Amigo," they created flexible occupational spaces for fun and participation in different types of play, whether in groups or solely. Sensory integration equipment became part of the whole space. They created a program called "Play is a serious thing" for children who had communication problems at school. For the families they organized educational and counseling sessions. Within this playful context, their main interventions were facilitation of exploration, MOHO-based skill teaching, participatory education and occupational counseling with families, and, most importantly, participation in meaningful occupations related to play and school assignments. The MOHO assessments used were the SCOPE, the PVQ, the Assessment of Communication and Interaction Skills (ACIS) the Child Occupational Self-Assessment, the Pediatric Interest Profile, and the School Setting Interview. As teachers and directors of the schools became convinced of the benefits of using MOHO together with therapists, the "Terapeuta Amigo" team decided that they had to design another parallel timeline to address public policy work with education-related political agendas. With the families' and the teachers' support, and evidence from program outcomes, they were now clear how to approach and work with these new social groups in order to make substantial changes in the educational system.

PROGRAM DESIGN AND ORGANIZATION

Program design and organization must respect the core and specific principles of MOHO to be a good fit with the needs assessed and established goals. Therapists, together with the group, can select, adapt, and enrich any MOHO-specific interventions, therapeutic strategies, and protocols of intervention to facilitate the creation of meaningful social contexts for occupational change. It is in this stage of program development where therapists must reason and plan to incorporate an intervention approach that addresses the needs of the collective as a group at the same time as those of the unique individuals who are part of it. Organizing a MOHO-based program involves considering the above-mentioned implications for the therapist and the unique dynamic generated by the program itself. These will directly impact the process of change for each participant and for the collective as a whole, generating an ascending spiral of ideas, initiatives, and collective and individual occupational projects.

Also in this stage, it is necessary to develop a feasible evaluation system, by selecting the MOHO assessment tools that are most likely to be used with a particular group during their process of change. For example, therapists working in residences with older adults who have severe cognitive and physical problems may choose the VQ as the most useful structured methods to understand the participants' participation in occupation, and to guide action plans delivered by the team. In other programs, a combination of different types of MOHO evaluation methods has been chosen according to the main goals of the group (Braveman et al., 2002, 2008; de las Heras, 2015; Kielhofner, 2009; Melton et al., 2008). In still more program settings, it has been determined that a MOHO assessment may be used in conjunction with a non-MOHO assessment. For example, in programs open to little children with cerebral palsy and their families, the SCOPE and PVQ have been identified as the MOHO assessments that are part of a package with Sensory Integration or Motor Control assessments (Abelenda, 2015; Calderón, 2010).

MOHO Problem-Solver Case: Adult Survivors of Sexual Abuse

The Multidisciplinary Center for sexually abused women and men (Haifa, Israel) is run by the Bnei-Zion Medical Center, Haifa municipality, and the Ministry of Social Affairs. It offers women and men who were sexually abused subsidized psychological treatment and an array of therapeutic groups in order to help them rebuild their lives after their traumatic experience. One of the groups offered is an Occupational Therapy group.

The Occupational Therapy group is a year-long program that takes place once a week during a 2-hour session. Every year there is a screening and intake process with women who are interested in participating in the group, in which the occupational therapist uses the Occupational Case Interview and Rating Scale (OCAIRS) and the OSA. She selected both assessments because they allowed her to get a broad yet detailed understanding of the occupational participation and subjective perception of the interviewee. In addition, the OSA gave her an understanding about the way women saw themselves as occupational beings. Each woman was assessed individually and the results of the assessment were discussed together in a separate meeting.

The group has been run as a peer-support educational group and is based on 3 years of ongoing development. Every year, the group decides together with the occupational therapist what goals to work on. In the first year, the group decided to work on building healthy life routines and learning how to manage time effectively. In the second year, the group chose to work on personal goal-setting and the planning and implementation of the different activities and tasks needed to achieve them. During this year, the therapist began to realize "that something was missing." "I saw that the whole occupational discourse was lacking because we addressed issues like habits and performance skills, but I didn't pay attention to the important dimension of volition that I had considered during the initial evaluation. I was not including it as a key aspect to integrate with the other dimensions during the intervention process." "What a mistake—I was not applying MOHO!"

Closing the year, the therapist explained MOHO to the group members and the rationale behind it. She gave them the opportunity to share how their lives had been shaped using MOHO concepts. The group began to understand their process of change better and they could explain to the therapist that their common need was to feel competent again. Following this experience, the therapist offered the group a chance to explore their own individual values during their third-year meetings. The group readily accepted the occupational therapist's proposition. At the end of the year, every participant was able to state their own values and reflect on how important the opportunity had been to explore them. They described themselves as being more confident, empowered, and satisfied with their occupational participation and routines.

Designing and planning an occupational therapy program based on MOHO allowed the therapist to offer clients a more holistic and comprehensive view of themselves as occupational beings and supported them to make a significant change in their thinking patterns, decision making, and well-being. Moreover, presenting the model and work program to the team resulted in a better understanding and a growing appreciation of the profession.

PROGRAM IMPLEMENTATION AND EVALUATION

In addition to respecting MOHO principles and selecting significant interventions when organizing the program design, therapists need to nurture flexibility in their therapeutic reasoning. This allows them to adapt, improve, or change the types of intervention once the program has been implemented. Changes may be made based on an ongoing assessment of the fit between the design and organization on the one hand, and the progress made by the collective and its constituents on the other. Thus the goal of program evaluation is to improve the action plan by refining, adapting, strengthening, or even discontinuing particular program components. According to MOHO theory and principles, program evaluation entails living the process of program change together with the collective.

Program development could be viewed following a continuum of implementation stages. It begins with an exploratory stage, or pilot program, where the design and implementation's efficacy and efficiency might be assessed after a 2- to 3-month period. Subsequently, a competency stage evolves, consisting of sustained practice, where the program is adjusted and run based on the outcomes of the assessment performed during the exploratory stage. Finally, the program reaches an achievement stage, or stage of coalescence of strategies and procedures, where innovation and expansion take place. Prioritizing timely interventions with both the group of participants and with all the relevant agencies involved makes the process of change a mutually rewarding process for all concerned (de las Heras, 2011, 2015).

Program evaluation may utilize and integrate different procedures according to the specific program context. In general, regularly held meetings of all participants and stakeholders will ensure the smooth life in progress of the program, allowing for joint problem solving and decision making on a variety of emerging issues (Table 24-1). Keeping records of

Table 24-1 Summary of Reassessment Procedures of a MOHO-Based Program

Types of Evaluation	Procedures
Evaluation of program components and global program	• *Focus groups*: Assessment of environmental impact, subjective impressions of program dynamics, global outcomes assessment of goals established in Gantt chart, goal planning based on feedback, problem solving, and decision making. • *Regularly held meetings* with all participants and stakeholders as part of the program's dynamic (general assemblies). • Meetings with participants of each program component as a routine procedure. • *Conversations* with key group *members* and social groups. • *Participant observation:* Ongoing evaluation of the volitional process, environmental impact, and individual and group participation. • Participatory action research. • Experimental research.
Evaluation of individual and group outcomes and approximate accomplishment of global objectives	• Assessment of goal attainment with each person, recording information using agreed outcome measures. • Percentage calculation of the sum of individual results, as a way to keep track of the global program value. • Program outcomes evaluation through application of MOHO selected assessments with the entire group.
Evaluation of job satisfaction and outlook of the facilitating team	• *Regularly held team meetings* to coordinate actions and evaluate program's procedures and implementation outcomes. • *Team meetings using* the WEIS (Moore-Corner et al., 1998) as individual self-assessment, followed by reflection of members of the team, feedback, problem solving, and planning of opportunities for satisfactory occupational participation in work and other relevant contexts.

Adapted from de las Heras (2015), p. 228.

conclusions reached during these meetings provides invaluable sources for enhancing MOHO programs and for the generation of evidence for practice. Further evaluation procedures may also be conducted, and may even form the basis of experimental research to determine the effectiveness of MOHO programs (Shinohara et al., 2012; Yamada et al., 2010).

DYNAMICS OF A MOHO-BASED PROGRAM

The dynamics of a MOHO-based program refer to the cohesion between goals, types of interventions, and the social climate created in such a way to allow the optimal environmental impact on the process of change for the participants and for the program as a whole. The basic dynamic of a MOHO-based program is accomplished through the implementation of meaningful occupational opportunities and through the exchanges and interactions among the participants. The former offers significant opportunities for individual and social participation in a smooth routine, which is then enriched by the active contribution of each member. Occupational counseling, peer-support educational groups, and self-help groups also enrich and supplement the dynamics, as they are focused on reflecting and processing the experience of daily participation in relevant occupational contexts with another or with others. This enhances motivation for continuing the collective and individual occupational journeys.

OCCUPATIONAL OPPORTUNITIES

Occupational opportunities refer to spaces that invite people to participate in significant occupations. These spaces are diverse in nature and need to be compatible with the work context and occupational needs of the collective.

When offering occupational opportunities, the therapist using MOHO considers the group members' occupational needs that have been assessed, acknowledging the critical importance of their culture, recognizing the relevance of occupations for their life in progress, and the personal and social meanings they are imbued with. Occupational opportunities are meant to fulfill common and individual goals in the continuity of time, be it to satisfy daily needs, to contribute to the preparation of a social event, to explore skills and practice the skills needed for supported or independent living or work, or to develop a hobby. This meaning renders them very different from other purposeful activities, which may be undertaken simply to fill in time without any intention to participate in them over the longer term.

Occupational opportunities must contribute to individual and collective needs by offering a variety of alternatives of doing that are compatible with the dimensions of participation sought by each participant. It should be remembered that they need to provide opportunities for meaningful participation by persons with a wide range of volitional and performance characteristics, who have come together to share common interests or goals. In addition, these opportunities should be as natural as possible. That is to say, they should be organized and implemented as far as possible in the manner that they take place in the ordinary daily life of the society and culture to which the group or collective belongs. This encourages shared exploration and learning, decision making, agreement, and negotiation among the group members and the therapist regarding optimal ways to carry out the intended activities and tasks that have been chosen to accomplish common and individual goals. In this context, rules, structures, and role expectations are derived automatically from natural life experience. This allows people to become more expressive and spontaneous when participating (either verbally or nonverbally) and more able to contribute their interests and skills within the group context (de las Heras, 2010, 2015).

For example, in Israel, a program was developed to support soldiers with combat stress to promote a rapid return to optimal occupational participation. Based on soldiers' occupational needs, therapists proposed an intervention aiming to enhance functioning by facilitating soldiers' engagement, as a group, in meaningful activities and tasks pertaining to their military roles. These were active roles that were needed to support projects in the military system. Participation in these activities and tasks has supported their military identity, fostering performance and increasing perceived competency. The program design is congruent with the Israeli Defense Force (IDF) and US *modus operandi*, emphasizing the development of a comfortable climate based on client-centered and occupation-based practice within a military environment. Occupational therapists participate in interdisciplinary work focused on recovering functional abilities and identified roles that were valued by participants, improving and preserving their occupational skills, as well as maintaining participation and promoting performance patterns (habits and routines; Gindi et al., 2015).

Properties and Ways of Participation in Occupational Opportunities

For a successful implementation of a MOHO-based program, occupational opportunities need to respect three properties: diversity, flexibility, and continuity (de las Heras, 2010, 2015).

Diversity refers to the variety of occupations available that meet the group's interests, values, and goals and varied opportunities to participate in them. Having a diversity of options enhances a sense of personal meaning, through exploration of motivational aspects, making choices and decisions, and developing a broader sense of capacity. Options for occupational participation include opportunities provided in the context of the program itself, in the context of the wider community networks, and in the private contexts of the group's participants.

Flexibility refers to the constant innovation of occupational opportunities because of the dynamic nature of the process of change for individuals and the group. Innovation may occur in response to goal attainment, a need for a higher challenge, or to emerging events or obstacles. To keep flexibility within occupational opportunities, it is necessary that they are carefully planned and assessed by the occupational therapist and the participants on an ongoing basis, deciding on the creation of new occupational projects, completing or ending others, or developing new procedures for attaining goals. Flexibility reproduces the experience of dynamism that is inherent in daily occupations, and is necessary for the development of initiative, a sense of capacity and efficacy, skills for planning, problem solving, decision making and social participation, and a sense of belonging as a contributor to the social group.

Continuity refers to the lifetime of occupational opportunities, which, if meaningful to the group, must offer continuity over time and grow as the group develops and individual projects expand. This is not to say that occupations cannot be discontinued if it is so decided by the therapist and participants based on their assessment, but new occupations will take their place. Essentially, continuity enables each new participant to join and collaborate with existing initiatives, either offering new ideas to the ongoing projects or helping to generate new ones at any given moment. In this way, continuity of occupational opportunities facilitates the exploration of a sense of the real temporal dynamism of participation, in occupations that are part of a routine. In sum, continuity fully allows participants' volitional and habituation processes to unfold.

MOHO-based programs benefit from offering three ways of participation in occupational opportunities: participating in collective projects, participating in personal projects, and participating through exploring (de las Heras, 2006, 2010, 2015).

Collective projects refer to undertaking a series of activities and tasks to achieve an occupational goal for a group. During the development of group occupational projects, the therapist encourages members' participation according to their personal occupational needs and those of the group as a whole. The following example illustrates this concept.

The Long Life Club

The Long Life Club was a program developed with older adults who had complex physical and mental conditions and were residents of specialized wards in a public psychiatric hospital. This club was formed by a group of men and women whose goals were to maintain their abilities and skills, and to offer others the practical knowledge they had acquired during their lives. The group, together with the occupational therapist, organized this occupational space based on the strengths they had as a group and individually. They had meetings where they shared and discussed about their interests and anecdotal experiences of events that represented the values and occupations that formed their lives when they were younger. Based on these stories, the therapist invited them to give ideas of which projects they would like to undertake within the hospital. They voted for the most popular ideas, selected a musical project, and wrote a newsletter to disseminate their culture to the staff and younger patients at the hospital.

Some of the members who had musical talents organized a time to rehearse singing songs from their era once a week. They also gathered recordings from the radio and resources for recording their own singing. Their goal was to give presentations at celebration events that were periodically organized by other groups at the hospital, and to forge alliances with the nursing staff on various wards. In order to do this they adopted and assigned people to a number of roles: social relations officer; time keeper; secretary in charge of getting copies of songs; song writers; singers; and musical director. In addition, they had a planning meeting with a nursing aide each week, where they discussed the timing for rehearsals, clothing for presentations, and coordinated the recording and playing of music to have for events and their musical representations on the wards.

The newsletter, called the "Good Old Times," was a common project for everyone, and members participated twice a week to plan and prepare content and pictures for it. They had different sections for the newsletter, with four corresponding subgroups being responsible for them. One section described how they continued to use old objects in their daily activities, another presented their personal stories and the emotional legacies they left, another featured poetry, and one contained cooking recipes. The newsletter was produced in the business center and members took on different roles according to their abilities and interests, with some of the residents using the computers, and one of them becoming the editor of the newsletter to coordinate the writing and final edits. They produced four newsletters a year. These projects led to other ones, including volunteering. Fund-raising was needed to sustain their projects over time, and they started selling baked products made by three of the club's members to the hospital cafeteria.

Planning and carrying out meaningful common occupational projects across time affords and demands a collaborative effort that fully encourages participation in roles and the development of commitment and social responsibility. More than this, it affords the exploration and development of communication and interaction skills, discovery of one's unique abilities, sense of efficacy, new habits, and self-knowledge as a social being. It also provides the initial spark for participating in personal projects, and negotiating internal and external role expectations.

Personal projects refer to undertaking a series of activities and related tasks to accomplish a meaningful occupational goal for an individual. These projects are selected by the person during his or her process of change and emerge from the assessment of personal needs reflected upon in collaboration with the therapist, or from his or her own experience of the occupational participation process. In general, undertaking *vital personal projects* is more challenging than taking part in a group project because they represent a personal challenge, drawing on one's own resources for problem solving and decision making regarding the options for accomplishing the desired goal. Participation in personal occupational projects imbues occupational participation and performance with personal meaning. It requires initiative for setting goals across time, increased commitment to fulfill them, systematic skills development, and methodical occupational performance to make them happen. In addition, it can afford the unique sense of contributing to social context and bolstering occupational identity and competence.

Exploratory participation refers to a person's initial and sometimes sole participation in occupations, with the goal of discovering, sampling, and reasserting a sense and knowledge of capacity. Exploratory participation can take place while participating in activities related to a group project, completing some of the steps, or performing the actions needed. This may be done either in close proximity to others or in a separate space, according to the volitional process and capacities of the person. Therapists and other members of the group need to be open to this type of participation, in order to facilitate volitional experience guided by the Remotivation Process (de las Heras, Llerena, & Kielhofner, 2003). The motivation and participation of others who are in more advanced states of change are invariably a valuable source of support and reaffirmation of the initiative and emerging exploratory feelings (Deegan, 1988; de las Heras et al., 2003).

Dynamics of Participation in and within Occupational Opportunities

Participation in *personal and collective* projects can intertwine if a person can participate in a group project while having a personal goal within it. Indeed, a group project may well afford the first opportunity for exploration of a possible personal project, as a person begins to attribute a personal meaning to the shared occupation. The perceived demands or expectations of personal performance and habits while participating and the environmental support required are unique to each person, but similar to those of the rest of the group in that they will relate to common goals, rules, and roles previously agreed upon by the group or collective. Each person is therefore able to carry out stages of his or her own project in a parallel fashion to a group project that is taking place in the same context, entering and coming out of group projects in different moments, or cooperating with the group projects through his or her own project (Fig. 24-1).

MOHO-Based Programs in Diverse Contexts

Each program has unique features arising from the groups' assessed occupational needs. As discussed in the introduction to this chapter, MOHO can be used in a wide variety of practice settings, ranging from the community at large to enclosed institutions. Each of

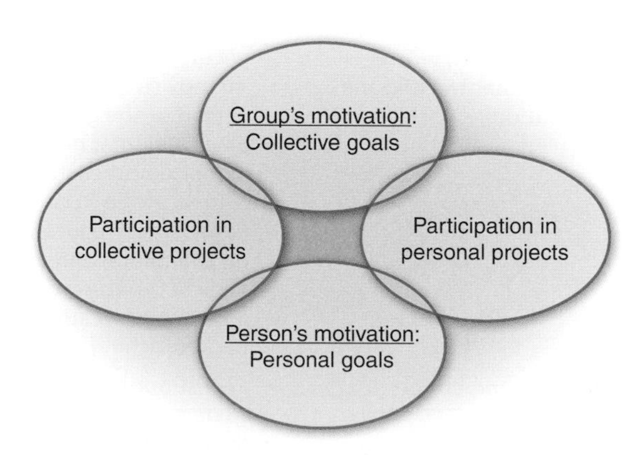

FIGURE 24-1 MOHO-Based Programs: Dynamics in and within Occupational Opportunities.

these has specific physical, social, cultural, financial, and political characteristics that differently impact the program goals and the roles the occupational therapist can assume in their midst.

ENCLOSED INSTITUTIONS

When working in short-term acute settings or rehabilitation settings (10–15 days) with persons across their lifespan, environmental management is of great importance. Environmental management may be used for organizing and arranging common spaces, such as the day room, or for making objects accessible to promote free-time activity choices and the opportunity to be in a group or alone according to the cultural needs and social preferences of each person in the moment. The arrangement of furniture (couches, chairs, tables, shelves) and the arrangement of meaningful objects are both key for facilitating participation. In the ideal situation, they allow a day room to become an elective space, where persons go to find a moment of entertainment, conversation, or respite from their bedrooms and medical treatments. The organization and layout of common spaces must therefore be such that they "call out" inviting a person to use them in the same way that they would in their daily lives beyond the medical setting (de las Heras, 2011; de las Heras et al., 1993; Table 24-2).

During this period of time, therapists need to utilize flexible methods of assessment if the assessment process is to be feasible. It is not possible to get to know the natural occupational participation of a person when he or she is undergoing the acute stage of an illness, which interferes significantly with his or her regular doing. In these situations the medical treatment is paramount. However, MOHO's occupational participation profiles and volitional questionnaire use observation as an information gathering method, and this allows therapists to work in cooperation with medical teams to research the impact of symptoms (objective aspects of performance capacity) on current occupational participation. Besides adding significantly to understanding the severity of the impact that an illness has on an

Table 24-2 Possible Interventions in a Short-Stay Inpatient Setting

Interventions	Description
Evaluation process	• Unstructured methods. • If possible to use: SCOPE or MOHOST; VQ or PVQ. • Administration of the REIS. • Narrative interview guided by OPHI-II, with integration of family's perspective. • Parents' interview based on SCOPE guidelines.
Addressing persons' lived body	• *Company and empathy:* Active listening, *validating* feelings and thoughts, *structuring* environment for sense of safety.
Supporting individual participation in occupational routines	• Accompany persons while performing activities of daily living as needed. • According to the state of each person's abilities and volition, support or assist occupational performance. • According to the state of each person's abilities and volition, advise or coach on key aspects that would be useful after discharge. • Most used strategies: validating, encouraging, structuring.
Education and environmental management within the institution	• *Participatory education* of staff members regarding occupational needs, expectations for performance, and any relevant information on occupational therapy strategies that may make their relationship and their work with each person or the group more effective and efficient. • *Environmental management:* Organization of physical and social environments alongside other staff according to conclusions obtained through the administration of the REIS. • *Participatory education* with the professional team, sharing information based on evaluation and assessment results, advocating for an extension of the admission if necessary. • *Most frequent strategies:* validating, negotiating, encouraging, giving feedback, coaching, structuring.
Group Intervention	• *Peer support educational groups*, regarding discharge issues, with persons able to participate. • *Share and facilitate participation* while being in day rooms or other common spaces, as needed. • Most frequent strategies: validating, advising, encouraging, giving feedback.

Table 24-2 Possible Interventions in a Short-Stay Inpatient Setting (*continued*)

Interventions	Description
Family education, counseling, and support	• *Participatory education* sessions and *occupational counseling* with families, either privately or collectively. • Distribution of brochures and other information on social networks as needed. • Distribution of written materials as needed. • Invitation to prepare a diary to share feelings, thoughts, and experiences with family members if desired. Using this diary as a springboard to offer feedback, information, and to guide counseling or education. • Share assessment report and discuss problem solving and decision making on best alternatives. • Most frequent strategies: validating, advising, encouraging, giving feedback.
Coordination with community networks and referral if warranted	• Establish contacts with community networks according to needs and agreements reached with individuals and family members. MOHO-based report is needed when referral is made by the institution's therapist to occupational therapists or people in charge of community networks.

Adapted from de las Heras (2015), pp. 238–239.

individual, observational assessments can also be used to track the course of recovery, manifested in increasingly satisfying daily engagement (Parkinson, Chester, Cratchley, & Rowbottom, 2008).

When persons require mid-term hospitalizations (1–2 months), the injuries or symptoms that originally interfered with occupational participation tend to stabilize. This allows occupational therapists to broaden the scope of their assessment and intervention processes (illustrated in Table 24-2) and to establish priorities as needed. MOHO-based programs in long-term hospitalization have been shown to initiate a process of progressive transformation of the culture and services in the hospitals, changing them into places where occupational participation is facilitated along a continuum that culminates in community integration (Abeydeera et al., 2006; Borell et al., 1994; Cifuentes, 2011; de las Heras et al., 1993; Dion et al., 1996; Lee & Harris, 2010; Melton et al., 2008; Olson & Kielhofner, 1998). These processes have been possible thanks to the interdisciplinary work led by occupational therapists who embrace the MOHO vision and hold the belief that a person's journey of recovery is accomplished across their lifetime, with the involvement of everyone in and outside of the institution.

In these settings, it is possible to carry out a comprehensive assessment process as well as intervention programs where collective and individually specific interventions can be integrated across time. The management of the physical environment remains critical, and so changing the arrangement of furniture and the decoration of spaces according to persons' volition, culture, and autonomy needs is to be encouraged. The social environment can also be shaped, by promoting and implementing projects for family participatory education, systematic participatory educational meetings with staff members, the development of a support network within the institution and in the community, and the establishment of a progressive system for community integration. This will involve establishing connections, exchanges, and referrals to community centers on an ongoing basis, as well as implementing common projects and events, encouraging regular visits to community facilities, and the progressive participation of the persons in community activities. The *Remotivation Process* (de las Heras et al., 2003) details how this can be accomplished with individuals, by working with all staff members to deliver an environmental climate that facilitates motivation for doing.

COMMUNITY CENTERS

Diverse MOHO-based experiences of community centers have been key to community integration for individuals from a wide range of ages and with a variety of occupational circumstances produced by incremental, transformational, or catastrophic changes in their lives. Some examples are: *Reencuentros* and *Senderos* in Chile (Braveman et al., 2002; de las Heras, 2006; Kielhofner, 2004, 2008, 2009); *Rumbos* in Argentina (Polleti, 2010, 2015); *Employment Options* in the United States (Braveman et al., 2002, 2008; Kielhofner, Braveman, & Finlayson, 2004); *Terapeuta Amigo* in Venezuela and *Uutchi* in Spain (de las Heras, 2015). Other initiatives have been developed in an array of private practice settings, such as day centers for older adults, family health care centers, and community-based mental health and physical rehabilitation centers run by national or local health initiatives (de las Heras, 2015, Echeverría, 2014; Fig. 24-2).

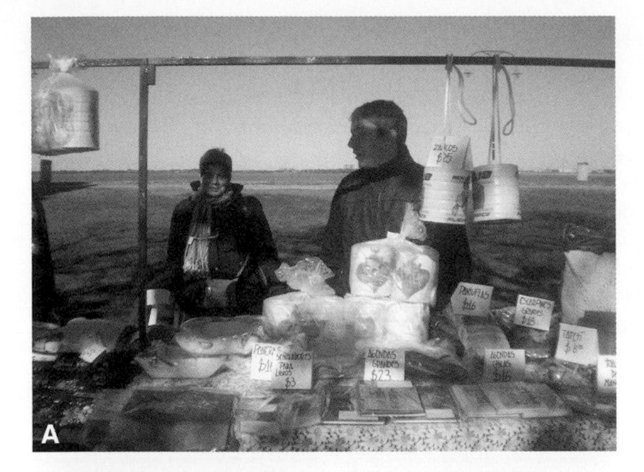

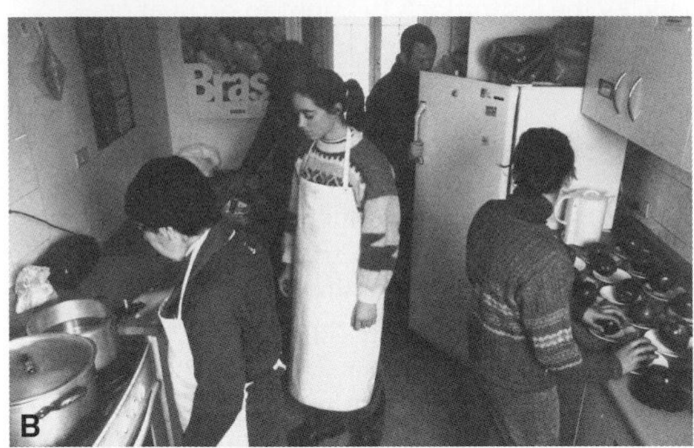

FIGURE 24-2 **A.** One of "Rumbos" Collective Projects: Producing Products and Selling at Fairs in Santa Fe, Argentina. **B.** One of the Five Collective Projects of the Kitchen (Occupational Space) at Reencuentros, Chile: Preparing Daily Lunch.

Community centers enable long-term work with people, thus making it possible to integrate a variety of specific interventions and protocols of intervention described in this book, beginning with a comprehensive assessment and continuing with the implementation of collective and individually specific interventions within the center and in the wider community. Possibilities of intervention are wide, including:

- formal and informal participatory community education;
- direct intervention in meaningful occupational contexts during the integration process;
- implementing specific programs to facilitate people's integration in valued roles;
- formal and informal training to other professionals and staff;
- program coordination and integration with other community networks;
- participatory education and negotiation with political entities; and
- promotion of equal participation opportunities in diverse occupational settings (de las Heras, 2015, Kielhofner et al., 2011).

The following example shows one of the initiatives mentioned above.

CASE EXAMPLE: NEEDS ASSESSMENT

In her informal conversations with the parents of children she was supporting through private practice, an occupational therapist came to realize the true impact of her work. She started to notice that many of them expressed that the greatest transformation during the therapeutic process had happened within them. Some said, "The greatest change this year has been my own," or "I have learned to relate to my child in a different way." Some families were able to articulate their transformation experiences, and even felt grateful to their children with disabilities for enabling them to discover strengths they had been unaware of. Other families did not express this with so much clarity, but the therapist saw them "transforming themselves in front of her very eyes." These nonstructured observations led her to confirm like Winnicott did (1960, p. 587), that "there is no such thing as an infant" and there is no such thing as *a* child. In other words, it is not possible to work with one without taking into account the family and multiple environments in which the child participates day to day. That is why she created a private clinic: Uutchi Desarrollo Infantil (Uutchi, Children Development).

What is Uutchi? Program Planning and Implementation

Uutchi is a space where the whole family can learn to know themselves better in order to accomplish more effective and satisfactory occupational participation. Uutchi supports families and their children in the development of skills and abilities needed for their full participation in their meaningful occupational settings, such as home, school, and the community. Children from birth to adolescence and their families can come to Uutchi once or twice a week, depending on their needs and prospects. Uutchi is part of the community occupational settings. Families are referred by acquaintances or family members, through connections in the community or through advice from the schools where the children attend. Most families have children with some type of developmental disorder, such as autism spectrum disorder, developmental delays, or genetic syndromes. Some children do not have any clear medical diagnosis, but their families have identified occupational participation challenges.

What Models Does Uutchi Use? Theoretical Foundation

Based on the specific needs of the families attending this program, three practice models guide the therapeutic reasoning and intervention: DIR/DIRFloortime (Greenspan & Wieder, 2007), Ayres Sensory Integration (ASI; Parham et al., 2011; Schaaf & Mailloux, 2015), and the MOHO (Kielhofner, 2008). The first one is an interdisciplinary model concerned with promoting the functional social–emotional developmental capacities to relate, communicate, and think in the context of natural and playful interactions between child and caregiver throughout the day, and in the therapeutic context. This approach encourages the development of connection, trust, flexibility in play, and increasingly longer and complex chains of interactions. The second, ASI, is an approach that promotes the child's processing and integration of sensory information from his or her body and the environment through active, self-directed participation in vigorous sensory-rich activities, enabling more effective and efficient participation in daily occupations.

These two models offer individual interventions tailored to either the child's sensorimotor or social–emotional profiles while they follow the child's interests. Both models share a belief that, given the opportunity, the child has the capability to reach his or her highest potential and seek what is best for him or her. Their common components are seamlessly framed within the MOHO. In addition, MOHO offers a deep understanding of the volitional indicators described in the PVQ (Basu et al., 2008) and specific intervention strategies detailed in by the Remotivation Process (de las Heras et al., 2003). These indicators allow the therapist to comprehend the volitional state of the children and to recognize where the children find themselves in terms of the volitional process. She can then decide if it is appropriate to increase a challenge, or if it is necessary to maintain exploration and enjoyment. It is also helpful to share these observations with parents, allowing them an entry point to understand their children better.

How Does the Program Work? Program Design and Organization

Sessions with the child and family members use different environmental contexts generated by the therapist, which foster the development of the child's confidence and sense of pleasure (volition), performance in play and basic ADL (occupational skills), and sensorimotor and emotional abilities (performance capacity). In Uutchi, spaces and objects are carefully planned (environmental management) so that the physical environment "speaks" of the affordances and possibilities it offers. The waiting room was designed as a transition space between the world outside and the world of Uutchi: a warm and comfortable space that invites dialogue, relaxation, and reflection. Books for adults, toys for children, a comfortable carpet to sit down and paint on are part of the space. The big room, or gym, offers the necessary equipment for sensory integration intervention, with swings for vestibular work, textured materials for tactile exploration, and plenty of opportunities to climb, push, and pull, to enhance body awareness while playing. There are also plenty of cushions to lie down on—places to think and reflect that encourage an exchange of ideas and conversation—plus dolls, a dollhouse, costumes, and fabrics to encourage symbolic play. Every space in Uutchi can be flexibly used in a therapeutic manner, according to the arising needs of children and their families.

What Makes This Program a Success? Program Evaluation

Following MOHO and DIR/DIRFloortime principles of working as a team with families is the key to success. Families have an active role in the sessions, and whenever possible, intervention is carried out through the families, facilitating their exploration of alternatives shared, and implementing participatory education using validation, feedback, and coaching strategies. Active participation in the sessions and the collaboration in the establishment of goals foster a sense of empowerment in the families, and strong sense of being an actor in their children's development.

COMMUNITY-BASED INTERVENTION

The role of an occupational therapist working in community intervention is closely linked with that of the therapist working in community program settings using MOHO to foster *joint development of collective life projects*. These include: microenterprises, projects of advocacy for equal occupational participation opportunities, community education projects with a variety of social groups, projects aiming to explore and expand social networks, joint implementation of participatory education groups and peer support educational groups for wellness, the programming and application of interventions in diverse occupational settings such as preschools, schools, work sites, residencies, sociocultural settings, neighborhoods, and directly in the streets; as well as joint negotiation with organizations and political and legal agencies. All types of MOHO-specific interventions and protocols of interventions (refer to Chapter 14) can be used in community intervention (Abelenda et al., 2005; Avrech Bar, Labock-Gal, & Jarus, 2011; Avrech Bar, Jarus, & Wada, 2015;

de las Heras, 2015; de las Heras et al., 2013; D'Angello, 1998; Du Toit, 2008; Girardi, 2010; Kielhofner et al., 2011; Margaría & Weidmann, 2008; Parkinson, 2014; Solomon, O'Brien, & Cohn, 2013; Yazdani, 2008; Ziv & Roitman, 2008).

Several community initiatives based on MOHO have been undertaken through partnerships between occupational therapy academic programs and community agencies (such as schools, departments of work affairs), or directly with community representatives, to develop interventions at occupational settings with children, adolescents, adults, and older adults. These projects have increased lately both within community-based rehabilitation teams and with populations who are going through incremental changes and facing severe environmental restrictions. The examples below provide an illustration of these projects, developed in Chile and the United States.

CASE EXAMPLE: COMMUNITY-BASED INTERVENTION

Since 2012, as part of the second year's courses on Human Occupation, a class of occupational therapy students and their professors from the University of Los Andes in Santiago participate in giving direct services to promote the satisfactory occupational participation of children who are living in poverty. Some of the children might get services at preschool or primary school public settings if there is somebody in the family to take them, but many spend the majority of their time without protection on the streets, where they are constantly exposed to community violence and drug addiction. The program on the streets aims to enhance opportunities for the children to play and relate safely. A need was identified by the older children and the community residents' representative for a place where the children could come together. A soccer field and a chapel were lent for this purpose. Every Friday afternoon, the students go through the streets with a professor, inviting the children to come along. Older children bring their little siblings and others go by themselves knowing now that it is their space to play.

The students decided to have two subgroups, one for little children (up to 6 years old) and another for older children from of 7 to 14 years old. Based on the children's interests, they organize and implement a series of sequenced, semi-structured, and free-play activities which are carefully selected according to culture and age, graded in complexity according to the children's volition, and implemented dynamically according to children's ideas and decisions made about the direction that play routine may take. In addition, they create simple informational flyers, which the children take to their caregivers to invite families for celebratory events.

Friday afternoon is also a special time for those children (3–5 years old) who can access preschool and school sites, having also a space for playing and doing other motivating activities. In these settings, occupational therapy students work with children in the classes and in schools' yards with one of their educators. They also engage in participatory education with teachers, sharing responsibilities and different approaches based on MOHO for students who are considered difficult to work with, to educate the teachers about their students' occupational needs and discover ways to facilitate their satisfactory participation.

The volitional questionnaires (VQ and PVQ) and the ACIS (refer to Chapter 15) are frequently used while implementing these programs, to identify changing needs and to act as outcome measures. Assessments are also shared with teachers who have become very interested after seeing positive results on children's participation in school.

Facilitating exploration and participation in play, providing participatory education (both formally and informally), and implementing environmental management strategies have given new opportunities for these children, their teachers, and some of the caregivers involved, to increase their confidence and satisfaction with their occupational participation. Every Friday, after the activities have concluded, students and professors follow an evaluation protocol of the day. They process together their professor team's work, their strengths and challenges as a group, and apply therapeutic reasoning with MOHO to gain a better personal understanding of the children's experiences and their own. Professors validate, and provide feedback and advice to students.

Taking on these group projects has resulted in the students learning diverse competencies as occupational therapists and as individuals. It has also built their confidence and trust in occupational therapy. Overall, this program has become one that fosters satisfactory occupational participation for everyone involved (de las Heras et al., 2013).

CASE EXAMPLE: COMMUNITY-BASED INTERVENTION

*F*itness, yo*U*, and *N*utrition (FUN) is an 8-week after-school MOHO-based program aimed at *increasing awareness and participation in physical and nutritional activity, to develop healthy habits and routines*. Over 100 children of similar age, in the third and fourth grades at a local elementary school in Maine, and their families, participated in the 3-year program. The FUN program was framed on exploring and discovering motivating, interesting, and valuable activities to develop a belief in their skills and abilities (sense of capacity and efficacy). Each weekly session included free play, warm-up, nutritional activities, physical activities, an educational piece, and a program wrap-up. The intent of each session was to develop a better understanding of a healthy lifestyle and to encourage children to want to make healthy physical and nutritional choices.

Nutritional activities were developed based on the food pyramid. Weekly topics included learning the food pyramid, portion size, water versus soda, healthy choices (avoiding fat, sodium, and hidden calories), eating for physical activity (carbohydrates and protein, bone growth (dairy)), and expanding one's food choices. Each session incorporated a healthy snack that reinforced the concept of the day. Physical activities were developed to encourage movement in fun and interesting ways. Children participated in sports (e.g., basketball, soccer), relay races, dances, recreational competitions (e.g., hula hoop contest) as well as nature walks and other outdoor activities (weather permitting). Activities were adapted according to children's abilities and ensured children participated within an exploratory context.

In addition, children were *encouraged* to complete daily activity journals of their nutritional and physical activity outside of the FUN program. Children did complete these journals and were assigned fun and challenging activities to complete during the week as "homework" to practice healthy habits and routines. For example, they were reminded to "drink water" instead of soda 1 week and improve their hula hoop skills. The program provided take-home materials (e.g., hula hoops, Frisbees) and healthy food and recipes each week. In this way children received family support and increased chance of generalizing the information that supported the necessary continuity of participation to make a lifestyle change.

Overall, children reported decreased time watching television or playing video games; increased overall playing time; wanting to participate in the FUN program again; and felt that they now eat healthier. Parents' surveys expressed that their children increased nutritional choices, were more active, and carried over educational portion to the entire family. While reviewing the individual child and parent questionnaires, the responses were overwhelmingly positive. Children not only expressed a change after the program, but parents supported their answers and were hopeful toward a healthier lifestyle for the entire family.

Increasing children's motivation toward participation in a variety of physical activities, which enhance their self-confidence (personal causation), may lead to lifelong participation or engagement in activities. Children who are obese frequently experience decreased volition, which leads to poor nutritional choices, which may then cause low self-esteem resulting in a more sedentary lifestyle. Helping children and families participate in motivational activities enables them to feel empowered and motivates continued involvement. Therefore, programs that stimulate a child's volition or motivation can serve to increase one's sense of self and lead to wellness (Kielhofner, 2008).

Encouraging children to partake in games and activities that require skill development within an exploratory context allows each child the same opportunities for success. Bringing children of similar age and play skills together to practice physical activities in fun ways (e.g., jump-rope, hula hoop, tag) increases skills and may lead to higher levels of participation, ultimately increasing healthy lifestyle choices (Solomon et al., 2013; Fig. 24-3)

Conclusion

Diverse programs, in diverse practice settings, can be developed based on MOHO. This chapter outlined a process of program development that responds to issues faced by occupational therapists in their daily practice. The chapter summarized principles, critical considerations, and procedures that can be followed in a flexible way in each step of the program development process. The chapter also illustrates the program development process with examples of some of the initiatives that occupational therapists had taken in different countries and cultures. Finally, the chapter shows that MOHO-based programs can be developed with groups of all ages and of diverse occupational needs.

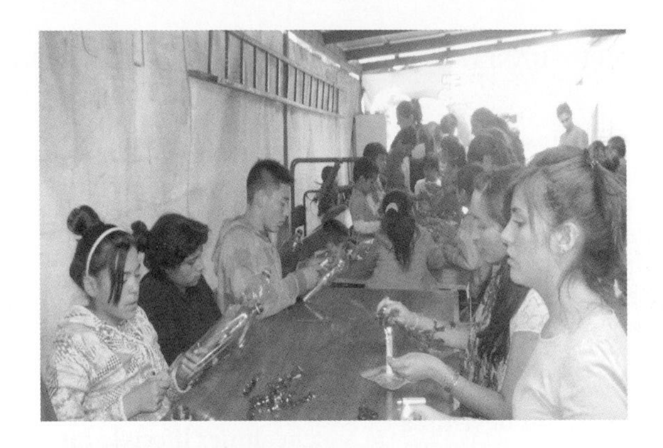

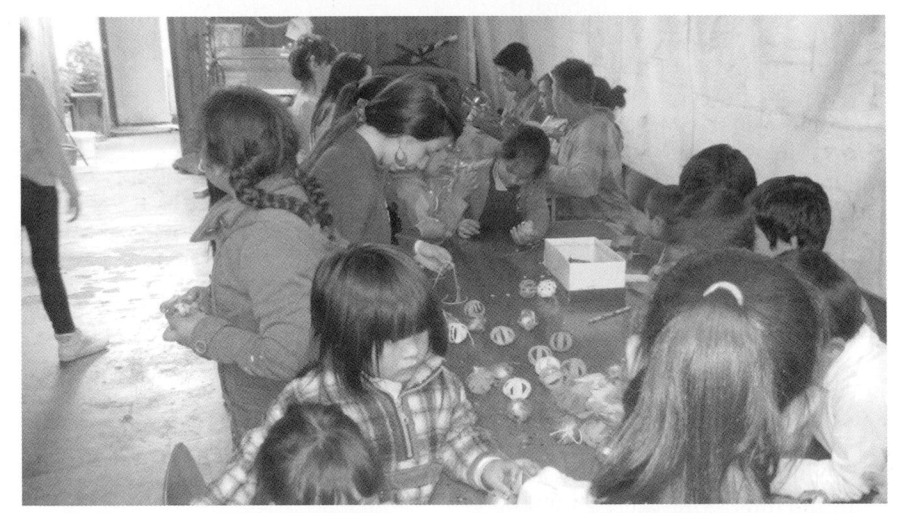

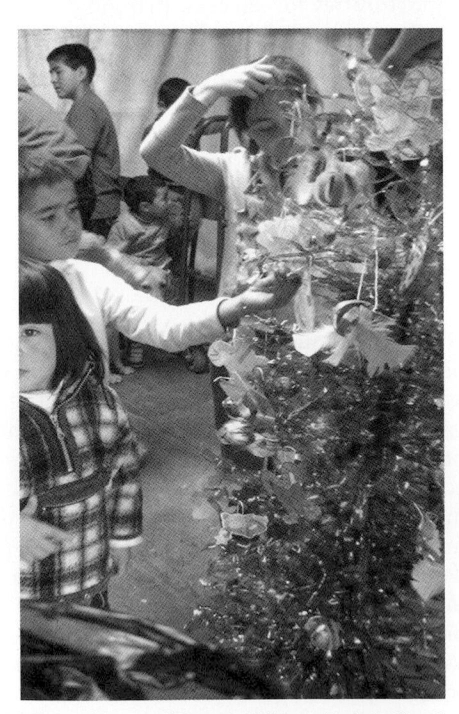

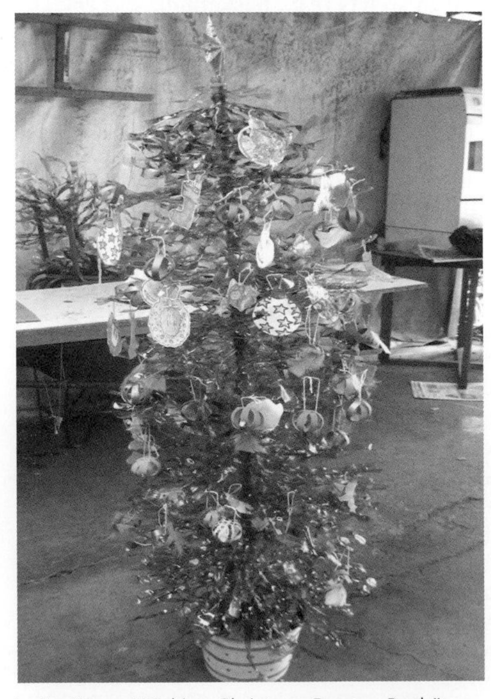

FIGURE 24-3 Students and Street Children in their Play Space in Santiago: "Making Christmas Dreams Real."

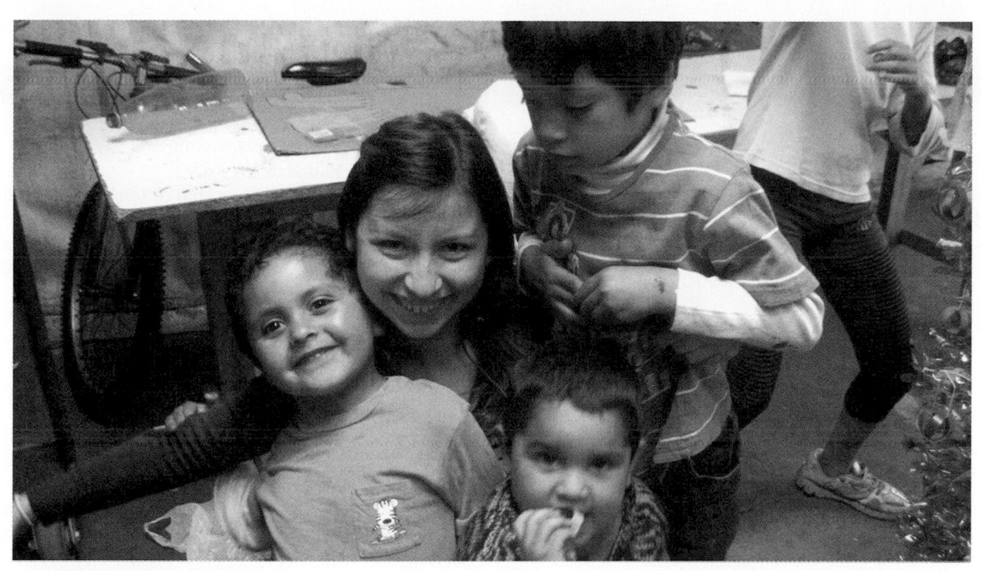

FIGURE 24-3 (continued)

Chapter 24 Review Questions

1. MOHO-based programs involve created social spaces—true or false?
2. Define the immersion process and justify its importance when doing a needs assessment.
3. Name a nonstructured needs assessment method.
4. Name the three properties of occupational opportunities required for successful implementation of a MOHO-based program.

HOMEWORK ASSIGNMENTS

What factors should occupational therapists consider when offering occupational opportunities?

Think about a program you are part of, or a program you know:

1. What are the principles underpinning the program?
2. How was the program developed and evaluated?
3. Has the program evolved?
4. Could the program be replicated in other settings?
5. How have therapists overcome difficulties?

thePoint® For additional resources and exercises, visit http://thePoint.lww.com

Key Terms

Collective projects: Undertaking of a series of activities and tasks to achieve an occupational goal for a group.

Continuity: The life time of occupational opportunities, which if meaningful to the group must offer continuity over time and grow as the group develops and individual or collective projects expand.

Diversity: The variety of occupations available that meet the group's interests, values, and goals, and varied opportunities to participate in them.

Exploratory participation: A person's initial and sometimes sole participation in occupations, with the goal of discovering, sampling, and reasserting a sense and knowledge of capacity.

Flexibility: The constant innovation of occupational opportunities because of the dynamic nature of the process of change for individuals and the group.

Occupational opportunities: Spaces that invite people to participate in significant occupations.

Personal projects: Undertaking a series of activities and related tasks to accomplish a meaningful occupational goal for an individual.

REFERENCES

Abelenda, J. (2015). Espacio para niños y sus Familias, Utchii. In C. G. de las Heras (Ed.), *Modelo de Ocupación Humana* (Chapter 14). Madrid, Spain: Editorial Síntesis.

Abelenda, J., & Helfrich, C. (2003). Family resilience and mental illness: The role of occupational therapy. *Occupational Therapy in Mental Health, 19*, 25–39.

Abelenda, J., Kielhofner, G., & Suarez-Balcazar, Y. (2005). The model of human occupation as a conceptual tool to understand and approach occupational apartheid. In F. Kronenberg, S. Simó Algado, & N. Pollard (Eds.), *Occupational therapy without borders: Learning from the spirit of survivors* (pp. 83–196). London, United Kingdom: Elsevier.

Abeydeera, K., Willis, S., & Forsyth, K. (2006). Occupation focused assessment and intervention for clients with anorexia. *International Journal of Therapy and Rehabilitation, 13*, 296.

Avrech Bar, M., & Jarus, T. (2015). The effect of engagement in everyday occupations, role overload and social support on health and life satisfaction among mothers. *International Journal of Environmental Research and Public Health, 12*, 6045–6065.

Avrech Bar, M., Jarus, T., Wada, M., Rechtman, L., & Noy, E. (2016). Male-to-female transitions: Implications for occupational performance history, health, and life satisfaction. *Canadian Journal of Occupational Therapy, 83*(2), 72–82. doi:10.1177/0008417415576185

Avrech Bar, M., Labock-Gal, D., & Jarus, T. (2011). Occupational performance, social support and life satisfaction in single mothers compared with married mothers. *The Israeli Journal of Occupational Therapy, 20*, 195–218.

Basu, S, Kafkes, A., Schatz, R., Kiraly, A., & Kielhofner, G. (2008). *Pediatric volitional questionnaire, version 2.1*. Chicago: Model of Human Occupation Clearinghouse, Department of Occupational Therapy, University of Illinois at Chicago.

Borell, L., Gustavsson, A., Sandman, P., & Kielhofner, K. (1994). Occupational programming in a day hospital for patients with dementia. *Occupational Therapy Journal of Research, 14*, 219–238.

Braveman, B., Kielhofner, G., & Bélanger, R. (2008). Program development. In G. Kielhofner (Ed.), *Model of human occupation: Theory and application* (4th ed., pp. 442–465). Philadelphia, PA: Lippincott Williams & Wilkins.

Braveman, B., Kielhofner, G., Bélanger, R., de las Heras, C. G., & Llerena, V. (2002). Program development. In G. Kielhofner (Ed.), *A model of human occupation: Theory and application* (3rd ed., pp. 553–586). Baltimore, MD: Lippincott Williams &Wilkins.

Briand, C., Bélanger, R., Hammel, V., Nicole, L., Stip, E., Reinharz, D., et al. (2005). Implantation multisite du programme Integrated Psychosocial Treatment (IPT) pour le personnes soufrant de schizophrénie: Élaboration dune version renouvelée. *Santé Mentale du Québec, 30*, 73–75.

Calderón, D. (2010, May). *Benefits of using the model of human occupation assessments: Promoting occupational participation in children and their families*. Paper presented at the World Federation of Occupational Therapy Congress, Santiago, Chile.

Catalán, S., & Cavieres, C. (2014). *Occupational therapy program in a closed penitentiary unit, at Gendarmería de Chile*. Final project to fulfill the requirements of post graduate Advanced Certificate on Model of Human Occupation, Universidad de los Andes, Santiago, Chile.

Chateau, C., Etchebarne, J., & Rubilar, T. (2013). *Occupational needs assessment for improving environmental conditions and programming with 66 older adults at a nursing home*. Santiago, Chile: Universidad de los Andes.

Cifuentes, D. (2011). *Working with children who have cancer and their families: Program development in a treatment setting*. Final project to fulfill the requirements of post graduate Advanced Certificate on Model of Human Occupation, Universidad Católica de Santa Fe, Santa Fe, Argentina.

D'Angello, M. (1998, July). *The soccer ball*. Paper presented at the Seventh Chilean Congress of Occupational Therapy, Santiago, Chile.

Deegan, P. (1988). Recovery: The lived experience of rehabilitation. *Psychosocial Rehabilitation Journal, 11*(4), 11–19.

de las Heras de Pablo, C. G. (2006, Printemps). Le processus de remotivation: De la pratique à la théorie et de la théorie à la pratique. *Le Paternaire Journal, 13*(2), 4–11.

de las Heras de Pablo, C. G. (2010). *Modelo de ocupación humana: Teoría e intervención actualizada*. Santiago, Chile: Autora.

de las Heras de Pablo, C. G. (2011). Promotion of occupational participation: Integration of the model of human occupation in practice. *The Israeli Journal of Occupational Therapy, 20*(3), E67–E88.

de las Heras de Pablo, C. G. (2015). *Modelo de Ocupación Humana*. Madrid, Spain: Editorial Síntesis.

de las Heras de Pablo, C. G., & Cantero Garlito, P. A. (2009). Dentro del modelo siempre se ha considerado el rescate del sentir, no solo del pensar y actuar. *TOG (A Coruña) [Revista por Internet]*, *6*(9), 11. Retrieved from www.revistatog.com/n9/pdfs/maestros.pdf

de las Heras de Pablo, C. G., Dion, G. L., & Walsh, D. (1993). Application of rehabilitation modes in a state psychiatric hospital. *Occupational Therapy in Mental Health, 12*(3), 1–32.

de las Heras de Pablo, C. G., Llerena, V., & Kielhofner G. (2003). *Remotivation process: Progressive intervention for persons with severe volitional challenges: Users' manual*. Chicago: The Model of Human Occupation Clearinghouse, Department of Occupational Therapy, College of Applied Health Sciences, University of Illinois at Chicago.

de las Heras de Pablo, C. G., Manghi, P., Acevedo, M. J., & Prieto, C. (2013). Promotion of occupational participation with children at risk in Lo Barnechea: An integrative academic program. In *Occupational therapy curriculum: Human occupation II and III*. Santiago, Chile: School of Occupational Therapy, Faculty of Medicine, Universidad de los Andes.

de las Heras de Pablo, C. G., Sanz Valer, P., & Robio Ortega, C. (2012). Sobre el arte de nuestra práctica [Revista por Internet], *TOG (A Coruña), 9*(16), 11. Retrieved from http://www.revistatog.com/n16/pdfs/historia3.pdf

Dion, G. L., Skerry, M., & Lovely, S. (1996). A comprehensive psychiatric rehabilitation approach to severe and persistent mental illness in the public sector: The Worcester State Hospital Experience. In S. M. Soreff (Ed.), *Handbook for the treatment of severely mentally ill*. Boston, MA: Hogrefe & Huber Publishers.

Du Toit, S. (2008). Using the model of human occupation to conceptualize an occupational program for blind persons in South Africa. *Occupational Therapy in Health Care, 22*, 51–61.

Echeverría, A. (2014). *Older adults' wellness program: A community center to promote participation in significant routines*. Final project to fulfill the requirements of post graduate "Advanced Certification on Model of Human Occupation," Universidad de los Andes, Santiago, Chile.

Gindi, S., Galili, G., Adir, S., Magen, O., & Volovic-Shushan, S. (2015). An occupational therapy model for treating combat reaction within a military unit. *The Israeli Journal of Occupational Therapy, 24*(3), E103, E104.

Girardi, A. (2010). *Promotion of occupational participation in adolescents of Santiago de Chile' high economic class who undergo a mental illness and occupational privation.* Paper presented at the World Federation of Occupational Therapy (WFOT) Congress, Santiago, Chile.

Greenspan, S. I., & Wieder, S. (2007). *Infant and early childhood mental health: A comprehensive developmental approach to assessment and intervention.* Arlington, VA: American Psychiatric Publishing.

Helfrich, C. (Ed.) (2001). *Domestic abuse through lifespan: The role of occupational therapy.* Binghamton, NY: The Haworth Press.

Kielhofner, G. (1983). *Health through occupation: Theory and practice in occupational therapy.* Philadelphia, PA: F. A. Davis.

Kielhofner, G. (2002). *Model of human occupation: Theory and application* (3rd ed.). Philadelphia, PA: Lippincott Williams & Wilkins.

Kielhofner, G. (2004). *Conceptual foundations of occupational therapy* (3rd ed.). Philadelphia, PA: F. A. Davis.

Kielhofner, G. (2008). *Model of human occupation: Theory and application* (4th ed.). Philadelphia, PA: Lippincott Williams & Wilkins.

Kielhofner, G. (2009). *Conceptual foundations of occupational therapy practice* (4th ed.). Philadelphia, PA: F. A. Davis.

Kielhofner, G., Braveman, B., Finlayson, M., Paul-Ward, A., Goldbaum, L., & Goldstein, K. (2004). Outcomes of a vocational program for persons with AIDS. *The American Journal of Occupational Therapy, 58*(1), 64–72.

Kielhofner, G., de las Heras, C. G., & Suarez Balcazar, Y. (2011). Human occupation as a tool for understanding and promoting social justice. In F. Kronemberg, N. Pollard, & D. Sakellariu (Eds.), *Occupational therapies without borders: Towards an ecology of occupation based practices* (Vol. 2, pp. 269–277). Edinburg, Scotland: Elsevier.

Lee, S., & Harris, M. (2010). The development of an effective occupational therapy assessment and treatment pathway for women with a diagnosis of borderline personality disorder in an inpatient setting: Implementing the model of human occupation. *British Journal of Occupational Therapy, 73*(11), 559–563.

Margaría, S., & Weidmann, E. (2011). *El Galpón: An alternative for children at risk to progresive integration to schools.* Final project as prerequisite for post graduate "Advanced Certification on the Model of Human Occupation," Universidad Católica de Santa Fe, Argentina.

Melton, J., Forsyth, K., Metherall, A., Robinson, J., Hill, J., & Quick, L. (2008). Program redesign based on the model of human occupation: Inpatient services for people experiencing acute mental illness in the UK. *Occupational Therapy in Health Care, 22,* 37–50.

Olson, L., & Kielhofner, G. (1998). *Work readiness day treatment for persons with chronic disabilities. A companion manual for the videotape "Proud of me".* Chicago: The Model of Human Occupation Clearinghouse, Department of Occupational Therapy, College of Applied Health Sciences, University of Illinois at Chicago. Retrieved from www.cade.uic/moho/productDetails.aspx?iid=2

Parham, L. D., Roley, S. S., May-Benson, T. A., Koomar, J., Brett-Green, B., Burke, J. P., et al. (2011). Development of a fidelity measure for research on the effectiveness of the ayres sensory integration intervention. *The American Journal of Occupational Therapy, 65*(2), 133–142.

Parkinson, S. (2014). *Recovery through activity: Increasing participation in everyday life.* London, United Kingdom: Speechmark.

Parkinson, S., Chester, A., Cratchley, S., & Rowbottom, J. (2008). Application of the Model of Human Occupation Screening Tool (MOHOST assessment) in an acute psychiatric setting. *Occupational Therapy in Health Care,* 22(2/3), 63–75.

Parkinson, S., Cooper J. R., de las Heras de Pablo, C. G., & Forsyth, K. (2014). Measuring the effectiveness of interventions when occupational performance is severely impaired. *British Journal of Occupational Therapy, 77*(2), 78–81.

Poletti, L. (2015). *Rumbos: Centro de Integración Comunitaria (Santa Fe, Argentina).* In C. G. de las Heras de Pablo (Ed.), *Modelo de ocupación humana.* Madrid, Spain: Editorial Síntesis.

Quick, L., Melton, J., Critchley, A., Loveridge, N., & Forsyth, K. (2012, October). *Remotivation process for occupation program.* Paper presented at the Third Model of Human Occupation Institute, Stockholm, Sweden.

Schaaf, R., & Mailloux, Z. (2015). *Clinician's guide for implementing Ayres Sensory Integration (R).* Bethesda, MD: AOTA Press.

Shinohara, K., Yamada, T., Kobayashi, N., & Forsyth, K. (2012). The model of human occupation-based intervention for patients with stroke: A randomised trial. *Hong Kong Journal of Occupational Therapy, 22*(2), 60–69. doi:10.1016/j.hkjot.2012.09.001

Solomon, J., O'Brien, J., & Cohn, J. (2013). Emerging occupational therapy practice areas. In J. O'Brien & J. Solomon (Eds.), *Occupational analysis and group process* (pp. 140–142). St. Louis, MO: Elsevier.

Vera, F. (2014). *A program design for school children with special needs.* Final project to fulfill the requirements of the post graduate "Advanced Certification on MOHO," Universidad de los Andes, Santiago, Chile.

Winnicott, D. W. (1960). The theory of the parent-infant relationship. *International Journal of Psychoanalysis, 41*(6), 585–595.

Yamada, T., Kawamata, H., Kobayashi, N., Kielhofner, G., & Taylor, R. R. (2010, November). A randomized clinical trial of a wellness programme for healthy older people. *British Journal of Occupational Therapy, 73*(11), 540–554.

Yazdani, F., Jibril, M., & Kielhofner, G. (2008). A study of the relationship between variables from the model of human occupation and subjective well-being among university students in Jordan. *Occupational Therapy in Health Care, 22*(2/3), 125–138.

Ziv, N., & Roitman, D. (2008). Addressing the needs of elderly clients whose lives have been compounded by traumatic histories. *Occupational Therapy in Heath Care, 22,* 85–93.

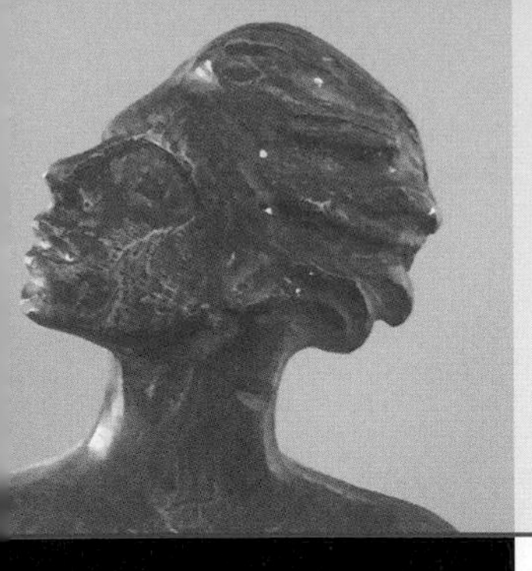

Evidence for Practice from the Model of Human Occupation

Patricia Bowyer and Jessica Kramer

CHAPTER 25

EXPECTED LEARNING OUTCOMES

Upon completion of this chapter, readers will be able to:

1. Understand the contributions of model of human occupation (MOHO) research in terms of explaining the occupational lives and needs of people with disabilities.
2. Recall evidence for the dependability and utility of MOHO-based assessments.
3. Describe practice based on MOHO.
4. Summarize the evidence with respect to positive clinical outcomes of MOHO-based interventions.
5. Grasp the perspective of clients with respect to their participation in MOHO-based services.
6. Explain how the therapeutic reasoning process is implemented.

Occupational therapists are increasingly under pressure from both within and outside the profession to deliver evidence-based practice (Copley & Allen, 2009; Law & Baum, 1998; Lloyd et al., 2004; McCluskey & Cusick, 2002). This means that therapists are expected to identify, critique, synthesize, and use evidence as a guide and justification for what they do in practice (Lin, Murphy, & Robinson, 2010; Roberts & Barber, 2001; Taylor, 1997).

To a large extent, practicing therapists agree with the importance of evidence-based practice (Bennett et al., 2003; Humphries et al., 2000; Metcalfe et al., 2001; Novak & McIntyre, 2010; Thomas & Law, 2013). However, practitioners express concerns about the practicality of using research to guide practice (Burke & Gitlin, 2012; Dysart & Tomlin, 2002; McCluskey, 2003; McCluskey & Cusick, 2002). Practitioners report that research often lacks real-life significance, addresses topics not relevant to practice, and fails to present findings in ways that facilitated their application (Dubouloz, Egan, Vallerand, & Von Zweck, 1999; Sudsawad, 2003).

The aim of this chapter is to streamline the process of identifying commonly sought evidence for practice. Some of the most typical questions for which practitioners seek evidence have been identified and synthesized with all the currently available evidence. The resources in this chapter should never completely substitute for other evidence-based strategies. Since the model of human occupation (MOHO) literature grows substantially each year, it is likely that there will be evidence beyond that included in this chapter upon publication. Moreover, because critique is part of the process of using evidence, therapists are encouraged to go beyond the brief descriptions provided here and directly examine the literature they summarize. Finally, this chapter focuses exclusively on evidence generated from published studies. However, there are also other sources of useful evidence. This includes evidence available in the literature such as case examples and program descriptions. The MOHO Web site provides access to the expertise of occupational therapists who use MOHO through archived listserv discussions coded by topic.

The Kinds of Evidence Needed to Support Practice

Evidence-based practice is the judicious use of the best available evidence to guide decision making in practice (Sackett et al., 1996). As this definition implies, the kind of evidence that is needed will differ depending on what decision a therapist is making (Tickle-Degnen & Bedell, 2003; Tse, Blackwood, & Penman, 2001). The definition above also indicates that therapists must work with available evidence. In cases where there is no or little evidence available from research studies, therapists will need to rely on other forms of evidence. Thus, relevant evidence for practice may include controlled studies of outcomes of services, clinical knowledge presented in case studies, research that explores and develops theory, the expertise of professional peers, and the perspectives of clients (Polatajko & Craik, 2006, Sudswad, 2006).

MOHO Evidence

The MOHO was published over three decades ago. Over that period, a substantial body of evidence has accumulated. Because MOHO was developed as a practice model, research has always tended to focus on topics relevant to practice. Moreover, in the past decade MOHO developers have embraced the scholarship of practice approach that focuses research on solving practice problems and that looks to practice for questions to be addressed through research (Kielhofner, 2005a, 2005b; Taylor, Fisher, & Kielhofner, 2006). Consequently, most recent MOHO studies have grown out of partnerships between practitioners and researchers assuring that the findings are of use to practice settings.

Finding MOHO Evidence

Therapists looking for evidence on a particular topic within the MOHO literature could easily find themselves searching through hundreds of articles and chapters. Although it is relatively easy to identify some types of evidence relevant to a topic or question, other relevant evidence may be less apparent. Thus, searching comprehensively for evidence is often a daunting task. To facilitate the location of evidence, the MOHO Clearinghouse Web site includes an evidence-based search engine that enables practitioners to locate citations relevant to practice topics. This search engine is explained in more detail in the Appendix. Although the search engine helps identify relevant literature, therapists must still locate the articles and sift through them for the desired evidence.

The Occupational Lives and Needs of People with Disabilities

From its inception, MOHO research has focused on understanding how both personal and environmental factors impact occupational participation. A large number of researchers who use MOHO as a framework for their research have examined the volition, habituation, performance capacity, and/or environments of persons with disabilities in their research, as well as the process of occupational adaptation via development of occupational competence and occupational identity. MOHO was the first occupational therapy model to incorporate the environment as a major variable in determining occupational participation, and MOHO-based research has sought to better illustrate the concept of environmental impact.

These studies include research that aims to explore or test MOHO concepts, research that seeks to identify challenges and needs of disabled persons, and research that asks about client or environmental characteristics and their relationship to how clients respond to services and what outcomes they achieve. This type of evidence can be helpful to practitioners in the following ways:

- It can identify factors that are particularly challenging for clients and that should be addressed in therapy
- It can identify factors that impact on the client's involvement in therapy that should be considered when giving services
- It can identify factors associated with positive or negative outcomes of therapy that should be recognized as liabilities or strengths and addressed accordingly.

Tables 25-1 through 25-3 list and summarize this research according to the major concepts of MOHO (volition, habitation, and environment).

Table 25-1 Clients' Characteristics Related to Volition

Citation	Outcomes/Findings
Asmundsdottir (2004)	Psychiatric clients reported a low sense of personal causation and self-efficacy as barriers to return to work.
Aubin, Hachey, and Mercier (1999)	Pleasure (an aspect of volition) in work and rest is positively correlated with subjective Quality of Life for outpatient psychiatric clients.
Barrett, Beer, and Kielhofner (1999)	A person's volitional narrative reveals influences of how he/she will participate in and benefit from therapy.
Barris, Dickie, and Baron (1988)	Young adults with eating disorders were more external on dimensions of self-control, young adults with chronic conditions were more internal on dimensions of self-control, and adolescents with psychiatric conditions were more external on dimensions of social control, compared to community-dwelling adolescents without disabilities.

(continued)

Table 25-1 Clients' Characteristics Related to Volition (*continued*)

Citation	Outcomes/Findings
Barris et al. (1986)	• Volitional aspects such as locus of control, importance and value of roles and activities, interests, and enjoyment impact occupational adaptation of adolescents with psychiatric conditions, psychophysiological conditions, and adolescents without disabilities.
Bridle, Lynch, and Quesenberry (1990)	2–8 years after spinal cord injury, persons report difficulty with volition, including less adaptive interests, fewer values and goals, and less adaptive perceptions of abilities and responsibilities.
Chen, Neufeld, Feely, and Skinner (1999)	Volition, specifically perceived self-efficacy, is a main predictor of compliance with home exercise programs among clients with upper extremity impairments and injuries.
Crowe, VanLeit, Berghmans, and Mann (1997)	There were no significant difference in the values reported for various roles by mothers of children with multiple disabilities, mothers of children with Down's Syndrome, and mothers of typically developing children.
Dickerson and Oakely (1995)	Clients with physical and psychosocial disabilities differed in the value assigned to present and future roles compared to persons without disabilities.
Ebb, Coster, and Duncombe (1989)	The total number of strong interests discriminated between adolescents with psychosocial disabilities staying in hospitals and community-dwelling adolescents without disabilities.
Ekbladh, Haglund, and Thorell (2004)	Persons who returned to work had significantly higher scores on the volitional construct of personal causation (as measured by the Worker Role Interview [WRI]) compared to persons who did not return to work.
Hachey, Boyer, and Mercier (2001)	Canadian adults with schizophrenia report most value for present roles of friend, worker, and family member, whereas they anticipate they will most value roles of friend, family member, home maintainer, and hobbyist in the future.
Hakansson, Eklund, Lidfeldt, Nerbrand, Samsioe, and Nilsson (2005)	Women who maintain employment report a significantly greater value for worker role and higher sense of well-being compared to women who report discontinuity in work related to illness.
Helfrich, Kielhofner, and Mattingly (1994)	People with disabilities perceive their lives and behavior according to their own narrative account of their lives and how the disability has influenced that life.
Jacobshagen (1990)	Interruptions during engagement in craft occupations can impact a person's sense of personal causation and competence for that activity.
Jonsson, Josephsson, and Kielhofner (2001)	Volitional narratives are plastic, and interactions between narratives and actual life events can alter the meaning and motivation for engaging in occupations.
Jonsson, Josephsson, and Kielhofner (2000)	Volitional narratives are not set scripts for action, but represent an active or passive orientation to act in a particular manner depending on the circumstances of an event.
Jonsson, Kielhofner, and Borell (1997)	A person's anticipated future narrative, whether progressive, stable, or regressive, is influenced by how the person currently experiences and interprets their involvement in occupations.
Katz, Josman, and Steinmetz (1988)	• Adolescents hospitalized with psychiatric disabilities expressed more interest in ADLs and less interest in cultural/educational and social/recreational activities compared to community-dwelling adolescents. • Locus of control did not differentiate between hospitalized and nonhospitalized adolescents.

Table 25-1 Clients' Characteristics Related to Volition (*continued*)

Citation	Outcomes/Findings
Katz, Giladi, and Peretz (1988)	• Israeli adult psychiatric clients are more interested in ALDs (all clients with psychiatric disabilities) and manual skills (those clients diagnosed with schizophrenia) compared to adults without disabilities.
Lederer, Kielhofner, and Watts (1985)	• Fewer incarcerated adolescents reported value for the student, worker, volunteer, and home maintainer role compared to adolescents in the community. • Incarcerated adolescents often reported value for roles related to risk-taking behavior and self-expression.
Morgan and Jongbloed (1990)	Volitional factors such as meaningfulness of an activities, personal standards for performance in an activity, and range of interests impacted person's participation in leisure activities after a stroke.
Neville-Jan (1994)	For clients in psychiatric inpatient hospitals, volitional aspects of pleasure and locus of control were significantly related to occupational adaptation when controlling and not controlling for depression.
Oakley, Kielhofner, and Barris (1985)	Clients with mental health problems had more external locus of control compared to persons in the community, but still reported strong interests.
Peterson et al. (1999)	Sense of self-efficacy related to falls was related to interference with participation and restriction of participation in social and leisure activities in older persons.
Rust, Barris, and Hooper (1987)	Leisure values and personal causation for exercise are predictive of women's exercise behavior.
Scaffa (1991)	Persons attending a program for alcohol abuse reported less participation in cultural/educational interests and fewer avocational interests compared to persons not in treatment for alcohol abuse.
Scheelar (2002)	Volition, including interests, personal satisfaction, and value for career, impacts an injured firefighter's decision to return to work.
Smith, Kielhofner, and Watts (1986)	Interests, values, and personal causation are positively correlated with life satisfaction for older adults living in the community and nursing home settings.
Smyntek, Barris, and Kielhofner (1985)	Adolescents hospitalized with psychosocial problems presented with different volition patterns compared to community-dwelling adolescents, including lower self-esteem, more external locus of control, decreased competence for rest, and less value assigned to roles.
Tham and Borell (1996)	Clients have a strong sense of self-efficacy for engaging in leisure and self-care activities regardless of the extent of unilateral neglect experienced post-CVA.
Watson and Ager (1991)	For adults aged 50 and up living in the community, value for the student role and religious participant roles was negatively related to life satisfaction, whereas value for home maintainer role was positively related to life satisfaction.
Widen-Holmqvist et al. (1993)	Adults living at home poststroke report a sense of personal causation, values, and interests that are similar to what other adults living in the community report.
Zimmerer-Branum and Nelson (1994)	Nursing home residents were more likely to choose an occupationally embedded exercise over a rote exercise, and those who chose occupation-based activities had increased level of engagement in the activity as demonstrated in the number of repetitions completed.

Table 25-2 Clients' Characteristics Related to Habituation

Citation	Outcomes/Findings
Baker, Curbow, and Wingard (1991)	Role change and role loss were reported by bone marrow transplant survivors, although roles of family member, friend, and home maintainer changed the least before and after the transplant. Retaining any roles, as well as retaining important roles, was significantly and positively correlated with satisfaction with life. Retaining roles and important roles was significantly and negatively correlated with negative mood. For men, loss of worker role, family role, and community role was associated with negative quality of life, affect, or mood variables. For women, loss of worker role was associated with decreased quality of life.
Barris, Dickie, and Baron (1988)	Young adults with eating disorders, young adults with chronic conditions, and adolescents with psychiatric disorders anticipated fewer future roles compared to community-dwelling young persons without disabilities. Adolescents with psychiatric disorders had fewer past roles compared to community-dwelling young persons without disabilities.
Barris et al. (1986)	Aspects of habituation, such as number of past roles and time spent in ADLs/work/play activities, impact the occupational adaptation of adolescents with psychiatric disabilities, psychophysiological conditions, and adolescents without disabilities.
Branholm and Fugl-Meyer (1992)	Across age cohorts and gender, involvement in family, leisure, and vocational roles was related to life satisfaction. Persons experienced changes in role engagement based on gender- and age-related life circumstances according to social and cultural customs.
Bridle et al. (1990)	2–8 years after spinal cord injury, persons report difficulty with habituation, including less adaptive organization of daily routines and less adaptive life roles.
Crowe, VanLeit, Berghmans, and Mann (1997)	Role engagement, complexity, and related expectations may change over time for mothers of children with and without disabilities. Mothers of children with Down's Syndrome and mothers of children with multiple disabilities reported engagement in fewer present roles compared to mothers of typically developing children. However, mothers of all children report role loss upon the birth of their children, although mothers of children with Down's Syndrome report the most role loss.
Davies Hallet, Zasler, Maurer, and Cash (1994)	Persons with traumatic brain injuries (TBIs) experience role changes after injury, including role loss (worker and hobby roles) and role gain. There was a significant relationship between the number of role changes and a score on a disability scale.
Dickerson and Oakely (1995)	• Clients with physical and psychosocial disabilities had differing patterns of role involvement compared to community-dwelling persons without disabilities. • Clients with physical and psychosocial disabilities reported engagement in fewer present role which may be indicative of their inpatient status. • Clients with psychosocial disabilities do not differ in anticipated patterns of future role engagement from community-dwelling persons, but clients with physical disabilities report a significantly different anticipated future role engagement, particularly in worker and hobbyist roles.
Duellman, Barris, and Kielhofner (1986)	There is a significant, positive relationship between the number of organized activities offered by the nursing home and the number of present and future roles reported by older adults living in nursing homes.
Ebb, Coster, and Duncombe (1989)	The total number of reported current and future roles discriminates between adolescents with psychosocial disabilities staying in the hospital and community-dwelling adolescents without disabilities.
Ekbladh et al. (2004)	Persons who return to work were better able to appraise their work expectations related to the worker role compared to persons who did not return to work.

Table 25-2 Clients' Characteristics Related to Habituation

Citation	Outcomes/Findings
Eklund (2001)	Roles, such as friend, hobbyist, family member, worker, and caregiver, are associated with quality of life for clients with mental health problems at admission, discharge, or follow-up.
Elliott and Barris (1987)	There is a significant, positive relationship between the number of roles and the meaningfulness of those roles and life satisfaction for community-dwelling adults. Involvement in meaningful roles leads to a sense of satisfaction with life, and enables persons to fulfill their need for mastery as well as meet expectations of society.
Frosch et al. (1997)	Caregivers of persons who experienced a traumatic brain injury reported significant changes in engagement in roles from the past to the present. There was a positive trend between number of role changes and the behavioral effects of the TBI survivor, and an inverse trend between the number of role changes and caregiver use of support systems.
Hachey, Boyer, and Mercier (2001)	Adults with schizophrenia report more involvement in roles in the past than in the present, but anticipate they will be involved in more roles in the future. Adults with schizophrenia also report more role loss than role gain from past to present. Roles of family member, friend, home maintainer, and hobbyist were the most frequently reported roles engaged in by the adults.
Hammel (1999)	For people with disabilities, roles are entered, developed, and exited over time on an individual basis, and the meaning, importance, and definition of roles can change according to an individual's role development process.
Horne, Corr, and Earle (2005)	First-time mothers report a change in roles and routines, resulting in periods of occupational imbalance after the birth of their first child.
Katz, Giladi, and Peretz (1988)	There are significant differences in role performance between Israeli adult psychiatric clients and adults without disabilities with regard to their patterns of engagement in a profession and patterns of engagement in ADL/play/recreation/rest/sleep.
Katz, Josman, and Steinmetz (1988)	Role engagement was significantly different between adolescents hospitalized with psychiatric conditions and community-dwelling adolescents, where hospitalized adolescents were more likely to engage in social activities and recreation at home, and were more likely to change schools because of problems associated with their hospitalization.
Lee, Strauss, Wittman, Jackson, and Carstens (2001)	Caregiving role and value for the caregiving role is associated with feelings of sorrow when caregivers care for adults with mental health problems at the time of the person's diagnosis and in the present. However, high levels of engagement in the hobbyist role are associated with lower levels of sorrow at the time of the person's diagnosis.
Morgan and Jongbloed (1990)	Clients returning home after a stroke report a shift in role balance and routine and report that they altered roles because of changed performance capacity. This included engagement in leisure roles.
Munoz, Karmosky, Gaugler, Lang, and Stayduhar (1999)	Although parents undergo role adaptation when parenting a child with a disability, this role shift does not inherently result in a strain on roles and occurs differently for mothers and fathers. Role adaptations could include a loss of roles (worker, friend), an expansion of roles (caregiver), or the acquisition of new roles (religious participant, advocate). Fathers reported less role disruption than mothers.
Oakley, Kielhofner, and Barris (1985)	Clients with mental health conditions report fewer roles and more role disruption compared to people without disabilities.
Rosenfeld (1989)	There is a disruption in occupational routines and changes in task pressures after a disaster such as a house fire.

(*continued*)

Table 25-2 Clients' Characteristics Related to Habituation

Citation	Outcomes/Findings
Rust, Barris, and Hooper (1987)	Women's exercise behavior can be predicted by the number of roles they are engaged in, the internalization of the exerciser role, and their exercise habits.
Scaffa (1991)	Persons attending a program for alcohol abuse reported less time engaged in work activities, more time engaged in alcohol activities, and less hours awake compared to persons living in the community.
Smith, Kielhofner, and Watts (1986)	The amount of time spent engaged in occupations of work and recreation is positively correlated with life satisfaction for older adults living in nursing homes and the community.
Smyntek, Barris, and Kielhofner (1985)	Adolescents hospitalized with psychosocial problems reported fewer present roles and less time spent doing ADL tasks compared to community adolescents on a typical Saturday, which may be related to the hospital environment.
Watson and Ager (1991)	Frequency of engagement in the home maintainer role was positively correlated with life satisfaction for adults aged 50 and up living in the community.
Weeder (1986)	People with schizophrenia attending a day program have different patterns of occupational engagement in daily activities such as sleep, leisure, and work during weekdays and weekends compared to people living in the community.
Widen-Holmqvist et al. (1993)	For adults living in the community after a stroke, engagement in activities was limited to home-based leisure activities and self-care activities.

Table 25.3 Clients' Characteristics Related to Environment

Citation	Outcomes and Findings
Ay-Woan, Sarah, Lylnn, Tsyn-Jang, and Ping-Chaun (2006)	Environmental assessment should be considered for clients experiencing depression, as the environmental aspects of the OSA predicted quality of life for adult Taiwanese clients with mental health disabilities.
Bridle et al. (1990)	2–8 years after a spinal cord injury, persons report less adaptive environmental influences that then impact occupational adaptation, mainly within the physical environment.
Duellman et al. (1986)	The environment of a nursing home, particularly the number of organized activities provided by the home, is positively correlated with older adults' perception of engagement in roles. People perceive themselves as actively engaged in their environment when opportunities to participate are provided.
Ekbladh et al. (2004)	Persons who returned to work perceived the physical work setting to be more supportive of return to work than persons who did not return to work.
Hemmingsson, Borell, and Gustavsson (1999)	Task expectations and demands of schoolteachers associated with their classroom management style can influence a student's ability to participate in school tasks independently.
Kjellberg (2002)	The environment, including national legislation, attitudes, and forms of routines and activities, was a barrier or a support to participation for persons with intellectual disabilities.
Molyneaux-Smith, Townsend, and Guernsey (2003)	The environment (including objects, social environment, and government policies) can be a barrier or a support to reengagement in vocational roles after injury.
Scheelar (2002)	The work social environment can affect an injured firefighter's willingness and ability to return to work.
Tham and Kielhofner (2003)	Social support and cues from the environment enable women with left neglect to engage in occupations and support participation.

Evidence Concerning the Dependability and Utility of MOHO Assessments

Most of the MOHO-based assessments have been extensively researched. Although the approach to developing MOHO-based assessments has changed over the years, the contemporary approach is to use item response theory (Velozo, Forsyth, & Kielhofner, 2006) as a basis for establishing the internal validity and measurement soundness. This process which ordinarily takes upward of 3 years results in the creation of key forms that allow the ordinal data obtained from rating scales to be converted into interval data (Kielhofner, Dobria, Forsyth, & Basu, 2005; Velozo et al., 2006). Traditional psychometric approaches (Kielhofner, 2006) are also used to test the reliability and validity of MOHO-based assessments. Finally, because MOHO research emphasizes the scholarship of practice, research often aims to examine the utility of the assessment from a practitioner and consumer perspective. Tables 25-4 through 25-19 present and summarize the research underlying each assessment. Research is presented in chronological order to illustrate the development of each assessment over time.

Table 25-4 Assessment of Communication and Interaction Skills (ACIS) Evidence Summary

Citation	Findings
Forsyth, Lai, and Kielhofner (1999)	ACIS items are a valid representation of the construct of communication and interaction skills, clients with mental health problems are measured in a valid way using the ACIS (although not clients with autism), and therapists use the ACIS in a consistent and interchangeable manner. The ACIS can be administered in a range of social situations in a valid manner.
Kjellberg (2002)	ACIS scores did not have a systematic relationship with a person's level of intellectual impairment or their level of dependence/interdependence/independence in work or leisure.
Haglund and Henriksson (2003)	Expert panel judged 60% of the ACIS items to be aligned with items in the ICIDH-2; 30% of the ACIS items had a correlation of at least 0.60 with the aligned ICIDH-2 items.
Kjellberg, Haglund, Forsyth, and Kielhofner (2003)	The items and rating scale in a Swedish translation of the AICS validly represent construct of communication and interaction and met the fit criteria. The continuum of communication and interaction skills as represented by the items replicates previous findings in the English version. Therapists assessed clients with learning disabilities, mental health disabilities, and neurological disorders in a consistent and interchangeable manner.
Haglund and Thorell (2004)	The study confirms that communication and interaction skills are context dependent for clients with schizophrenia and mood disorders, as clients had at least one item rating that changed across settings. There did not appear to be a relationship between the importance or inherent fun of each activity setting and the ACIS ratings as reported by the clients.
Hsu, Pan, and Chen (2008)	The Chinese version of the ACIS (ACIS-C) was examined in this study. A convenience sample of 101 participants diagnosed with psychiatric disabilities was recruited from four centers in Taiwan. The ACIS-C items were found to measure the concept of communication/interaction and the results support that the tool is sensitive and valid.
Petersen and Bente (2008)	This study validated the Danish translation of the ACIS and OSA. The study consisted of a four-step process by occupational therapists. The therapists tested pilot versions in practice, provided peer review and back-translation. The study found the Danish version of the ACIS to be valid.

Table 25-5 Assessment of Occupational Functioning (AOF) Evidence Summary

Citation	Findings
Watts, Kielhofner, Bauer, Gregory, and Valentine (1986)	The AOF can be used in a reliable way with older adult clients with mental health conditions and community-dwelling older adults. The AOF has evidence of concurrent validity and can discriminate between clients in institutions and community-dwelling older adults.
Brollier, Watts, Bauer, and Schmidt (1988a)	The AOF has concurrent validity with the Global Assessment Scale when used with clients diagnosed with schizophrenia. The AOF may be sensitive to a client's socioeconomic status.
Brollier, Watts, Bauer, and Schmidt (1988b)	A panel of OT experts determined that the AOF had content validity and covered the domain of content for six MOHO components.
Watts, Brollier, Bauer, and Schmidt (1989)	The AOF has concurrent validity with the OCAIRS when used with clients diagnosed with schizophrenia.
Viik, Watts, Madigan, and Bauer (1990)	AOF can discriminate between adult clients just entering rehabilitation for alcohol abuse and persons with 1 year of sobriety.
Lycett (1992)	The Occupational Assessment identified important information when used as an evaluation method with 9 of 16 elderly clients. The Occupational Assessment influenced five of the elderly client's treatment plans. The Occupational Assessment was rated as most useful by clients who had experienced a stroke and who required longer treatment stays.
Widen-Holmqvist et al. (1993)	The AOF can be used by adults living in the community in Stockholm after a stroke to report their sense of volition.
Grogan (1994)	The AOF can be used with adult clients with mental health conditions to show change related to engagement in OT intervention as well as changes related to symptomatology.
Eklund (1996a)	• AOF components of volition, habituation, and performance are all clustered on the "health" side of a continuum of wellness of the *x*-axis of a PCS analysis. • On the *y*-axis, AOF component of habituation appeared in the middle of the cluster of health variables. Volition appeared at the top of the cluster of health variables. The AOF concept of performance appeared most removed from the other health variables.
Eklund (1996b)	The AOF can be used to assess intervention outcomes for Swedish clients with mental health disabilities.
Eklund and Hansson (1997)	The AOF can be used to assess the long-term impact of occupational therapy service on everyday occupational functioning of clients with mental health disabilities 1 year after discharge from therapy.
Eklund (1999)	AOF can be used to demonstrate outcomes after an occupational therapy intervention in volition, habituation, and communication/interaction skills, for adult clients with mental health conditions.

Table 25-6 The Child Occupational Self Assessment (COSA) and its predecessor, the Child Self Assessment of Occupational Functioning (SAOF) Evidence Summary

Citation	Findings
Keller, Kafkes, and Kielhofner (2005)	COSA items coalesce to form a valid construct of occupational competence. Clients aged 8–17 who received OT and did not receive OT both used the competence scale in a reliable and valid way, but did not frequently use the lowest rating category. COSA items also coalesce to form a valid construct of Value (importance) of occupations. Again, clients used the value scale in a reliable and valid way, but did not frequently use the lowest rating scale category. Recommend revision of rating scale.

Table 25-6 The Child Occupational Self Assessment (COSA) and its predecessor, the Child Self Assessment of Occupational Functioning (SAOF) Evidence Summary (*continued*)

Citation	Findings
Keller and Kielhofner (2005)	With a revised 4-point scale, COSA items represent a valid and more sensitive construct of occupational competence. Clients aged 8–17, with neurological, mental health, orthopedic, medical, and developmental diagnosis were able to use the competence scale in a valid and reliable manner. With a revised 4-point scale, 20 of the 24 COSA items are part of a valid and more sensitive construct of Value (importance) of occupations. Clients were able to use the value scale in a valid and reliable manner. Item hierarchies or the continuum of occupational competence and value items replicated content of hierarchies in previous study. Recommend future research on revised items.
Knis-Matthews, Richard, Marquez, and Mevawala (2005)	Adolescent females with mental health problems can use the Children's Self-Assessment of Occupational Functioning to identify priorities for therapy, including family concerns, health, and wellness.
Ayuso and Kramer (2009)	This study examined the psychometric properties of the Spanish version of the COSA. The COSA is a self-report of occupational competence and value for activities.
Kramer, Kielhofner, and Smith (2010)	Rasch Partial Credit Model and parametric and nonparametric statistics to obtain validity evidence. The COSA was found to have good content, structural and substantive validity.
Kramer (2011)	A pilot process of triangulating multiple methods to evaluate an assessment of social validity was tested on the COSA. Steps in the process are described.
Kramer, Walker, Cohn, Mermelstein, Olsen, O'Brien, et al. (2012)	Examination of the "tridactic" relationship and how a self-report, such as the COSA, can be used to foster the partnership.

Table 25-7 Interest Checklist Evidence Summary

Citation	Findings
Rogers, Weinstein, and Figone (1978)	When high school students from the United Sates use the NPI interest checklist, four constructs emerge: ADLs, manual skills, cultural/educational, and physical sports. Social/ recreational items are distributed throughout, signifying a more complex theoretical construct.
Oakley, Kielhofner, and Barris (1985)	Adults with mental health problems and adults living in the community can use the interest checklist to report interests as one part of a battery of assessments to measure MOHO concepts of volition and habituation.
Katz (1988)	When adult psychiatric clients from Israel completed the Role Checklist, four constructs emerged that explained most of the variance in their responses: sports and physical tasks, intellectual and musical activities, social activities, and finally motor manual tasks and housekeeping.
Katz, Giladi, and Peretz (1988)	Israeli adults in both psychiatric hospitals and living in the community can use the interest checklist to report their patterns of interests, and the interest checklist reveals different patterns of interests between the two groups.
Katz, Josman, and Steinmetz (1988)	Israeli adolescents hospitalized for psychiatric conditions and community-dwelling adolescents used the interest checklist to report their patterns of interests.

(*continued*)

Table 25-7 Interest Checklist Evidence Summary (*continued*)

Citation	Findings
Ebb, Coster, and Duncombe 1989	The interest checklist was used with male adolescents with psychosocial disabilities and without disabilities. The interest checklist differentiated between the two groups on number of strong interests.
Scaffa (1991)	The interest checklist was used with a adults with alcoholism attending a substance abuse program and community-dwelling adults without identified substance abuse problems. The interest checklist found significant differences between the groups in frequency of engagement in interest and range of interests.
Widen-Holmqvist et al. (1993)	Adults living in the community after experiencing a stroke used the interest checklist to compare engagement in interests and leisure activities pre- and poststoke.
Heasman and Atwal (2004)	Interest checklist was used as part of an individualized intervention program for adults with psychiatric disabilities to create an action plan to being engagement in one new leisure activity.
Horne, Corr, and Earle (2005)	New mothers used the interest checklist to report changes in patterns of engagement in interests after the birth of their first child.
Nakamura-Thomas and Yamada (2011)	The study examined the factorial structure of the Japanese Interest Checklist (JICE). 967 healthy older adults completed the JICE. The study found that the JICE can capture the interests of older Japanese people.
Nakamura-Thomas and Yamada (2008)	The JICE was administered to 65 participants. Upon completion the participants were interviewed to examine reasons behind levels of interest.

Table 25-8 Model of Human Occupation Screening Tool (MOHOST) and Short Child Occupational Profile (SCOPE) Evidence Summary

Citation	Findings
Kielhofner, Fogg, Braveman, Forsyth, and Rappenhagen (2006)	The MOHOST can be described as representing a six-dimensional model of occupational adaptation—volition, habitation, process skills, motor skills, communication/interaction skills, and the environment.
Bowyer, Kielhofner, Kramer, Maziero Barbosa, and Girolami (2007)	The items on the SCOPE represent a valid construct of occupational participation. The SCOPE can be used by occupational therapists, physical therapists, and speech language pathologists to rate young clients with disabilities aged 2–21 years with a range of disabilities in a similar and reliable manner.
Parkinson, Chester, Cratchley, and Rowbottom (2008)	A descriptive article including a case study and discussions with occupational therapists on use of the MOHOST in practice.
Kramer, Bowyer, Kielhofner, O'Brien, and Maziero-Barbosa (2009)	A multifaceted Rasch analysis was conducted using data from 39 practitioners working in eight practice sites. One hundred and sixty eight clients' de-identified data were shared. The findings suggest that a variety of methods can be used to learn to administer the SCOPE appropriately.
Kramer, Bowyer, O'Brien, Kielhofner, and Maziero-Barbosa (2009)	Identified process used to select assessment tools and strategies to assess clients.
Kielhofner, Fogg, Braveman, Forsyth, Kramer, and Duncan (2009)	Confirmatory factorial analyses were conducted to examine whether there was evidence that the items of the MOHOST cluster in meaningful theoretical subconstructs. Nine occupational therapists in the United States and the United Kingdom used the MOHOST with 166 clients. The study confirmed that the MOHOST captures the six subconstructs of volition, habituation, motor skills, process skills, communication/interaction skills, and the environment.

Table 25-8 Model of Human Occupation Screening Tool (MOHOST) and Short Child Occupational Profile (SCOPE) Evidence Summary (*continued*)

Citation	Findings
Kramer, Kielhofner, Lee, Ashpole, and Castle (2009)	This study examined the utility of the MOHOST as an outcome measure. A retrospective design was used to gather admission and discharge MOHOST ratings from an inpatient rehabilitation unit over a 20-month period. The study indicates that the MOHOST, with minimal training, can be used in a consistent and interchangeable manner to measure occupational participation changes in clients.
Lee and Harris (2010)	This article describes a process used to adopt a conceptual model of practice to guide assessment and treatment pathway for women with borderline personality disorders.
Bowyer, Lee, Kramer, Taylor, and Kielhofner (2012)	A process to study the clinical utility of assessments. The process was used with the SCOPE.
Pan, Fan, Chung, Chen, Kielhofner, Wu, et al. (2011)	This study examined the psychometric properties of the MOHOST (Chinese version). Both item response theory and classical test theory were used. One hundred and one clients with mental health problems aged 18–65 participated. Rasch analysis and correlational analysis were used. The MOHOST-C was found to be valid when used with clients with mental health problems.
Hawes and Houlder (2010)	This was a preliminary 6-month study examining use of the MOHOST with a community learning disability service. The study demonstrated that the MOHOST provides a format for concise and professional reports while supporting use of a practice model.
Forsyth, Parkinson, Kielhofner, Kramer, Summerfield Mann, and Duncan (2011)	Nine occupational therapists used the MOHOST with 163 clients in the United States and the United Kingdom. Data were compiled to examine the psychometric properties of the MOHOST. A many-faceted Rasch analysis results support that the MOHOST can accurately measure the construct of occupational participation.
Lee, Forsyth, Morley, Garnham, Heasman, and Taylor (2013)	A retrospective study was conducted to develop care packages in England; 675 individuals from two organizations in England serving individuals with mental health disorders participated. Occupational groupings were established using a two-step cluster. The six subscales of the MOHOST were analyzed using the multivariate analysis of variance to examine the mean scores. Then, the occupational groupings were compared to the participants' membership in the payment-by-results clusters. Three categories were found: high-, middle-, or low-functioning occupational groupings. The results suggest that the mental health clustering tool and MOHOST target different aspects of service needs.
Notoh, Yamada, Kobayashi, Ishii, Forsyth (2014)	This study examined the construct validity of the Japanese version of the MOHOST using Rasch analysis and confirmatory factor analysis. The results found the Japanese version of the MOHOST to be a valid tool for measuring occupational participation.
Smith and Mairs (2014)	This study was a practice analysis examining use of global MOHO assessments in community mental health in the UK. The main assessment used by the ten occupational therapists participating in the study was the MOHOST. Second most commonly used MOHO assessment was the OCAIRS. Results found service users have different ranges of occupational difficulties and that MOHO assessments are not necessarily routinely used. The study did not establish the reason for the variability in use of MOHO assessments.

Table 25-9 Occupational Circumstances Assessment Interview and Rating Scale (OCAIRS) Evidence Summary

Citation	Findings
Kaplan (1984)	The OCAIRS has almost perfect interrater reliability overall, and there was a strong relationship between sum of component ratings and sum of global assessment ratings.
Brollier, Watts, Bauer, and Schmidt (1988)	Evidence for the concurrent validity of the OCAIRS was provided by the assessment's correlation with the Global Assessment Scale when used with clients with schizophrenia. OCAIRS may be sensitive to SES as correlations were lower when SES was controlled for.
Watts, Brollier, Bauer, and Schmidt (1989)	Evidence for criterion validity of the OCAIRS was provided by the assessment's high correlation with a similar MOHO-based assessment, the Assessment of Occupational Functioning (AOF), when used with clients with schizophrenia.
Haglund and Henriksson (1994)	Evidence of content validity of the Swedish version of the OCAIRS is provided by at least 60% agreement of therapists when matching items to domains. Interrater reliability of six occupational therapists for rating inpatient psychiatric clients and community-dwelling clients with chronic muscular pain exceeded 60% for 14 OCAIRS domains. Variance among raters and client scores is high, and only some OCAIRS items differentiate between inpatient psychiatric and community-dwelling chronic pain clients.
Henriksson(1995a)	OCAIRS interview can be used internationally (Sweden and USA) with women with fibromyalgia to better understand their encounters within the health care system, interactions with others, and consequences of living with fibromyalgia.
Henriksson (1995b)	OCAIRS interview can be used internationally (Sweden and USA) to understand the strategies women with fibromyalgia use to cope with pain and ADLs, including adjusting routines, changing their life situation and their attitudes.
Henriksson and Burckhardt (1996)	The OCAIRS has a stable meaning across two countries, as the mean scores for women with fibromyalgia from either USA or Sweden were almost identical, although women in the USA working full time reported more stress, more exhaustion, and less satisfaction compared to the Swedish women.
Haglund (1996)	There was no significant difference between 38 Swedish occupational therapists' decision to include/exclude a videotaped client from therapy services based on results of a standard interview vs. OCAIRS interview. For therapists who had worked in psychiatry for over 1.5 years, there was no significant difference in the recommendation for therapy.
Haglund, Thorell, and Walinder (1998a)	A revised version of the Swedish OCAIRS improved interrater agreement when used with Swedish psychiatry clients. Low to moderate intercorrelations between components of the OCAIRS also indicate the instrument assesses different domains of participation.
Haglund, Thorell, and Walinder (1998b)	The Swedish OCAIRS may discriminate between the occupational participation of clients with different mental health conditions, as the ratings from the Swedish version of the OCAIRS are significantly different for clients with depression, schizophrenia, and bipolar disorder and as clients with depression having the highest occupational participation scores.
Lai, Haglund, and Kielhofner (1999)	Most items on the OCAIRS represent a valid construct of occupational adaptation and can differentiate between clients with different levels of occupational adaptation (clients with unipolar affective disorder tended to be more adaptive, and clients with schizophrenia tended to be less adapted). Although five of six therapists did not differ significantly from each other when rating clients using the OCAIRS, the meaning of the 5-point rating varied across items.
Heasman and Atwal (2004)	The OCAIRS can be used as an initial interview to identify leisure goals for young adult clients (ages 20+) with mental health disabilities attending a day program.

Table 25-10 Occupational Performance History Interview (OPHI-II) Evidence Summary

Citation	Findings
Kielhofner, Harlan, Bauer, and Maurer (1986)	The OPHI had acceptable overall interrater and test–retest reliability when used with clients with disabilities seen in inpatient and outpatient settings. The OPHI may also be able to detect change over time.
Kielhofner and Henry (1988)	The OPHI had moderate test–retest and interrater reliability when used by therapists in the USA and Canada to rate adolescent, adult, and older adult clients with psychiatric and physical disabilities. Past and present scales appear to represent two different constructs. Therapists indicated they would use the OPHI interview regularly or for some clients.
Bridle et al. (1990)	The OPHI can be used to reveal changes in occupational adaptation (in roles and routines, volition, and environment) 2–8 years after spinal cord injury.
Kielhofner, Henry, Walens, and Rogers (1991)	Therapists using an eclectic approach and therapists using a MOHO approach interpreted the OPHI scales in a similar and dependable manner when rating psychiatric clients after attending a workshop on the assessment. One exception was that therapists using a MOHO approach did not use the OPHI present scale in an acceptable manner.
Lynch and Bridle (1993)	The OPHI had acceptable construct validity (and covaried with the Multidimensional Pain Inventory Scales (MPI) and the Center for Epidemiological Studies Depression Scale [CES-D]), and the OPHI can reveal changes in occupational performance over time as a result of a spinal cord injury.
Neistadt (1995)	13% of 269 directors of adult physical disability settings that served adolescents, adults, and older adults reported that therapists used the OPHI to identify client priorities (in a total of 35 facilities).
Kielhofner and Mallinson (1995)	The types of questions asked by therapists conducting an OPHI interview influenced the type of client response, where questions about change, motives, and specific circumstances elicited narrative responses. Therapists who let the OPHI interview go where the client's responses led, who asked clients to elaborate their responses, who waited until clients finished their responses, and who showed a genuine interest in a client's response were better able to elicit narrative during the OPHI interview.
Mallinson, Kielhofner, and Mattingly (1996)	The OPHI interview can be used with men and women with mental health disabilities to elicit metaphors that explain their life history.
Fossey (1996)	The OPHI can be used with English clients attending a psychiatric day program to identify turning points in their life narrative, and the narrative summary can be used to convey information about the client's life history to other professionals.
Mallinson, Mahaffey, and Kielhofner (1998)	Analysis of the OPHI items reveals three constructs of occupational adaptation—occupational competence, occupational identity, and environments/settings. Items rearranged into these three constructs demonstrate good psychometric properties. Revisions to the OPHI are recommended, and new items should be added to strengthen each construct.
Kielhofner, Mallinson, Forsyth, and Lai (2001)	• The items of each OPHI-II scale validly measure the underlying constructs of occupational competence, occupational identity, and occupational behavior settings (environment) for an international sample of people with physical, psychiatric, or no known disabilities. • The OPHI-II validly measures the occupational adaptation of persons and is sensitive enough to detect differences in occupational adaptation among persons. • An international group of therapists can use the OPHI-II in a valid way by using the administration manual.
Buning, Angelo, and Schmeler (2001)	The OPHI-II can be used to capture the positive changes in past to present occupational performance of adults who use powered mobility devices.

(*continued*)

Table 25-10 Occupational Performance History Interview (OPHI-II) Evidence Summary (*continued*)

Citation	Findings
Braveman and Helfrich (2001)	The OPHI-II can be used to better understand the experiences and sense of occupational competence and occupational identity of men returning to work with AIDS.
Graff, Vernooij-Dassen, Hoefnagels, Dekker, and de Witte (2003)	The OPHI-II was used to gather information from older adults with cognitive impairments regarding their past and present needs, interests, habits, and roles as part of an intervention to support older adults with cognitive impairments living at home and their caregivers.
Gray and Fossey (2003)	The OPHI-II can be used to understand the experiences of Australian men and women living with chronic fatigue syndrome.
Levin and Helfrich (2004)	The OPHI-II can be used to understand the experiences of homeless teenage mothers in the USA. The OPHI-II explicated the identity of homeless adolescent mothers and found their identity was influenced by their development, role choices, and their future desire to engage in the mother role.
Goldstein, Kielhofner, and Paul-Ward (2004)	The OPHI-II can be used to explore the narratives of men with AIDS participating in a return to work program.
Chan (2004)	The OPHI-II interview can be used to understand how Chinese men with chronic obstructive pulmonary disease experience the disease process and engagement in occupations.
Farnworth, Nihitin, and Fossey (2004)	The OPHI-II interview was used to elicit the perspectives of clients in a forensic setting regarding their life on the ward.
Braveman, Helfrich, Kielhofner, and Albrecht (2004)	The OPHI was used to better understand how men with AIDS experienced returning to work over a 12-month period when they were engaged in a return to work study program.
Chaffey and Fossey (2004)	Mothers who were caregivers of adult sons with schizophrenia described their experiences and the meaning of their caregiving using the OPHI-II interview.
Kielhofner et al. (2004)	The OPHI-II narrative slope predicted outcomes of clients with AIDS (and other difficulties such as mental health conditions and substance abuse) who participated in a return to work program. Clients with progressive narrative slopes were twice as likely to have a successful outcome in the program of employment, school, or volunteer work.
Ingvarsson and Theodorsdottir (2004)	The OPHI-II can be used as part of individualized, vocational rehabilitation program for clients in order to better understand client strengths and problems and to set individualized goals.
Apte, Kielhofner, Paul-Ward, and Braveman (2005)	Therapists and most clients view the OPHI-II interview and narrative slope as a meaningful and rapport-building part of the therapy process.
Kielhofner, Dobria, Forsyth, and Basu (2005)	The OPHI-II key forms, developed using an international sample of over 700 people with physical, psychiatric, or no known disabilities, allow therapists to derive a corresponding calibration, or measure, for each OPHI-II total raw score, derived for each of the three OPHI-II scales.

Table 25-11 The Occupational Questionnaire (OQ) and the NIH Activity Record (ACTRE) Evidence Summary

Citation	Findings
Smyntek, Barris, and Kielhofner (1985)	The OQ was used to assess the self efficacy and habits of nonpsychotic adolescents with psychiatric disabilities and adolescents living in the community.
Furst, Gerber, Smith, Fisher, and Schulman (1987)	This study modified the OQ to create the NIH Activity Record (ACTRE) that was used with adults with rheumatoid arthritis to assess changes in patterns of physical activity and rest.

Table 25-11 The Occupational Questionnaire (OQ) and the NIH Activity Record (ACTRE) Evidence Summary (*continued*)

Citation	Findings
Ebb, Coster, and Duncombe (1989)	The OQ was used with male adolescents with disabilities and without disabilities to talk about their typical routines. The OQ did not differentiate differences in typical days between groups.
Keilhofner and Brinson (1989)	The OQ can be used to identify client goals as part of a MOHO-based intervention program that transition young people discharged from psychiatric hospitalizations back to the community.
Aubin, Hachey, and Mercier (1999)	French translation of OQ was successfully used with clients with schizophrenia and similar diagnosis to report feelings of competence in everyday activities.
Gerber and Furst (1992)	The NIH Activity Record (ACTRE) is a valid measure of adult's perceptions of arthritis symptoms during participation in daily activities.
Aubin, Hachey, and Mercier (2002)	The French translation of the OQ can be used by adult clients with severe mental health problems to assess the importance of and enjoyment for their daily activities and routine.
Pentland, Harvey, and Walker (2006)	Canadian men with spinal cord injuries used the OQ to report their use of time in occupational areas of sleep, personal care, productive activities, and leisure.
Henry, Costa, Ladd, Robertson, Rollins, and Roy (1996)	The OQ can be used to have US college students report their patterns of time use and feelings about time use.
Smith, Kielhofner, and Watts (1986)	The OQ can be successfully used to analyze relationship between volition and engagement in everyday occupations and quality of life for older adults living in nursing homes and community settings.
Widen-Holmqvist et al. (1993)	Adults living in the community after a stroke can use the OQ to report their engagement in interests, leisure activities, and social activities.
Packer, Foster, and Brouwer (1997)	The NIH Activity Record can be used to examine differences in the daily routines of Canadians with and without chronic fatigue syndrome.
Leidy and Knebel (1999)	A modified version of the NIH Activity Record can be used by adults with COPD, chronic bronchitis, or emphysema to assess their daily routines and performance in activities.

Table 25-12 Pediatric Interest Profile (PIP) Evidence Summary

Citation	Findings
Hann, Regele, Walsh, Fontana, and Bentley (1994)[a]	The 80-item checklist pilot study version of the Adolescent Leisure Interest Profile had items that are meaningful to students in junior and high school in the USA.
Andrews et al. (1995)[a]	A series of studies were used to develop the items for the Kid Play Profile and the Preteen Play Profile by having children between the ages of 6 and 12 complete the profiles and through an expert OT review.
Beck et al. (1996)[a]	Young children in the USA successfully completed a 19-item pilot study version of the Kid Play Profile with pictures and used the assessment in a consistent manner.
Henry (2000)	In the pilot study, children aged 9–11 completed a 53-item version of the Preteen Play Profile with pictures, with questions about frequency and feelings of competence in a consistent manner.
Budd et al. (1997)[a]	The Kid Play Profile items can be used reliably over time by children aged 6–9.
Henry (2000)	The Preteen Play Profile can be used reliably over time by children aged 9 and 10.
Brophy et al. (1995)[a]	The Adolescent Leisure Interest Profile can be used reliably over time by adolescents aged 14–19.

[a]As reported in Henry (2000).

Table 25-13 Pediatric Volitional Questionnaire (PVQ) Evidence Summary

Citation	Findings
Andersen, Kielhofner, and Lai (2005)	The PVQ items represent a valid construct of volition and reflect a volitional continuum of exploration, competency, and achievement. The PVQ can be used to validly measure young client's volition. Environments of classroom, playground, and playroom are appropriate contexts to assess volition. Therapists may not be interchangeable when rating young clients with the PVQ.
Harris and Reid (2005)	The PVQ can be used in a meaningful way to assess the volition children with CP exhibit when engaged in therapeutic activities, such as a virtual reality game environment.
Reid (2005)	The PVQ can be used to measure volition of children with CP engaged in therapeutic activities, such as a virtual reality game environment. In addition, average PVQ scores are significantly correlated with the Test of Playfulness average motivation scores. Scores for the PVQ items "Stays engaged," "Tries to produce effects," "Is task directed," "Initiates actions," "Shows preferences," "Expresses mastery pleasure," and "Organizes and modifies environment" were significantly correlated with Test of Playfulness average motivation score.

Table 25-14 Residential Environment Impact Survey (REIS) and REIS Short Form (REIS-SF) Evidence Summary

Citation	Findings
Parkinson, Fisher, and Fisher (2011)	This article describes the development of the REIS and REIS-SF, a nonstandardized, semi-structured assessment and consulting instrument for examining quality of residential homes rather than private homes.
Fisher and Kayhan (2012)	A survey on use of the REIS and REIS-SF was used to gather information from international (non-US) users to find out how the tools were being used and how they could be improved. The data complied will be used to alter the tools to better meet the needs of users.

Table 25-15 Role Checklist Evidence Summary

Citation	Findings
Lederer, Kielhofner, and Watts (1985)	Incarcerated adolescents and adolescents living in the community used the Role Checklist to report the value for roles. The Role Checklist was able to capture different patterns of value for roles between the two groups.
Oakley, Kielhofner, and Barris (1985)	Adult clients with mental health problems can use the Role Checklist to effectively report on role continuity and role disruption.
Smyntek, Barris, and Kielhofner (1985)	The Role Checklist can be used with adolescents with psychosocial problems and adolescents without problems to assess differences in role engagement and value for roles in the two groups.
Barris et al. (1986)	The Role Checklist is one assessment that can be used to examine differing patterns of occupational engagement (including role engagement) between adolescents with psychophysiological diagnoses, psychiatric diagnoses, and adolescents without disabilities.
Duellman, Barris, and Kielhofner (1986)	The Role Checklist can be used by older adults in nursing homes to report the number of anticipated future roles in order to better understand their sense of occupational engagement while in the nursing home.
Oakley, Kielhofner, Barris, and Reichler (1986)	OT experts confirmed that the Role Checklist has content validity. The Role Checklist has good reliability, although older person's responses to sections I and II of the Role Checklist may be more consistent.

Table 25-15 Role Checklist Evidence Summary (*continued*)

Citation	Findings
Elliott and Barris (1987)	Role Checklist was used by older adults without disabilities living in the community to report past and present role engagement. The Role Checklist was able to capture changes in role engagement over time.
Rust, Barris, and Hooper (1987)	The Role Checklist and a Modified Role Checklist can be used by college women to report engagement in exercise and related roles.
Barris, Dickie, and Baron, (1988)	The Role Checklist can be used to assess different patterns of past and future role engagement between female young adults with eating disorders and their matched peer groups, adolescents with psychiatric disabilities and their matched peer groups, and young adults with chronic conditions and their matched peer groups.
Ebb, Coster, and Duncombe (1989)	Adolescent males with psychosocial disabilities and adolescents living in the community without disabilities can use the Role Checklist to report role engagement. The Role Checklist can be used to discriminate between the two groups of adolescents.
Branholm and Fugl-Meyer (1992)	The Role Checklist can be used effectively across age cohorts and by males and females living in Sweden to examine differences in role engagement with respect to age and gender.
Baker, Curbow, and Wingard (1991)	Role Checklist was used to have survivors of bone marrow transplant (BMT) report if they engaged in roles before and after BMT, and also to rate importance of each role.
Watson and Ager (1991)	Role Checklist was modified to include ratings of role importance and frequency of engagement, and change in values for roles over time and used by older adults in the community in several age cohorts effectively.
Egan, Warren, Hessel, and Gilewich (1992)	The Role Checklist was completed by Canadian older adults posthip fracture before and 3 weeks after discharge to assess participation and performance.
Hallett, Zasler, Maurer, and Cash (1994)	People living in the community after experiencing a brain injury can use the Role Checklist to report role loss and value for roles.
Dickerson and Oakley (1995)	The Role Checklist was used by adults with physical disabilities, psychosocial disabilities, and adults without disabilities living in the community to report on role engagement. Role Checklist was able to detect difference between all the groups on the number of roles engaged in the present and future, and difference in value for roles.
Hachey, Jummoorty, and Mercier (1995)	French translation of the Role Checklist was translated using parallel back translation, and the instrument had moderate interlanguage and intralanguage test–retest reliability when used with bilingual psychiatric clients in Canada.
Kusznir, Scott, Cooke, and Young (1996)	A modified version of the Role Checklist was used effectively by adults seen in a bipolar clinic to report on involvement in life roles and the importance of those roles.
Larsson and Branholm (1996)	Role Checklist was used by Swedish adults in a neurological rehab center to identify goals for therapy.
Crowe, VanLeit, Berghmans, and Mann (1997)	The Role Checklist was used by mothers of children with multiple disabilities, mothers of children with Down's Syndrome, and mothers of typically developing children to report changes in role engagement after the birth of their child.
Frosch et al. (1997)	The Role Checklist was used only to detect changes in role engagement in past and in present roles for caregivers of persons with traumatic brain injury.
Munoz et al. (1999)	In part of a qualitative study, the Role Checklist was used to examine parents' of children with cerebral palsy perceptions of role involvement and role meaningfulness.
Eklund (2001)	The Role Checklist was used with OT clients with psychotic and nonpsychotic conditions to report on role engagement and value for roles over time, including at admission, discharge, and 1-year follow-up.

(*continued*)

Table 25-15 Role Checklist Evidence Summary (*continued*)

Citation	Findings
Lee, Strauss, Wittman, Jackson, and Carstens (2001)	Role Checklist was used by caregivers of adults with mental illness to illuminate relationship between role engagement in past and present and caregiver sorrow.
Hachey, Boyer, and Mercier (2001)	The French version of the Role Checklist can be used to explore engagement in and value for roles for persons with schizophrenia.
Colon and Haertlein (2002)	Spanish translation of the Role Checklist had acceptable intralanguage test–retest reliability.
Corr and Wilmer (2003)	The Role Checklist was used by participants aged 34–55 who experienced a stroke. The Role Checklist revealed that work was important to these individuals.
Corr, Phillips, and Walker (2004)	Adults who experienced a stroke and who attended a day program used the Role Checklist to assess role engagement.
Schindler (2004)	The Role Checklist was used within a larger study to identify incarcerated or recently released men's engagement in roles and to identify roles to develop during an intervention.
Horne, Corr, and Earle (2005)	Used Role Checklist with first-time mothers to report changes in role engagement after birth of their first child.
Schindler and Baldwin (2005)	Role Checklist was used by adult psychiatric clients to identify roles to address while engaged in an intervention to acquire roles.
Hakansson et al. (2005)	The Role Checklist can be used to discern difference in value for the worker role between Swedish women who are continuously healthy and working, and women who report discontinuity in work related to illness.
Cordeiro, Camelier, Oakley, and Jardim (n.d.)	The Brazilian Portuguese translation of the Role Checklist can be used in a reliable manner to gather information about occupational role engagement and the value of those roles.

Table 25-16 School Setting Interview (SSI) Evidence Summary

Citation	Findings
Hemmingsson and Borell (1996)	The SSI content areas are sensitive and specific and can be used to appropriately identify accommodation needs of students with physical disabilities in regular and special classrooms. Interrater reliability of SSI is acceptable, and expert review clarified relevant content areas.
Hemmingsso and Borell (2000)	The SSI can be used to determine the accommodation needs and unmet needs of students with physical disabilities in Sweden, where 98% of students reported a need for accommodations, and 83.3% of students reported an unmet need. Accommodations most frequently needed were in the areas of writing, classroom work, and personal assistance, and most frequently reported unmet needs were in the areas of reading, remembering, and speaking.
Prellwitz and Tham (2000)	Using the SSI interview, students with restricted mobility reported few major difficulties with the physical environment of their Swedish primary schools, but had difficulties with the social environment, such as teaching situations, social contact with peers, dealing with their personal assistant, and bullying.
Hemmingsson and Borell (2002)	Swedish students aged 10–19 with physical disabilities identified unmet needs using the SSI, and these unmet needs were categorized according to MOHO environmental concepts of spaces, objects, occupational forms, and social groups. SSI revealed differences in needs and unmet needs among students with and without personal assistants, and younger and older students.
Hemmingsson, Kottorp, and Bernspang (2004)	The SSI items represent a valid construct of student–environment fit and need for accommodations when used with students with physical disabilities aged 8–19 in regular and special education classrooms. Items do not fully cover the range of student environment fit and needs of students who are most able; however, most students were validly measured by the SSI.

Table 25-17 Volitional Questionnaire (VQ) Evidence Summary

Citation	Findings
Chern, Kielhofner, de las Heras, and Magalhaes (1996)	Series of two studies: *Study One:* Items are a valid representation of construct of volition, but require further development to reflect the volitional continuum. Can be used to measure volition of clients with psychiatric disabilities or developmental delays. *Study Two:* Revised VQ items are a valid representation of the construct of volition and are distributed along the volitional continuum. VQ can be used to assess volition of clients with psychiatric disabilities and developmental delays, but may not accurately measure clients with high levels of volition.
Reid (2003)	The Volitional Questionnaire can be used to assess the volition of older adult stroke survivors while engaged in intervention and leisure activities, such as a virtual reality experience.
Li and Kielhofner (2004)	The VQ items coalesce to represent a valid, sensitive construct of volition and represent a volitional continuum of exploration, competency, and achievement. The VQ can be used to measure the volition of clients with psychiatric disabilities and HIV/AIDS in a valid manner. Therapists use the VQ rating scale in a consistent and valid manner but are not interchangeable when assessing client's volition using the VQ.
Agren and Kjellberg (2008)	This study examined the utility and content validity of the Swedish version of the Volitional Questionnaire (VQ-S). Thirteen occupational therapists familiar with the MOHO and who worked with clients (intellectual impairments) for whom the VQ-S was appropriate were selected for the study. The VQ-S was administered six times and after each use a questionnaire was completed concerning the utility and validity of the VQ-S. Upon analysis of the data from the questionnaires and the VQ-S assessment forms the results support that the VQ-S has clinical relevance and content validity.

Table 25-18 Work Environment Impact Scale (WEIS) Evidence Summary

Citation	Findings
Corner, Kielhofner, and Lin (1997)	The WEIS items coalesce to represent a valid construct of the impact of the work environment on worker performance. The WEIS can be used to assess the impact of the environment on the performance of workers with psychiatric disabilities in a valid and reliable way.
Kielhofner, Lai, Olson, Haglund, Ekbadh, and Hedlund (1999)	WEIS items: coalesce to represent a valid construct environmental impact on work performance, can be used to assess clients in a valid manner, and can be used in a valid and reliable way by therapists across cultures (USA and Sweden).
Ekbladh, Fan, Sandqvist, Hemmingson, and Taylor (2014)	This study examined the psychometric properties of the Swedish version of the WEIS. The results provide evidence that the Swedish version of the WEIS is psychometrically sound across diagnoses and occupations.

Table 25-19 Worker Role Interview (WRI) Evidence Summary

Citation	Findings
Biernacki (1993)	When using the WRI to evaluate clients with UE injuries, OTs with experience in rehab demonstrated high test–retest reliability. However, some WRI items did not meet standards for reliability and further development of the assessment was recommended.

(*continued*)

Table 25-19 Worker Role Interview (WRI) Evidence Summary (*continued*)

Citation	Findings
Haglund, Karlsson, and Kielhofner (1997)	The items and rating scale on a Swedish translation of the WRI can be used in a valid manner and represent a continuum of ability to return to work. However, environmental items should be revised to ensure they validly represent the construct of return to work.
Velozo, Kielhofner, Gern, Lin, Lai, and Fischer (1999)	A series of three studies: *Study One:* WRI items represent a valid, sensitive construct of return to work, represent a continuum of ability to return to work, and can measure clients in a valid way. However, environmental items should be revised to ensure they validly represent the construct of return to work. *Study Two:* Revised WRI items represent a valid, increasingly sensitive construct of return to work, measure an increased number of clients in a valid manner, including clients with diverse physical injuries. Only one environmental item continues to not have acceptable statistics. Items represent continuum of return to work, and replicate past item hierarchies. *Study Three:* When the WRI was used with clients with back injuries, no variables were significant predictors of return to work.
Ekbladh et al. (2004)	For a variety of Swedish clients with musculoskeletal, connective tissue and mood disorders, WRI personal causation items ("Assess abilities and limitations," "Expectations of job success," and "Takes responsibility"), one role item ("Appraises work expectations"), and one environmental item ("Perception of work setting") have tentative predictive validity for return to work.
Jackson, Harkess, and Ellis (2004)	The use of two standardized work assessment, the WRI or the Valpar Component Work Samples assessment, by skilled occupational therapists with clients with physical and mental health disabilities improved the reporting of clients' work abilities across 12 domains that include physical demands, environment, and personal characteristics.
Asmundsdottir (2004)	The WRI can be used with psychiatric clients who are looking to return to work to enable them to express their attitudes and opinions about work. Findings from WRI interviews can be used to inform work rehabilitation program service provision.
Ingvarsson and Theodorsdottir (2004)	The WRI can be used as an initial evaluation that considers psychosocial and environmental factors that impact return to work as part of a successful vocational rehabilitation program for clients with a variety of disabilities.
Fenger and Kramer (2004)	The items and rating scale in an Icelandic translation of the WRI coalesce to represent a valid and sensitive construct of return to work, measure clients in a valid manner, and can be used by therapists in a valid manner. Items represent continuum of return to work, and replicate past item hierarchies. However, two environmental items may not represent the contrast of ability to return to work, and therapists are not interchangeable when using the WRI-IS.
Forsyth, Braveman, Kielhofner, Ekbladh, Haglund, Fenger, et al. (2006)	Across countries (USA, Iceland, and Sweden), the WRI items work well to validly define the construct of psychosocial ability to return to work. Items represent continuum of return to work, and replicate past item hierarchies. Most clients are validly measured by the WRI across countries, and the WRI is a sensitive instrument across countries. Therapists across countries can use the WRI consistently to assess clients. All four environmental items on the WRI exceed acceptable statistics and may represent a separate construct of return to work.
Kielhofner, Braveman, Finlayson, Paul-Ward, Goldbaum, and Goldstein (2004)	The WRI can be used as part of an initial evaluation in a successful return to work program based on MOHO for individuals with AIDS.
Codd, Stapleton, Veale, FitzGerald, and Bresnihan (2010)	This study examined the impact of rheumatoid arthritis (RA) on employment 2 years postdiagnosis. The WRI was used as the tool to collect the data.

Evidence Concerning the Nature of MOHO Practice

A few studies have focused on the process of therapy based on MOHO. These studies provide evidence about the dynamics of therapy and about factors that may contribute to positive outcomes of therapy. The publications are summarized in Table 25-20. Another source of information about what MOHO practice looks like is the many articles and chapters that describe programs based on MOHO or that present case examples that illustrate the use of MOHO.

Table 25-20 Evidence Concerning the Nature of MOHO Practice

Citation	Outcome/Findings/Implications
Apte, Kielhofner, Paul-Ward, and Braveman (2005)	Therapists reported that the OPHI-II interview and narrative slope was a rapport-building process that can be adjusted according to characteristics of client and their current life situation in order to engage clients in collaborative goal setting.
Barrett, Beer, and Kielhofner (1999)	• Therapy is more effective when therapists are aware of clients' narrative and the related meaning of change to their client and respect that narrative in the therapy process.
Braveman, Helfrich, Kielhofner, and Albrecht (2004)	For adults with AIDS, returning to work is a individualized, personal decision about what is best for that person's future, and requires individualized service and ongoing support. Even clients with many concerns can be supported to return to work.
Daniels et al. (2011)	A program based on MOHO constructs which is focused on disability prevention in frail older people. The program includes six steps: screening, assessment, analysis and preliminary action plan, agreement on an action plan, execution of action plan, and evaluation/follow-up.
Desiron, Donceel, de Rijk, and Van Hoof (2013)	An examination of occupational therapy models to aid return to work (RTW) for clients with breast cancer was explored. The basis for the exploration was to identify a model that could enhance RTW interventions for the breast cancer population. Of the nine models initially identified MOHO was found to have the highest compliance rate for inclusion. Furthermore, MOHO was the only model which provides tools and instruments focused on RTW. MOHO needs to be adapted to address the needs of this population's RTW needs.
Alcorn and Broome (2014)	A literature review designed to explore the role of occupational therapy in wellness and prevention. MOHO constructs aligned with how healthy lifestyle behavior can have personal factors, which are barriers or facilitators of this type of lifestyle. Emphasis is on the role of coaching in changing occupational performance.
Eklund (1996)	• Psychological engagement in a day program intervention, as rated by staff, was positively related to client's volition and habituation.
Folland and Forsyth (2011)	Development of an academic/practice partnership to support government policy to address the need for evidence of clinical effectiveness. The National Health Service (NHS) in the UK chose to adopt the MOHO as the overarching conceptual practice model. Using MOHO to guide practice promotes the government policy in the UK.
Goldstein, Kielhofner, and Paul-Ward (2004)	Therapists should adjust their approach based on a client's occupational narrative. Clients with a progressive narrative may require support and structure to reach their goals, whereas clients with a regressive narrative need support to identify attainable goals that they can successfully achieve.

(continued)

Table 25-20 Evidence Concerning the Nature of MOHO Practice (*continued*)

Citation	Outcome/Findings/Implications
Gregitis, Gelpi, Moore, and Dees (2010)	A case study design was used to examine and describe the Occupation-Based Self-Determination (OBSD) program. The program is designed to increase adolescents' motivation and desire to set personal goals, undertake and complete meaningful tasks, pursue significant roles while transitioning into adulthood, and develop resiliency. The program uses theoretical concepts from MOHO and the Self-Determination Model.
Heasman and Morley (2011)	In the UK government policy requires occupational therapists to demonstrate clinical effectiveness. The electronic case records (ECRs) are used to aid in tracking. A multifaceted practice development program to train, support, and monitor the effective use of assessment tools based on MOHO.
Helfrich and Kielhofner (1994)	Clients perceive occupational therapy intervention as relevant or meaningful based on their own volitional narratives and life events prior to beginning therapy. Client views of OT and its meaning may be incompatible with therapists' views of OT.
Jones (2008)	Occupational therapists in the UK provide a range of physical activities as a standard intervention for clients with mental health problems such as badminton, swimming, soccer, pool, table tennis, and yoga. Community and local parks near clients' homes are the venues for the activities.
Kielhofner and Barrett (1998)	• The occupational forms used in therapy must relate them to the larger context of the client's life. Misunderstanding can occur in goal setting when an implied progressive therapy narrative does not match client's volitional narrative.
Kimball-Carpenter and Smith (2013)	Based on the concepts of MOHO an occupational therapist developed an interprofessional activity group for a geriatric psychiatry clinic. The program allowed the occupational therapists to have a positive impact on clients and increased the visibility of occupational therapy with the interdisciplinary team members.
Lim and Rodger (2008)	Use of MOHO as an overarching occupation theory to guide practice with children with difficulties in social participation can be effective. MOHO cannot be used alone, rather can be used with other congruent models to determine each child's challenges.
Liu and Ng (2008)	Use of the MOHO (a Western theory) in Hong Kong (an Eastern context) can be useful with problem identification and intervention planning. Two cases demonstrate the insights that can be achieved in practice and influence participation of clients with disabilities in the Chinese culture.
Mallinson, Kielhofner, and Mattingly (1996)	Clients use deep metaphors to explain and interpret their life circumstances and guide their actions during life history interviews. For example, metaphors of momentum evoke images of speed, inertia, and deceleration to describe progression and direction of life, whereas metaphors of entrapment describe feelings of restriction and confinement and reveal a conflict between desires and reality.
Melton, Forsyth, Metherall, Hill, Quick (2008)	Occupation-focused program redesign using the MOHO in the UK with acute care inpatient hospitals.
Morgan and Long (2012)	A literature analysis was conducted to examine the effectiveness of motor interventions for children with developmental coordination disorder (DCD). MOHO was used as a guide to structure the findings. The findings suggest that using an overarching occupation model to aid in interpretation of multiple sources of evidence can aid in the interpretation and therapeutic reasoning process.
Munoz, Lawlor, and Kielhofner (1993)	Therapists feel that MOHO is an occupation-focused and well-developed model, and they use main MOHO concepts to guide the therapy process and convey the purpose of OT to others.

Table 25-20 Evidence Concerning the Nature of MOHO Practice (*continued*)

Citation	Outcome/Findings/Implications
Parkinson, Lowe, and Vecsey (2011)	A horticulture program was evaluated for aspects contributing the greatest therapeutic benefit. The positive effects of a horticulture program are not a given. Personal factors have to be taken into consideration such as gender preferences and social needs.
Pepin, Guerette, Lefebvre, and Jacques (2008)	Use of the Remotivation Process, based on MOHO, was found to have a positive impact on individuals experiencing depression.
Raber, Teitelman, Watts, and Kielhofner (2010)	An exploration of volition in people with moderate dementia living in a memory-supported assisted living. Eight older people participated. Understanding volition is highly significant to support better engagement in meaningful occupations.
Rothberg, Coopoo, Burns, and Franzsen (2009)	A MOHO-based individualized employee fitness program was developed. An in-house program was found to have benefits for some of the participants in the program.
Tham and Borell (1996)	• Motivation to engage in training and intervention may be related to how aligned the intervention is with the client's personal view of their situation. An individual's view of the future and the presence of goals may motivate them to participate in intervention.
Tham and Kielhofner (2003)	Women in rehabilitation with left neglect relied on the social environment to negotiate their new experiences and to move forward with their rehabilitation.
Toit (2008)	A program developed based on MOHO for adults who are blind and unemployed was found to achieve many of its aims.
Turner and Lydon (2008)	A MOHO-based intervention program developed for mental health was found to be beneficial in the areas of volition, habituation, and skills.
Wimpenny, Forsyth, Jones, Matheson, Colley (2010)	Implementation of MOHO concepts in mental health service. A structured program was provided over a 2-year period.
Ziv, Roitman (2008)	A community-based group for elderly women in Israel to address problems of aging.
Durand, Vachon, Loisel, and Berthelette (2003)	Work rehabilitation programs based on MOHO concepts can be successfully implemented and can enable clients to meet program goals.

Evidence Concerning the Outcomes of MOHO-Based Practice

One of the most important kinds of evidence concerns client outcomes that result from services based on MOHO. Table 25-21 includes the results of studies published to date. This type of research is one of the fastest growing areas of MOHO research, so therapists looking for evidence should also check the literature or the MOHO Clearinghouse Web site for the most recent studies. Also, outcomes research is the most challenging and costly to conduct, so such studies may not be available for a particular population. In this instance, other forms of evidence, such as the expertise of occupational therapists as documented in descriptions of programs and case examples, are the next best sources of evidence for practice.

Client Perspectives on MOHO Services

Client satisfaction with service is an important indicator of the quality of services. Disabled scholars have critiqued occupational therapists' approaches to practice and interpretation of practice outcomes (Abberley, 1995; Giangreco, 1999). Disabled persons have also asserted that health care professionals' imagined experience of disability is quite different from the reality of living with a disability. As a result, the evidence base for practice may be flawed if research lacks the assessment of outcomes that are meaningful to people with disabilities (Basnett, 2001). Similarly, clients who were recipients of occupational therapy services have stressed that listening to their concerns would lead to better provision of services (Corring & Cook, 1999). The evidence generated by occupational therapy clients regarding their experience with MOHO-based therapy services is summarized in Table 25-22.

Table 25.21 MOHO Research on Outcomes: Intervention Studies

Reference	Type of Study	Sample Info	Description of Intervention	Findings and Clinical Implications
Brown and Carmichael (1992)	Group study; quasi-experimental.	33 Canadian clients from a large psychiatric hospital Diagnosis: 18 schizophrenia, 7 personality disorders, 8 affective disorders. 16 females and 17 males.	• Assertiveness training sought to improve communication/interaction skills. Influence of volition and environment was also considered. • Session topics included asking questions, self-esteem, assertiveness techniques, nonverbal communication, and making requests. • Group met 2 times a week for 1½-hour session over a 7-week period. Average group size was eight clients with two OT coleaders. Assessments completed during initial and final session of intervention program.	Participation in an assertiveness training intervention based on MOHO increases client assertiveness and self-esteem.
Corcoran and Gitlin (2001)	Quasi-experimental. Random assignment to intervention group.	100 caregivers of persons with dementia in the United States. Caregivers were aged 23–87, mean age 59.3 years. 77% of caregivers were Caucasian. 73% of caregivers were female. Those being cared for: mean age 78.5, had moderate impairments in self-care, and had an average of 20 behavioral difficulties as reported by caregivers.	• Intervention was based on conception of environment as objects, social tasks, and culture (as defined by MOHO), and focused on ADLs, toileting, leisure and IADLs, safety, mobility, wandering, communication, catastrophic reactions, and caregiver center concerns (fatigue). • Five 90-minute home visits over 2 months. Therapist and caregiver worked together to identify environmental strategies to resolve behavioral concerns. • First three sessions focused on education on interaction between person and environment and problem solving. Last two sessions reinforced techniques and helped to generalize new skills to emerging problem areas.	An individualized intervention focused on the environment, as described by MOHO, can generate useful strategies to decrease problem behaviors of people with dementia living at home. • 220 problem areas identified by caregivers were addressed in the intervention • Caregivers tried a total of 1068 strategies, and used 869 successfully. • Of the strategies used, 343 were modifications at the task level, 200 at the object level, and 326 at the social group level.

Corr et al. (2004)	Randomized cross-over design.	Group A: nine clients who experienced a stroke day program over 6 months. Average age 49 years (*SD* = 5). 11 males, 3 females. Average time since stroke 26 months (*SD* = 40). 57% right side affected by stroke. Group B: Wait to attend. Seven clients who had experienced a stroke. 4 males, 8 females. Average age 46 years (*SD* = 8). Average 14 months since stroke (*SD* = 19). 67% right side affected by stroke.	Day program service provided 1 day a week for people who had experienced a stroke. Assessments included the Role Checklist, COPM, and the SF-36. Meeting space included kitchen, practical activities area, social area, computers, small meeting room, and toilet facilities. Arts and crafts, outings, and other activities run by a paid nonhealth care employee.	Participation in a day service intervention any time after experiencing a stroke may increase ability to carry out occupations, especially kitchen tasks, increase satisfaction with performance, and increase number of leisure activities. Attending a day service intervention does not appear to impact depression or anxiety.
Daniels et al. (2011)	Literature review and description of current services through focus group	16 researchers in elderly care	Program developed to prevent disability in community-dwelling frail older persons. Includes screening, individualized assessment, analyses and action plan (multidisciplinary), home visit, execution of plan, evaluation of plan, and follow-up. Program is based on the Behavioral Change Model and the Model of Human Occupation.	Additional empirical evidence is needed to examine the full effectiveness of this program.
DeForest, Watts, and Madigan (1991)	Pretest, intervention, posttest. No control group.	Six adolescent males in a US juvenile corrections residential facility. 4 African American, 2 Caucasian. Ages 13–15.	• Participation in three craft activities (leather, wood, and clay) for total of 12 hours over 6 days. • 3 days between each pretest and intervention, and 3 days between each intervention and posttest.	Participation in craft activities increases youth's personal causation and belief in skill for engaging in occupations.
Fitzgerald (2011)	Pretest, posttest, between-group comparison	Social Inclusion Program (SIP) group: *n* = 24; 21 males, 3 females Treatment as usual (TAU) group: *n* = 19; 15 males, 4 females	Purpose was to evaluate occupational functioning difference between service users attending SIP and receiving TAU and those who received only TAU at a low-secure rehabilitation forensic service. The program included graded community engagement and one-on-one goal planning with a unit-based OT along with TAU.	The overall mean preintervention and postintervention scores showed a mean increase for the SIP group. The MOHOST found little difference between the SIP and TAU groups before intervention and significant difference in the SIP group after intervention.

(*continued*)

Table 25.21 MOHO Research on Outcomes: Intervention Studies (*continued*)

Reference	Type of Study	Sample Info	Description of Intervention	Findings and Clinical Implications
Gitlin et al. (2003)	Pretest, intervention, posttest with control group. Stratified, random assignment to group.	89 caregivers in experimental group. Mean age 60.4 (*SD* = 13.6 years). 42.7% Caucasian, 53.9% African American, 3.4% other. 24.7% male, 75.3% female. 41.9% of group had education beyond high school. Mean age of care recipient was 80.2 years, 71.9% female. 101 caregivers in control group. No significant difference between groups at baseline.	The Environmental Skill Building Program seeks to provide caregivers with strategies and problem-solving skills to modify environment (as conceptualized on a MOHO concept of physical, task, and social layers) to make caregiving easier and reduce care recipient problem behaviors.	An individualized intervention focused on the environment, as described by MOHO, can improve the experience of giving care to a person with dementia in the home. This includes decrease in assistance needed from others in caregiving, less upset, improved ability to manage caregiving, and less time spent in caregiving. Outcomes differ according to the gender of the caregiver.
Graff et al. (2003)	Single-group pretest–posttest design.	12 older individuals and their caregivers from the Netherlands who were returning home or to a residential home from the hospital. Older adults were aged 69–88, average age 79.9 years. 8 females, 4 males. Primary caregivers: 8 females, 3 males.	• Intervention guidelines, based on MOHO and Canadian Model of Occupational Performance, identified clients' needs, interests, beliefs, habit, roles, skills, and environmental supports and barriers. • Intervention occurred twice a week for 2 weeks in the hospital, and twice a week for 5 weeks at home. Same therapist at hospital and at home OT sessions. • Intervention used environmental strategies as well as education, problem solving, and coping strategies.	Participation in home-based interventions based on occupation-based models of practice, such as MOHO, can improve older adults' motor and process skills, decrease need for assistance, increase sense of competence and satisfaction when performing everyday activities, and increase caregiver competence.

Ingvarsson and Theodorsdottir (2004)	Program evaluation	70 individuals have attended the program since its beginning in 2000. 45 women and 25 men, with a range of disabilities. Age range is 18–59 years (mean age of 39 years). Five clients discharged themselves for various reasons, without completing the program.	Day program in outpatient clinic based on MOHO, Canadian Model of Occupational Performance, and Cognitive Behavioral approaches. Participants attend average of 8–16 weeks. Initial assessment with COPM, WRI, further assessment as needed with OPHI-II, AMPS, and standardized measures of strength, dexterity, and depression. Goals set with client and program is individualized for client. First 2 weeks are education and training in seminars on ergonomics. Morning, clients participate in 3-hour continuous work (work hardening) of their choice (office or workshop). Afternoon, clients attend groups or individual therapy. Groups include stress management seminar, goal-setting group, self-awareness group (who am I?), and relaxation.	The results from the first 6-month follow-up after discharge with 39 clients: 25% were attending adult education, 25% were employed, 20% were looking for work, and 10% currently received disability benefits.
Josephsson et al. (1993)	Single-subject case design.	• Four clients at the psychogeriatric day care unit of a Swedish geriatric hospital. • Three diagnosed with Alzheimer's and one with multi-infarct dementia. • 3 females and 1 male. • Ages 65–74.	• An individualized program, based on MOHO concepts, was developed for each client that would rely on procedural motor skills rather than higher order cognitive functions. • One ADL that was motivating and a habitual part of their routine, and that the client was beginning to have difficulty participating in, was chosen. • Subjects were trained for nine sessions with environmental support (external, verbal, and physical support).	Individualized ADL training for clients with dementia that relies on procedural motor skills may improve process skills when environmental support is provided. • One client showed no changes. • Two clients showed improved performance in process skills • One client demonstrated an improvement in process skills with and without environmental support and at 2-month follow-up.

(*continued*)

Table 25.21 MOHO Research on Outcomes: Intervention Studies (*continued*)

Reference	Type of Study	Sample Info	Description of Intervention	Findings and Clinical Implications
Kielhofner et al. (2004)	Quasi-experimental.	Convenience sample of 129 persons with AIDS. Ages 24–61 years, mean age 41. 82.2% male, 16.3% female, 1.5% transgender. 39.5% Caucasian, 44.2% African American, 10.8% Hispanic, 5.5% other. Client history: 44% substance abuse, 84% mental illness, 26% physical disability.	Four-phase intervention based on MOHO to address volition, habitation, performance capacity, and community and workplace environments: • Phase 1: 8 weeks. Initial screening with OPHI-II, WRI, and OSA. Provide opportunities to self-assess and refine vocation choice, develop job skills, gather information, and experience support. Weekly group sessions, peer support, and work task experiences. • Phase 2: Experience productive roles through volunteering, internship, and temp positions. Job coaching provided as needed. Continued participation in some group programming. • Phase 3: Job placement or support for job application. Job coaching, individual support, and employer education provided as needed. Individual meetings with staff. • Phase 4: Long-term follow-up and support with peers and staff to sustain employment.	Participating in a community-based return to work program based on MOHO leads to productive outcomes. • 67% of participants who completed the program were involved in work, volunteering, or school. • Persons with progressive narrative slopes were twice as likely to have a successful outcome.
Kielhofner and Brinson (1989)	Posttest only. Random assignment to experimental or control group. Program evaluation.	• 34 clients ending inpatient hospitalization in the USA, and previously had at least two psychiatric hospitalizations. • Experimental group had 16 participants, control group had 14 participants.	• 12-week-long program, total 36 sessions. 1½–2 hour sessions, three times a week. Modules occurred throughout that were based on MOHO. • First month of program involved exploration of roles, skills, and interests. Participants also set long-term goal in areas of self-care, leisure, and productivity. • Second month of program involved practicing skills in community settings. Goal setting and achieving goals continued in groups and during "homework." • In the third month clients selected a group work activity to raise money for group outing.	• Participation in intervention based on MOHO that supports transition to the community decreases recidivism and increases time engaged in work activities. • Interventions delivered in small group formats are supportive to clients. • To maximize client goal achievement, interventions should be flexible to meet the needs of the clients.

Kielhofner, Braveman, Fogg, and Levin (2008)	Pre- and posttest; control group study.	Participants were from four supportive living facilities for adults living with HIV/AIDS. • $n = 38$ for the ESD program; $n = 27$ for the standard care program • Total of 52 males and 13 females • Had to be a legal adult and have a diagnosis of HIV/AIDS	• Eight 1-hour weekly sessions were held at each participating site. Two sites implemented a model program, the Enabling Self-Determination (ESD), and two offered the standard care programESD • program: • Individual sessions were used for ongoing assessment and consultation and activities • Up to 9 months of service could be received • The ESD program utilized peer mentoring • Standard care program: • Held group sessions and provided written materials or referrals to community resources -offered monthly presentations on topic related to employment and productivity • Could also have individual sessions and receive additional information	The participants in the ESD program were found to sustain productive participation over time; 72% of the ESD participants had productive outcomes (52% employed); the favorable outcomes of the ESD program may be because: • ESD program was systematic in considering the clients' needs; • based on MOHO and Social Model of Disability (addressed volition, habituation, and performance capacity along with environmental barriers); • the ESD program was tailored to the unique needs of each client using in-depth and collaborative evaluation using MOHO-based assessments; services were tailored to clients' desires.
Kurokawa, Yabuwaki, and Kobyashi (2013)	Cross-sectional study	Participants were chosen from the Organ Transplant Tracking Record database. $n = 144$ randomly selected out of 530 in the database. • Inclusion criteria: adult, first graft renal transplant recipient between 2003 and 2008; 18–65 years at time of transplant, read and comprehend English, no diagnosed cognitive impairment • Exclusion criteria: second transplant or had a renal transplant in combination with another organ. Average age was 49.4 years and majority were male (68.3%).	In January 2010 an introductory letter with the questionnaire was mailed to all eligible participants with a self-addressed stamped envelope for return. Nonresponders received a second mailing package 1 month after the initial mailing. A three-digit code was assigned to each participant to maintain confidentiality and nonidentifying information was included in the questionnaire. There were 60 returned questionnaires (41.7% return rate).	The rate of employment decreased significantly (68.3% pre- to 38.3% posttransplant, retirement rates increased significantly from 8.3% pre- to 18.3% posttransplant. Person- and work-related factor impacted return to work. Return to work after a transplant is multifaceted and complex. Facilitating return to work after a transplant is important to allow recipients to resume valued life activities.

(continued)

Table 25.21 MOHO Research on Outcomes: Intervention Studies (*continued*)

Reference	Type of Study	Sample Info	Description of Intervention	Findings and Clinical Implications
Lee et al. (2012)	Descriptive study	Purposive sample of occupational therapists working in mental health settings in the UK. Inpatient and outpatient mental health settings Six National Heath Trusts; selected because of relationship with UK-CORE. 429 therapists were invited to participate; 262 completed the survey. (61.07% response rate). Eighty-five percent were female	A survey was posted on the Web using SurveyMonkey. Potential respondents received an e-mail to participate; the e-mail provided a link to the survey. The request to participate e-mail was sent out three times over a 3-week period.	The majority of therapists reported a positive impact on their ability to assess clients, set treatment goals, do relevant interventions, conduct occupation-focused practice, satisfy clients and achieve positive outcomes when using MOHO as their guiding theory.
Morley et al. (2011)	Three-phase study: • Phase 1: retrospective study • Phase 2: online survey • Phase 3: action research study	Three-phase study: • Phase 1: analyzed deidentified data that had already been collected as part of the course of normal clinical work; 352 females, 273 males • Phase 2: online survey to six mental health trusts in the United Kingdom; 262 out of 429 invited therapists participated in the study. • Phase 3: Seven English mental health organizations participated in the action research; 300 reflective responses were received	The purpose of the three phases was to identify specific OT interventions. Care packages were developed. They included the following topics: assessment of self-care, productivity and leisure activities, challenges for engaging in self-care, productivity and leisure activities; outcome of therapeutic encounter, intervention, skill/level, contact, resources, added value.	The OT indicative care packages are viewed as templates setting out potential OT assessment, intervention and outcomes for service users of the care clusters. The clusters included: nonpsychotic problems, psychosis, and cognitive impairment. The study provided evidence of occupational need for each of the care clusters and led to the development of the OT care packages. Based on the studies local care pathways for service users will be created.

Nour, Heck, and Ross (2014)	Cross-sectional design	Eligible sample from the Canadian Transplant Centre $n = 530$; selected for study $n = 144$; not selected for the study $n = 386$. Average age of respondents was 49.4 years and the majority were male (68.3%).	A questionnaire based on the framework of MOHO was mailed to the randomly selected recipients. Sixty questionnaires were returned of 144 sent for a 41.7% response rate.	The rate of employment decreased significantly from 68.3% pre- to 38.3% posttransplant, retirement rates increased from 8.3% pre- to 18.3% posttransplant. Those who were not employed were most likely living alone and had lower level of education. Person and work-related factors impacted return to work posttransplant. Enabling factors were positive employer attitude toward medical history, change from heavy physical demands to sedentary work, allowance to take time off for medical appointments. There was a recommendation for development of a rehabilitation program focused on working and consulting with transplant recipients' employers to enable further successful reintegration.
Nygren, Sandlund, Bernspång, and Fisher (2013)	Repeated measures using the Occupational Self-Assessment (OSA)	Ninety-one clients enrolled in the Individual Placement and Support (IPS) program for rehabilitation to work for persons with mental illness. Inclusion criteria: mental illness, motivation to work, inclusion in one of the two IPS programs. Entered the program between March 2007 and November 2008. $n = 45$; between ages 19 and 55 years; most lived alone; gender distribution was relatively even.	The study examined participant perceptions of occupational competence and occupational value as participants were involved in the IPS program. Measures were taken at baseline, 12 months, and 24 months using the OSA. Data collection lasted from 60 to 120 minutes. The OSA is a self-report assessment which measures occupational competence and occupational value.	The items on the OSA found by the participants to be easiest to perceive as being performed well were: taking care of myself, getting where I need to go, getting along with others. There were nine items that were hard to be perceived as being performed well, ranging from getting done what I need to do to handling my responsibilities. The results of the study demonstrate it is easier for participants to value the OSA items as important than to perceive them as being well performed.
Parkinson, Morley, Stewart, and Brockbank (2012)	Survey	$n = 51$ occupational therapists	A survey of a local National Health Services (NHS) in the United Kingdom participating in a national study of six NHS. OTs were asked to record treatment aims for a sample of up to 10 clients receiving OT and to indicate the key factors that influenced the aims using MOHO concepts.	The national and local study show ways MOHO can be integrated into practice and research to articulate the focus of OT. The local study showed MOHO can be used to analyze the strengths and weaknesses of their clients and it supported many of the national study findings. The differences in the national and local survey results were that the local survey sample had a smaller percentage of nonpsychotic clients.

(continued)

Table 25.21 MOHO Research on Outcomes: Intervention Studies (*continued*)

Reference	Type of Study	Sample Info	Description of Intervention	Findings and Clinical Implications
Taylor et al. (2009)	Single-subject A-B-B design. Each participant served as his/her own control.	Convenience sample of three children enrolled in a hippotherapy treatment program • Ages 4–6 years • Boys and girls included • No other medical or psychiatric diagnosis besides autism	Consisted of 18 sessions. Prior to beginning hippotherapy each child was observed and videotaped • Standardized play protocol was used to evaluate baseline motivation • The same play protocol was used after eight sessions and then 16 sessions (all sessions were videotaped) • Participated in weekly 45-minute hippotherapy sessions • Each session and child used same 12-year-old American Quarter horse Sessions were under the direction of a pediatric physical therapist with extensive training and certification in hippotherapy • Parents were present in arena Children mounted the horse via a portable mounting ramp and dismounted to the ground Same therapy procedures used; each rider was accompanied by one trained horse leader, two trained side walkers, and one therapist—this was the same for every session • Pediatric Volitional Questionnaire used as measure (baseline, eighth week, at end of program) • Videotaped sessions were viewed and rated by two trained observers	The results indicate that all three participants increased in volition from baseline to the time three observation • Change was unique to each child participant • Hippotherapy has an impact on volition in children with autism
Todorova (2008)	Needs Assessment Interviews	15 second-year students in Bulgaria with a mean age of 18 years; 12 females and 3 males	Development of work-related program for Bulgarian youths with intellectual disabilities who are socially disadvantaged.	Findings will guide the development of a work-related job skills program.

Table 25-22 Evidence Concerning Client Perspectives on MOHO-Based Services

Citation	Findings
Apte, Kielhofner, Paul-Ward, and Braveman (2005)	Most clients with AIDS participating in a return to work program report that the OPHI interview enables them to communicate with their therapists and allows the therapist to better understand their circumstances. Clients found the narrative slope helpful and motivating, and some expressed a desire to personally create the narrative slope and/or keep a copy of the narrative slope as a visual motivator.
Asmundsdottir (2009)	Data were collected using in-depth interviews with participants between 2001 and 2005. The aim of the study was to use the data gathered to improve policies and practice in mental health in Iceland based on users' perspective. All interviews were audiotaped and transcribed. Additionally, two focus groups and participant observations (recorded as filed notes) added additional data. Triangulation was utilized to ensure validity. Convenience sample was used. The participants were selected by senior personnel in mental health aftercare services. There were 25 participants (15 women and 10 men) aged 21–59 years with a mean age of 37 years. One-third had severe chronic depression; another third had personality disorders. (five with schizophrenia, four with bipolar disorder). A grounded theory approach was used. Data were coded to identify themes. Internal and external factors impact participants' recovery. Taking control was often enabled by a combination of personal traits and social interaction. Based on MOHO concepts, it was found that the recovery process began when volition was enforced by the performance of tasks participants enjoyed and valued. New services were created using this information. Overcoming stigma and taking responsibility; roles; support from families, peers, friends; medication; services; different demands and helping professions
Ecklund (1996)	• Clients' positive perceptions of the relationship between them and their main therapist in a psychiatric day program was associated with better mental health and MOHO-based outcomes. • Clients who reported that their relationship with their therapist improved during the course of intervention had significant differences in global mental health and habituation scores compared to clients who reported that their relationship with their therapist declined. • Clients' perceptions of their relationship with their main therapist were positively related to global mental health, volition, habituation, and communication and interaction skills.
Farnworth, Nihitin, and Fossey (2004)	Clients in forensic mental health wards created challenges for themselves to keep themselves occupied, found their own personal meanings in occupations, and enjoyed OT groups that had an outcome (i.e., cooking group).
Fisher and Savin-Baden (2001)	MOHO is a person-centered framework that facilitates integrated service models that are acceptable to young adults, mental health consumers, and their families. These clients felt supported and that they had a voice in their services.
Heasman and Atwal (2004)	About 50% of adult clients with mental illness achieved leisure goals when attending a day program based on MOHO. Clients reported that lack of follow-up, lack of motivation, and lack of social support were barriers to successful achievement of leisure goals.
Linddahl, Norrby, and Bellner (2003)	For clients with psychiatric disabilities in a Swedish work rehabilitation program, the hardest volitional related item on a MOHO-based assessment was regarding saying "no" when there is something you do not want to do. Clients felt that the hardest habituation-related item on a MOHO-based assessment was taking a leadership role in a group. Clients felt that the hardest communication/interaction skill–related item on a MOHO-based assessment was keeping up a conversation. Client felt the hardest process skill–related item on a MOHO-based assessment was working against the clock. Clients felt the hardest motor skill–related item on a MOHO-based assessment was maintaining physical persistence while performing activities.

Conclusion

This chapter provided summaries of much of the MOHO-related evidence available to support practice. As noted earlier, this chapter focused on research evidence and there are many other sources of relevant and useful evidence. Additionally, the resources in this chapter are designed to give the reader a quick and accessible overview of what evidence exists. We have not critiqued the rigor of the studies, which is an important step in evidence-based practice. Therapists who wish to use evidence summarized in this chapter should access the original research in order to form their own opinions about the extent of confidence that should be placed in each study.

thePoint® For additional resources and exercises, visit http://thePoint.lww.com

REFERENCES

Abelenda, J., & Helfrich, C. (2003). Family resilience and mental illness: The role of occupational therapy. *Occupational Therapy in Mental Health, 19*(1), 25–39.

Abelenda, J., Kielhofner, G., Suarez-Balcazar, Y., & Kielhofner, K. (2005). The Model of Human Occupation as a conceptual tool for understanding and addressing occupational apartheid. In F. Kronenberg, S. Simo-Algado, & N. Pollard (Eds.), *Occupational therapy without borders: Learning from the spirit of survivors* (pp. 183–196). London, United Kingdom: Elsevier Churchill Livingstone.

Adelstein, L. A., Barnes, M. A., Murray-Jensen, F., & Skaggs, C. B. (1989). A broadening frontier: Occupational therapy in mental health programs for children and adolescents. *Mental Health Special Interest Section Newsletter, 12,* 2–4.

Affleck, A., Bianchi, E., Cleckley, M., Donaldson, K., McCormack, G., & Polon, J. (1984). Stress management as a component of occupational therapy in acute care settings. *Occupational Therapy in Health Care, 1*(3), 17–41.

Ågren, K., & Kjellberg, A. (2008). Utilization and content validity of the Swedish version of the Volitional Questionnaire (VQ-S). *Occupational Therapy in Health Care, 22*(2/3), 163–176.

Alcorn, K., & Broome, K. (2014). Occupational performance coaching for chronic conditions: A review of literature. *New Zealand Journal of Occupational Therapy, 62*(3), 49–56.

Andersen, S., Kielhofner, G., & Lai, J. (2005). An examination of the measurement properties of the Pediatric Volitional Questionnaire. *Physical & Occupational Therapy in Pediatrics, 25*(1/2), 39–57.

Andrews, P. M., Bleecher, R., Genoa, A. M., Molloy, P., Monahan, K., & Sargent, J. (1995). *Leisure interests of children.* Unpublished manuscript, Worcester State College, Worcester, MA.

Apte, A., Kielhofner, G., Paul-Ward, A., & Braveman, B. (2005). Therapists' and clients' perceptions of the occupational performance history interview. *Occupational Therapy in Health Care, 19,* 173–192.

Arnsten, S. M. (1990). Intrinsic motivation. *The American Journal of Occupational Therapy, 44,* 462–463.

Asgari, A., & Kramer, J. (2008). Construct validity and factor structure of the Persian Occupational Self-Assessment (OSA) with Iranian students. *Occupational Therapy in Health Care, 22*(2/3), 187–200.

Ásmundsdóttir, E. E. (2004). The worker role interview: A powerful tool in Icelandic work rehabilitation. *Work: A Journal of Prevention, Assessment, and Rehabilitation, 22*(1), 21–26.

Ásmundsdóttir, E. E. (2009). Creation of new services: Collaboration between mental health consumers and occupational therapists. *Occupational Therapy in Mental Health, 25,* 115–126.

Aubin, G., Hachey, R., & Mercier, C. (1999). Meaning of daily activities and subjective quality of life in people with severe mental illness. *Scandinavian Journal of Occupational Therapy, 6,* 53–62.

Aubin, G., Hachey, R., & Mercier, C. (2002). The significance of daily activities in persons with severe mental disorders [in French]. *Canadian Journal of Occupational Therapy, 69,* 218–228.

Ayuso, D., & Kramer, J. (2009). Using the Spanish Child Occupational Self-Assessment (COSA) with children with ADHD. *Occupational Therapy in Mental Health, 25,* 101–114.

Ay-Woan, P., Sarah, C. P., Lylnn, C., Tsyr-Jang, C., & Ping-Chuan, H. (2006). Quality of life in depression: Predictive models. *Quality of Life Research, 15,* 39–48.

Baker, F., Curbow, B., & Wingard, J. R. (1991). Role retention and quality of life of bone marrow transplant survivors. *Social Science and Medicine, 32,* 697–704.

Banks, S., Bell, E., & Smits, E. (2000). Integration tutorials and seminars: Examining the integration of academic and fieldwork learning by student occupational therapists. *Canadian Journal of Occupational Therapy, 67,* 93–100.

Baron, K. (1987). The Model of Human Occupation: A newspaper treatment group for adolescents with a diagnosis of conduct disorder. *Occupational Therapy in Mental Health, 7*(2), 89–104.

Baron, K. (1989). Occupational therapy: A program for child psychiatry. *Mental Health Special Interest Section Newsletter, 12,* 6–7.

Baron, K. (1991). The use of play in child psychiatry: Reframing the therapeutic environment. *Occupational Therapy in Mental Health, 11*(213), 37–56.

Baron, K., Kielhofner, G., lyenger, A., Goldhammer, V., & Wolenski, J. (2006). *The Occupational Self-Assessment (OSA)* [Version 2.2]. Chicago: Model of Human Occupation Clearinghouse, Department of Occupational Therapy, College of Applied Health Sciences, University of Illinois at Chicago.

Baron, K., & Littleton, M. J. (1999). The model of human occupation: A return to work case study. *Work: A Journal of Prevention, Assessment, and Rehabilitation, 12,* 37–46.

Barrett, L., Beer, D., & Kielhofner, G. (1999). The importance of volitional narrative in treatment: An ethnographic case study in a work program. *Work: A Journal of Prevention, Assessment, and Rehabilitation, 12,* 79–92.

Barris, R. (1982). Environmental interactions: An extension of the Model of Human Occupation. *The American Journal of Occupational Therapy, 36,* 637–644.

Barris, R. (1986). Activity: The interface between person and environment. *Physical and Occupational Therapy in Geriatrics, 5*(2), 39–49.

Barris, R. (1986). Occupational dysfunction and eating disorders: Theory and approach to treatment. *Occupational Therapy in Mental Health, 6*(1), 27–45.

Barris, R., Dickie, V., & Baron, K. (1988). A comparison of psychiatric patients and normal subjects based on the Model of Human Occupation. *Occupational Therapy Journal of Research, 8* (1), 3–37.

Barris, R., Kielhofner, G., Burch, R. M., Gelinas, I., Klement, M., & Schultz, B. (1986). Occupational function and dysfunction in three groups of adolescents. *Occupational Therapy Journal of Research, 6,* 301–317.

Barris, R., Oakley, F., & Kielhofner, G. (1988). The Role Checklist. In B.J. Hemphill (Ed.), *Mental Health Assessment in Occupational Therapy: An integrative approach to the evaluative process* (pp. 73–91). Thorofare, NJ: Slack.

Barrows, C. (1996). Clinical interpretation of "Predictors of functional outcome among adolescents and young adults with psychotic disorders." *The American Journal of Occupational Therapy, 50,* 182–183.

Basu, S., Jacobson, L., & Keller, J. (2004). Child-centered tools: Using the model of human occupation fr11mework. *School System Special Interest Section Quarterly, 11*(2), 1–3.

Basu, S., Kafkes, A., Geist, R., & Kielhofner, G. (2002). *The Pediatric Volitional Questionnaire (PVQ)* [Version 2.0]. Chicago: Model of Human Occupation Clearinghouse, Department of Occupational Therapy, College of Applied Health Sciences, University of Illinois at Chicago.

Bavaro, S. M. (1991). Occupational therapy and obsessive compulsive disorder. *The American Journal of Occupational Therapy, 45,* 456–458.

Beck, D., Benson, S., Curet, J., Froehlich, D., McCrary, L., Rasmussen, L., et al. (1996). Pilot study of a child's play interest profile. Unpublished manuscript, Worcester State College, Worcester, MA.

Bennett, S., Tooth, L., McKenna, K., Rodger, S., Strong, J., Ziviani, J., et al. (2003). Perceptions of evidence-based practice: A survey of Australian occupational therapists. *Australian Journal of Occupational Therapy*, 50, 13–22.

Bentler, P. (1990). Comparative fit indexes in structural models. *Psychological Bulletin, 107,* 238–246.

Bernspang, B., & Fisher, A. (1995). Differences between persons with right or left cerebral vascular accident on the Assessment of Motor and Process Skills. *Archives of Physical Medicine and Rehabilitation, 76,* 1144–1151.

Biernacki, S. D. (1993). Reliability of the worker role interview. *The American Journal of Occupational Therapy, 47,* 797–803.

Bjorklund, A., & Henriksson, M. (2003). On the context of elderly persons' occupational performance [Journal Article, Research, Tables/Charts] *Physical and Occupational Therapy in Geriatrics, 21*(3), 49–58.

Blakeney, A. (1985). Adolescent development: An application to the Model of Human Occupation. *Occupational Therapy in Health Care, 2*(3), 19–40.

Boisvert, R. A. (2004, May 31). Enhancing substance dependence intervention. *Occupational Therapy Practice*, 11–16.

Borell, L., Gustavsson, A., Sandman, P., & Kielhofner, G. (1994). Occupational programming in a day hospital for patients with dementia. *Occupational Therapy Journal of Research, 14*(4), 219–238.

Borell, L., Sandman, P., & Kielhofner, G. (1991). Clinical decision making in Alzheimer's disease. *Occupational Therapy in Mental Health, 11*(4), 111–124.

Bourland, E., Neville, M., & Pickens, N. (2011). Loss, gain, and the reframing of perspectives in long-term stroke survivors: a dynamic experience of quality of life. *Topics in Stroke Rehabilitation, 18*(5), 437–449.

Bowyer, P., Kielhofner, G., Kramer, J., Maziero Barbosa, V., & Girolami, G. (2007.). The measurement properties of the Short Child Occupational Profile (SCOPE). *Physical and Occupational Therapy in Pediatrics, 27*(4), 67–85.

Bowyer, P., Lee, J., Kramer, J., Taylor, R., & Kielhofner, G. (2012). Determining the clinical utility of the Short Child Occupational Profile (SCOPE). *The British Journal of Occupational Therapy, 75*(1), 19–28.

Bowyer, P., Ross, M., Schwartz, O., Kielhofner, G., & Kramer, J. (2005). *The Short Child Occupational Profile (SCOPE)* [Version 2.1]. Chicago: Model of Human Occupation Clearinghouse, Department of Occupational Therapy, College of Applied Health Sciences, University of Illinois at Chicago.

Branholm, I., & Fugl-Meyer, A. R. (1992). Occupational role preferences and life satisfaction. *Occupational Therapy Journal of Research, 12*(3), 159–171.

Braveman, B. (1999). The model of human occupation and prediction of return to work: A review of related empirical research. *WORK, 12,* 13–23.

Braveman, B. (2001). Development of a community-based return to work program for people with AIDS. *Occupational Therapy in Health Care, 13*(314), 113–131.

Braveman, B. (Ed.). (2005). *Leading and managing occupational therapy services: An evidence-based approach* (pp. 215–244). Philadelphia, PA: F. A. Davis.

Braveman, B., & Helfrich, C. A. (2001). Occupational identity: Exploring the narratives of three men living with AIDS. *Journal of Occupational Science, 8*(2), 25–31.

Braveman, B., Helfrich, C., Kielhofner, G., & Albrecht, G. (2004). The experiences of 12 men with AIDS who attempted to return to work. *The Israel Journal of Occupational Therapy, 13,* E69–E83.

Braveman, B., & Kielhofner, G. (2006). Developing evidence-based occupational therapy programming. In B. Braveman, C. Helfrich, & G. Kielhofner (2003). The narratives of 12 men with AIDS: Exploring return to work. *The Journal of Occupational Rehabilitation, 13*(3), 143–157.

Braveman, B., Kielhofner, G., Albrecht, G., & Helfrich, C. (2006). Occupational identity, occupational competence, and occupational settings (environment): Influence on return to work in men living with HIV/AIDS. *WORK*, 27(3), 267–276.

Braveman, B., Robson, M., Velozo, C., Kielhofner, G., Fisher, G., Forsyth, K., & Kerschbaum, J. (2005). *Worker Role Interview (WR/)* [Version 10.0]. Chicago: Model of Human Occupation Clearinghouse, Department of Occupational Therapy, College of Applied Health Sciences, University of Illinois at Chicago.

Braveman, B., Sen, S., & Kielhofner, G. (2001). Community-based vocational rehabilitation pro grams. In M. Scaffa (Ed.), *Occupational therapy in community-based practice settings* (pp. 139–162). Philadelphia, PA: F. A. Davis.

Briand, C., Belanger, R., Hamel, V., Nicole, L., Stip, E., Reinharz, D., Lalonde, P., & Lesage, A. O. (2005). Implantation multisite du programme Integrated Psychological Treatment (IPT) pour les personnes souffrant de schizophrenie. Elaboration d'une version renouvelee. *Sante mentale au Quebec, 30,* 73–95.

Bridgett, B. (1993). Occupational therapy evaluation for patients with eating disorders. *Occupational Therapy in Mental Health, 12*(2), 79–89.

Bridle, M. J., Lynch, K. B., & Quesenberry, C. M. (1990). Long term function following the central cord syndrome. *Paraplegia, 28,* 178–185.

Broadley, H. (1991). Assessment guidelines based on the Model of Human Occupation. *World Federation of Occupational Therapists: Bulletin, 23,* 34–35.

Brollier, C., Watts, J. H., Bauer, O., & Schmidt, W. (1988). A concurrent validity study of two occupational therapy evaluation instruments: The AOF and OCAIRS. *Occupational Therapy in Mental Health, 8*(4), 49–59.

Brollier C., Watts, J. H., Bauer, D., & Schmidt, W. (1988). A content validity study of the Assessment of Occupational Functioning. *Occupational Therapy in Mental Health, 8*(4), 29–47.

Brophy, P., Caizzi, D., Crete, B., Jachym, T., Kobus, M., & Sainz, C. (1995). Preliminary reliability study of the Adolescent Leisure Interest Profile. Unpublished manuscript, Worcester State College, Worcester, MA.

Brown, C. H. & Cudeck, R. (1993) Alternative ways of assessing model fit. In K. A. Bollen & J. S. Long (Eds.). *Testing Structural Equation Models.* Newbury Park, CA: Sage, 136–162.

Brown, G. T., Brown, A., & Roever, C. (2005). Paediatric occupational therapy university programme curricula in the United Kingdom. *British Journal of Occupational Therapy, 68,* 457–466.

Brown, G. T., & Carmichael, K. (1992). Assertiveness training for clients with a psychiatric illness: a pilot study. *British Journal of Occupational Therapy, 55*(4), 137–140.

Bruce, M., & Borg, B. (1993). The Model of Human Occupation. In *Psychosocial Occupational Therapy: Frames of Reference for Intervention* (2nd ed., pp. 145–175). Thorofare, NJ: Slack.

Budd, P., Ferraro, D., Lovely, A., McNeil, T., Owanisian, L., Parker, J., et al. (1997). Pilot study of the revised child's play interest profile. Unpublished manuscript, Worcester State College, Worcester, MA.

Buning, M. E., Angelo, J. A., & Schmeler, M. R. (2001). Occupational performance and the transition to powered mobility: A pilot study. *The American Journal of Occupational Therapy, 55*, 339–344.

Burke, J. P. (1998). Commentary: Combining the model of human occupation with cognitive disability theory. *Occupational Therapy in Mental Health, 8,* xi-xiii.

Burke, J. P., Clark, F., Dodd, C., & Kawamoto, T. (1987). Maternal role preparation: A program using sensory integration, infant-motor attachment, and occupational behavior perspectives. *Occupational Therapy in Health Care, 4,* 9–21.

Burke, J. P., & Gitlin, L. (2012). How do we change practice when we have the evidence? *The American Journal of Occupational Therapy, 66,* E85–E88.

Burrows, E. (1989). Clinical practice: An approach to the assessment of clinical competencies. *British Journal of Occupational Therapy, 52,* 222–226.

Burton, J. E. (1989). The model of human occupation and occupational therapy practice with elderly patients, Part 1: Characteristics of aging. *British Journal of Occupational Therapy, 52,* 215–218.

Burton, J. E. (1989). The model of human occupation and occupational therapy practice with elderly patients, Part 2: Application. *British Journal of Occupational Therapy, 52,* 219–221.

Byrne, B. M. (1989). *A primer of LISREL: Basic applications and programming for confirmatory factor analysis models.* New York, NY: Springer-Verlag.

Cermak, S. A., & Murray, E. (1992). Nonverbal learning disabilities in the adult framed in the Model of Human Occupation. In N. Katz (Ed.), *Cognitive rehabilitation: Models for intervention in occupational therapy* (pp. 258–291). Boston, MA: Andover Medical Publishers.

Chaffey, L., & Fossey, E. (2004). Caring and daily life: Occupational experiences of women living with sons diagnosed with schizophrenia. *Australian Occupational Therapy Journal, 51*(4), 199–207.

Chan, S. C. (2004). Chronic obstructive pulmonary disease and engagement in occupation. *The American Journal of Occupational Therapy, 58*(4), 408–415.

Chen, C., Neufeld, P. S., Feely, C. A., & Skinner, C. S. (1999). Factors influencing compliance with home exercise programs among patients with upper-extremity impairment. *The American Journal of Occupational Therapy, 53*(2), 171–180.

Chern, J., Kielhofner, G., de las Heras, G., & Magalhaes, L. C. (1996). The Volitional Questionnaire: Psychometric development and practical use. *The American Journal of Occupational Therapy, 50,* 516–525.

Codd, Y., Stapleton, T., Veale, D., Fitzgerald, O., & Bresnihan, B. (2010). A qualitative study of work participation in early rheumatoid arthritis. *International Journal of Therapy and Rehabilitation, 17*(7), 24–33.

Cole, F. (2010). Physical activity for its mental health benefits: Conceptualising participation within the Model of Human Occupation. *The British Journal of Occupational Therapy, 73*(12), 607–615.

Cole, M. (1998). A model of human occupation approach. In *Group dynamics in occupational therapy: The theoretical basis and practice application of group treatment* (2nd ed., pp. 268–290). Thorofare, NJ: Slack.

Colon, H., & Haertlein, C. (2002). Spanish translation of the Role Checklist. *The American Journal of Occupational Therapy, 56*(5), 586–589.

Conroy, M. (1997) "Why are you doing that?" A project to look for evidence of efficacy within occupational therapy. *British Journal of Occupational Therapy, 60,* 487–490.

Copley, J., & Allen, S. (2009). Using all the available evidence: Perceptions of paediatric occupational therapists about how to increase evidence-based practice. *International Journal of Evidence-Based Healthcare, 7,* 193–200.

Corcoran, M. A., & Gitlin, L. A. (2001). Family caregiver acceptance and use of environmental strategies provided in an occupational therapy intervention. *Physical and Occupational Therapy in Geriatrics, 19*(1), 1–20.

Cordeiro, J. R., Camelier, A., Oakley, F., & Jardim, J. R. (2007). Cross-cultural reproducibility of the Brazilian Portuguese Version of the role checklist for persons with chronic obstructive pulmonary disease. *The American Journal of Occupational Therapy, 61*(1), 33–40.

Corner, R., Kielhofner, G., & Lin, F. L. (1997). Construct validity of a work environment impact scale. *Work, 9*(1), 21–34.

Corr, S., Phillips, C. J., & Walker, M. (2004). Evaluation of a pilot service designed to provide support following stroke: A randomized cross-over design study. *Clinical Rehabilitation, 18* (1), 69–75.

Corr, S., & Wilmer, S. (2003). Returning to work after a stroke: An important but neglected area. *British Journal of Occupational Therapy,* 66, 186–192.

Costa, A., & Othero, M. (2012). Palliative care, terminal illness, and the model of human occupation. *Physical & Occupational Therapy in Geriatrics, 30*(4), 316–327.

Coster, W. J., & Jaffe, L. E. (1991). Current concepts of children's perceptions of control. *The American Journal of Occupational Therapy, 45,* 19–25.

Creek, J., & Ilott, I. (2002). *Scoping study of occupational therapy research and development activity in Scotland, Northern Ireland and Wales: Executive summary.* London, United Kingdom: College of Occupational Therapists.

Crist, P., Fairman, A ., Munoz, J. P., Hansen, A. M. W., Sciulli, J., & Eggers, M. (2005). Education and practice collaborations: A pilot case study between a university faculty and county jail practitioners. *Occupational Therapy in Health Care, 19* (112), 193–210.

Crowe, T. K., Vanleit, B., Berghmans, K. K., & Mann, P. (1997). Role perceptions of mothers with young children: The impact of a child's disability. *The American Journal of Occupational Therapy, 51,* 651–661.

Cubie, S., & Kaplan, K. (1982). A case analysis method for the model of human occupation. *The American Journal of Occupational Therapy, 36,* 645–656.

Cull, G. (1989). Anorexia nervosa: A review of theory approaches to treatment. *Journal of New Zealand Association of Occupational Therapists, 40*(2), 3–6.

Curtin, C. (1990). Research on the Model of Human Occupation. *Mental Health-Special Interest Section Newsletter, 13*(2), 3–5.

Curtin, C. (1991). Psychosocial intervention with an adolescent with diabetes using the Model of Human Occupation. *Occupational Therapy in Mental Health, 11*(213), 23–36.

Daniels, R., Rossum, E., Metzelthin, S., Sipers, W., Habets, H., Hobma, S., et al. (2011). A disability prevention programme for community-dwelling frail older persons. *Clinical Rehabilitation, 25*(11), 963–974.

Davies Hallet, J., Zasler, N., Maurer, P., & Cash, S. (1994). Role change after traumatic brain injury in adults. *The American Journal of Occupational Therapy, 48*(3), 241–246.

DeForest, D., Watts, J. H., & Madigan, M. J. (1991). Resonation in the model of human occupation: a pilot study. *Occupational Therapy in Mental Health, 11*(2/3), 57–71.

de las Heras, C. G., Dion, G. L., & Walsh, D. (1993). Application of rehabilitation models in a state psychiatric hospital. *Occupational Therapy in Mental Health, 12*(3), 1–32.

de las Heras, C. G., Geist, R., Kielhofner, G., & Li, Y. (2003). *The Volitional Questionnaire (VQ)* [Version 4.0]. Chicago: Model of Human Occupation Clearinghouse, Department of Occupational Therapy, College of Applied Health Sciences, University of Illinois at Chicago.

de las Heras, C. G., Llerena,V., & Kielhofner, G. (2003). *Remotivation process: Progressive intervention for individuals with severe volitional challenges.* [Version 1.0]. Chicago: Department of Occupational Therapy, University of Illinois at Chicago.

DePoy, E. (1990). The TBIIM: An intervention for the treatment of individuals with traumatic brain injury. *Occupational Therapy in Health Care, 7*(1), 55–67.

DePoy, E., & Burke, J. P. (1992). Viewing cognition through the lens of the model of human occupation. In N. Katz (Ed.), Cognitive Rehabilitation: Models for intervention in occupational therapy (pp. 240–257). Stoneham, MA: Butterworth-Heinemann.

Désiron, H., Donceel, P., Rijk, A., & Hoof, E. (2013). A conceptual-practice model for occupational therapy to facilitate return to work in breast cancer patients. *Journal of Occupational Rehabilitation, 23,* 516–526.

Dickerson, A. E., & Oakley, F. (1995). Comparing the roles of community-living persons and patient population. *The American Journal of Occupational Therapy, 49,* 221–228.

Dion, G. L., Lovely, S., & Skerry, M. (1996). A comprehensive psychiatric rehabilitation approach to severe and persistent mental illness in the public sector. In S. M. Soreff (Ed.), Handbook for the treatment of the seriously mentally ill. Seattle, WA: Hogrete & Huber.

Doble, S. (1991). Test-retest and inter-rater reliability of a process skills assessment. *Occupational Therapy Journal of Research, 11*(1), 8–23.

Doble, S. (1988). Intrinsic motivation and clinical practice: The key to understanding the unmotivated client. *Canadian Journal of Occupational Therapy, 55,* 75–81.

Doughton, K. J. (1996). Hidden talents. *O. T. Week, 10*(26), 19–20.

Dubouloz, C., Egan, M., Vallerand, J., & VonZweck, C. (1999). Occupational therapists' perceptions of evidence based practice. *The American Journal of Occupational Therapy, 53,* 445–453.

Duellman, M. K., Barris, R., & Kielhofner, G. (1986). Organized activity and the adaptive status of nursing home residents. *The American Journal of Occupational Therapy, 40,* 618–622.

Dugow, H., & Connolly, D. (2012). Exploring impact of independent living programme on activity participation of elderly people with chronic conditions. *International Journal of Therapy and Rehabilitation, 19*(3), 154–162.

Duran, L. J., & Fisher, A. G. (1996). Male and female performance on the assessment of motor and process skills. *Archives of Physical Medicine and Rehabilitation, 77,* 1019–1024.

Dyck, I. (1992). The daily routines of mothers with young children: Using a sociopolitical model in research. *Occupational Therapy Journal of Research, 12*(1), 17–34.

Dysart, A. M. & Tomlin, G. S. (2002). Factors related to evidence-based practice among US occupational therapy clinicians. *The American Journal of Occupational Therapy, 56*(3), 275–284.

Early, M., & Pedretti, L. (1998). A frame of reference and practice models for physical dysfunction. In M. Early (Ed.), *Physical dysfunction practice skills for the occupational therapy assistant.* (pp. 17–30). St. Louis, MO: Mosby.

Ebb, E. W., Coster, W. J., & Duncombe, L. (1989). Comparison of normal and psychosocially dysfunctional male adolescents. *Occupational Therapy in Mental Health, 9*(2), 53–74.

Ecklund, M. (1996). Working relationship, participation, and outcome in a psychiatric day care unit based on occupational therapy. *Scandinavian Journal of Occupational Therapy, 3,* 106–113.

Egan, M., Warren, S. A., Hessel, P. A., & Gilewich, G. (1992). Activities of daily living after hip fracture: Pre- and post discharge. *Occupational Therapy Journal of Research, 12,* 342–356.

Ekbladh, E., Haglund, L., & Thorell, L. (2004). The Worker Role Interview: Preliminary data on the predictive validity of return to work clients after an insurance medicine investigation. *Journal of Occupational Rehabilitation, 14,* 131–141.

Ekbladh, E., Fan, C. W., Sandqvist, J., Hemmingsson, H., Taylor, R. (2014). Work environment impact scale: Testing the psychometric properties of the Swedish version. *Work, 47,* 213–219.

Eklund, M. (1996a). Patient experiences and outcome of treatment in psychiatric occupational therapy-three cases. *Occupational Therapy International, 3*(3):212–239.

Eklund, M. (1996b). Working relationship, participation, and outcome in a psychiatric day care unit based on occupational therapy. *Scandinavian Journal of Occupational Therapy, 3,* 106–113.

Eklund, M. (1999). Outcome of occupational therapy in a psychiatric day care unit for long-term mentally ill patients. *Occupational Therapy in Mental Health, 14*(4), 21–45.

Eklund, M. (2001). Psychiatric patients' occupational roles: changes over time and associations with self-rated quality of life. *Scandinavian Journal of Occupational Therapy, 8*(3), 125–130.

Eklund, M., & Hansson, L. (1997). Stability of improvement in patients receiving psychiatric occupational therapy: A one-year follow-up. *Scandinavian Journal of Occupational Therapy, 4*(1–4), 15–122.

Elliott, M., & Barris, R. (1987). Occupational role performance and life satisfaction in elderly persons. *Occupational Therapy Journal of Research, 7,* 215–224.

Ennals, P., & Fossey, E. (2007). The occupational performance history interview in community mental health case management: Consumer and occupational therapists perspectives. *Australian Occupational Therapy Journal, 54,* 11–21.

Esdaile, S. A. (1996). A play-focused intervention involving mothers of preschoolers. *The American Journal of Occupational Therapy, 50,* 113–123.

Esdaile, S. A., & Madill, H. M. (1993). Causal attributions: Theoretical considerations and their relevance to occupational therapy practice and education. *British Journal of Occupational Therapy, 56,* 330–334.

Evans, J., & Salim, A. A. (1992). A cross-cultural test of the validity of occupational therapy assessments with patients with schizophrenia. *The American Journal of Occupational Therapy, 46,* 695.

Farnworth, L., Nikitin, L., & Fossey, E. (2004). Being in a secure forensic psychiatry unit: Every day is the same, killing time to making the most of it. *British Journal of Occupational Therapy, 67,* 1–9.

Fenger, K., & Kramer, J. M. (2007). Worker role interview: Testing the psychometric properties of the Icelandic version. *Scandinavian Journal of Occupational Therapy, 14*(3), 160–172.

Fisher, A., & Savin-Baden, M. (2001). The benefits to young people experiencing psychosis, and their families, of an early intervention programme: evaluating a service from the consumers' and the providers' perspectives. *British Journal of Occupational Therapy, 64*(2), 58–65.

Fisher, A. G. (1993). The assessment of IADL motor skills: An application of many-faceted Rasch analysis. *The American Journal of Occupational Therapy, 47,* 319–329.

Fisher, A. G. (1999). *Assessment of motor and process skills* (3rd ed.). Ft. Collins, CO: Three Star Press.

Fisher, A. G., & Kielhofner, G. (1995). *Skills in occupational performance. A model of human occupation: Theory and application* (2nd ed.). Baltimore, MD: Williams & Wilkins.

Fisher, A. G., Liu, Y., Velozo, C. A., & Pan, A. W. (1992). Cross-cultural assessment of process skills. *The American Journal of Occupational Therapy, 46,* 876–885.

Fisher, G. (2004). The residential environment impact survey. *Developmental Disabilities Special Interest Section Quarterly, 27*(3), 1–4.

Fisher, G. S. (1999). Administration and application of the Worker Role Interview: Looking beyond functional capacity. *Work, 12,* 25–36.

Fisher, G., & Kayhan, E. (2012). Developing the residential environment impact survey instruments through faculty–practitioner collaboration. *Occupational Therapy Health Occupational Therapy in Health Care, 26*(4), 224–239.

Fitzgerland, L., Ferlie E., Hawkins C. (2003). Innovations in healthcare: how does credible evidence influence professionals? *Health and Social Care in the Community, 11*(3): 219–228.

Fitzgerald, M. (2011). An evaluation of the impact of a social inclusion programme on occupational functioning for forensic service users. *The British Journal of Occupational Therapy, 74*(10), 465–472.

Folland, J., & Forsyth, K. (2011). UKCORE practice development: using an innovative approach to transforming occupational therapy services. *Mental Health Occupational Therapy, 16*(1), 12–14.

Forsyth, K., Braveman, B., Kielhofner, G., Ekbladh, H., Haglund, H., Fenger, K., et al. (2006). Psychometric properties of the Worker Role Interview. *Work, 27*, 313–318.

Forsyth, K., Deshpande, S., Kielhofner, G., Henriksson, C., Haglund, l., Olson, l., et al. (2005). *The Occupational Circumstances Assessment Interview and Rating Scale (OCAIRS)* [Version 4.0]. Chicago: Model of Human Occupation Clearinghouse, Department of Occupational Therapy, College of Applied Health Sciences, University of Illinois at Chicago.

Forsyth, K., Duncan, E. A. S., & Mann, L. S. (2005). Scholarship of practice in the United Kingdom: An occupational therapy service case study. *Occupational Therapy in Health Care, 19*, 17–29.

Forsyth, K., & Kielhofner, G. (1999). Validity of the assessment of communication and interaction skills. *British Journal of Occupational Therapy, 62*, 69–74.

Forsyth, K., & Kielhofner, G. (2003). Model of human occupation. In: P. Kramer, J. Hinojosa, & C. Royeen, (Eds.), *Human occupation: Participation in life* (pp. 45–86). Philadelphia, PA: Lippincott Williams & Wilkins.

Forsyth, K., Lai, J., & Kielhofner, G. (1999). The Assessment of Communication and Interaction Skills (ACIS): Measurement properties. *British Journal of Occupational Therapy, 62*(2), 69–74.

Forsyth, K., Melton, J., & Mann, L. S. (2005). Achieving evidence-based practice: A process of continuing education through practitioner-academic partnership. *Occupational Therapy in Health Care, 19*(112), 211–227.

Forsyth, K., Parkinson, S., Kielhofner, G., Kramer, J., Mann, L., Summerfield, et al. (2011). The measurement properties of the model of human occupation screening tool and implications for practice. *New Zealand Journal of Occupational Therapy, 58*(2), 5–13.

Forsyth, K., Salamy, M., Simon, S., & Kielhofner, G. (1997). *Assessment of communication and interaction skills*. Chicago: University of Illinois at Chicago, Model of Human Occupation Clearinghouse.

Forsyth, K., Salamy, M., Simon, S., & Kielhofner, G. (1998). *The assessment of communication and interaction skills* [Version 4.0]. Chicago: Department of Occupational Therapy, University of Illinois at Chicago.

Forsyth, K., Summerfield-Mann, L., & Kielhofner, G. (2005). A Scholarship of practice: Making occupation-focused, theory-driven, evidence-based practice a reality. *British Journal of Occupational Therapy, 68*, 261–268.

Fossey, E. (1996). Using the occupational performance history interview (OPHI): Therapists' reflections. *British Journal of Occupational Therapy, 59*(5), 223–228.

Fougeyrollas, P., Noreau, l., & Boschen, K. A. (2002). Interaction of environment with individual characteristics and social participation: Theoretical perspectives and applications in persons with spinal cord injury. *Topics in Spinal Cord Injury Rehabilitation, 7*, 1–16.

Foundation of Nursing Studies (2001). *Taking action: Moving towards evidence-based practice*. London, UK: FoNS.

Froelich, J. (1992). Occupational therapy interventions with survivors of sexual abuse. *Occupational Therapy in Health Care, 8*(213), 1–25.

Frosch, S., Gruber, A., Jones, C., Myers, S., Noel, E., Westerlund, A., et al. (1997). The long term effects of traumatic brain injury on the roles of caregivers. *Brain Injury, 11*, 891–906.

Furst, G., Gerber, L., Smith, C., Fisher, S., & Schulman, B. (1987). A program for improving energy conservation behaviors in adults with rheumatoid arthritis. *The American Journal of Occupational Therapy, 41*, 102–111.

Gerardi, S. M. (1996). The management of battle fatigued soldiers: An occupational therapy model. *Military Medicine, 161*, 483–488.

Gerber, L., & Furst, G. (1992). Scoring methods and application of the Activity Record (ACTRE) for patients with musculoskeletal disorders. *Arthritis Care and Research, 5*(3), 151–156.

Gerber, L., & Furst, G. (1992). Validation of the NIH Activity Record: A quantitative measure of life activities. *Arthritis Care and Research, 5*, 81–86.

Gerish, K., & Clayton, J. (2004). Promoting evidence-based practice: an organizational approach. *Journal of Nursing Management, 12*, 114–123.

Gillard, M., & Segal, M. E. (2002). Social roles and subjective well-being in a population of nondisabled older people. Proceedings of Habits 2 Conference. *Occupational Therapy Journal of Research, 22*(suppl 1), 96S.

Gitlin, L. N., Winter, L., Corcoran, M., Dennis, M. P., Schinfeld, S., & Hauck, W. W. (2003). Effects of the Home Environmental Skill-Building Program on the caregiver-care recipient dyad: 6-month outcomes from the Philadelphia REACH initiative. *The Gerontologist, 43*, 532–546.

Gloucestershire Health Authority. (2001). "Meeting the Challenge - Proposals for Developing Health services in Gloucestershire, Consultation Document"

Goldstein, K., Kielhofner, G., & Paul-Ward, A. (2004). Occupational narratives and the therapeutic process. *Australian Occupational Therapy Journal, 51*, 119–124.

Gorde, M. W., Helfrich, C. A., & Finlayson, M. L. (2004). Trauma symptoms and life skill needs of domestic violence victims. *Journal of Interpersonal Violence, 19*(6): 691–708.

Graff, M. J. L., Vernooij-Dassen, M. J. F. J., Hoefnagels, J. D., Dekker, J. & de Witte, L. P. (2003). Occupational therapy at home for older individuals with mild to moderate cognitive impairments and their primary caregivers: A pilot study. *Occupational Therapy Journal of Research, 23* (4), 155–163.

Gray, M. L., & Fossey, E. M. (2003). Illness experience and occupations of people with chronic fatigue syndrome. *Australian Occupational Therapy Journal, 50*, 127–136.

Gregitis, S., Gelpi, T., Moore, B., & Dees, M. (2010). Self-Determination skills of adolescents enrolled in special education: An analysis of four cases. *Occupational Therapy in Mental Health, 26*, 67–84.

Gregory, M. (1983). Occupational behavior and life satisfaction among retirees. *The American Journal of Occupational Therapy, 37*(8), 548–553

Grogan, G. (1991). Anger management: A perspective for occupational therapy (part 1). *Occupational Therapy in Mental Health, 11*(213), 135–148.

Grogan, G. (1994). The personal computer: A treatment tool for increasing sense of competence. *Occupational Therapy in Mental Health, 12*, 47–60.

Guidetti, S., & Tham, K. (2005). Therapeutic strategies used by occupational therapists in self-care training: A qualitative study. *Occupational Therapy International, 9*, 257–276.

Gusich, R. L. (1984). Occupational therapy for chronic pain: A clinical application of the model of human occupation. *Occupational Therapy in Mental Health, 4* (3), 59–73.

Gusich, R. L., & Silverman, A. L. (1991). Basava day clinic: The model of human occupation as applied to psychiatric day hospitalization. *Occupational Therapy in Mental Health, 11* (213), 113–134.

Hachey, R., Boyer, G., & Mercier, C. (2001). Perceived and valued roles of adults with severe mental health problems. *Canadian Journal of Occupational Therapy, 68*(2), 112–120.

Hachey, R., Jummoorty, J., & Mercier, C. (1995). Methodology for validating the translation of test measurements applied to occupational therapy. *Occupational Therapy International, 2* (3), 190–203.

Haglund, L. (2000). Assessment in general psychiatric care. *Occupational Therapy in Mental Health, 15*, 35–47.

Haglund, L., Ekbladh, E., Lars-Hakan, T., & Hallberg, I. R. (2000). Practice models in Swedish psychiatric occupational therapy. *Scandinavian Journal of Occupational Therapy, 7*, 107–113.

Haglund, L., & Henriksson, C. (1994). Testing a Swedish version of OCAIRS on two different patient groups. *Scandinavian Journal of Caring Sciences, 8*, 223 230.

Haglund, L., & Henriksson, C. (1995). Activity: From action to activity. *Scandinavian Journal of Caring Sciences, 9*, 227–234.

Haglund, L., & Henriksson, C. (2003). Concepts in occupational therapy in relation to the ICF. *Occupational Therapy International, 10*(4), 253–268.

Haglund, L., Karlsson, G., & Kielhofner, G. (1997). Validity of the Swedish version of the Worker Role Interview. *Physical and Occupational Therapy in Geriatrics, 4*(1–4), 23–29.

Haglund, L., & Kjellberg, A. (1999). A critical analysis of the model of human occupation. *Canadian Journal of Occupational Therapy, 66*, 102–108.

Haglund, L., & Thorell, L. (2004). Clinical perspective on the Swedish version of the assessment of communication and interaction skills: Stability of assessments. *Scandinavian Journal of Caring Sciences, 18*, 417–423.

Haglund, L., Thorell, L., & Walinder, J. (1998a). Assessment of occupational functioning for screening of patients to occupational therapy in general psychiatric care. *Occupational Therapy Journal of Research, 18*(4), 193–206.

Haglund, L., Thorell, L., & Walinder, J. (1998b). Occupational Functioning in relation to psychiatric diagnoses; Schizophrenia and Mood Disorders. *Journal of Psychiatry, 52*(3), 223–229.

Hahn-Markowitz, J. (2004). Advancing practice through scholarship. *The Israel Journal of Occupational Therapy, 13*, E130 E134.

Hakansson, C., Eklund, M., Lidfeldt, J., Nerbrand, C., Samsioe, G., & Nilsson, P. M. (2005). Well-being and occupational roles among middle-aged women. *Work, 24*(4), 341–351.

Hallett, J. D., & Zasler, N. D., Maurer, P., & Cash, S. (1994). Role change after traumatic brain injury in adults. *The American Journal of Occupational Therapy, 48*, 241–246.

Hammel, J. (1999). The life rope: A transactional approach to exploring worker and life role develop ment. *WORK, 12*, 47–60.

Hammel, J., Finlayson, M., & Lastowski, S. (2003). Using participatory action research to create a shared assistive technology alternative financing outcomes database and to effect social action systems change. *Journal of Disability Policy Studies, 14* (2), 109–118.

Harris, K., & Reid, D. (2005). The influence of virtual reality play on children's motivation. *Canadian Journal of Occupational Therapy, 72*, 21–29.

Harrison, H., & Kielhofner, G. (1986). Examining reliability and validity of the Preschool Play Scale with handicapped children. *The American Journal of Occupational Therapy, 40*, 167–173.

Harrison, M., & Forsyth, K. (2005). Developing a vision for therapists working within child and adolescent mental health services: Poised of paused for action? *British Journal of Occupational Therapy, 68*, 1–5.

Hawes, D., & Houlder, D. (2010). Reflections on using the Model of Human Occupation Screening Tool in a joint learning disability team. *The British Journal of Occupational Therapy, 73*(11), 564–567.

Heasman, D., & Atwal, A. (2004). The Active Advice pilot project: leisure enhancement and social inclusion for people with severe mental health problems. *British Journal of Occupational Therapy, 67*(11), 511–514.

Heasman, D., & Morly, M. (2011). Using the Model of Human Occupation assessment tools to deliver clinical outcomes in mental health. *Mental Health Occupational Therapy, 16*(1), 3–7.

HEFCE. (2001). Promoting research in nursing and the allied health professions. Report to Task group 3 to HEFCE and the Department of Health. London: HEFCE.

Helfrich, C., & Aviles, A. (2001). Occupational therapy's role with domestic violence: Assessment and intervention. *Occupational Therapy in Mental Health, 16*(314), 53–70.

Helfrich, C., & Kielhofner, G. (1994). Volitional narratives and the meaning of occupational therapy. *The American Journal of Occupational Therapy, 48*, 319–326.

Helfrich, C., Kielhofner, G., & Mattingly, C. (1994). Volition as narrative: understanding motivation in chronic illness. *The American Journal of Occupational Therapy, 48*(4), 311–317.

Hemmingsson, H., Borell, L., & Gustavsson, A. (1999). Temporal aspects of teaching and learning: Implications for pupils with physical disabilities. *Scandinavian Journal of Disability Research, 1*, 26–43.

Hemmingsson, H., & Borell, L. (1996). The development of an assessment of adjustment needs in the school setting for use with physically disabled students. *Scandinavian Journal of Occupational Therapy, 3*, 156–162.

Hemmingsson, H., & Borell, L. (2000). Accommodation needs and student- environment fit in upper secondary school for students with severe physical disabilities. *Canadian Journal of Occupational Therapy, 67*, 162–173.

Hemmingsson, H., & Borell, L. (2002). Environmental barriers in mainstream schools. *Child Care, Health, and Development, 28* (1), 57–63.

Hemmingsson, H., Egilson, S., Hoffman, O., & Kielhofner, G. (2005). *School Setting Interview (SSI)* [Version 3.0]. Nacka, Sweden: Swedish Association of Occupational Therapists.

Hemmingsson, H., Kottorp, A., & Bernspang, B. (2004). Validity of the School Setting Interview: An assessment of the student-environment fit. *Scandinavian Journal of Occupational Therapy, 11*, 171–178.

Henriksson, C., & Burckhardt, C. (1996). Impact of fibromyalgia on everyday life: A study of women in the USA and Sweden. *Disability and Rehabilitation, 18*, 241–248.

Henriksson, C., Gundmark, I., Bengtsson, A., & Ek, A. C. (1992). Living with fibromyalgia. *Clinical Journal of Pain, 8*, 138–144.

Henriksson, C. M. (1995). Living with continuous muscular pain: Patient perspectives: part I. *Scandinavian Journal of Caring Sciences, 9*, 67–76.

Henriksson, C. M. (1995). Living with continuous muscular pain: Patient perspectives: part II. *Scandinavian Journal of Caring Sciences, 9*, 77–86.

Henriksson, C. M. (1995a). Living with continuous muscular pain: Patient perspectives. Part I: encounters and consequences. *Scandinavian Journal of Caring Sciences, 9*(2), 67–76.

Henriksson, C. M. (1995b). Living with continuous muscular pain: Patient perspectives Part II: Strategies for daily life. *Scandinavian Journal of Caring Sciences, 9*, 77–86.

Henry, A. (1998). Development of a measure of adolescent leisure interests. *The American Journal of Occupational Therapy, 52*(7), 531–539.

Henry, A. D. (1998). Development of a measure of adolescent leisure interests. *The American Journal of Occupational Therapy, 52*, 531–539.

Henry, A. D. (2000). *The Pediatric Interest Profiles: Surveys of play for children and adolescents.* Unpublished manuscript, Model of Human Occupation Clearinghouse, Department of Occupational Therapy, University of Illinois at Chicago.

Henry, A. D., Baron, K. B., Mouradian, L., & Curtin, C. (1999). Reliability and validity of the self-assessment of occupational functioning. *The American Journal of Occupational Therapy, 53*(5), 482–488.

Henry, A. D., Costa, C., Ladd, D., Robertson, C., Rollins, J., & Roy, L. (1996). Time use, time management and academic achievement among occupational therapy students. *Work, 6*(2), 115–126.

Henry, A. D., Costa, C., Ladd, D., Robertson, C., Rollins, J., & Roy, L. (2006). Time use, time management and academic achievement among occupational therapy students. *Work, 6*, 115–126.

Henry, A. D., & Coster, W. J. (1996). Predictors of functional outcome among adolescents and young adults with psychotic disorders. *The American Journal of Occupational Therapy, 50*, 171–181.

Henry, A. D., & Coster, W. J. (1997). Competency beliefs and occupational role behavior among adolescents: Explication of the personal causation construct. *The American Journal of Occupational Therapy, 51*, 267–276.

Hocking, C. (1989). Anger management. *Journal of New Zealand Association of Occupational Therapists, 40*(2), 12–17.

Hocking, C. (1994). Objects in the environment: A critique of the model of human occupation dimensions. *Scandinavian Journal of Occupational Therapy, 1*, 77–84.

Horne, J., Corr, S., & Earle, S. (2005). Becoming a mother: occupational change in first time motherhood. *Journal of Occupational Science, 12*(3), 176–183.

Howie, L., Coulter, M., & Feldman, S. (2004). Crafting the self: Older persons' narratives of occupational identity. *The American Journal of Occupational Therapy, 58*, 446–454.

Hubbard, S. (1991). Towards a truly holistic approach to occupational therapy. *British Journal of Occupational Therapy, 54*, 415–418.

Humphries, D. (1998). Managing knowledge into practice. *Manual Therapy, 3*(3), 153–158.

Humphries, D., Littlejohns, P., Victor, C., O'Halloran, P., & Peacock, J. (2000). Implementing evidence-based practice: Factors that influence the use of research evidence by occupational therapists. *British Journal of Occupational Therapy, 63*(11), 516–522.

Hurff, J. M. (1984). Visualization: A decision-making tool for assessment and treatment planning. *Occupational Therapy in Health Care, 1*(2), 3–23.

Ingvarsson, L., & Theodorsdottir, M. H. (2004). Vocational rehabilitation at Reykjalundur rehabilitation Center in Iceland. *WORK, 22*(1), 17–19.

Ishikawa, Y., & Okamura, H. (2008). Factors that impede the discharge of long-term schizophrenic inpatients. *Scandinavian Journal of Occupational Therapy, 15*, 230–235.

Jackoway, I., Rogers, J., & Snow, T. (1987). The role change assessment: An interview tool for evaluating older adults. *Occupational Therapy in Mental Health, 7*(1), 17–37.

Jackson, M., Harkess, J., & Ellis, J. (2004). Reporting patients' work abilities: How the use of standardised work assessments improved clinical practice in Fife. *British Journal of Occupational Therapy, 67*(3), 129–132.

Jacobshagen, I. (1990). The effect of interruption of activity on affect. *Occupational Therapy in Mental Health, 10* (20), 35–45.

Jones, L. (2008). Promoting physical activity in acute mental health. *The British Journal of Occupational Therapy, 71*(77), 499–502.

Jongbloed, L. (1994). Adaptation to a stroke: The experience of one couple. *The American Journal of Occupational Therapy, 48*, 1006–1013.

Jonsson, H. (1993). The retirement process in an occupational perspective: A review of literature and theories. *Physical and Occupational Therapy in Geriatrics, 11*(4), 15–34.

Jonsson, H., Borell, L., & Sadlo, G. (2000). Retirement: An occupational transition with consequences, temporality, balance, and meaning of occupations. *Journal of Occupational Science, 7*(1), 29–37.

Jonsson, H., Kielhofner, G., & Borell, L. (1997). Anticipating retirement: The formation of narratives concerning an occupational transition. *The American Journal of Occupational Therapy, 51*, 49–56.

Jonsson, H., Josephsson, S., & Kielhofner, G. (2000). Evolving narratives in the course of retirement: A longitudinal study. *The American Journal of Occupational Therapy, 54*(5), 463–470.

Jonsson, H., Josephsson, S., & Kielhofner, G. (2001). Narratives and experiences in an occupational transition: A longitudinal study of the retirement process. *The American Journal of Occupational Therapy, 55*(4), 424–432.

Jonsson, H., Kielhofner, G., & Borell, L. (1997). Anticipating retirement: Narratives concerning an occupational transition. *The American Journal of Occupational Therapy, 51*(1), 49–56.

Josephsson, S., Backman, L., Borell, L., Bernspang, B., Nygard, L., & Ronnberg, L. (1993). Supporting everyday activities in dementia: An intervention study. *International Journal of Geriatric Psychiatry, 8*, 395–400.

Josephsson, S., Backman, L., Borell, L., Hygard, L., & Bernspang, B. (1995). Effectiveness of an intervention to improve occupational performance in dementia. *Occupational Therapy Journal of Research, 15*(1), 36–49.

Jungersen, K. (1992). Culture, theory, and the practice of occupational therapy in New Zealand/Aotearoa. *The American Journal of Occupational Therapy, 46*, 745–750.

Kåhlin, I., & Haglund, L. (2009). Psychosocial strengths and challenges related to work among persons with intellectual disabilities. *Occupational Therapy in Mental Health, 25*, 151–163.

Kaner, E., Steven, A., Cassidy, P., & Vardy, C. (2003). Implementation of a model for service delivery and organization in mental healthcare: a qualitative exploration of service provider views. *Health and Social Care in the Community, 11*(6), 519–527.

Kaplan, K. (1984). Short-term assessment: The need and a response. *Occupational Therapy in Mental Health, 4*(3), 29–45.

Kaplan, K. (1986). The directive group: Short term treatment for psychiatric patients with a minimal level of functioning. *The American Journal of Occupational Therapy, 40*, 474–481.

Kaplan, K. (1988). *Directive group therapy: Innovative mental health treatment.* Thorofare, NJ: Slack.

Kaplan, K., & Eskow, K. G. (1987). Teaching psychosocial theory and practice: The model of human occupation as the medium and the message. *Mental Health Special Interest Section Newsletter, 10*(1), 1–5.

Kaplan, K., & Kielhofner, G. (1989). *Occupational Case Analysis Interview and rating scale.* Thorofare, NJ: Slack.

Katz, N. (1988). Introduction to the collection (MOHO). *Occupational Therapy in Mental Health, 8*(1), 1–6.

Katz, N. (1985). Occupational therapy's domain of concern: Reconsidered. *The American Journal of Occupational Therapy, 39*, 518–524.

Katz, N. (1988). Interest Checklist: A factor analytical study. *Occupational Therapy in Mental Health, 8*(1), 45–55.

Katz, N., Giladi, N., & Peretz, C. (1988). Cross- cultural application of occupational therapy assessments: Human occupation with psychiatric inpatients and controls in Israel. *Occupational Therapy in Mental Health, 8*(1), 7–30.

Katz, N., Josman, N., & Steinmetz, N. (1988). Relationship between cognitive disability theory and the model of human occupation in the assessment of psychiatric and nonpsychiatric adolescents. *Occupational Therapy in Mental Health, 8*(1), 31–43.

Kavanagh, J., & Fares, J. (1995). Using the model of human occupation with homeless mentally ill patients. *British Journal of Occupational Therapy, 58*, 419–422.

Kavanagh, M. R. (1990). Way station: A model community support program for persons with serious mental illness. *Mental Health-Special Interest Section Newsletter, 13*(1), 6–8.

Keller, J., & Forsyth, K. (2004). The model of human occupation in practice. *The Israel Journal of Occupational Therapy. 13*, E99–E106.

Keller, J., Kafkes, A., & Kielhofner, G. (2005). Psychometric characteristics of the Child Occupational Self Assessment (COSA), part 1: An initial examination of psychometric properties. *Scandinavian Journal of Occupational Therapy, 12*, 118–127.

Keller, J., Kafkes, A., Basu, S., Federico, J., & Kielhofner, G. (2005). *The Child Occupational Self Assessment* [Version 2.1]. Chicago: Model of Human Occupation Clearinghouse, Department of Occupational Therapy, College of Applied Health Sciences, University of Illinois at Chicago.

Keller, J., & Kielhofner, G. (2005). Psychometric characteristics of the child occupational self-assessment (COSA), part two: Refining the psychometric properties. *Scandinavian Journal of Occupational Therapy, 12*, 147–158.

Kelly, L. (1995). What occupational therapists can learn from tradtional healers. *British Journal of Occupational Therapy, 58*, 111–114.

Keponen, R., & Kielhofner, G. (2006) Occupation and meaning in the lives of women with chronic pain. *Scandinavian Journal of Occupational Therapy, 13*(4), 211–220.

Keponen, R., & Launiainen, H. (2008). Using the model of human occupation to nurture an occupational focus in the clinical reasoning of experienced therapists. *Occupational Therapy in Health Care, 22*(2–3), 95–104.

Khoo, S. W., & Renwick, R. M. (1989). A model of human occupation perspective on mental health of immigrant women in Canada. *Occupational Therapy in Mental Health, 9*(3), 31–49.

Kielhofner, G. (1980). A model of human occupation, part 2: Ontogenesis from the perspective of temporal adaptation. *The American Journal of Occupational Therapy, 34*, 657–663.

Kielhofner, G. (1980). A model of human occupation, part 3: Benign and vicious cycles. *The American Journal of Occupational Therapy, 34*, 731–737.

Kielhofner, G. (1984). An overview of research on the model of human occupation. *Canadian Journal of Occupational Therapy, 51*, 59–67.

Kielhofner, G. (1985). *A model of human occupation: Theory and application* (2nd ed.). Baltimore, MD: Williams & Wilkins.

Kielhofner, G. (1986). A review of research on the model of human occupation: part 1. *Canadian Journal of Occupational Therapy, 53*, 69–74.

Kielhofner, G. (1986). A review of research on the model of human occupation: part 2. *Canadian Journal of Occupational Therapy, 53*, 129–134.

Kielhofner, G. (1992). The future of the profession of occupational therapy: Requirements for developing the field's knowledge base. *Journal of Japanese Association of Occupational Therapists, 11*, 112–129.

Kielhofner, G. (1993). Functional assessment: Toward a dialectical view of person environment relations. *The American Journal of Occupational Therapy, 47*, 248–251.

Kielhofner, G. (1995). A meditation on the use of hands. *Scandinavian Journal of Caring Sciences, 2*, 153–166.

Kielhofner, G. (1995). *A model of human occupation: Theory and application* (2nd ed.) Philadelphia, PA: Lippincott Williams & Wilkins.

Kielhofner, G. (1999). Guest editorial. *Work, 12*, 1.

Kielhofner, G. (2002). *A model of human occupation: Theory and application* (3rd ed.). Baltimore, MD: Williams & Wilkins.

Kielhofner, G. (2004). *Conceptual foundations of occupational therapy* (3rd ed.). Philadelphia, PA: F. A. Davis.

Kielhofner, G. (2004). The model of human occupation. In G. Kielhofner (Ed.), *Conceptual foundations of occupational therapy* (3rd ed., pp. 147–170). Philadelphia, PA: F. A. Davis.

Kielhofner, G. (2005a). A scholarship of practice: Creating discourse between theory, research and practice. *Occupational Therapy in Health Care, 19*(112), 7–17.

Kielhofner, G. (2005b). Scholarship and practice: Bridging the divide. *The American Journal of Occupational Therapy, 59*, 231–239.

Kielhofner, G., & Barrett, L. (1998). Meaning and misunderstanding in occupational forms: A study of therapeutic goal setting. *The American Journal of Occupational Therapy, 52*, 345–353.

Kielhofner, G., & Barrett, L. (1998). Theories derived from occupational behavior perspectives. In M. E. Neistadt & E. B. Crepeau (Eds.), *Willard and Spackman's occupational therapy* (9th ed., pp. 525–535). Philadelphia, PA: Lippincott.

Kielhofner, G., & Brinson, M. (1989). Development and evaluation of an aftercare program for young and chronic psychiatrically disabled adults. *Occupational Therapy in Mental Health, 9*(2), 1–25.

Kielhofner, G., & Burke, J. P. (1980). A model of human occupation, part 1: Conceptual framework and content. *The American Journal of Occupational Therapy, 34*, 572–581.

Kielhofner, G., Burke, J. P., & Heard, I. C. (1980). A model of human occupation, part 4. Assessment and intervention. *The American Journal of Occupational Therapy, 34*, 777–788.

Kielhofner, G., & Fisher, A. (1991). Mind-brain relationships. In A. Fisher, E. Murray, & A. C. Bundy (Eds.), *Sensory integration: theory and practice* (pp. 27–45). Philadelphia: F. A. Davis.

Kielhofner, G., & Forsyth, K. (1997). The model of human occupation: An overview of current concepts. *British Journal of Occupational Therapy, 60*, 103–110.

Kielhofner, G., & Forsyth, K. (2001). Measurement properties of a client self-report for treatment planning and documenting therapy outcomes. *Scandinavian Journal of Occupational Therapy, 8*(3), 131–139.

Kielhofner, G., & Forsyth, K. (2001). Measurement properties of a client self -report for treatment planning and documenting therapy outcomes. *Scandinavian Journal of Occupational Therapy, 8*(3), 131–139.

Kielhofner, G., & Henry, A. D. (1988). Development and investigation of the Occupational Performance History Interview. *The American Journal of Occupational Therapy, 42*, 489–498.

Kielhofner, G., & Mallinson, T. (1995). Gathering narrative data through interviews: Empirical observations and suggested guidelines. *Scandinavian Journal of Occupational Therapy, 2*, 63–68.

Kielhofner, G., & Neville, A. (1983). *The modified interest checklist*. Unpublished manuscript, Model of Human Occupation Clearinghouse, Department of Occupational Therapy, University of Illinois at Chicago.

Kielhofner, G., & Nicol, M. (1989). The model of human occupation: A developing conceptual tool for clinicians. *British Journal of Occupational Therapy, 52*, 210–214.

Kielhofner, G., Barris, R., & Watts, J. H. (1982). Habits and habit dysfunction: A clinical perspective for psychosocial occupational therapy. *Occupational Therapy in Mental Health, 2* (2), 1–21.

Kielhofner, G., Braveman, B., Baron, K., Fischer, G., Hammel, J., & Littleton, M. J. (1999). The model of human occupation: Understanding the worker who is injured or disabled. *Work, 12*, 3–11.

Kielhofner, G., Braveman, B., Finlayson, M., Paul-Ward, A., Goldbaum, L., & Goldstein, K. (2004). Outcomes of a vocational program for persons with AIDS. *The American Journal of Occupational Therapy, 58* (1), 64–72.

Kielhofner, G., Braveman, B., Fogg, L., & Levin, M. (2008). A controlled study of services to enhance productive participation among people with HIV/AIDS. *The American Journal of Occupational Therapy, 62*(1), 36–45.

Kielhofner, G., Dobria, L., Forsyth, K., & Basu, S. (2005). The construction of key forms for obtaining instantaneous measures from the occupational performance history interview rating scales. *Occupational Therapy Journal of Research, 25*, 23–32.

Kielhofner, G., Fogg, L., Braveman, B., Forsyth, K., Kramer, J., & Duncan, E. (2009). A factor analytic study of the model of human occupation screening tool of hypothesized variables. *Occupational Therapy in Mental Health, 25*, 127–137.

Kielhofner, G., Hammel, J., Helfrich, C., Finlayson, M., & Taylor, R. (2004). Studying practice and its outcomes: A conceptual approach. *The American Journal of Occupational Therapy, 58*, 15–23.

Kielhofner, G., Harlan, B., Bauer, D., & Maurer, P. (1986). The reliability of a historical interview with physically disabled respondents. *The American Journal of Occupational Therapy*. 40, 551–556.

Kielhofner, G., Henry, A. D., Walens, D., & Rogers, E. S. (1991). A generalizability study of the Occupational Performance History Interview. *Occupational Therapy Journal of Research, 11*, 292–306.

Kielhofner, G., Henry, A. D., Walens, D., & Rogers, E. S. (1991). A generalizability study of the Occupational Performance History Interview. *Occupational Therapy Journal of Research, 11*, 292–306.

Kielhofner, G., Lai, J. S., Olson, L., Haglund, L., Ekbadh, E., & Hedlund, M. (1999). Psychometric properties of the work environment impact scale: a cross-cultural study. *Work, 12*(1), 71–77.

Kielhofner, G., Lai, J., Olson, L., Haglund, L., Ekbadh, E., & Hedlund, M. (1999). Psychometric properties of the work environment impact scale: a cross-cultural study. *WORK, 12*, 71–77.

Kielhofner, G., Mallinson, T., Crawford, C., Nowak, M., Rigby, M., Henry, A., & Walens, D. (2004). *Occupational Performance History Interview-I/ (OPHl-11)* [Version 2.1]. Chicago: Model of Human Occupation Clearinghouse, Department of Occupational Therapy, College of Applied Health Sciences, University of Illinois at Chicago.

Kielhofner, G., Mallinson, T., Forsyth, K., & Lai, J. S. (2001). Psychometric properties of the second version of the Occupational Performance History Interview (OPHl-11). *The American Journal of Occupational Therapy, 55*, 260–267.

Kielhofner. G. (1999). From doing in to doing with: The role of environment in performance and disability. *Toimintaterapeutti, 1*, 3–9.

Kielhofner. G., Dobria, L., Forsyth, K., & Basu, S. (2005). The construction of key forms for obtaining instantaneous measures from the occupational performance history interview rating scales. *Occupational Therapy Journal of Research, 25*(1), 23–32.

Kimball-Carpenter, A., & Smith, M. (2013). An occupational therapist's interdisciplinary approach to a geriatric psychiatry activity group: A case study. *Occupational Therapy in Mental Health, 29*, 293–298.

Kjellberg, A. (2002). More or less independent. *Disability and Rehabilitation, 24*(16), 828–840.

Kjellberg, A., Haglund, L., Forsyth, K., & Kielhofner, G. (2003). The measurement properties of the Swedish version of the assessment of communication and interaction skills. *Scandinavian Journal of Caring Sciences, 1*, 271–277.

Knis-Matthews, L., Richard, L., Marquez, L., & Mevawala, N. (2005). Implementation of occupational therapy services for an adolescent residence program. *Occupational Therapy in Mental Health, 21*, (1), 57–72.

Kramer, J. (2011). Using mixed methods to establish the social validity of a self-report assessment: An illustration using the Child Occupational Self-Assessment (COSA). *Journal of Mixed Methods Research, 5*(1), 52–76.

Kramer, J., Bowyer, P., Kielhofner, G., O'Brien, J. (2009). Examining rater behavior on revised version of the short Child occupational profile (SCOPE). *Occupation Participation Health, 29*(2), 88–96.

Kramer, J., Bowyer, P., Kielhofner, G., O'Brien, J., & Maziero-Barbosa, V. (2009). Examining rater behavior on a revised version of the Short Child Occupational Profile (SCOPE). *Occupation, Participation, Health, 29*(2), 88–96.

Kramer, J., Bowyer, P., O'Brien, J., Kielhofner, G., & Maziero-Barbosa, V. (2009). How interdisciplinary pediatric practitioners choose assessments. *Canadian Journal of Occupational Therapy, 76*(1), 56–64.

Kramer, J., Kielhofner, G., Lee, S., Ashpole, E., & Castle, L. (2009). Utility of the model of human occupation screening tool for detecting client change. *Occupational Therapy in Mental Health, 25*, 181–191.

Kramer, J., Kielhofner, G., & Smith, E. (2010). Validity evidence for the child occupational self assessment. *The American Journal of Occupational Therapy, 64*, 621–632.

Kramer, J., Smith, E., & Kielhofner, G. (2009). Rating scale use by children with disabilities on a self-report of everyday activities. *Archives of Physical Medicine and Rehabilitation, 90*, 2047–2053.

Kramer, J., Walker, R., Cohn, E., Mermelstein, M., Olsen, S., O'Brien, J., & Bowyer, P. (2012). Striving for shared understandings: Therapists' perspectives of the benefits and dilemmas of using a child self-assessment. *Occupation, Participation, Health, 32*(1), S48–S58.

Krefting, L. (1985). The use of conceptual models in clinical practice. *Canadian Journal of Occupational Therapy, 52*, 173–178.

Kurokawa, H., Yabuwaki, K., & Kobavashi, R. (2013). Factor structure of "personhood" for elderly healthcare services: a questionnaire survey of long-term care facilities in Japan. *Disability and Rehabilitation, 35*(7), 551–556.

Kusznir, A., Scott, E., Cooke, R. G., & Young, L. T. (1996). Functional consequences of bipolar affective disorder: an occupational therapy perspective. *Canadian Journal of Occupational Therapy, 63*, 313–322.

Kyle, T., & Wright, S. (1996). Reflecting the model of human occupation in occupational therapy documentation. *Canadian Journal of Occupational Therapy, 63*, 192–196.

Lai, J. S., Haglund, L., & Kielhofner, G. (1999). Occupational case analysis interview and rating scale. *Scandinavian Journal of Caring Sciences, 13*, 276–273.

Lancaster, J. M. (1991). Occupational therapy treatment goals, objectives, and activities for improving low self-esteem in adolescents with behavioral disorders. *Occupational Therapy in Mental Health, 11*(213), 3–22.

Larsson, M., & Branholm, I. (1996). An approach to goal-planning in occupational therapy and rehabilitation. *Scandinavian Journal of Occupational Therapy, 3*(1), 14–19.

Law, M., & Baum, C. (1998). Evidence-based practice occupational therapy. *Canadian Journal of Occupational Therapy, 65*, 131–135.

Lederer, J., Kielhofner, G., & Watts, J. H. (1985). Values, personal causation and skills of delinquents and non delinquents. *Occupational Therapy in Mental Health, 5*(2), 59–77.

Lee, A. L., Strauss, L., Wittman, P., Jackson, B., & Carstens, A. (2001). The effects of chronic illness on roles and emotions of caregivers. *Occupational Therapy in Health Care, 14*(1), 47–60.

Lee, C. J., & Miller, L. T. (2003). The process of evidence-based clinical decision making in occupational therapy. *The American Journal of Occupational Therapy, 57*, 473–477.

Lee, S., Forsyth, K., Morley, M., Garnham, M., Heasman, D., & Taylor, R. (2013). Mental health payment-by-results clusters and the model of human occupation screening tool. *Occupation, Participation, Health, 33*(1), 40–49.

Lee, S., & Harris, M. (2010). The development of an effective occupational therapy assessment and treatment pathway for women with a diagnosis of borderline personality disorder in an inpatient setting: Implementing the Model of Human Occupation. *The British Journal of Occupational Therapy, 73*(11), 559–563.

Lee, S., Kielhofner, G., Morley, M., Heasman, D., Garnham, M., Willis, S., et al. (2012). Impact of using the Model of Human Occupation: A survey of occupational therapy mental health practitioners' perceptions. *Scandinavian Journal of Occupational Therapy, 19*, 450–456.

Lee, S., Taylor, R. R., Keilhofner, G., & Fisher, G. (2008).Theory use in practice: A national survey of therapists who use the model of human occupation. *The American Journal of Occupational Therapy, 62*(1), 106–117.

Leidy, N. K., & Knebel, A. R. (1999).Clinical validation of the functional performance inventory in patients with chronic obstructive pulmonary disease. *Respiratory Care, 44*, 932–939.

Levin, M., & Helfrich, C. (2004). Mothering role identity and competence among parenting and pregnant homeless adolescents, *Journal of Occupational Science, 11*(5), 95–104.

Levin, M., Kielhofner, G., Braveman, B., & Fogg, L. (2007). Narrative slope as a predictor of return to work and other occupational participation. *Scandinavian Journal of Occupational Therapy, 14*(4), 258–264.

Levine, R. (1984).The cultural aspects of home care de livery. *The American Journal of Occupational Therapy, 38*, 734–738.

Levine, R., & Gitlin, L. N. (1990). Home adaptations for persons with chronic disabilities: An educational model. *The American Journal of Occupational Therapy, 44*, 923–929.

Levine, R., & Gitlin, L. N. (1993). A model to promote activity competence in elders. *The American Journal of Occupational Therapy, 47*, 147–153.

Lexell, E., Lund, M., & Iwarsson, S. (2009). Constantly changing lives: experiences of people with multiple sclerosis. *The American Journal of Occupational Therapy, 63*(6), 772–781.

Li, Y., & Kielhofner, G. (2004). Psychometric properties of the volitional questionnaire. *The Israel Journal of Occupational Therapy, 13*, E85–E98.

Lim, S., & Rodger, S. (2008). An occupational perspective on the assessment of social competence in children. *The British Journal of Occupational Therapy, 71*(11), 469–481.

Lin, S., Murphy, S., & Robinson, J. (2010). Facilitating evidence-based practice: process, strategies, and resources. *The American Journal of Occupational Therapy, 64*, 164–171.

Linddahl, I., Norrby, E., & Bellner, A. (2003). Construct validity of the instrument DOA: a dialogue about ability related to work. *WORK, 20*(3), 215–224.

Liu, K., & Ng, B. (2008). Usefulness of the model of human occupation in the Hong Kong Chinese context. *Occupational Therapy in Health Care, 22*(2–3), 25–36.

Lloyd, C, Basset, H, King, R. (2004). Occupational Therapy and evidence-based practice in mental health, *British Journal of Occupational Therapy, 67*(2), 83–88.

Lloyd, C., King, R., & Bassett, H. (2002). Evidence-based practice in occupational therapy—Why the jury is still out. *New Zealand Journal of Occupational Therapy, 49*, 10–14.

lngvarsson, L., & Theodorsdottir, M. H. (2004). Vocational rehabilitation at Reykjalundur rehabilitation center in Iceland. *Work, 22*, 17–19.

Locock, L., Dopson, S., Chamber, D., & Gabbay, J. (2001) Understanding opinion leaders roles. *Social Science and Medicine, 53*, 745–757.

Lycett, R. (1992). Evaluating the use of an occupational assessment with elderly rehabilitation patients. *British Journal of Occupational Therapy, 55*(9), 343–346.

Lynch, K., & Bridle, M. (1993). Construct validity of the Occupational Performance Interview. *Occupational Therapy Journal of Research, 13*, 231–240.

Lyons, M. (1984). *Shapingup: The model of human occupation as a guide to practice.* Proceedings of the 13th Federal Conference of the Australian Association of Occupational Therapists, 2, pp. 95–100.

Mackenzie, L. (1997). An application of the model of human occupation to fieldwork supervision and fieldwork issues in New South Wales. *Australian Occupational Therapy Journal, 44*, 71–80.

Mallinson, T., Kielhofner, G., & Mattingly, C. (1996). Metaphor and meaning in a clinical interview. *The American Journal of Occupational Therapy, 50*, 338–346.

Mallinson, T., LaPlante, D., & Hollman-Smith, J. (1998). *Work rehabilitation in mental health programs.* Chicago: Model of Human Occupation Clearinghouse, Department of Occupational Therapy, College of Applied Health Sciences, University of Illinois at Chicago.

Mallinson, T., Mahaffey, L., & Kielhofner, G. (1998). The occupational performance history interview: Evidence for three underlying constructs of occupational adaptation. *Canadian Journal of Occupational Therapy, 65*(4), 219–228.

Marsh, H. W., & Hocevar, D. (1985) Application of confirmatory factor analysis of self-concept: First- and higher-order factor models and their invariance across groups. *Psychological Bulletin, 97*, 562–582.

Maynard, M. (1987). An experiential learning approach: Utilizing historical interview and an occupational inventory. *Physical and Occupational Therapy in Geriatrics, 5*(2), 51–69.

McCluskey, A. (2003). Occupational therapists report a low level of knowledge, skill and involvement in evidence-based practice. *Australian Occupational Therapy Journal, 50*(1), 3–12.

McCluskey, A., & Cusick, A. (2002). Strategies for introducing evidence-based practice and changing clinical behaviour: A manager's toolbox. *Australian Occupational Therapy Journal, 49*(2), 63–70.

Medina, D., Haltiwanger, E., & Funk, K. (2011). The experience of chronically ill elderly Mexican-American men with spouses as caregivers. *Physical & Occupational Therapy in Geriatrics, 29*(3), 189–201.

Melton. (2002). *Occupational Therapy Service Strategy for Service Development and Research Programme.* Gloucestershire Partnership NHS Trust

Melton, J., Forsyth, K., & Freeth, D. (2010). A practice development programme to promote the use of the Model of Human Occupation: Contexts, influential mechanisms and levels of engagement amongst occupational therapists. *The British Journal of Occupational Therapy, 73*(11), 549–558.

Melton, J., Forsyth, K., Metherall, A., Robinson, J., Hill, J., & Quick, L. (2008). Program redesign based on the model of human occupation: inpatient services for people experiencing acute mental illness in the UK. *Occupational Therapy in Health Care, 22*(2–3), 37–50.

Mentrup, C., Niehous, A., & Kielhofner, G. (1999). Applying the model of human occupation in work-focused rehabilitation: A case illustration. *Work: A Journal of Prevention, Assessment, and Rehabilitation*, 12, 61–70.

Metcalf, C., Perry, S., Bannigan, K., Lewin, R. J. P., Wisher, S., Klaber Moffatt, J. (2001). Barriers to implementing the evidence base in four NHS therapies. *Physiotherapy, 87*(8), 433–441.

Metcalfe, C., Lewin, R., Wisher, S., Perry, S., Bannigan, K., & Moffett, J. K. (2001). Barriers to implementing the evidence base in four NHS therapies: Dietitians, occupational therapists, physiotherapists, speech and language therapists. *Physiotherapy, 87*(8), 433–441.

Michael, P. S. (1991). Occupational therapy in a prison? You must be kidding! *Mental Health-Special Interest Section Newsletter, 14*, 3–4.

Misko, A., Nelson, D., & Duggan, J. (2015). Three case studies of community occupational therapy for individuals with human immunodeficiency virus. *Occupational Therapy in Health Care, 29*(11), 11–26.

Mocellin, G. (1992). An overview of occupational therapy in the context of the American influence on the profession: part 2. *British Journal of Occupational Therapy, 55*, 55–60.

Mocellin, G. (1992). An overview of occupational therapy in the context of the American influence on the profession: part 1. *British Journal of Occupational Therapy, 55*, 7–12.

Molyneaux-Smith, L., Townsend, E., & Guernsey, J. R. (2003). Occupation disrupted: Impacts, challenges, and coping strategies for farmers with disabilities. *Journal of Occupational Science, 10*, 14–20.

Moore-Corner, R., Kielhofner, G., & Olson, L. (1998). *Work Environment Impact Scale (WEIS)* [Version 2.0]. Chicago: Model of Human Occupation Clearinghouse, Department of

Occupational Therapy, College of Applied Health Sciences, University of Illinois at Chicago.

Morgan, D., & Jongbloed, L. (1990). Factors influencing leisure activities following a stroke: an exploratory study. *Canadian Journal of Occupational Therapy, 57*(4), 223–229.

Morgan, R., & Long, T. (2012). The effectiveness of occupational therapy for children with developmental coordination disorder: A review of the qualitative literature. *The British Journal of Occupational Therapy, 75*(1), 10–18.

Morley, M., Garnham, M., Forsyth, K., Lee, SW., Taylor, R. R., & Kielhofner, G. (2011). Developing occupational therapy indicative care packages in preparation for mental health Payment by Results. *Mental Health Occupational Therapy*, 16(1), 15–19.

Munoz, J. P., Karmosky, A., Gaugler, J., Lang, K., and Stayduhar, M. (1999). Perceived role changes in parents of children with cerebral palsy. *Mental Health Special Interest Section Quarterly, 22*(4), 1–3.

Munoz, J. P. (1988). A program for acute inpatient psychiatry. *Mental Health-Special Interest Section Newsletter, 11*, 3–4.

Munoz, J. P., Lawlor, M., & Kielhofner, G. (1993). Use of the model of human occupation: A survey of therapists in psychiatric practice. *Occupational Therapy Journal of Research, 13*, 117–139.

Nakamura-Thomas, H., & Yamada, T. (2008). Assessing interests in Japanese elders: a descriptive study. *Occupational Therapy in Health Care, 22*(2–3), 151–162.

Nakamura-Thomas, H., & Yamada, T. (2011). A factor analytic study of the Japanese Interest Checklist for the Elderly. *The British Journal of Occupational Therapy, 74*(2), 86–91.

Nave, J., Helfrich, C., & Aviles, A. (2001). Child witnesses of domestic violence: A case study using the OTPAL. *Occupational Therapy in Mental Health*, 16, 127–140.

Neistadt, M. E. (1995). Methods of assessing clients' priorities: a survey of adult physical dysfunction settings. *The American Journal of Occupational Therapy, 49*(5), 428–436.

Neville, A. (1985). The model of human occupation and depression. *Mental Health-Special Interest Section Newsletter, 8*(1), 1–4.

Neville-Jan, A. (1994). The relationship of volition to adaptive occupational behavior among individuals with varying degrees of depression. *Occupational Therapy in Mental Health, 12*(4), 1–18.

Neville-Jan, A., Bradley, M., Bunn, C., & Gheri, B. (1991). The model of human occupational and individuals with co-dependency problems. *Occupational Therapy in Mental Health, 11*(213), 73–97.

NHS Centre for review and Dissemination. (1999). *Effective Health care, getting evidence into practice*. The Royal Society of Medicine Press, University of York.

Notoh, H., Yamada, T., Kobayashi, N., Ishii, Y., & Forsyth, K. (2014). Examining the structural aspect of the construct validity of the Japanese version of the Model of Human Occupation Screening Tool. *British Journal of Occupational Therapy, 77*(10), 516–525.

Nour, N., Heck, C., & Ross, H. (2015). Factors related to participation in paid work after organ transplantation: perceptions of kidney transplant recipients. *Journal of Occupational Rehabilitation, 25*, 38–51.

Novak, I., & Mcintyre, S. (2010). The effect of Education with workplace supports on practitioners' evidence-based practice knowledge and implementation behaviours. *Australian Occupational Therapy Journal, 57*, 386–393.

Nygren, U., Sandlund, M., Bernspång, B., & Fisher, A. (2013). Exploring perceptions of occupational competence among participants in Individual Placement and Support (IPS). *Scandinavian Journal of Occupational Therapy, 20*, 429–437.

Oakley, F. (1987). Clinical application of the model of human occupation in dementia of the Alzheimer's type. *Occupational Therapy in Mental Health, 7*(4), 37–50.

Oakley, F., Kielhofner, G., & Barris R. (1985). An occupational therapy approach to assessing psychiatric patients' adaptative functioning. *The American Journal of Occupational Therapy, 39*, 147–154.

Oakley, F., Kielhofner, G., Barris, R., & Reichler, R. K. (1986). The Role Checklist: Development and empirical assessment of reliability. *Occupational Therapy Journal of Research, 6*, 157–170.

O'Brien, J., Asselin, E., Fortier, K., Janzegers, R., Lagueux, B., & Silcox, C. (2010). Using therapeutic reasoning to apply the model of human occupation in pediatric occupational therapy practice. *Journal of Occupational Therapy, Schools, & Early Intervention, 3*, 348–365.

Olin, D. (1984). Assessing and assisting the person with dementia: An occupational behavior perspective. *Physical and Occupational Therapy in Geriatrics, 3*(4), 25–32.

Olson, L. M., & Kielhofner, G. (1998). *Work readiness: Day treatment for persons with chronic disabilities*. Chicago: Model of Human Occupation Clearinghouse, Department of Occupational Therapy, College of Applied Health Sciences, University of Illinois at Chicago.

Osterholm, J., Bjork, M., & Hakansson, C. (2013). Factors of importance for maintaining work as perceived by men with arthritis. *Annals of the Rheumatic Diseases, 45*, 439–448.

Ottenbacher, K. J., Barris, R., Van Deusen, J. (1986). Some issues related to research utilization in occupational therapy. *The American Journal of Occupational Therapy, 40*, 111–116.

Packer, T. L., Foster, D. M., & Brouwer, B. (1997). Fatigue and activity patterns of people with chronic fatigue syndrome. *Occupational Therapy Journal of Research, 17*(3), 186–199.

Padilla, R. (1998). Application of occupational therapy theories with elders. In H. Lohman, R. Padilla, & S. Byers-Connon (Eds.), *Occupational therapy with elders: Strategies for the certified occupational therapist assistant*. (pp. 63–79). St. Louis, MO: Mosby.

Padilla, R., & Bianchi, E. M. (1990). Occupational therapy for chronic pain: Applying the model of human occupation to clinical practice. *Occupational Therapy Practice, 2*, 47–52.

Pan, A., Fan, C., Chung, L., Chen, T., Kielhofner, G., Wu, M., & Chen, Y. (2011). Examining the validity of the Model of Human Occupation Screening Tool: Using classical test theory and item response theory. *The British Journal of Occupational Therapy, 74*(1), 34–40.

Parkinson, S., Chester, A., Cratchley, S., & Rowbottom, J. (2008). Application of the Model of Human Occupation Screening Tool (MOHOST Assessment) in an Acute Psychiatric Setting. *Occupational Therapy in Health Care, 22*(2–3), 63–75.

Parkinson, S., Fisher, G., & Fisher, J. (2011). Development of an occupation-focused home assessment for use in mental health services. *Mental Health Occupational Therapy,* 16(1), 8–11.

Parkinson, S., Forsyth, K., & Kielhofner, G. (2006). *The Model of Human Occupation Screening Tool* [Version 2.0]. Chicago: University of Illinois at Chiacgo.

Parkinson, S., Lowe, C., & Vecsey, T. (2011). The therapeutic benefits of horticulture in a mental health service. *The British Journal of Occupational Therapy, 74*(11), 525–534.

Parkinson, S., Morley, M., Stewart, L., & Brockbank, H. (2012). Meeting the occupational needs of mental health service users: Indicative care packages and actual practice. *The British Journal of Occupational Therapy, 75*(8), 384–389.

Patomella, A., Kottorp, A., & Nygård, L. (2013). Design and management features of everyday technology that challenge older adults. *The British Journal of Occupational Therapy, 76*(9), 390–398.

Paul-Ward, A., Braveman, B., Kielhofner, G., & Levin, M. (2005). Developing employment services for individuals with HIV/AIDS: Participatory action strategies at work. *Journal of Vocational Rehabilitation, 22*, 85–93.

Peloquin, S. M., & Abreu, B. C. (1996). The academia and clinical worlds: Shall we make meaningful connections? *The American Journal of Occupational Therapy, 50*(7), 588–591.

Peloquin, S. M. (2002). Confluence: Moving forward with affective strength. *The American Journal of Occupational Therapy, 56*(1), 69–77.

Pentland, W., Harvey, A. S., & Walker, J. (2006). The relationships between time use and health and well being in men with spinal cord injury. *Journal of Occupational Science, 5*(1), 14–25.

Pépin, G., Guérette, F., Lefebvre, B., & Jacques, P. (2008). Canadian therapists' experiences while implementing the model of human occupation remotivation process. *Occupational Therapy in Health Care, 22*(2–3), 115–124.

Petersen, K., & Hartvig, B. (2008). A process for translating and validating model of human occupation assessments in the Danish context. *Occup Ther Health Occupational Therapy in Health Care, 22*(2–3), 139–149.

Peterson, E., Howland, J., Kielhofner, G., Lachman, M.E., Assmann, S., Cote, J., et al. (1999). Falls self-efficacy and occupational adaptation among elders. *Physical and Occupational Therapy in Geriatrics, 16*(1/2), 1–16.

Pizur-Barnekow, K., & Erickson, S. (2011). Perinatal posttraumatic stress disorder: Implications for occupational therapy in early intervention practice. *Occupational Therapy in Mental Health, 27*, 126–139.

Pizzi, M. A. (1984). Occupational therapy in hospice care. *The American Journal of Occupational Therapy, 38*, 257.

Pizzi, M. A. (1990). The model of human occupation and adults with HIV infection and AIDS. *The American Journal of Occupational Therapy, 44*, 257–264.

Pizzi, M. A. (1989). Occupational therapy: Creating possibilities for adults with HIV infection, ARC and AIDS. *AIDS Patient Care, 3*, 18–23.

Pizzi, M. A. (1990). Occupational therapy: Creating possibilities for adults with human immunodeficiency virus infection, AIDS related complex, and acquired immunodeficiency syndrome. *Occupational Therapy in Health Care, 7*(21314), 125–137.

Platts, L. (1993). Social role valorisation and the model of human occupation: A comparative analysis for work with learning disability in the community. *British Journal of Occupational Therapy, 56*, 278–282.

Polatajko, H. J., & Craik, J. (2006). Editorial: In search of evidence: strategies for an evidence-based practice process. *Occupation, Participation, and Health, 26*(1), 2–3.

Prellwitz, M., & Tham, M. (2000). How children with restricted mobility perceive their school environment. *Scandinavian Journal of Occupational Therapy, 7*, 165–173.

Provident, I. M., & Joyce-Gaguzis, K. (2005). Brief report: Creating an occupational therapy level field work experience in a county jail setting. *The American Journal of Occupational Therapy, 59*, 101–106.

Raber, C., Teitelman, J., Watts, J., & Kielhofner, G. (2010). A phenomenological study of volition in everyday occupations of older people with dementia. *The British Journal of Occupational Therapy, 73*(11), 498–506.

Rappolt, S. (2003). The role of professional expertise in evidence-based occupational therapy. *The American Journal of Occupational Therapy, 57*, 589–593.

Reekmans, M., & Kielhofner, G. (1998). Defining occupational therapy services in child psychiatry: An application of the model of human occupation. *Ergotherapie, 5*, 6–11.

Reid, D. (2003). The influence of a virtual reality leisure intervention program on the motivation of older adult stroke survivors: a pilot study. *Physical & Occupational Therapy in Geriatrics, 21*(4), 1–19.

Reid, D. T. (2005). Correlation of the pediatric volitional questionnaire with the test of playfulness in a virtual environment: The power of engagement. *Early Child Development and Care, 175*(2), 153–164.

Reid, C. L., & Reid J. K. (2000). Care giving as an occupational role in the dying process. *Occupational Therapy in Health Care, 12* (213), 87–93.

Restall, G., & Magill-Evans, J. (1994). Play and preschool children with autism. *The American Journal of Occupational Therapy, 48* (2), 113–120.

Roberts, A. E. (2002). Advancing practice through continuing education: the case for reflection. *British Journal of Occupational Therapy, 65*(5), 237–241.

Roberts, A. E. K., & Barber, G. (2001). Applying research evidence to practice. *British Journal of Occupational Therapy, 64*, 223–227.

Rogers, J., Weinstein, J., & Figone, J. (1978). The Interest Checklist: An empirical assessment. *The American Journal of Occupational Therapy, 32*, 628–630.

Roitman, D. M., & Ziv, N. (2004). Application of the Model of Human Occupation in a geriatric population in Israel: Two case studies. *Israeli Journal of Occupational Therapy, 13*, E24–E28.

Rosenfeld, M. S. (1989). Occupational disruption and adaptation: A study of house fire victims. *The American Journal of Occupational Therapy, 43*, 89–96.

Rothberg, A., Coopoo, Y., Burns, C., & Franzsen, D. (2009). Uptake and drop-out from a corporate health-promotion programme for employees with health risks. *South African Journal of Occupational Therapy*, 39(1), 26–31.

Rubin, D. (1987). *Multiple Imputation for Nonresponse in Surveys*. New York, NY: John Wiley and Sons.

Rust, K., Barris, R., & Hooper, F. (1987). Use of the model of human occupation to predict women's exercise behavior. *Occupational Therapy Journal of Research, 7*, 23–35.

Sackett, D. L., Rosenberg, W. M. C., Muir Gray, J. A., Haynes, R. B., Richardson, W. S. (1996). Evidence based medicine: what it is and what it isn't. *British Medical Journal, 312*, 71–72.

Salz, C. (1983). A theoretical approach to the treatment of work difficulties in borderline personalities. *Occupational Therapy in Mental Health, 3*(3), 33–46.

Scaffa, M. E. (1991). Alcoholism: an occupational behavior perspective. *Occupational Therapy in Mental Health, 11*, 99–111.

Scarth, P. P.(1983). Services for chemically dependent adolescents. *Mental Health Special Interest Section Newsletter, 13*, 7–8.

Schaff, R. C., & Mulrooney, L. L. (1989). Occupational therapy in early intervention: A family centered approach. *The American Journal of Occupational Therapy, 43*, 745–754.

Scheelar, J. F. (2002). A return to the worker role after injury: Firefighters seriously injured on the job and the decision to return to high-risk work. *Work, 19*(2), 181–184.

Schindler, V. P. (1990). AIDS in a correctional setting. *Occupational Therapy in Health Care, 7*,171–183.

Schindler, V. J. (1988). Psychosocial occupational therapy intervention with AIDS patients. *The American Journal of Occupational Therapy, 42*, 507–512.

Schindler, V. P. (2004). Evaluating the effectiveness of role development: Quantitative Data. *Occupational Therapy in Mental Health, 20*(3/4), 79–104.

Schindler, V. P. (2004). *Occupational therapy in forensic psychiatry: Role development and schizophrenia. Occupational Therapy in Mental Health, 20*, 57–104.

Schindler, V. P., & Baldwin, S. A. M. (2005). Role development: Application to community-based clients. *The Israel Journal of Occupational Therapy, 14*, E3–E18.

Scott, P. (2011). Occupational therapy services to enable liver patients to thrive following transplantation. *Occupational Therapy in Health Care, 25*(4), 240–256.

Scottish Executive. (2002). *Building on success: Future directions for the allied health professions in Scotland*. Edinburgh, Scotland: Author.

Sepiol, J. M., & Froehlich, J. (1990). Use of the role checklist with the patient with multiple personality disorder. *The American Journal of Occupational Therapy, 44*, 1008–1012.

Series, C. (1992). The long-term needs of people with head injury: A role for the community occupational therapist? *British Journal of Occupational Therapy, 55*, 94–98.

Shimp, S. L. (1989). A family-style meal group: Short term treatment for eating disorder patients with a high level of functioning. *Mental Health Special Interest Section Newsletter, 12* (3), 1–3.

Shimp, S. L. (1990). Debunking the myths of aging. *Occupational Therapy in Mental Health, 10*(3), 101–111.

Sholle-Martin, S. (1987). Application of the model of human occupation: Assessment in child and adolescent psychiatry. *Occupational Therapy in Mental Health, 7*(2), 3–22.

Sholle-Martin, S., & Alessi, N. E. (1990). Formulating a role for occupational therapy in child psychiatry: A clinical application. *The American Journal of Occupational Therapy, 44*, 871–881.

Simmons, D. (1999). The psychological system in adolescence. In S.M. Porr & E.B. Rainville (Eds.), *Pediatric therapy: A systems approach* (pp. 430–432). Philadelphia, PA: F. A. Davis.

Simo-Algado, S., & Cardona, C. E. (2005). The return of the corn men. In F. Kronenberg, S. Simo-Algado, & N. Pollard (Eds.), *Occupational therapy without borders: Learning from the spirit of survivors* (pp. 336–350). London, UK: Elsevier Churchill Livingstone.

Simo-Algado, S., Mehta, N., Kronenberg, F., Cockburn, L., & Kirsh, B. (2002). Occupational therapy intervention with children survivors of war. *Canadian Journal of Occupational Therapy, 69*, 205–217.

Skold, A., Josephsson, S., & Eliasson, A. C. (2004). Performing bimanual activities: The experiences of young persons with hemiplegic cerebral palsy. *The American Journal of Occupational Therapy, 58*, 416–425.

Sleep, J., Page, S., and Tamblin, L. (2002) Achieving clinical excellence through evidence-based practice: report of an educational initiative. *Journal of Nursing Management, 10*, 139–143.

Smith, H. (1987). Mastery and achievement: Guidelines using clinical problem solving with depressed elderly clients. *Physical and Occupational Therapy in Geriatrics*, 5, 35–46.

Smith, J., & Mairs, H. (2014). Use and Results of MOHO Global Assessments in Community Mental Health: A Practice Analysis. *Occupational Therapy in Mental Health, 30*, 381–389.

Smith, N., Kielhofner, G., & Watts, J. (1986). The relationship between volition, activity pattern and life satisfaction in the elderly. *The American Journal of Occupational Therapy, 40*, 278–283.

Smith, R. O. (1992). The science of occupational therapy assessment. *Occupational Therapy Journal of Research, 12*(1), 3–15.

Smith, T., Drefus, A., & Hersch, G. (2011). Habits, routines, and roles of graduate students: Effects of hurricane Ike. *Occupational Therapy in Health Care, 25*(4), 283–297.

Smyntek L. Barris R. Kielhofner G. (1985). The model of human occupation applied to psychosocially functional and dysfunctional adolescents. Occupational Therapy in Mental Health, 5(1), 21–39.

Spadone, R. A. (1992). Internal-external control and temporal orientation among Southeast Asians and white Americans. *The American Journal of Occupational Therapy, 46*(8), 713–719.

Stamm, T. A., Cieza, A., Machold, K., Smolen, J. S., & Stucki, G. (2006). Exploration of the link between conceptual occupational therapy models and the International Classification of Functioning, Disability and Health. *Australian Occupational Therapy Journal, 53*, 9–17.

Stein, F., & Cutler, S. (1998). Theoretical models underlying the clinical practices of psychosocial occupational therapy. In: F. Stein & S. K. Cutler, (Eds.), *Psychological occupational therapy: A holistic approach* (pp. 150–152). San Diego, CA: Singular.

Stofell, V. (1992). The Americans with Disabilities Act of 1990 as applied to an adult with alcohol dependence. *The American Journal of Occupational Therapy, 46*, 640–644.

Sudsawad, P. (2003, October 24). *Rehabilitation practitioners' perspectives on research utilization for evidence-based practice.* Paper presented at the American Congress of Rehabilitation Medicine conference, Tucson, AZ.

Sviden, G. A., Tham, K., & Borell, L. (2004). Elderly participants of social and rehabilitative day centres. *Scandinavian Journal of Caring Sciences, 18*(4), 402–409.

Tatham, M. (1992). Leisure facilitator: The role of the occupational therapist in senior housing. *Journal of Housing for the Elderly, 10*(112), 125–138.

Tayar, S. G. (2004). Description of a substance abuse relapse prevention program conducted by occupational therapy and psychology graduate students in a United States women's prison. *British Journal of Occupational Therapy, 67*, 159–166.

Taylor, M. C. (1997). What is evidence-based practice? *British Journal of Occupational Therapy, 60*, 470–474.

Taylor, R., Kielhofner, G., Smith, C., Butler, S., Cahill, S., Ciukaj, M., et al. (2009). Volitional change in children with autism: A single-case design study of the impact of hippotherapy on motivation. *Occupational Therapy in Mental Health, 25*, 192–200.

Taylor, R., O'Brien, J., Kielhofner, G., Lee, S., Katz, B., & Mears, C. (2010). The occupational and quality of life consequences of chronic fatigue syndrome/myalgic encephalomyelitis in young people. *The British Journal of Occupational Therapy, 73*(11), 524–530.

Taylor, R. R., Fisher, G., & Kielhofner, G. (2005). Synthesizing research, education, and practice according to the scholarship of practice model: Two faculty examples. *Occupational Therapy in Health Care, 19*(112), 107–122. R. R., Fisher, G., & Kielhofner, G. (2006). Synthesizing research, education, and practice according to the scholarship of practice model: two faculty examples. *Occupational Therapy in Health Care,* 107–122.

Taylor, R. R., Fisher, G., & Kielhofner, G. (2006). Synthesizing research, education, and practice according to the scholarship of practice model: two faculty examples. *Occupational Therapy in Health Care,* 107–122.

Taylor, R. R., Kielhofner, G., Abelenda, J., Colantuono, K., Fong, R., & Heredia, R. (2003). An approach to persons with chronic fatigue syndrome based on the Model of Human Occupation, part 1: Impact on occupational performance and participation. *Occupational Therapy in Health Care, 17*, 47–62.

Taylor, R. R., & Kielhofner, G. W. (2003). An occupational therapy approach to persons with chronic fatigue syndrome, part 2: Assessment and intervention. *Occupational Therapy in Health Care, 17*, 63–88.

Tham, K., & Borell, L. (1996). Motivation for training: a case study of four persons with unilateral neglect. *Occupational Therapy in Health Care, 10*(3), 65–79.

Tham, K., & Kielhofner, G. (2003). Impact of the social environment on occupational experience and performance among persons with unilateral neglect. *The American Journal of Occupational Therapy, 57*, 403–412.

Tham, K., Borell, L., & Gustavsson, A. (2000). The discovery of disability: A phenomenological study of unilateral neglect. *The American Journal of Occupational Therapy, 54*, 398–406.

Thomas, A., & Law, M. (2013). Research utilization and evidence-based practice in occupational therapy: A scoping study. *The American Journal of Occupational Therapy, 67*(4), E55–E65.

Tickle-Degnen, L., & Bedell, G. (2003). Heterarchy and hierarchy: A critical appraisal of the "levels of evidence" as a tool for clinical decision-making. *The American Journal of Occupational Therapy, 57*, 234–237.

Todorova, L. (2008). Assessing employment needs of Bulgarian youths with intellectual impairments. *Occupational Therapy in Health Care, 22*(2–3), 77–84.

Toit, S. (2008). Using the model of human occupation to conceptualize an occupational therapy program for blind persons in South Africa. *Occupational Therapy in Health Care, 22*(2–3), 51–61.

Townsend, S. C., Carey, P. D., Hollins, N. L., Helfrich, C., Blondis, M., Hoffman, A., et al. (2001). *The Occupational Therapy Psychosocial Assessment of Learning (OT PAL)* [Version 1.0]. Chicago: Model of Human Occupation Clearinghouse, Department of Occupational Therapy, University of Illinois at Chicago.

Tse, S., Blackwood, K., & Penman, M. (2001). From rhetoric to reality: Use of randomised controlled trials in evidence-based occupational therapy. *Australian Occupational Therapy Journal, 47*, 181–185.

Turner, N., & Lydon, C. (2008). Psychosocial programming in Ireland based on the model of human occupation: a program evaluation study. *Occupational Therapy in Health Care, 22*(2–3), 105–114.

Velozo, C. A. (1993). Work evaluations: Critique of the state of the art of functional assessment of work. *The American Journal of Occupational Therapy, 47*, 203–209.

Velozo, C. A., Kielhofner, G., Gern, A., Lin, F. L., Lai, J., & Fischer, G. (1999). Worker role interview: Toward validation of a psychosocial work-related measure. *Journal of Occupational Rehabilitation, 9*, 153–168.

Venable, E., Hanson, C., Shechtman, O., & Dasler, P. (2000). The effects of exercise on occupational functioning in the well elderly. *Physical and Occupational Therapy in Geriatrics, 17* (4), 29–42.

Viik, M. K., Watts, J., Madigan, M. J., & Bauer, D. (1990). Preliminary validation of the Assessment of Occupational Functioning with an alcoholic population. *Occupational Therapy in Mental Health, 70*(2), 19–33.

Wallenbert, I., & Jonsson, H. (2005). Waiting to get better: A dilemma regarding habits in daily occupations after stroke. *The American Journal of Occupational Therapy, 59*, 218–224.

Watson, M.A., & Ager, C. L. (1991). The impact of role valuation and performance on life satisfaction in old age. *Physical and Occupational Therapy in Geriatrics, 10*(1), 27–48.

Watts, J. H., Brollier, C., Bauer, D., & Schmidt, W. (1989). A comparison of two evaluation instruments used with psychiatric patients in occupational therapy. *Occupational Therapy in Mental Health, 8*, 7–27.

Watts, J. H., Hinson, R., Madigan, M. J., McGuigan, P. M., & Newman, S. M. (1999). The Assessment of Occupational Functioning: Collaborative version. In B. J. Hempill-Pearson (Ed.), *Assessments in occupational therapy in mental health*. Thorofare, NJ: Slack.

Watts, J., Brollier, C., Bauer, D., & Schmidt, W. (1989). The Assessment of Occupational Functioning: The second revision. *Occupational Therapy in Mental Health*, 8 (4), 61–87.

Watts, J. H., Brollier, C., Bauer, D., & Schmidt, W. (1989). A comparison of two evaluation instruments used with psychiatric patients in occupational therapy. *Occupational Therapy in Mental Health, 8*, 7–27.

Watts, J. H., Kielhofner, G., Bauer, D., Gregory, M., & Valentine, D. (1986). The assessment of occupational functioning: A screening tool for use in long- term care. *The American Journal of Occupational Therapy, 40*(4), 231–240.

Weeder, T. (1986). Comparison of temporal patterns and meaningfulness of the daily activities of schizophrenic and normal adults. *Occupational Therapy in Mental Health, 6*(4), 27 45.

Wei-Ling, H., Ay-Woan, P., & Tsyr-Jang, C. (2008). A psychometric study of the Chinese version of the assessment of communication and interaction skills. *Occupational Therapy in Health Care, 22*(2–3), 177–185.

Weissenberg, R., & Giladi, W. (1989). Home economics day: A program for disturbed adolescents to pro mote acquisition of habits and skills. *Occupational Therapy in Mental Health, 9*(2), 89–103.

Widen-Holmqvist, L., de Pedro-Cuesta, J., Holm, M., Sandsrom, B., Hellblom, A., Stawiarz, L., et al. (1993). Stroke rehabilitation in Stockholm. Basis for late intervention in patients living at home. *Scandinavian Journal of Rehabilitation Medicine, 25*(4), 173–181.

Wienringa, N., & McColl, M. (1987). Implications of the model of human occupation for intervention with native Canadians. *Occupational Therapy in Health Care, 4*(1), 73–91.

Williams, A., Fossey, E., & Harvey, C. (2010). Sustaining employment in a social firm: Use of the Work Environment Impact Scale v2.0 to explore views of employees with psychiatric disabilities. *The British Journal of Occupational Therapy, 73*(11), 531–539.

Wimpenny, K., Forsyth, K., Jones, C., Matheson, L., & Colley, J. (2010). Implementing the Model of Human Occupation across a mental health occupational therapy service: Communities of practice and a participatory change process. *The British Journal of Occupational Therapy, 73*(11), 507–516.

Woodrum, S. C. (1993). A treatment approach for attention deficit hyperactivity disorder using the model of human occupation. *Developmental Disabilities Special Interest Section Newsletter, 16*(1), 5–12.

Yamada, T., Kawamata, H., Kobayashi, N., Kielhofner, G., & Taylor, R. (2010). A randomised clinical trial of a wellness programme for healthy older people. *The British Journal of Occupational Therapy, 73*(11), 540–548.

Yazdani, F. (2011). How students with low level subjective wellbeing perceive the impact of the environment on occupational behaviour. *International Journal of Therapy and Rehabilitation*, 18(8), 462–469.

Yazdani, F., Jibril, M., & Kielhofner, G. (2008). A study of the relationship between variables from the model of human occupation and subjective well-being among university students in Jordan. *Occupational Therapy in Health Care, 22*(2–3), 125–138.

Yeager, J. (2000). Functional implications of substance use disorders. *Occupational Therapy Practice, 5*, 36–39.

Yelton, D., & Nielson, C. (1991). Understanding Appalachian values. Implications for occupational therapists. *Occupational Therapy in Mental Health, 11*(213), 173–195.

Yong, A., & Price, L. (2014). The human occupational impact of partner and close family caregiving in dementia: A meta-synthesis of the qualitative research, using a bespoke quality appraisal tool. *The British Journal of Occupational Therapy, 77*(8), 410–421.

Zimmerer-Branum, S., & Nelson, D. (1994). Occupationally embedded exercise versus rote exercise: A choice between occupational forms by elderly nursing home residents. *The American Journal of Occupational Therapy, 49*(5), 397–402.

Ziv, N., & Roitman, D. (2008). Addressing the needs of elderly clients whose lives have been compounded by traumatic histories. *Occup Ther Health Occupational Therapy in Health Care, 22*(2–3), 85–93.

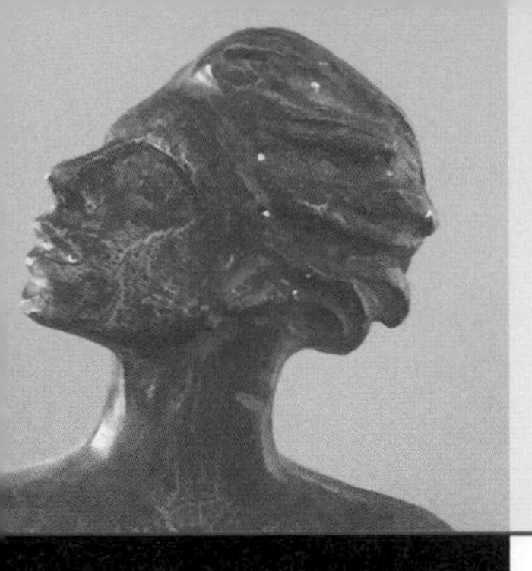

The Model of Human Occupation, the ICF, and the Occupational Therapy Practice Framework: Connections to Support Best Practice around the World

Lena Haglund, Patricia Bowyer, Patricia J. Scott, and Renée R. Taylor

CHAPTER 26

EXPECTED LEARNING OUTCOMES

Upon completion of this chapter, readers will be able to:

1. Compare and contrast elements of the Model of Human Occupation (MOHO) with the International Classification of Functioning, Disability and Health (ICF).
2. Understand the elements of MOHO that are incorporated into the American Occupational Therapy Association's Occupational Therapy Practice Framework.
3. Understand critical points of divergence between a conceptual practice model and a framework for classification.
4. Link elements from the ICF and MOHO with a range of other assessments based on MOHO, including the Model of Human Occupation Screening Tool, the Short Child Occupational Profile, and the Role Checklist Version 3.

Almost since its inception, the Model of Human Occupation (MOHO) has been used by international therapists working in a variety of contexts. These therapists work in settings that may also use classification frameworks to organize rehabilitation and/or occupational therapy service provision. Two of the most widely influential frameworks within the field of occupational therapy are:

- the International Classification of Functioning, Disability and Health (ICF) and
- the American Occupational Therapy Association's (AOTA) Occupational Therapy Practice Framework.

This chapter briefly describes the ICF and the AOTA Occupational Therapy Practice Framework and discusses how MOHO is aligned with them to support practitioners who use MOHO along with these frameworks. It also demonstrates how MOHO concepts and assessments may be used to deepen and inform aspects of these frameworks. The given examples can serve as suggestions on how to implement MOHO in conjunction with these classification frameworks.

In the case of the ICF, the framework has been decided through consensus of a team of professionals at the workplace or by the health care service providers and organizers. In the case of the OT Practice Framework, similarities would be drawn within the field of occupational therapy. Despite the differences, a therapist choosing to use MOHO needs to develop an awareness of how MOHO is related to these classification frameworks and how it offers some practical tools to use with clients. Therefore, it is the purpose of this chapter to demonstrate how to think about MOHO in relation to classification frameworks, providing pragmatic ideas that facilitate the practice of occupational therapy using MOHO in settings that ascribe to a predetermined classification framework.

The International Classification of Function, Disability and Health

The development of the international classification was started by the World Health Organization (WHO) in 1973 and, in 2001, the most recent final draft was adopted by the WHO with the title "International Classification of Function, Disability and Health (ICF)."

The ICF defines health and health-related components of well-being. The aim is to provide a common basis for both understanding health conditions and a language that can be used between different professions in the social and health care area. The ICF is intended for use by a myriad of stakeholders including researchers, policy makers, and persons with disabilities. It enables international comparison of health conditions. Furthermore, it is intended for application at both the individual and population levels. The ICF is complementary to the *ICD-10* (*International Classification of Diseases*, 10th revision, 2015). Where the *ICD-10* classifies health conditions such as diseases and disorders, ICF classifies functioning and disability. They both belong to the WHO family of international classifications.

In contrast to other major approaches, such as the medical model, which understands disability as being caused by illness and requiring medical care, and the social model, which sees disability as a socially created problem, the ICF integrates aspects of these two opposing models. The ICF uses a biopsychosocial approach. A person's health condition and its consequences, for example, specific activities, are understood through a dynamic interaction between personal health factors and contextual factors.

Since the ICF is a classification framework, it is well structured in the way it is organized. It comprises two parts, each with two components. The first part provides information concerning functioning and disability. It contains the components "Body Functions and Body Structures" and "Activities and Participation." Body Functions are the physiological functions of the body, including psychological functions, and Body Structures are the anatomical parts of the body. Activities represent the execution of actions and tasks by the person, and Participation describes involvement in a life situation.

The second part covers the contextual factors and contains the components "Environmental Factors" and "Personal Factors." Environmental Factors include the physical, social, and attitudinal environment around the person. The Personal Factors include gender, race, age, lifestyle, habits, etc. However, Personal Factors are not classified in the current version of ICF despite their significant influence on health conditions. If needed, the users of the ICF can decide to incorporate them in their applications of ICF (Table 26-1).

The components are divided into chapters, domains, and categories. The component "Activities and Participation" includes, for example, nine chapters. The component "Environmental Factors" includes five chapters. The ICF comprises over 1800 categories describing different health-related states, which are structured at domains and different levels in accordance with their different components. Except for Body Structures, every category has a written definition.

The classification is built based on the specific component code; b = body functions, s = body structures, d = activities and participation, and e = environment. Each code is followed by a numeric code representing the chapter number. Additional levels of specification are represented with digits for each level, as shown in Table 26-2.

Each category can also be provided with a qualifier, which describes the extent to which a problem exists or not. The qualifiers vary depending on the component, but all components use the same generic scale: No, Mild, Moderate, Severe, and Complete problem. There are two additional qualifiers for "Unspecified" and "Not applicable." Without using qualifiers, the information of the categories is reduced according to the WHO. It will only provide a definition of the categories included. However, sometimes, that is enough. The vocabulary of ICF gives the professions and the client a language to use. Using such a classification can avoid many misunderstandings in communication, both written and verbal, when all of the providers serving the client have the opportunity to have the same interpretation of central concepts related to health. Furthermore, the ICF does not measure or classify a person; it is a classification and description of health and health-related states in the context in which the person lives.

The ICF is very complex to use in practice. The daily work of practitioners does not require the use of all categories defined in the ICF when describing the clients' health conditions. Therefore, Core Sets have been developed (ICF-CSs). In a Core Set, the most relevant categories that are characteristic for a special condition or diagnosis have been selected by a systematic process such as a Delphi process, or through experts and/or consensus conference. More than 30 core sets are available that are related to different diagnoses such as depression, low back pain, and children and youth with cerebral palsy. Core sets are available for vocational rehabilitation as well (Core Sets, 2015).

The WHO has started to develop the International Classification of Health Interventions (ICHI). The ICHI is a systematic way to describe health interventions covering surgical and other health-related care services. It covered a wide range of interventions taken for investigative, curative, and preventive purposes.

Table 26-1 Term and Structure in ICF

Part 1 Function and Disability		Part 2 Contextual Factor	
Body structures Body functions	Activities and participation	Environmental factors	Personal factors

Table 26-2 Example of the ICF structure from the Component, Activities and Participation

Code	Description
d5	Chapter 5, Self-care
d510	Washing oneself
d5100	Washing body parts
d5101	Washing whole body
d5102	Drying oneself

The ICHI is professions neutral. The classification also includes occupational therapy interventions. It belongs to the WHO family of international classifications and is complementary to the ICF. The interventions are described using three axes: target, action, and means (International Classification of Health Interventions, 2015).

The ICF has been used for more than 15 years and many countries have adopted it. It has been used in research and, in many countries, health care service providers and organizers have decided to use the ICF as the common documentation language for medical record systems. In Sweden, the National Board of Health and Welfare recommends that the professionals evaluating eligibility for sickness/disability benefits use selected categories from the ICF when describing the clients' situation. It is not always enough to have a diagnosed disease on the certification.

ICF: LIMITATIONS

Even if it is shown that the ICF is a useful tool, it is important to consider its limitations. Some have argued that the ICF lacks focus on the subjective experience of meaning that affects the individual's experience of autonomy and self-determination, which are important aspects of the experience of participation (Hemmingsson & Jonsson, 2005; Nordenfelt, 2006). However, it is mentioned in the classification that a qualifier in which the clients themselves express their experience and subjective satisfaction with, for example, "Activities and Participation" can be developed. Such a development has been done in a pilot study in the mental health area with supported results (Haglund & Fältman, 2012). Nordenfelt also expresses skepticism of the qualifier of performance. The person's willingness to perform the activities is lacking, and since human activity is always carried out in a context, and the environment influences whether or not the performance is successful, he suggests a qualifier of *opportunity* instead of *performance*.

Furthermore, it is important to reduce the risk that the ICF will only be used from the perspective of the professional. One main limitation is that the ICF does not prescribe how to collect information in order to describe health and health-related states. By using different methods for gathering information such as observation, interviews, and self-assessment, a broad perspective on the clients' health states can be collected. The ICF would need to be applied in occupational therapy in such a way that the subjective meaning of each individual is incorporated. A client-centered approach must always be prioritized. Any classification would need to be a tool that is easily used by both the occupational therapist and the client.

Another limitation is that the ICF includes the two concepts of "Activities and Participation" in the same component. The component contains activities at many levels of complexity, with some being much more demanding than the others. The classification is formed according to a structure built on categories rather than on the complexity of the actions and activities. Additionally, there is no clarity on how to distinguish between activities and participation for each category in the component.

Furthermore, from an occupational therapy perspective, the environment is regarded as multifaceted and complex, and its influence on the individual is a crucial issue (Hemmingsson & Jonsson, 2005). It cannot, as in the ICF, be seen as a facilitator or barrier. It might be both for one person at the same time. And, the last concern, gender, habits, and social background are among the factors that influence human occupation. Because these and other personal variables are not classified in the ICF, occupational therapists must add that kind of knowledge into their therapeutic reasoning.

THE RELATIONSHIP BETWEEN MOHO AND ICF

There are many health assessments developed over the years, some more generic and some more specific, including a wide range of occupational therapy assessments. To understand the relationship between any assessment and the ICF, a linking approach can be used. The aim with such an approach is to identify how the central concepts in an assessment correspond to components, domains, and category/categories of the ICF.

As described above, the ICF is a common framework in the social and health sectors, promoting a common language in order to improve interprofessional communication. Therefore, it is important to clarify how conceptual practice models and assessments that occupational therapist use in their daily work are related to the ICF. Cieza et al. (2005) described a structured method of linking the concepts between frameworks along with the quality of the relationship. By using a linking approach, occupational therapy practice using MOHO and MOHO-based assessments facilitates understanding and increased acceptance of MOHO by professionals outside occupational therapy.

There are several similarities between MOHO and the ICF. Some ways in which the MOHO and ICF are aligned include:

- Both MOHO and the ICF recognize the centrality of participation and activity as an outcome.
- Both MOHO and the ICF recognize that health conditions can alter a person's activity and participation.

- Both MOHO and the ICF recognize that individual characteristics and the environment determine participation and activity.
- Both MOHO and the ICF recognize that these various factors influence each other in a dynamic and nonlinear way.

MOHO concepts align with the ICF in different ways and at different levels of specificity. The relationship between chapters, domains, and categories is listed next to complementary MOHO concepts in Table 26-3. As noted in the table, the MOHO concept, *volition*, is aligned with the ICF category "b.1301 Motivation" in Chapter 1, "Mental functions, Body Functions." Motivation, which the ICF defines as the "incentive to act" and "the conscious or unconscious driving force for action," shares some similarities with the MOHO concept of a volitional drive to act. In other cases, it is more than one category in the ICF that corresponds to MOHO. For example, "Communication and Interaction Skills" corresponds to two components: "Body Functions" and "Activities and Participation." It can also be hard to find adequate and reasonable relationships. As Stamm, Cieza, Machold, Smolen, and Stucki (2006) and Kielhofner (2008) identified, MOHO is not perfectly aligned with the ICF. However, this is not surprising. MOHO is an occupational therapy–based practice model aiming to offer an understanding of the nature of human occupation. It emphasizes the understanding of how, when, and why humans engage in occupations. The ICF is a classification system for describing health and health-related states. Despite the different purposes and applications of MOHO and the ICF, occupational therapists need to be prepared to work in an ICF context, particularly in countries where it is used more frequently.

The profession-specific model of MOHO and its related assessments and occupational therapy language cannot be replaced by using the ICF classification (Haglund & Henriksson, 2003). The profession-specific language should be used as a complement to the ICF. Also, Schell, Gillen, and Scaffe (2014) stress the use of occupational therapy language when applying the ICF. As the ICF is most likely going to be a common language, occupational therapists should be well acquainted with the categories in the ICF that pertain to their special areas of practice. It is important to note that the ICF lacks certain categories to describe what occupational therapists need to communicate

Table 26-3 ICF Components, Domains, and Categories Related to MOHO Concepts

ICF Components	ICF Domains and Categories	MOHO Concepts
Body functions	*Chapter 1. Mental functions*	
	b1140 Orientation to time	Habituation
	b117 Intellectual functions	Performance capacity
	b1266 Confidence	Personal causation
	b1301 Motivation	Volition
	b122 Global psychosocial functions b140 Attention b164 Higher-level cognitive functions b167 Mental functions of language	Communication and interaction skills
	b164 Higher-level cognitive functions	Process skills
	b176 Mental functions of sequencing complex movements	Motor and process skills
	Chapter 2. Sensory functions and pain	Objective and subjective aspects of performance capacity
	Chapter 3. Voice and speech functions	
	b320 Articulation b330 Fluency and rhythm of speech b340 Alternative vocalization functions	Communication and interaction skills
	Chapter 7. Neuromusculoskeletal and movement-related functions	Objective aspects of performance capacity
	b760 Control of voluntary movement functions	Motor skills
Body structures		Objective aspects of performance capacity

(continued)

Table 26-3 ICF Components, Domains, and Categories Related to MOHO Concepts (*continued*)

ICF Components	ICF Domains and Categories	MOHO Concepts
Activities and Participation	*Chapter1. Learning and applying knowledge*	
	d110 Watching d115 Listening	Communication and interaction skills
	Applying knowledge (d160–d170)	Process skills
	Chapter 2. General tasks and demands	
	d210 Undertaking a single task d220 Undertaking multiple tasks	Process skills
	d2103 Undertaking a single task in a group d2203 Undertaking multiple tasks in a group	Communication and interaction skills Process skills Social and occupational demands of the environment
	d230 Carrying out daily routine d2400 Handling responsibilities	Habituation
	Chapter 3. Communication	
	d330 Speaking d335 Producing nonverbal messages d350 Conversation d355 Discussion d360 Using communication devices and techniques	Communication and interaction skills
	Chapter 4 Mobility	
	Changing and maintaining body position (d410–d429) Carrying, moving, and handling objects (d430–d449) Walking and moving (d450–d469)	Motor skills
	Moving around using transportation (d470–d489)	Occupational competence
	Chapter 5. Self-care	Occupational performance
	Chapter 6. Domestic life	Occupational performance Occupational competence Occupational identity
	d620 Acquisition of goods and services Household tasks (d630–d649) Caring for household objects and assisting others (d650–d669)	Skills (process, motor, and communication and interaction)
	Chapter 7. Interpersonal interactions and relationships	
	General interpersonal interactions (d710–d729) Particular interpersonal relationships (d730–d779)	Communication and interaction skills
	Particular interpersonal relationships (d730–d779)	Communication and interaction skills Roles
	Chapter 8. Major life areas	Occupational participation
	Chapter 9. Community, social, and civic life	
	d910 Community life d920 Recreation and leisure d930 Religion and spirituality d950 Political life and citizenship	Occupational participation Occupational competence Occupational identity

Table 26-3 ICF Components, Domains, and Categories Related to MOHO Concepts (*continued*)

ICF Components	ICF Domains and Categories	MOHO Concepts
Environmental Factors	*Chapter 1. Products and technology*	Physical environment (objects and spaces)
	Chapter 2. Natural environment and human-made changes to the environment	
	e210 Physical geography e220 Flora and fauna e225 Climate e240 Light e250 Sound e260 Air quality	Physical environment (objects and spaces)
	Chapter 3. Support and Relationships	Social environment (Social groups)
	Chapter 4. Attitudes	Social environment (Social groups)
	e460 Societal attitudes e465 Social norms, practices, and ideologies	Culture
	Chapter 5. Services, Systems, and Policies	Political conditions of the environment Economic conditions of the environment

to clients and colleagues and other professions in everyday practice.

Linking MOHO-Based Assessments to ICF

MOHO-based assessments allow for a good amount of consistency with the ICF. This may help occupational therapists to use and interpret results from MOHO-based assessments within the context of a multidisciplinary team that is using the ICF as a guiding framework.

LINKING THE ASSESSMENT OF COMMUNICATION AND INTERACTION SKILLS TO THE ICF

The Assessment of Communication and Interaction Skills

The Assessment of Communication and Interaction Skills (ACIS; Haglund & Kjellberg, 2012) is an observational assessment that measures a client's occupational performance within a social group. The assessment allows for the determination of the client's strengths and weaknesses when communicating and relating with others during the course of one or more daily occupations. More information about the ACIS is provided in Chapter 15, which covers observational assessments.

A linking project between the ACIS and the ICF was made by two occupational therapists in Sweden who knew the assessment, the MOHO and the ICF, well (Haglund & Kjellberg, 2012). First, they separately completed an analysis based on comparing the definitions of the 20 items in the ACIS with equivalent categories in the ICF. Subsequently, they discussed and compared the two analyses until a consensus was reached. The process for the linking was inspired by content analysis and the rules presented by Cieza and colleagues in 2005.

The linking of the ACIS to the ICF shows that the ACIS is related to the components "Body Functions and Activities" and "Participation." All skill items in the ACIS are represented similarly in the ICF (Table 26-4). Five of these items are linked to the ICF component "Body Function." Furthermore, "Focuses and Modulates" are linked to two ICF categories within the component "Activities and Participation," in which 18 ACIS items are linked. Two of them, Collaboration and Speaks, are linked to two ICF categories in the component. Furthermore, these two items are also related to categories in Body Functions. Concerning the ICF category d360, "Using Communication Devices and Techniques, information can be noted on the ACIS Summary form as background data. And, depending on whom the person is collaborating with within the domain, "d730 to d779," Particular Interpersonal Relationships, can be linked.

Since the ACIS includes skills items, it is easier to find and relate the ICF categories on more detailed levels than what is presented in Table 26-3. The additional specifications are presented in brackets in Table 26-4.

Similarities found within this linking exercise can be investigated more deeply, for example, by evaluating how well each category within the ICF and each

Table 26-4 Relation between ICF (Domains and Categories) and ACIS Items

ICF	ACIS
Body Functions	
Chapter 1 Mental functions	
b140 Attention functions	Focuses
b164 Higher-level cognitive functions	Collaborates Focuses
b167 Mental functions of language	Speaks
Chapter 3 Voice and speech functions	
b320 Articulation functions	Articulates
b330 Fluency and rhythm of speech functions	Modulates
b340 Alternative vocalization functions	Modulates
Activities and Participation	
Chapter 1 Learning and applying knowledge	
d110 Watching	Gazes
Chapter 2 General tasks and demands	
d2103 Undertaking a single task in a group	Collaborates Focuses
d2203 Undertaking multiple tasks in a group	Collaborates Focuses
Chapter 3 Communication	
d330 Speaking	Speaks
d335 Producing nonverbal messages	Gestures
d350 Conversation	Asks Engages (d3500 Starting a conversation) Speaks Sustains (d3501 Sustaining a conversation)
d355 Discussion	Asserts
d360 Using communication devices and techniques	Information about this is described on the Summary form in the ACIS
Chapter 7 Interpersonal interactions and relationships	
General interpersonal interactions, d710–d729	Contacts (d7105 Physical contact in relationships) Maneuvers (d7204 Social cues in relationships) Orients Postures Expresses Shares Conforms Relates (d7101 Appreciation in relationships) Respects
Particular interpersonal relationships, d730–d779	Depending on who the person is collaborating with, these categories may be relevant

corresponding ACIS item are related to each other by using a 4-point scale (The Sweden National Board of Health and Welfare, 2015).

The results of this linking exploration with the ACIS show that there are gaps between the definition of the skills items in the ACIS and related definitions of categories in the ICF. For example, the items, Collaboration and Speaks, in the ACIS are linked to two categories in the components, Activities and Participation, and Body Functions. It is possible that this result indicates that the ACIS offers a more specialized terminology than the ICF, reflecting the language of an underlying conceptual practice model that is specific to the field of occupational therapy. It can be argued that our profession needs this language in order to better observe and describe a person's skill level in terms of communicating and interacting with others.

The ACIS is an observational assessment where each item is assessed separately. However, it can be a little bit more difficult to compare and contrast an assessment that uses a semi-structure interviewing for gathering information. Additionally, assessments that measure the MOHO concepts, more broadly, are more difficult to link to the ICF. For example, the MOHO concept of volition includes the aspect of personal causation, which refers to one's sense of personal capacity and self-efficacy. During the interview, the client may talk about much more than only the concept of personal causation when one asks the recommended questions: "What is the most difficult thing for you at the moment?" In response, the client may not only provide information related to ICF category b1266 Confidence, but may also give information "Interpersonal interactions and relationships" (see Table 26-3). In such a case, ICF categories under Chapter 7 can be reported even if the aim was not to gather such information. This is another example of how MOHO and ICF are not interchangeable, but they have several similarities.

LINKING THE MODEL OF HUMAN OCCUPATIONAL SCREENING TOOL (MOHOST) TO THE ICF

Below another example of linking a MOHO-based assessment to the ICF is presented. In this case, the Swedish version of MOHOST has been used (Haglund, 2014). The MOHOST is a multidimensional measure that may be administered in semi-structured interview format or as an observational assessment. Responses may be recorded from the perspective of the client, caregiver, or provider. Information from chart notes may also be incorporated into the MOHOST. The MOHOST measures the client's occupational performance and participation from all dimensions of MOHO: volition (motivation for occupation), habituation (pattern of occupation), performance capacity (communication and interaction skills, process skills, and motor skills), and environment. Table 26-5 presents findings from a comparison between the ICF domains and categories and MOHOST items.

Table 26-5 Relation between ICF (Domains and Categories) and MOHOST Item

ICF	MOHOST
Body Functions	
Chapter 1 Mental functions	
b1400 Orientation to time	Routine
b117 Intellectual functions	Knowledge
b1266 Confidence	Appraisal of ability Expectation of success
b1301 Motivation	Appraisal of ability Expectation of success
b140 Attention	Timing
b164 Higher-level cognitive functions	Adaptability Timing Organization Problem-solving
b167 Mental functions of language	Conversation Vocal expression
b176 Mental functions of sequencing complex movements	Coordination
Chapter 3 Voice and speech functions	
b320 Articulation functions	Vocal expression
b330 Fluency and rhythm of speech functions	Vocal expression
b340 Alternative vocalization functions	Vocal expression

(continued)

Table 26-5 Relation between ICF (Domains and Categories) and MOHOST Item (*continued*)

ICF	MOHOST
Chapter 7. Neuromusculoskeletal and movement-related functions	
b760 Control of voluntary movement functions	Posture and mobility Coordination
Activities and Participation	
Chapter 1 Learning and applying knowledge	Adaptability Knowledge Timing Problem-solving
Chapter 2 General tasks and demands	
d210 Undertaking a single task	Knowledge Timing Organization Occupational demands
d2103 Undertaking a single task in a group	Relationships Knowledge Timing Organization Occupational demands
d220 Undertaking multiple tasks	Knowledge Timing Organization Coordination Occupational demands
d2203 Undertaking multiple tasks in a group	Relationships Knowledge Timing Organization Coordination Occupational demands
d230 Carrying out daily routine	Choices Routine Adaptability Responsibility
d2400 Handling responsibilities	Roles Responsibility
Chapter 3 Communication	
d350 Conversation	Conversation Vocal expression Relationships
Chapter 4 Mobility	
Changing and maintaining body position (d410–d429)	Posture and mobility
Carrying, moving, and handling objects (d430–d449)	Coordination Strength and effort Energy
Walking and moving (d450–d469)	Posture and mobility Coordination Energy
Chapter 5. Self-care	Depending on information gathering categories in this chapter can be used
Chapter 6. Domestic life	Depending on information gathering categories in this chapter can be used

Table 26-5 Relation between ICF (Domains and Categories) and MOHOST Item (*continued*)

ICF	MOHOST
Chapter 7 Interpersonal interactions and relationships	
General interpersonal interactions, d710–d729	Nonverbal skills Conversation Vocal expression Relationships
Particular interpersonal relationships, d730–d779	Nonverbal skills Conversation Vocal expression Relationships
Chapter 8. Major life areas	Depending on information gathering categories in this chapter can be used
Chapter 9. Community, social, and civic life	
d910 Community life	Interests Choices Roles Responsibility Social groups Occupation demands
d920 Recreation and leisure	Interests Choices Roles Responsibility Social groups Occupation demands
d930 Religion and spirituality	Interests Choices Roles Responsibility Social groups Occupation demands
d950 Political life and citizenship	Interests Choices Roles Responsibility Social groups Occupation demands
Environmental Factors	
Chapter 1. Products and technology	Physical space Physical resources
Chapter 2. Natural environment and human-made changes to the environment	
e210 Physical geography	Physical space
e220 Flora and fauna	Physical space
e225 Climate	Physical space
e240 Light	Physical space
e250 Sound	Physical space
e260 Air quality	Physical space
Chapter 3. Support and Relationships	Social groups
Chapter 4. Attitudes	
e460 Societal attitudes	Social groups Occupational demands
e465 Social norms, practices, and ideologies	Social groups Occupational demands
Chapter 5. Services, Systems, and Policies	Physical resources

In addition to drawing comparisons between the ICF and the broader aspects of MOHO, as reflected in the MOHOST, comparisons may be drawn between the ICF and other, more specific aspects of MOHO. For example, aspects of habituation, such as roles, can be compared.

LINKING THE ICF CONCEPT OF PARTICIPATION TO THE MOHO CONCEPT OF ROLE

The ICF considers participation or "involvement in a life situation" in the context of a person's environmental and personal factors. As mentioned previously, we recognize that the ICF and MOHO do not perfectly align; however, both in MOHO and the ICF, action and **activity** are essential for participation outcomes. MOHO describes how occupational skill and occupational performance underlie occupational participation, whereas the ICF discusses body functions and structures that underlie activities and participation.

Participation in occupational roles is an ideal way to capture "involvement with others in a life situation" (World Health Organization [WHO], 2001, p. 10) since roles represent the intersection of the individual's identity and societal status (Kielhofner, 2008). Although the definitions posed by the ICF and by the MOHO differ somewhat, they are complementary. This relationship between roles as a way to capture participation as defined by the ICF is supported in the literature (Scott, 2013). Given roles are the way we identify ourselves to the outside world, they convey a series of expectations and requirements for actions and carry with them an external and internal assessment of adequacy. People, for example, identify themselves to others, "I am a mother," "I am the brother of Henry," "I am a violinist." Take the role of a violinist. An individual may self-identify as a violinist and experience pride, yet others cringe when the person arrives at a social gathering with their instrument in tow. Alternatively, one may express a sense of inadequacy in their skill playing the violin, whereas others marvel at their skill and look forward to their performances. It is this self-assessment of performance, described earlier, that is problematic between the ICF and MOHO, as the model is inherently client centered, and the ICF strives to establish a common language that can be used to describe populations.

The Role Checklist (Oakley, Kielhofner, Barris, & Reichler, 1986) (refer to chapter 16 where information regarding Role Checklist can be found) measures role participation consistent with the MOHO. The Role Checklist was first published in 1986 and the ICF 15 years later, yet the relationship between the two is clear. Sections of Chapters 6 to 9 in the component Activities and Participation correspond directly to the ten roles included in the Role Checklist, that is, Chapter 6 Domestic Life corresponds to Caregiver and Home Maintainer; Chapter 7 Interpersonal Interactions and Relationships corresponds to Friend and Family Member; Chapter 8 Major Life Areas corresponds to Student, Worker, and Volunteer; and Chapter 9 Community, Social and Civic Life corresponds to Hobbyist, Participant in Organizations, and Religious Participant (Scott, McFadden, Yates, Baker, & McSoley, 2014). The Role Checklist provides a measure of the person's perception of past, present, and desired future role occupancy and the value associated with each of these ten roles.

Earlier we mentioned the lack of attention in the ICF to the client perspective, and how the client-centered MOHO values this self-perception of adequacy of performance. A second and now a third version of the Role Checklist, the Role Checklist Version 3 (RC v3), adds a measure of self-reported satisfaction with role performance and a way to identify unfulfilled roles the person currently wishes to be performing, thus strengthening it as a measure of participation. The RC v3 is discussed at length in Chapter 16.

CASE EXAMPLE: A YOUNG ADULT WITH PSYCHOSOCIAL CONCERNS

The RC v2:QP is relevant here to the case of Martin, as published by Aslaksen and colleagues (2014). Martin is a Norwegian male in his late 20s. Information from the patient record revealed that he lived with an aunt and had become gradually withdrawn over the last 2 years. He received a disability pension and had no particular occupations to structure his daily life. He had lost contact with his friends, and most of his time was spent at his computer where he engaged in online gaming and social media.

Martin completed the Role Checklist Version 3: Quality of Performance (RC v3:QP) with his occupational therapist, Maya. During the interview he provided elaborate answers and shared many experiences with the listed roles.

Martin had started but not completed secondary education because of social anxiety. Since then, he had gradually become more isolated, and during the last 2 years had not been outside his home except when he needed to go shopping. In this period of his life he moved in with his aunt for economic reasons. The aunt did most of the household chores, and he kept mostly to himself in his room. To achieve a certain level of social interaction he participated in social forums on

the Internet and had created several pseudonyms to be used in these. Because of things he had written in the Internet forums, he had a feeling that people disliked him and potentially would want to harm him. He had given up on leisure activities, like playing basketball. Eventually, he was afraid that he might accidentally run into friends and acquaintances, or that he might be recognized from his activities in social forums on the Internet.

Martin was motivated to change his lifestyle. He conveyed the desire to become more active with others around him, yet he was afraid that he would be disliked and dismissed. His RC v3 results are in Table 26-6. They revealed the following:

He considered that having the roles of student, volunteer, caregiver, and participant in organizations would be long-term goals, and thus, these roles were not addressed during his hospital stay. Martin indicated worker, friend, and hobbyist (sports participant) as roles he wanted to pursue now. He had arrived at an understanding of these roles as being crucial for his functioning in the valued role of participant in society. Martin did not want to commit to making serious changes in terms of his role participation, as making such changes was still too overwhelming. However, through the prioritization of roles on the RC v3, Martin successfully arranged for a meeting concerning future possibilities for work and he contacted some of his old friends and met with them twice during the following weeks. Maya was able to identify a ball-game group at the hospital as positive for Martin to participate in. However, as he had only been performing this role within the boundaries of the hospital, Maya and Martin discussed whether or not doing exercise activities at a local gym center might be an appropriate goal for him. This way, he could further develop his desired role of sports participant.

In the case of Martin, use of the RC v3 allowed Maya, his occupational therapist, to hone in on Martin's dissatisfaction with a valued and desired role: hobbyist. This role was important and he expressed dissatisfaction with it, thus rendering it safe. Martin's social phobia made it important to select a role that was familiar and valued—not too scary, and much desired. This illustrated how attention to a participation-focused approach enabled the occupational therapist to center treatment around the client goals.

Table 26-6 Martin's RC v3 Results and Implications for Therapeutic Intervention

Information Gathered from Parts 1 and 2 from the Role Checklist Version 3

Choices for Part 1—Satisfaction with Currently Performed Roles	Very dissatisfied	Somewhat dissatisfied	Satisfied	Very satisfied
Choices for Part 2—Desired participation for all roles not currently performing	Would like to be performing now	Satisfied waiting until later	No interest in this role	

Roles listed on RCV v3 with associated ICF areas	Response to Part 1 for currently performed roles or responses to Part 2 for all roles not currently performing	Therapeutic considerations and implications for treatment
Student (d8)	Satisfied waiting until later	Long-term goal
Worker (d8)	Satisfied waiting until later	Long-term goal
Volunteer (d8)	Satisfied waiting until later	Long-term goal
Caregiver (d6)	Satisfied waiting until later	Long-term goal
Home maintainer(d6)	Satisfied	Demands lowered while in the hospital
Friend (d7)	Would like to be performing now	Short-term goal
Family member (d7)	Satisfied	Reinforce
Hobbyist (d9)	Very dissatisfied	Needs to be focus of current intervention
Religious participant (d9)	Not interested	N/A
Participant in organizations(d9)	Satisfied waiting until later	Long-term goal

The AOTA Occupational Therapy Practice Framework and Its Relation to MOHO

The use of the AOTA Occupational Therapy Practice Framework (American Occupational Therapy Association [AOTA], 2014), hereinafter referred to as the *OTP Framework*, is to help occupational therapy practitioners have a formalized method to articulate the unique contributions of the profession for promotion of the health and well-being of populations and individuals served. The *OTP Framework* used concepts from MOHO to shape it. Therefore, MOHO is well aligned with it. This section defines the ways in which MOHO and the *OTP Framework* are aligned.

- The way the *OTP Framework* defines occupational therapy
- The specific practice domains for occupational therapists as defined by the OTP Framework

The *OTP Framework* has two major sections: *domain* and *process* and it states that occupational therapy consists of evaluation, intervention, and outcomes. This three-phase process corresponds with the MOHO therapeutic reasoning. MOHO's theory-driven method of therapeutic reasoning further supports occupational therapists in evaluation, intervention, and outcomes by describing specific actions that integrate theory into practice. The *OTP Framework* describes the actions practitioners undertake when working with populations and individuals. The process encompasses the evaluation, intervention, and targeted outcomes; it is client centered and focused on use of occupation. Table 26-7 shows how each step in the MOHO therapeutic reasoning is part of the larger occupational therapy process.

The *domain* outlines areas of practice as well as the areas of knowledge and expertise of the profession. Within the domain of occupational therapy there are *occupations*, *client factors*, *performance skills*, *performance patterns*, and *context or environments*. Each of these broad areas within the domain is aligned with the MOHO. Table 26-8 shows how central concepts

Table 26-7 Alignment of *OTP Framework Process* Steps and MOHO's Therapeutic Reasoning

OTP Framework Process Steps	MOHO Therapeutic Reasoning Steps
Evaluation	Use questions to guide information gathering
	Gather information on/with the client using structured and unstructured means
	Create a conceptualization of the client that includes strengths and challenges
Intervention	Generating goals and strategies for therapy
	Implementing and monitoring therapy
Outcomes	Determining outcomes of therapy

Table 26-8 Alignment of MOHO Concepts and *OTP Framework* Domains

OTP Framework Domain	Related MOHO Concept	Explanation of Alignment
Occupations	Occupational Participation Occupational Performance	The MOHO definition of participation mirrors the OTP Framework definition of performance in that they describe engagement in work, play, and leisure. However, MOHO additionally considers the tasks that support this engagement in larger life roles in the concept of occupational performance.
Performance skills, including: Communication/Interaction Skills Motor Skills Process Skills	Skills, including: Communication/Interaction Skills Motor Skills Process Skills	Both definitions define skill as something one does while engaging in a specific action. MOHO's definition more explicitly considers the impact the environment has on skill.

Table 26-8 Alignment of MOHO Concepts and OTP Framework Domains

OTP Framework Domain	Related MOHO Concept	Explanation of Alignment
Performance Patterns, including: Habits Roles	Habituation, including: Habits Internalized Role	Both definitions recognize routine and ritual as integral to performance patterns. Both MOHO and OTP Framework define habits as automatic responses that support performance. Both MOHO and OTP Framework recognize that roles are delineated by socially defined actions.
Context/Environment	Environment, including: Physical Environment Social Environment Tasks/Occupational Forms Environmental Impact Culture	MOHO considers the social and physical demands as an aspect of the environment, whereas the OTP Framework separates activity demands into its own domain separate from the environment. Both definitions recognize that the social groups, physical space, and culture influence the client context.
Client Factors	Performance capacity	MOHO concept of objective performance capacity is aligned with the OTP Framework' client factors. However, MOHO additionally considers the experience of living with specific capacities in the subjective performance capacity concept, lived body.

in the *OTP Framework* and MOHO are related to each other in order to facilitate understanding of the relationship. As can be seen the *OTP Framework* outlines five domains that occupational therapists may address to support participation in context.

Definitions of terms from the *OTP Framework* can be found in the glossary at the end of this chapter. Although MOHO concepts and the *OTP Framework* domains are highly similar because they share a focus on occupation and participation, the purpose of the *OTP Framework* is to describe the domain of practice, not to explain how and why occupational therapy clients have difficulty engaging in everyday life activities. As a result, MOHO definitions and *OTP Framework* domain definitions differ in their specificity, terminology, and scope. Therapists using MOHO can also use information from MOHO-based assessments to gather information relevant to the *OTP Framework* domains, as outlined in Table 26-9.

As MOHO-based assessments focus on participation rather than specific abilities, occupational therapists are able to evaluate the client's whole occupational performance and to better understand each client's unique occupational profile.

The *OTP Framework* calls for an approach that is guided by client-centered collaboration. Central to all other aspects of the *OTP Framework* is the client. The MOHO supports client centeredness because it views each client as a unique individual whose characteristics and context or environment determine the rationale and nature of therapy. Furthermore, Table 26-10 shows how each MOHO assessment allows for opportunities to support client-centered occupational therapy process.

Client-Centered Collaboration in the Assessment Process

When an assessment administration process requires the involvement of the client or the client's family or caregivers, an assessment can be said to support a formal collaboration. However, other MOHO assessments offer informal opportunities for occupational therapists to collaborate with clients, their family, and other professionals even if it is not a requirement for the assessment administration. This includes for example:

- Gathering additional information in interviews instead of relying only on observation during the administration of the MOHOST/Short Child Occupational Profile (SCOPE),
- Talking with a client and/or someone who cares about them in order to identify a meaningful

Table 26-9 Relation OTP Framework and MOHO-Based Assessments

Assessment	Occupational Performance	Occupational Skills	Performance Patterns	Context
ACIS	X	X		
AMPS	X	X		
Interest Checklist	X		X	
MOHOST/SCOPE	X	X	X	X
OCAIRS	X	X	X	X
OPHI-II	X		X	X
OQ/ACTRE	X		X	
OSA/COSA	X		X	X
OT PAL	X		X	
Role Checklist v3	X		X	
SSI	X			X
VQ/PVQ	X			X
WEIS	X			X
WRI	X		X	X

Table 26-10 Opportunities for Collaboration Using MOHO-Based Assessments

MOHO Assessment	Formal Collaboration Opportunities	Informal Collaboration Opportunities
ACIS		Selecting meaningful activity for observation with client
COSA	Client self-evaluation	Setting goals and intervention plan based on evaluation Sharing information with interdisciplinary team
MOHOST		Interview with client Interview with interdisciplinary team
OCAIRS	Interview with client	
OPHI-II	Interview with client	Creating narrative slope with client
OSA	Client self-evaluation, but may be administered Setting goals and intervention plan based on evaluation	Sharing information with interdisciplinary team
OT PAL	Teacher interview Parent take-home interview	Interview with student
PVQ		Working with interdisciplinary team to identify activities for observation
Role Checklist v3	Client self-evaluation	Collaborating with the client to describe participation. Sharing information with the interdisciplinary team
SCOPE	Teacher form Parent form	Interview with client Interview with parent Interview with classroom teacher Interview with interdisciplinary team

Table 26-10 Opportunities for Collaboration Using MOHO-Based Assessments (*continued*)

MOHO Assessment	Formal Collaboration Opportunities	Informal Collaboration Opportunities
SSI	Evaluation conducted in collaboration with student Interview with student Identifying solutions/accommodations with students	Working with interdisciplinary team to identify solutions/accommodations (i.e., teachers, other school support staff)
VQ		Working with interdisciplinary team to identify activities for observation
WEIS	Interview with client	Collaborate with client to request accommodations from employer
WRI	Interview with client	

activity that can be observed when administering the ACIS, and

- Sharing client self-report responses, such as OSA/COSA results, with other professionals during interdisciplinary meetings to ensure the client's voice is heard if they are absent.

Taking advantage of assessments that offer both formal and informal opportunities for collaboration supports best practice and ensures that the assessment and intervention planning process remains as client driven and centered as possible. Below, some example opportunities each assessment provides for collaboration are listed.

CASE EXAMPLE: A CHILD WITH BEHAVIORAL CONCERNS

Madge is a 6-year-old living in the United States with her mother, father, and four older siblings. She is in the first grade. When she began to work on writing letters and reading, it was noted that she refused to pick up a pencil and she would not open any books during reading. She would look out the window and become disruptive by trying to engage her classmate in conversation or play. The teacher is concerned because of this behavior. She has sought the assistant of the school occupational therapist because it appears the behavior is for no specific reason. The occupational therapist evaluated Madge using the Short Child Occupational Profile (SCOPE; Bowyer et al., 2008) in order to obtain an occupational profile on Madge. She observed her in the classroom, spoke with the teacher, and was able to send a parent from home to obtain information about how Madge functions outside the school environment.

Upon review of the data obtained from the teacher and parents as well as observations, the occupational therapist learned that at home Madge would attempt to pick up a pencil and write letters, but many of the letters were scribbles on a page and after a few scribbles Madge would throw the pencil down saying, "I don't want to do it." Or when her parents tried to help her read she would look at the pictures, point and name the pictures correctly, but would not attempt to read words. Madge would push the book away, begin to act silly, or jump up and run to play with her siblings or toys. This behavior was consistent with what the occupational therapist observed and was reported by the classroom teacher. Madge's parents and teacher are very concerned that Madge is falling behind and want to help her achieve the reading and writing goals expected of a first grader.

Based on the results of the SCOPE, the occupational therapist was able to determine that Madge was experiencing volitional issues with reading and writing, specifically with response to challenge. The occupational therapist decided to investigate this further by using a biomechanical assessment, Motor-Free Visual Perception Test and the Inventory of Reading of Occupations (Grajo, Candler, & Bowyer, 2015).

Using MOHO to guide therapeutic reasoning around occupational participation, the occupational therapist describes Madge as follows: Madge does not like to explore her writing or reading skills and does not respond well to challenges in these educational activities. She is beginning to exhibit behavioral issues when confronted with a reading or writing activity.

Using the OTP Framework, the following areas are impacted: Education-formal education participation and Social participation-community. Table 26-11 summarizes how this case fits with the MOHO and the OTP Framework.

Table 26-11 Results of Madge's Assessment Using MOHO and the *OTP Framework*

Madge's Problems	MOHO	OTP Framework
Reading	Performance capacity/ response to challenge	Education-formal education participation
Writing	Performance capacity/ response to challenge	Education-formal education participation
Loss of student role	Role loss	Social participation-community

CASE EXAMPLE: AN ELDERLY WOMAN WITH HEARING LOSS

Greta is 86 years old and has for the past 3 years experienced increased difficulties with hearing. She lives by herself in a small house in a suburb. She does not like to ask people repeat what they say. Therefore, in order to hear what people say she prefers close physical contact when interacting with others. However, she often perceives others to be uncomfortable with close physical contact. She finds that she has said "yes" even if she had not heard the question. She finds herself more and more alone, she does not invite friends to visit as she did before, and she is not visiting others either. She has stopped using the telephone.

Table 26-12 summarizes how Greta's problem can be described when using MOHO, ICF, or the OTP Framework.

Table 26-12 Using Different Framework for Describing Greta's Difficulties

Greta's Problems	MOHO	ICF	OTP Framework
Decline in hearing	Performance capacity	d115 Listening, d310 Communicating with—receiving—spoken messages, d350 Conversation, d360 Using communication devices and techniques, d710–d729 General interpersonal interactions	Client factors-hearing
Loss of friend	Role loss	d710–d729 General interpersonal interactions	Performance Skills—social interactions Performance patterns—roles Contexts—virtual Environment—social
Isolation	Lack of engagement in meaningful activities	e320 Friends	Performance Skills—social interactions Performance patterns—roles Contexts—virtual Environment—social
Socialization		d9205 Socializing	Performance Skills—social interactions Performance patterns—roles Contexts—virtual Environment—social
Daily schedule	Loss of habits and routines	d710–d729 General interpersonal interactions	Performance Skills—social interactions Performance patterns—roles Contexts—virtual Environment—social

Conclusion

In this chapter, we compared and contrasted MOHO and many of its assessments with two prominent classification frameworks within the field of occupational therapy: the International Classification of Functioning, Disability and Health (ICF) and the AOTA Occupational Therapy Practice Framework. It is important to recognize that, whereas these three approaches to describing clients share some conceptual and linguistic similarities, MOHO is unique in several important ways. First, MOHO is a conceptual practice framework designed to guide therapeutic reasoning during practice. It is client centered and occupation focused, requiring a deep empathetic understanding of the client's self-perception and innate experience of key aspects that incorporate both mind and body. Because MOHO is both simple and comprehensive, it offers a natural fit with much of the terminology and concepts used in popular frameworks such as the ICF and OT Practice Framework.

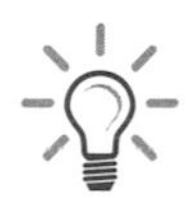

Chapter 26 Review Questions

1. Describe the underlying principles in ICF.
2. Which chapters, domains, and categories are most relevant to use when you are using MOHO as your frame of reference?
3. Why need occupational therapists to have an understanding of ICF?
4. What shortage can you identify with ICF from an occupational therapy perspective?
5. What is a shared tenant of MOHO and the OT Practice Framework?
6. What is a common core concept that provides individuals with an identity and a sense of competence in both MOHO and the OTP Framework?
7. Which domains of the OTP Framework are aligned with MOHO?

thePoint® For additional resources and exercises, visit http://thePoint.lww.com

ICF Key Terms

This glossary contains a selection of central glossary and definitions from the ICF in relation to MOHO. All definitions in the ICF can be found at http://www3.who.int/icf/onlinebrowser/icf.cfm.

Activity: The execution of a task or action by an individual.

Attitudes: Observable consequences of customs, practices, ideologies, values, norms, factual beliefs, and religious beliefs.

Body functions: Physiological functions of the body systems

Communication: General and specific features of communicating by language, signs, and symbols, including receiving and producing messages, carrying on conversations, and using communication devices and techniques.

Community, social, and civic life: Actions and tasks required to engage in organized social life outside the family, in community, social and civic areas of life.

Domestic life: Carrying out domestic and everyday actions and tasks. Areas of domestic life include acquiring a place to live, food, clothing and other necessities, household cleaning and repairing, caring for personal and other household objects, and assisting others.

Environmental factors: The physical, social, and attitudinal environment in which people live and conduct their lives.

General tasks and demands: General aspects of carrying out single or multiple tasks, organizing routines, and handling stress

Interpersonal interactions and relationships: Carrying out the actions and tasks required for basic and complex interactions with people (strangers, friends, relatives, family members, and partners) in a contextually and socially appropriate manner.

Learning and applying knowledge: Learning, applying the knowledge that is learned, thinking, solving problems, and making decisions.

Major life areas: Carrying out the tasks and actions required to engage in education, work, and employment and to conduct economic transactions.

Mental functions: Functions of the brain, both global mental functions, such as consciousness, energy and drive, orientation, and temperament and personality; and specific mental functions, such as attention, memory, organization and planning, language, and calculation of mental functions.

Participation: Involvement in a life situation.

Self-care: Caring for oneself, washing and drying oneself, caring for one's body and body parts, dressing, eating and drinking, and looking after one's health.

MOHO and the Occupational Therapy Practice Framework (OTPF)

This glossary contains a selection of central glossary and definitions from OTPF in relation to MOHO. These definitions can be found in the OT Practice Framework (AOTA, 2014).

Activity demands: The aspects of an activity, which include the objects, space, social demands, sequencing or timing, required actions, and required underlying body functioning and body structures needed to carry out the activity.

Client factors: Those factors that reside within the client and that may affect performance in areas of occupation. Client factors include body functions and body structures.

Communication/interaction skills: Conveying intentions and needs as well as coordinating social behavior to act together with people.

Context: Refers to a variety of interrelated conditions within and surrounding the client that influence performance.

Habits: Autonomic behavior that is integrated into more complex patterns that enable people to function on a day-to-day basis.

Motor skills: Skills in moving and interacting with task, objects, and environment.

Occupational performance: The ability to carry out activities of daily life. The accomplishment of the selected activity or occupation resulting from the dynamic transaction among the client, the context, and the activity.

Occupational roles: Activities and tasks, when combined, serve to enable performance in society.

Participation: Involvement in a life situation.

Performance patterns: Patterns of behavior related to daily life activities that are habitual or routine.

Performance skills: Features of what one does, not of what one has, related to observable elements of action that have implicit functional purposes.

Process skills: Skills used in managing and modifying actions en route to the completion of daily life tasks.

Role incumbency: The belief of a person that they perform a specified role.

Roles: A set of behaviors that have some socially agreed upon function and for which there is an accepted code of norms.

REFERENCES

Aslaksen, M., Scott, P. J., Haglund, L., & Ellingham, B. (2014). The Role Checklist Version 2: Quality of performance in the occupational therapy process in a mental health setting. *Ergoterapeuten,* (4), 38–45.

American Occupational Therapy Association. (2014). *Occupational Therapy Practice Framework: Domain & process* (3rd ed.). Bethesda, MD: Author.

Cieza, A., Geyh, S., Chatterji, S., Kostanjsek, N., Üstün, B., & Stucki, G. (2005). ICF linking rules: An update based lesson on learned. *Journal of Rehabilitation Medicine, 37,* 212–218.

Core Sets, International Classification of Functioning, Disability and Health, ICF, Research Branch. (2015). Retrieved from http://www.icf-research-branch.org/icf-core-sets-projects2

Bowyer, P., Kramer, J., Ploszaj, A., Ross, M., Schwartz, O., Kielhofner, G., et al. (2008). *The Short Child Occupational Profile (SCOPE)* [Version 2.2]. Chicago: The Model of Human Occupation Clearinghouse, University of Illinois.

Grajo, L., Candler, C., & Bowyer, P. (2015). *Inventory of Reading Occupations (IRO).* Unpublished manuscript.

Haglund, L. (2014). Screening av delaktighet i olika aktiviteter. In S. Parkinson, K. Forsyth, & Kielhofner, G. (Eds.), *MOHOST-S, Swedish version of the Model of Human Occupational Screening Tool (MOHOST), 2.0 (2006)* [in Swedish]. Nacka, Sweden: Förbundet Sveriges Arbetsterapeuter.

Haglund, L., & Fältman, S. (2012). Activity and participation—Self assessment according to the International Classification of Functioning: A study in mental health. *British Journal of Occupational Therapy, 75*(9), 412–418.

Haglund, L., & Henriksson, C. (2003). Concepts in occupational therapy in relation to the ICF. *Occupational Therapy International, 10*(4), 253–268.

Haglund, L., & Kjellberg, A. (2012). Bedömning av kommunikation och interaktionsfärdigheter. In K. Forsyth, M. Salamy, S. Simon, & Kielhofner, G. (Eds.), *ACIS-S, Swedish version of the Assessment of Communication and Interaction Skills (ACIS), 4.0 (1998)* [in Swedish]. Nacka, Sweden: Förbundet Sveriges Arbetsterapeuter.

Hemmingsson, H., & Jonsson, H. (2005). An occupational perspective on the concept of participation in the International Classification of Functioning, Disability and Health—Some critical remarks. *American Journal of Occupational Therapy, 59*(5), 569–576.

International Classification of Diseases (10th rev.). (2015). Retrieved from http://apps.who.int/classifications/icd10/browse/2015/en

International Classification of Health Interventions. (2015). Retrieved from http://www.who.int/classifications/ichi/en/

Kielhofner, G. (2008). *Model of human occupation: Theory and application* (4th ed). Philadelphia, PA: Lippincott Williams & Wilkins.

Nordenfelt, L. (2006). On health, ability and activity: Comments on some basic notions in the ICF. *Disability and Rehabilitation, 15,* 1461–1465.

Oakley, F., Kielhofner, G., Barris, R., & Reichler, R. K. (1986). The Role Checklist: Development and empirical assessment of reliability. *Occupational Therapy Journal of Research, 6*(3), 158–170.

Schell, B., Gillen, G., & Scaffe, M. (Eds.). (2014). *Willard and Spackman's occupational therapy* (12th ed.). Philadelphia, PA: J. B. Lippincott.

Scott, P. J. (2013). Measuring participation outcomes following life-saving medical interventions: The Role Checklist Version 2: Quality of performance. *Disability and Rehabilitation*, 1–5.

Scott, P. J., McFadden, R., Yates, K., Baker, S., & McSoley, S. (2014). The Role Checklist Version 2: Quality of performance: Reliability and validation of electronic administration. *British Journal of Occupational Therapy, 77*(2), 92–106.

Stamm, T., Cieza, A., Machold, K., Smolen, J., & Stucki, G. (2006). Exploration of the link between conceptual occupational therapy models and the International Classification of Functioning, Disability and Health. *Australian Occupational Therapy Journal, 53*, 9–17.

The Sweden National Board of Health and Welfare. (2015). Retrieved from http://www.socialstyrelsen.se/publikationer2011/utbildningsmaterial-om-icf-icfcy/sidor/default.aspx

World Health Organization. (2001). *International Classification of Functioning, Disability and Health (ICF)*. Geneva, Switzerland: Author.

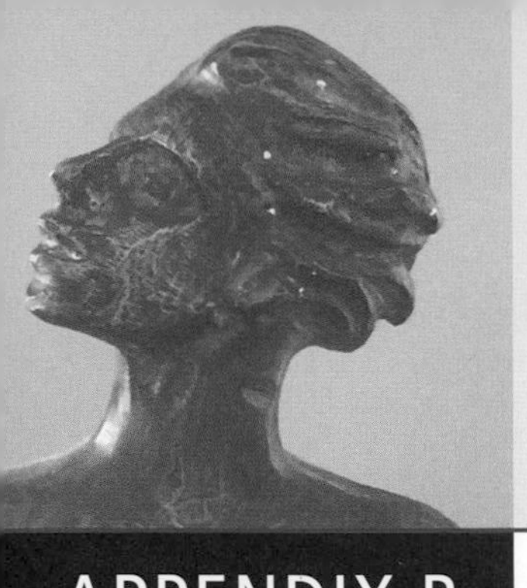

Introduction to the UIC MOHO Clearinghouse and MOHOWeb Website

Renée R. Taylor

APPENDIX B

UIC MOHO Clearinghouse

The MOHO Clearinghouse, located at the University of Illinois, Chicago (UIC), is an open, collaborative, international hub for *practice*-based communication and exchange focused on the Model of Human Occupation. It was established within the UIC Department of Occupational Therapy by the late Professor Gary Kielhofner in the late 1990s. Its mission is to serve the clinical and scientific communities as a center for exchange of research, scholarship, and clinical innovation concerning the broad application of MOHO across many specialty areas within the field of occupational therapy. Over the years, the UIC MOHO Clearinghouse has hosted numerous national and international scholars, postdocs, and undergraduate and graduate research assistants, as well as four international conferences (Figs. B-1–B-5).

Since its inception, the UIC MOHO Clearinghouse has grown to become an international distributor of 15 validated MOHO assessments, the Remotivation Process Intervention, and a range of additional assessments and resources that are currently under development or have not yet been tested in formal validation studies. Translations of these resources are offered in up to 21 different languages. Any scholar is welcome to post educational events related to MOHO on MOHOWeb (Fig. B-6), and to collaborate with

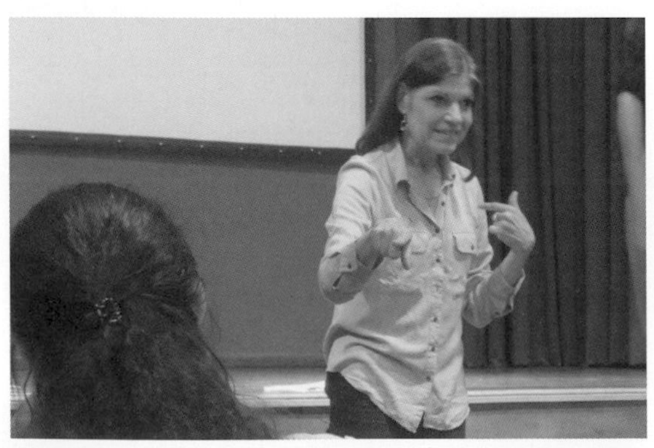

FIGURE B-1 Carmen Gloria de las Heras Lecturing about MOHO.

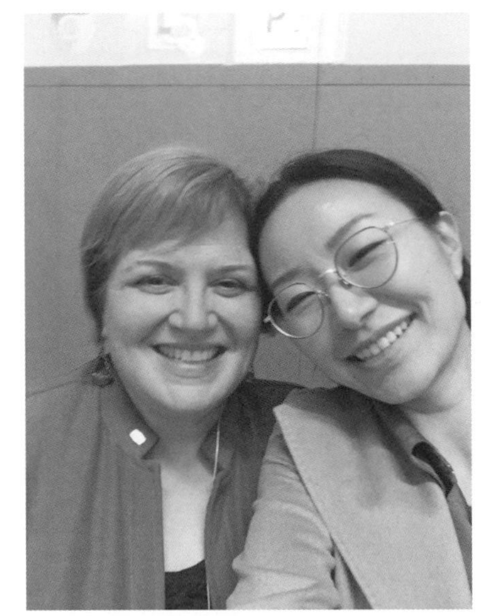

FIGURE B-2 Christine Raber and Sun Wook Lee at the Fourth International MOHO Institute on the Model of Human Occupation.

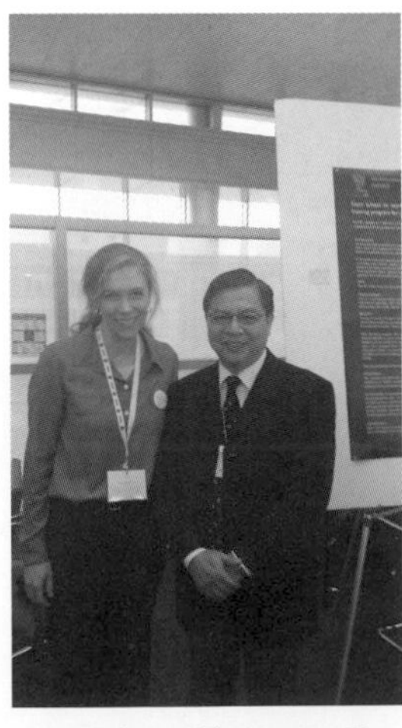

FIGURE B-3 Renée Taylor with Hector Tsang Presenting at the Fourth International MOHO Institute on the Model of Human Occupation.

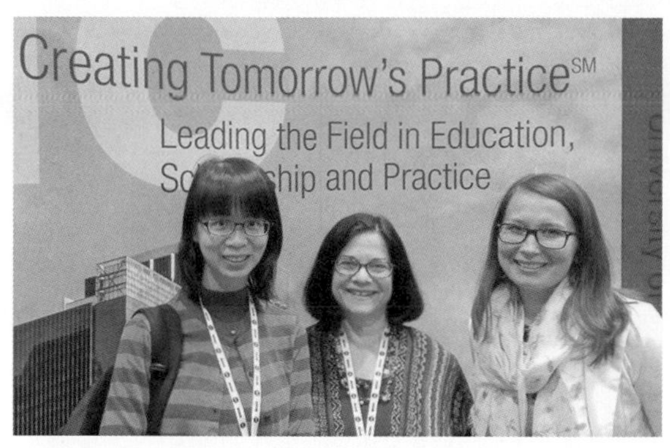

FIGURE B-4 Past and Present Members of the UIC MOHO Clearinghouse: Chia-Wei Fan, Gail Fisher, and Evguenia (Jenny) Popova at the AOTA UIC—MOHO Booth.

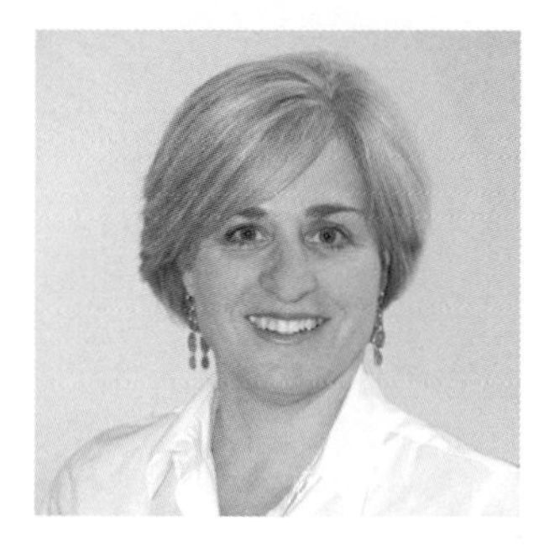

FIGURE B-5 Jane O'Brien Integrates MOHO in Obesity Research.

Clearinghouse staff to develop and test a needed resource that would enhance the growth and dissemination of MOHO (Figs. B-7 and B-8).

MOHOWeb

MOHOWeb is a central avenue for communication and exchange within the Clearinghouse (http://www.cade.uic.edu/moho/). As a public university resource, it is open to the public, with no subscription or membership fees. Specifically, if offers the following resources, most of which are free of charge:

- *Intro to MOHO.* This page summarizes the history of Dr. Gary Kielhofner's development of MOHO, along with a brief explanation of the model and its application in practice.
- *Practitioner Perspectives.* Testimonials on the application of MOHO from practitioners and scholars from around the world are presented in this section.
- *All of the Validated MOHO Assessments.* These are offered in two formats: Electronic Versions with Automatic Scoring and Digital PDF Fillable-forms, which are downloadable for printing.
- *Secure, Confidential Data Storage for Assessment Results.* (Free with purchase of the MOHO Assessments). MOHOWeb stores your deidentified data according to a unique ID that you assign within a secure web space for every assessment administered to every client you have.
- *MOHO Listserv.* With more than 3000 subscribers, this e-mail exchange is the central place for conversation among practitioners and scholars. Instructions for joining the listserv are provided on the MOHOWeb home page, and also under the "Resources" tab. All conversations are archived and available within MOHOWeb (Fig. B-9)
- *Educational Videos.* With more than 13,000 views for the *Introduction to the Model of Human Occupation* free YouTube video and more than 4000 views for the *MOHO in Motion* free YouTube video, the educational videos offer an introduction to practicing with MOHO and to the use of some of the most utilized MOHO assessments.
- *Programs and Interventions.* MOHO-based programs and interventions are described, along with a link to the e-store to purchase these products.
- *Evidence-Based Practice MOHO Search Engine.* Under the "Scholarship" tab, you will find a search engine that may be used to search for research articles and evidence briefs on a wide range of MOHO-related assessments and topics. MOHOWeb contains a comprehensive list of the scientific literature on MOHO. Users may narrow their search by criteria such as topic or practice setting.
- *ListServ Archives.* Under the "Resources" tab, you will find all of the discussions on the MOHO Listserv are archived and organized by topic area. One can search for past queries and responses.
- *MOHO Assessment and Product Translations.* Also under the "Resources" tab, you will find a list of the MOHO assessments and the languages into which these assessments have been translated. Current contact information for obtaining the translated resources is also provided.

Home | My MOHO | Products | Scholarship | Resources | FAQ | About MOHO | Contact Us

Model Of Human Occupation
THEORY AND APPLICATION

Welcome to MOHO Web

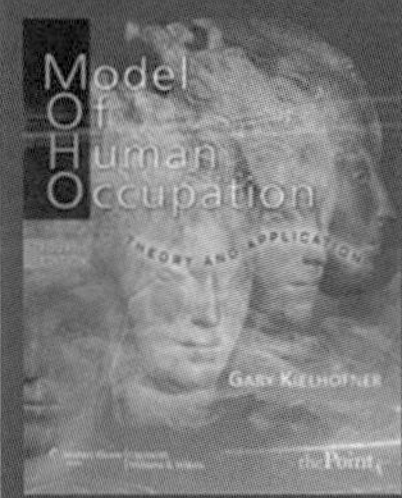

The Model of Human Occupation (MOHO) explains how occupations are motivated, patterned, and performed within everyday environments (Kielhofner, 2008). It has been argued that MOHO is the most widely-cited and utilized occupation-focused practice model in the world (Haglund, Ekbladh, Thorell, & Hallberg, 2000; Law & McColl, 1989; Lee, 2010; National Board for Certification in Occupational Therapy, 2004).

MOHO Web is a confidential online resource for occupational therapy practitioners, educators, students, and researchers. Here you may access and use all of the MOHO assessments and interventions that are supported for distribution through the University of Illinois at Chicago. Assessments for sale have been psychometrically validated using classical test theory and RASCH approaches. References to this research and other evidence for the use of MOHO throughout the world are available in the Scholarship section. Additionally, MOHO Web offers access to translated versions of the MOHO Assessments in 20 languages.

The Model of Human Occupation and its corresponding assessments and resources are the result of three decades of extensive contributions and collaborations from the late Dr. Gary Kielhofner, Professor and Head of the Department of Occupational Therapy at the University of Illinois at Chicago. MOHO Web is dedicated to his memory.

"It's not what you take when you leave this world behind you. It's what you leave behind you when you go." - Randy Travis.

[References]

MOHO News

Four new translations of the Introductory MOHO video are now available!

Chinese Japanese Korean Spanish

Join the conversation!

Subscribe to the MOHO ListServ and submit your questions to the MOHO community for discussion: listserv@listserv.uic.edu

MOHO is on the MOVE! Follow us on Facebook

Already have a MOHO Web account?

If you already have an account at MOHO Web, you can log in to create a new assessment, review previously entered assessments, run reports or purchase additional assessments.

Log in to My MOHO

What would you like to do next?

- Create an Account
- Find the right Assessment for my needs
- Purchase an Assessment
- Contact Us

More About MOHO Web

Check out MOHO on YouTube: Introduction to MOHO MOHO in Motion MOHO goes to AOTA 2015

We are excited to announce the following updates to MOHO Web:

- Residential Environment Impact Scale (REIS) Version 4.0, 2014 is available for purchase through MOHO Web.
- Child Occupational Self Assessment (COSA) Version 2.2, 2014 is available for purchase through MOHO Web. The assessment manual is available free of charge to all existing COSA users under "My MOHO" tab.
- Spanish Assessment and Intervention Package is available for purchase

UIC © Copyright 2016 University of Illinois Board of Trustees. Terms of use | Privacy Policy | Credits

FIGURE B-6 Screenshot of "MOHOWeb," Website of the UIC MOHO Clearinghouse.

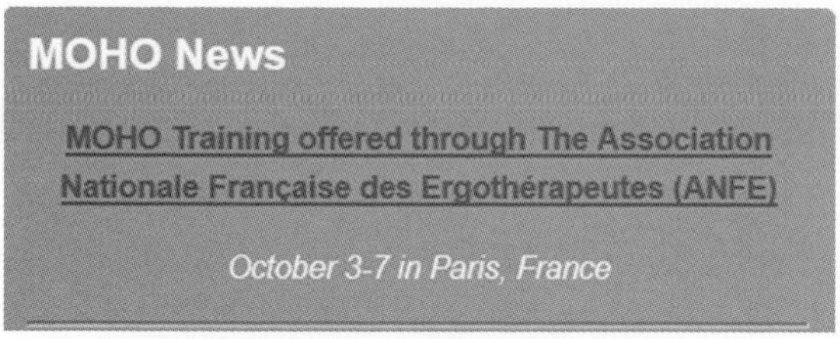

MOHO News

MOHO Training offered through The Association Nationale Française des Ergothérapeutes (ANFE)

October 3-7 in Paris, France

FIGURE B-7 MOHOWeb Announcement of an Upcoming Event.

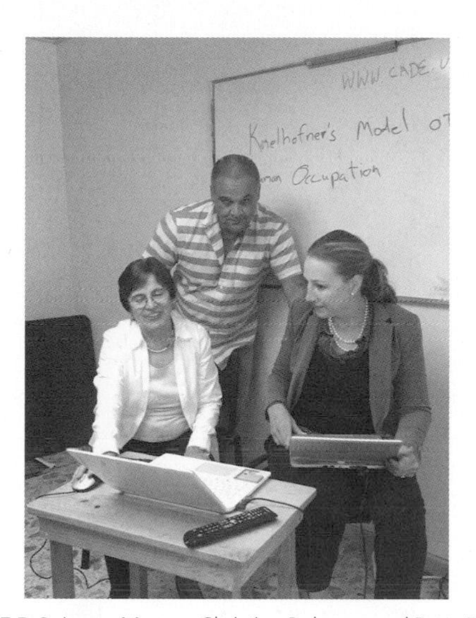

FIGURE B-8 Lauro Munoz, Christina Bolanos, and Patty Bowyer at the Occupational Therapy Institute in Mexico.

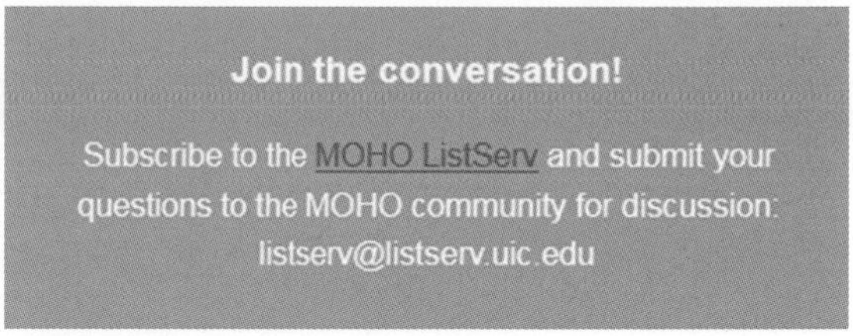

Join the conversation!

Subscribe to the MOHO ListServ and submit your questions to the MOHO community for discussion: listserv@listserv.uic.edu

FIGURE B-9 The UIC MOHO Listserv, Accessed through MOHOWeb.

Index

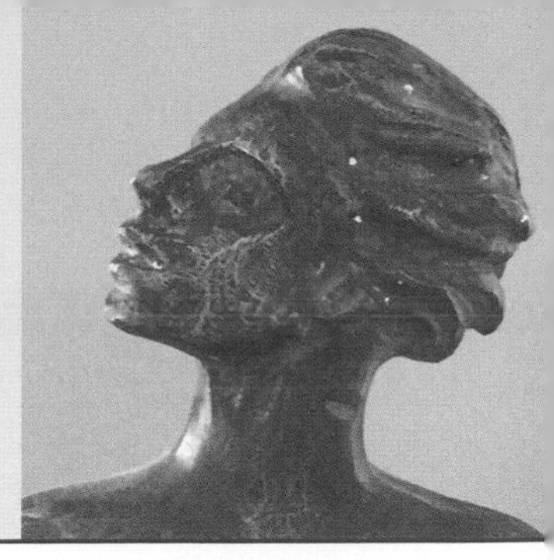

Note: Page numbers in *italics* refer to illustrations; page numbers followed by "*t*" refer to tables.

N

O